Gilbert VAES

AF738125

CANCER INVASION AND METASTASIS: BIOLOGIC AND THERAPEUTIC ASPECTS

The University of Texas
M. D. Anderson Hospital and Tumor Institute at Houston
36th Annual Symposium on Fundamental Cancer Research

Published for
The University of Texas
M. D. Anderson Hospital and Tumor Institute at Houston
Houston, Texas, by Raven Press, New York

The University of Texas
M. D. Anderson Hospital and Tumor Institute at Houston
36th Annual Symposium on Fundamental Cancer Research

Cancer Invasion and Metastasis: Biologic and Therapeutic Aspects

Edited by

Garth L. Nicolson, Ph.D.
Florence M. Thomas Professor of Cancer Research
Chairman, Department of Tumor Biology
The University of Texas
M. D. Anderson Hospital and Tumor Institute at Houston
Houston, Texas

Luka Milas, M.D., Ph.D.
Professor of Experimental Radiotherapy
Chairman, Department of Experimental Radiotherapy
The University of Texas
M. D. Anderson Hospital and Tumor Institute at Houston
Houston, Texas

Raven Press ■ New York

Raven Press, 1140 Avenue of the Americas, New York, New York 10036

Made in the United States of America

Library of Congress Cataloging in Publication Data

Symposium on Fundamental Cancer Research (36th : 1983 :
M. D. Anderson Hospital and Tumor Institute at Houston)
Cancer invasion and metastasis.
"Published for the University of Texas, M. D. Anderson Hospital and Tumor Institute at Houston, Houston, Texas."
Includes bibliographical references and index.
1. Cancer invasiveness—Congresses. 2. Metastasis—Congresses. I. Nicolson, Garth L. II. Milas, Luka. III. M. D. Anderson Hospital and Tumor Institute at Houston. IV. Title. [DNLM: 1. Neoplasm invasiveness—Congresses. 2. Neoplasm metastasis—Congresses. 3. Neoplasms—Therapy—Congresses. W3 SY5177 36th 1983c / QZ 202 S986 1983c
RC269.S9 1983 616.99'4 83-48667
ISBN 0-89004-896-7

This volume is a compilation of the proceedings of The University of Texas M. D. Anderson Hospital and Tumor Institute at Houston's 36th Annual Symposium on Fundamental Cancer Research, held February 28–March 3, 1983, in Houston, Texas.

The material contained in this volume was submitted as previously unpublished material, except in the instances in which credit has been given the source from which some of the illustrative material was derived.

Preface

Metastasis represents the most awesome characteristic of the neoplastic process. The ability of malignant cells to invade adjacent tissue and penetrate into the lymphatic or circulatory systems, or both, and spread to near and distant sites to form new metastatic colonies is receiving increasing attention in cancer research and is now important in cancer treatment. Although clinical procedures have dramatically increased the chances of surviving cancer in the remainder of this century, a major hurdle has yet to be overcome—the successful prevention and eradication of metastases that are often derived from completely controllable primary cancers. Thus, one of the major impediments to long-term cancer cures is metastasis, and until tumor metastasis can be prevented and metastatic cells selectively destroyed, the chances of increasing cure rates for many of the major classes of cancers will remain a difficult task. Since metastatic tumors often spread to distant sites where they involve major organs, existing conventional forms of therapy are quite limited in removing or destroying metastatic foci.

For these reasons, The University of Texas M. D. Anderson Hospital and Tumor Institute at Houston's 36th Annual Symposium on Fundamental Cancer Research addressed the phenomena of tumor invasion and metastasis. An important portion of the conference dealt with the diversity in cellular properties of metastatic cells including their cell surface components, enzymes, secreted components, antigens, adhesion and recognition components, chromosome markers, and hormone and growth factor receptors, as well as other properties. In addition to the biochemical diversity found in malignant cell subpopulations, heterogeneity in biologic characteristics, such as tissue and blood vessel invasion, vascularization, colonization at regional and distant sites, and sensitivity to chemotherapy, radiotherapy, and immunotherapy, were discussed. The uniqueness of the highly metastatic cells within a tumor is important in the design of new therapeutic approaches to blocking metastasis or selectively destroying established metastatic cells.

Tumor metastasis appears to be dependent on both host and tumor characteristics, a proposal that dates back to 1889 and the studies of S. Paget. Different symposium speakers dealt with host and tumor cell properties and their roles in metastasis. An important tool in studying these processes has been the development of animal tumor models that mimic human metastatic cancer. Various speakers presented information on the use of animal tumor models for elucidating the intricacies of tumor cell properties, as well as tumor-host interactions during the metastatic cascade.

The development of cell subpopulations within tumors possessing metastatic phenotypes is thought to be an important aspect of tumor progression. This phenomenon was thought by L. Foulds to be a series of permanent, irreversible changes that occurred uniquely in each tumor. That this phenomenon has a genetic basis was discussed during the symposium. It now appears, however, that in addition to changes in tumor cells that occur independently and lead to individual cells that gradually gain autonomy from host controls, there are interactions between different tumor cells that can result in a stabilization of phenotypes and possibly also stabilization of their interactions with host cells and other hemostatic controlling mechanisms.

If tumors are truly monoclonal in origin, then acquired phenotypic heterogeneity is probably the result of phenotypic drift of individual cell clones in the tumor cell population. Several symposium speakers discussed this extremely interesting aspect of cellular control. Unfortunately, its molecular or genetic basis remains elusive; it will continue to be one of the important problems of cancer biology in the next decade.

The ability of tumor cells to undergo change while acquiring differing properties with time is likely to contribute to our inability to completely destroy metastatic cells in a treatment setting. The success of cancer therapy could well depend upon the abilities of various therapeutic modalities to eliminate the rare, highly metastatic cell subpopulations that exist within a tumor or its metastases. The presence of heterogeneous cell subpopulations and their abilities to undergo rapid phenotypic change have important implications for the treatment of cancer. The management of highly malignant tumor cells could depend upon treatments that are able to circumvent the resistance of minor populations of malignant cells to various treatments, a resistance that results in survival after therapy.

In addition to tumor cell properties, a multitude of host factors affect the metastatic process in various ways. The ability of tumor cells to metastasize is greatly dependent on vascular hemodynamics, coagulation, capillary structure, and local tissue microenvironment, as well as various host resistance mechanisms. The identification of additional factors and an elucidation of how these influence the metastatic process will undoubtedly enhance our potential to interfere with such factors in order to prevent the formation of metastases and achieve successful therapy of established metastases.

The chapters presented in this monograph address many of the problems discussed above. We expect that the next decade will result in a relentless attack on metastatic cells and the process of metastasis.

Garth L. Nicolson
Luka Milas

Editors' Foreword

The topic of the 36th Annual Symposium on Fundamental Cancer Research, held in Houston, February 28–March 3, 1983, was "Cancer Invasion and Metastasis." Due to the fact that most cancer patients die of metastatic or disseminated malignant disease, tremendous interest was generated in this topic. Approximately 750 scientists from around the world attended the conference and poster sessions, attesting to the importance of this symposium.

We would like to thank a number of individuals who unselfishly provided advice and assistance at every stage during the planning and execution of the symposium. The Symposium Organizing Committee members from The University of Texas M. D. Anderson Hospital and Tumor Institute at Houston, Drs. Frederick F. Becker, James M. Bowen, Robert C. Hickey, and Lester J. Peters, in addition to an external advisory committee composed of Drs. Isaiah J. Fidler, Bernard Fisher, Kurt Hellmann, and Gloria Heppner, are gratefully acknowledged. We also thank the session chairmen, Drs. Robert H. Baldwin, Isaiah J. Fidler, Bernard Fisher, Kurt Hellmann, and Irving Zeidman, for their expert guidance during the proceedings.

We owe special thanks and appreciation to Mr. Jeff Rasco of the U.T. M. D. Anderson Hospital Conference Services and his staff, as well as Ms. Frances Goff, for providing assistance throughout the symposium. Benefactors such as Bristol-Myers Company, Burroughs Wellcome Company, Smith Kline and French Laboratories, Syntex U.S.A., Inc., and the Upjohn Company provided funds for the meeting, and we express our sincere gratitude for their support. We are especially grateful to the National Cancer Institute and the Texas Division of the American Cancer Society for their continuing sponsorship. The symposium was conducted in cooperation with The University of Texas Health Science Center and The University of Texas Graduate School of Biomedical Sciences at Houston. In addition we would like to thank the Department of Scientific Publications and the Department of Public Information and Education at the U.T. M. D. Anderson Hospital for editing the manuscripts and producing the publication and announcements of the symposium. Finally, we express our special thanks to Mr. Walter J. Pagel of the Department of Scientific Publications, who edited and compiled the manuscripts for this monograph.

Contents

Tumor Invasion

Tumor Heterogeneity

Host Factors and Metastasis

Therapy of Metastasis

Contributors

Peter Alexander
Department of Medical Oncology
University of Southampton
Southampton General Hospital
Hants SO9 4XY England

Peter Altevogt
Institut für Immunologie und Genetik
Deutsches Krebsforschungszentrum
D-6900 Heidelberg, West Germany

Nicholas M. Armitage
Department of Surgery
University of Nottingham
Nottingham NG7 2RD England

Robert W. Baldwin
Cancer Research Campaign Laboratories
University of Nottingham
Nottingham NG7 2RD England

Sanford Barsky
Section of Tumor Invasion and Metastases
Laboratory of Pathology
National Cancer Institute
Bethesda, Maryland 20205

Stephen B. Baylin
The Oncology Center and Department of Medicine
The Johns Hopkins University Medical Institutions
Baltimore, Maryland 21205

Emil Bogenmann
Department of Pediatrics
Childrens Hospital of Los Angeles
Los Angeles, California 90027

Stephen K. Carter
Pharmaceutical Research and Development Division
Bristol-Myers Company
New York, New York 10022

Rachanee Cheingsong-Popov
Institut für Immunologie und Genetik
Deutsches Krebsforschungszentrum
D-6900 Heidelberg, West Germany

Steven Corwin
Smith Kline and French Laboratories
Philadelphia, Pennsylvania 19101

Patrick De Baetselier
Service of General Biology
Free University of Brussels
Brussels, Belgium

Yves A. DeClerck
Department of Pediatrics
Childrens Hospital of Los Angeles
Los Angeles, California 90027

James W. Dennis
present address:
Cancer Research Division
Department of Pathology
Queen's University
Kingston, Ontario, Canada K7L 3N6

Daniel L. Dexter
present address:
Du Pont Company
Glenolden Laboratories
Glenolden, Pennsylvania 19036

Terrence P. Donaghue
Cancer Research Division
Department of Pathology
Queen's University
Kingston, Ontario, Canada K7L 3N6

Donald J. Dykes
Chemotherapy Department
Southern Research Institute
Birmingham, Alabama 35205

Rule Dzarlieva
Institut für Biochemie
Deutsches Krebsforschungszentrum
D-6900 Heidelberg, West Germany

Suzanne A. Eccles
Institute of Cancer Research
Sutton, Surrey SM2 5PX England

Lea Eisenbach
Department of Cell Biology
The Weizmann Institute of Science
Rehovot, Israel 76100

M. Jim Embleton
Cancer Research Campaign Laboratories
University of Nottingham
Nottingham NG7 2RD England

Jaime Estrada
Department of Pediatrics
The University of Texas M. D. Anderson Hospital and Tumor Institute at Houston
Houston, Texas 77030

Paul A. Farrands
Department of Surgery
University of Nottingham
Nottingham NG7 2RD England

Michael Feldman
Department of Cell Biology
The Weizmann Institute of Science
Rehovot, Israel 76100

Isaiah J. Fidler
Cancer Metastasis and Treatment Laboratory
NCI-Frederick Cancer Research Facility
Frederick, Maryland 21701

Bernard Fisher
Department of Surgery
University of Pittsburgh
Pittsburgh, Pennsylvania 15261

Gilbert H. Fletcher
Division of Radiotherapy
The University of Texas M. D. Anderson Hospital and Tumor Institute at Houston
Houston, Texas 77030

Mina Fogel
Institut für Immunologie und Genetik
Deutsches Krebsforschungszentrum
D-6900 Heidelberg, West Germany

Judah Folkman
Department of Surgery
Children's Hospital Medical Center
Boston, Massachusetts 02115

Marie Claude Fulchignoni-Lataud
Department of Medical Genetics
Hospital for Sick Children
University of Toronto
Toronto, Ontario, Canada

Amy M. Fulton
Department of Immunology
Michigan Cancer Foundation
Detroit, Michigan 48201

Arnold H. Greenberg
Manitoba Institute of Cell Biology
University of Manitoba
Winnipeg, Manitoba, Canada R3E OV9

Russell Greig
Smith Kline and French Laboratories
Philadelphia, Pennsylvania 19101

Daniel P. Griswold, Jr.
Chemotherapy Department
Southern Research Institute
Birmingham, Alabama 35205

Janet Gross
Department of Cell Biology
New York University School of Medicine
New York, New York 10016

Nabil Hanna
Department of Immunology
Smith Kline and French Laboratories
Philadelphia, Pennsylvania 19101

Jack D. Hardcastle
Department of Surgery
University of Nottingham
Nottingham NG7 2RD England

Ian R. Hart
Cancer Metastasis and Treatment Laboratory
NCI-Frederick Cancer Research Facility
Frederick, Maryland 21701

Margaret Heisel
Department of Pediatrics
Childrens Hospital of Los Angeles
Los Angeles, California 90027

Gloria H. Heppner
Department of Immunology
Michigan Cancer Foundation
Detroit, Michigan 48201

Peter Hilgard
Asta-Werke AG Degussa Pharma Gruppe
D-4800 Bielefeld 14, West Germany

Kenneth V. Honn
Departments of Radiation Oncology, Radiology, and Biological Sciences
Wayne State University
Detroit, Michigan 48202

Tatsuro Irimura
Department of Tumor Biology
The University of Texas M. D. Anderson Hospital and Tumor Institute at Houston
Houston, Texas 77030

Hart Isaacs
Department of Pathology
Childrens Hospital of Los Angeles
Los Angeles, California 90027

Rebecca H. Jackson
The Oncology Center and Department of Medicine
The Johns Hopkins University Medical Institutions
Baltimore, Maryland 21205

Eric Jaffe
Department of Medicine
Cornell University School of Medicine
New York, New York 10021

Peter A. Jones
Departments of Biochemistry and Pediatrics
Childrens Hospital of Los Angeles
Los Angeles, California 90027

Borislav Kamenov
Department of Immunology
University of Alberta
Edmonton, Alberta, Canada T6G 2H7

Shulamit Katzav
Department of Cell Biology
The Weizmann Institute of Science
Rehovot, Israel 76100

Mark W. Kieran
Department of Immunology
University of Alberta
Edmonton, Alberta, Canada T6G 2H7

Robert S. Kerbel
Cancer Research Division
Department of Pathology
Queen's University
Kingston, Ontario, Canada K7L 3N6

Untae Kim
Department of Pathology
Roswell Park Memorial Institute
New York State Department of Health
Buffalo, New York 14263

Thomas Koestler
Smith Kline and French Laboratories
Philadelphia, Pennsylvania 19101

Michael Kramer
Institut für Immunologie and Genetik
Deutsches Krebsforschungszentrum
D-6900 Heidelberg, West Germany

Alain E. Lagarde
Cancer Research Division
Department of Pathology
Queen's University
Kingston, Ontario, Canada K7L 3N6

W. Russell Laster, Jr.
Chemotherapy Department
Southern Research Institute
Birmingham, Alabama 35205

Walter E. Laug
Department of Pediatrics
Childrens Hospital of Los Angeles
Los Angeles, California 90027

John Barrington Leigh
Department of Immunology
University of Alberta
Edmonton, Alberta, Canada T6G 2H7

William Lennarz, Jr.
The Oncology Center and Department of Medicine
The Johns Hopkins University Medical Institutions
Baltimore, Maryland 21205

Lance A. Liotta
Section of Tumor Invasion and Metastases
Laboratory of Pathology
National Cancer Institute
Bethesda, Maryland 20205

B. Michael Longenecker
Department of Immunology
University of Alberta
Edmonton, Alberta, Canada T6G 2H7

Scott E. Loveless
Department of Immunology
Michigan Cancer Foundation
Detroit, Michigan 48201

Keith H. Mahoney
Department of Immunology
Michigan Cancer Foundation
Detroit, Michigan 48201

David G. Menter
Department of Biological Sciences
Wayne State University
Detroit, Michigan 48202

Luka Milas
Division of Radiotherapy
The University of Texas M. D. Anderson Hospital and Tumor Institute at Houston
Houston, Texas 77030

Fred R. Miller
Department of Immunology
Michigan Cancer Foundation
Detroit, Michigan 48201

David Moscatelli
Department of Cell Biology
New York University School of Medicine
New York, New York 10016

Motowo Nakajima
Department of Tumor Biology
The University of Texas M. D. Anderson Hospital and Tumor Institute at Houston
Houston, Texas 77030

Fred P. Nestel
Cancer Research Division
Department of Pathology
Queen's University
Kingston, Ontario, Canada K7L 3N6

Harry B. Neustein
Department of Pathology
Childrens Hospital of Los Angeles
Los Angeles, California 90027

Garth L. Nicolson
Department of Tumor Biology
The University of Texas M. D. Anderson Hospital and Tumor Institute at Houston
Houston, Texas 77030

James M. Onoda
Department of Radiation Oncology
Wayne State University
Detroit, Michigan 48202

Alan Perkins
Medical Physics Department
University of Nottingham
Nottingham NG7 2RD England

Lester J. Peters
Division of Radiotherapy
The University of Texas M. D. Anderson Hospital and Tumor Institute at Houston
Houston, Texas 77030

Malcolm V. Pimm
Cancer Research Campaign Laboratories
University of Nottingham
Nottingham NG7 2RD England

George Poste
Department of Pathology and Laboratory Medicine
University of Pennsylvania
Philadelphia, Pennsylvania 19104

Nageswara C. Rao
Section of Tumor Invasion and Metastases
Laboratory of Pathology
National Cancer Institute
Bethesda, Maryland 20205

Daniel B. Rifkin
Department of Cell Biology
New York University School of Medicine
New York, New York 10016

Frank M. Schabel, Jr.
Chemotherapy Department
Southern Research Institute
Birmingham, Alabama 35205

Volker Schirrmacher
Institut für Immunologie und Genetik
Deutsches Krebsforschungszentrum
D-6900 Heidelberg, West Germany

Shraga Segal
Department of Microbiology
Ben-Gurion University of the Negev
Beer-Sheva, Israel

Joel H. Shaper
Department of Pharmacology and Experimental Therapeutics
The Johns Hopkins University Medical Institutions
Baltimore, Maryland 21205

Louis Siminovitch
Department of Medical Genetics
Hospital for Sick Children
University of Toronto
Toronto, Ontario, Canada

Bonnie F. Sloane
Departments of Radiation Oncology and Pharmacology
Wayne State University
Detroit, Michigan 48202

Georg F. Springer
Evanston Hospital
Northwestern University
Evanston, Illinois 60201

Dale A. Stringfellow
Cancer Research
Pharmaceutical Research and Development
Bristol-Myers Company
Syracuse, New York 13201

John D. Taylor
Departments of Radiation Oncology and Biological Sciences
Wayne State University
Detroit, Michigan 48202

Victor P. Terranova
Laboratory of Developmental Biology and Anomalies
National Institute of Dental Research
Bethesda, Maryland 20205

Unnur Thorgeirsson
Section of Tumor Invasion and Metastases
Laboratory of Pathology
National Cancer Institute
Bethesda, Maryland 20205

Mary W. Trader
Chemotherapy Department
Southern Research Institute
Birmingham, Alabama 35205

James Tzeng
Department of Pathology and Laboratory Medicine
University of Pennsylvania
Philadelphia, Pennsylvania 19104

Israel Vlodavsky
Department of Radiation and Clinical Oncology
The Hebrew University
Hadassah School of Medicine
Jerusalem, Israel

Catherine A. Waller
Institut für Immunologie und Genetik
Deutsches Krebsforschungszentrum
D-6900 Heidelberg, West Germany

CANCER INVASION AND METASTASIS: BIOLOGIC AND THERAPEUTIC ASPECTS

The University of Texas
M. D. Anderson Hospital and Tumor Institute at Houston
36th Annual Symposium on Fundamental Cancer Research

Cancer Invasion and Metastasis: Biologic and Therapeutic Aspects edited by Garth L. Nicolson and Luka Milas. Raven Press, New York © 1984.

An Introduction to Cancer Invasion and Metastasis

Garth L. Nicolson

Department of Tumor Biology, The University of Texas M. D. Anderson Hospital and Tumor Institute at Houston, Houston, Texas 77030

If detected early enough, most primary cancers of nondermal origin can be treated successfully by surgery, often in combination with chemotherapy, radiotherapy, or biological therapy. However, once cancers have spread from primary to near and distant metastatic sites, their complete eradication is much more difficult to achieve. By the time cancer has been diagnosed in many patients, they often possess multiple metastatic lesions, many of which are too small to be detected by currently available procedures. Even when small metastases are detected, their size, number, and frequently dispersed anatomic locations preclude use of most surgical procedures and make other types of therapy more difficult to administer. Multiple adjuvant therapies have thus evolved for routine use against cancers that possess high probabilities of metastasizing (see chapters by Griswold, Carter, and Peters).

It is now well known that malignant tumors contain cell subpopulations with widely different susceptibilities to the therapeutic treatments mentioned above. Since malignant cells can be highly unstable and change in their sensitivities to various therapeutic treatments with time, the procedures that reduce tumor bulk drastically may fail ultimately, if resistant cell subpopulations emerge that are refractory to further treatments. This extensive heterogeneity in the susceptibility of tumor cell subpopulations to therapy extends to other properties of malignant cells such as surface charge, morphology, karyotype, motility, degradative enzymes, recognition structures, antigens, glycoproteins, glycolipids, secretory products, and metabolism. These various properties and their relationship to metastasis formation are considered in detail in many of the contributions to this monograph and in several recent reviews (Table 1).

Cancer invasion and metastasis formation occur via a complex series of sequential steps in which malignant cells first invade and occupy adjacent tissues and penetrate into the lymphatics, blood circulatory systems, or body cavities. These events have been termed "primary invasion" to distinguish between invasion at primary and secondary or metastatic sites. Once malignant cells enter new compartments, such as the lymph or blood, they can separate or detach from the primary tumor mass and be transported to near and distant sites, where

TABLE 1. *Some recent reviews on metastasis formation and the properties of metastatic cells*

General reviews	Baldwin 1978, Hart and Fidler 1981, Fidler and Nicolson 1981, Fidler et al. 1978, Nicolson 1982a, Nicolson and Poste 1982, 1983a, 1983b, Poste 1982a, Poste and Fidler 1980, Sugarbaker 1979, 1981, Zeidman 1981, Weiss 1977, 1980
Cell surface properties	Fidler et al. 1978, Fidler and Nicolson 1981, Nicolson 1982a, 1982b, Nicolson and Poste 1982, 1983a, 1983b, Warren 1981, Turner 1982
Tumor invasion	Hart 1981, 1982, Mareel 1979, 1980, Nicolson 1982a, 1982b, Nicolson and Poste 1983b, Liotta et al. 1982, Liotta and Hart 1982, Varani 1982
Tumor heterogeneity	Poste 1982a, 1982b, Hart and Fidler 1981, Fidler and Hart 1982, Nicolson 1982a, Heppner 1982, Fidler and Poste 1982, Nicolson and Poste 1982, 1983b
Host factors	Kim 1970, Fidler and Nicolson 1981, Fidler et al. 1978, Hanna 1982, Nicolson 1982a, Nicolson and Poste 1983a, 1983b, Honn and Sloane 1983, Hart and Fidler 1981, Folkman 1974, 1975
Therapy	Sugarbaker 1981, Sugarbaker et al. 1982, Day et al. 1977, Poste 1982a, Nicolson and Poste 1983a, 1983b

they must then implant, invade surrounding tissues ("secondary invasion"), survive, and finally proliferate to form metastatic lesions. The overall success of this process ultimately depends on the proper interplay between several tumor cell and host properties that are important in metastasis (Tables 1 and 2).

It has been proposed that tumor metastasis is the end result of a highly selective process whereby each step of the metastatic cascade places selective restraints on tumor cell subpopulations. Only certain tumor cells that can successfully complete the entire sequence are selected, and these specialized cells give rise to metastatic lesions (Poste and Fidler 1980). It has also been argued that metastasis is an entirely random process, and every tumor cell has the

TABLE 2. *Tumor and host properties in metastasis formation*

Tumor properties	
1. Cell growth	5. Cell degradative enzymes
2. Mechanical and osmotic factors	6. Cell chemotactic substances
3. Cell adhesive and attachment properties	7. Cell cytolytic substances
4. Cell locomotion and taxis	8. Other cell secreted products
Host properties	
1. Tissue and stromal barriers to invasion	5. Specific and nonspecific immunological responses
2. Tissue cell cohesion	6. Vascularization
3. Serum and tissue enzyme inhibitors	7. Nutrition and oxygenation
4. Inflammatory and noninflammatory reactions	8. Serum and tissue growth stimulators and inhibitors

Modified from Nicolson and Poste 1983b.

capability to metastasize and is potentially a malignant neoplasm (Weiss 1980). Tumor cell survival at particular steps during the metastatic process can certainly be random, and in certain tumors, particularly in those animal tumors that have already undergone purposeful selection, the process of metastasis formation may appear random if the tumors already possess high metastatic capacities (Talmadge and Fidler 1982).

The purposeful selection of tumor cell subpopulations with enhanced metastatic and other properties in animal tumor systems has been especially helpful in the analysis of tumor and host characteristics important in metastasis formation (see reviews by Nicolson 1982a, Poste 1982a, 1982b, Nicolson and Poste 1982, 1983a, 1983b). Of course, when using these animal models, careful attention must be paid to the stabilities of tumor cell subpopulations (especially cell clones) in order to relate specific cellular properties to metastatic behavior. It is now well known that individual tumor cells can be unstable and undergo phenotypic drift in their properties (see reviews by Fidler and Hart 1982, Nicolson 1982a, Poste 1982a, Nicolson and Poste 1982).

The generation of tumor cell subpopulations with altered phenotypes (including metastatic behavior) is probably the most dangerous characteristic of malignant neoplasms. This characteristic could account for the successful survival of tumor cell subpopulations faced with multiple therapeutic pressures that would be expected to eliminate all cells within a tumor. In addition, with time tumor heterogeneity and the diversification of malignant cell phenotypes should also insure that some of the surviving cells, for example after therapy, would eventually have increased therapeutic resistance and metastatic potentials. It is the presence of these residual, resistant, unstable cells and further host selection processes that probably lead to the progression of tumors to more malignant neoplasms. Ultimately, phenotypic instability (probably due to genotypic instability) should insure that tumor cell subpopulations arise that will eventually metastasize and kill their host.

The chapters in this monograph deal with tumor and host characteristics important in metastasis, as well as the current forms of therapy that attempt to destroy malignant cells and prevent or inhibit metastasis formation.

REFERENCES

Baldwin, R. W., ed. 1978. Secondary Spread of Cancer. Academic Press, London, 244 pp.

Day, S. B., W. P. L. Myers, P. G. Stansly, S. Garattini, and M. G. Lewis, eds. 1977. Cancer Invasion and Metastasis: Biologic Mechanisms and Therapy. Raven Press, New York.

Fidler, I. J., D. M. Gersten, and I. R. Hart. 1978. The biology of cancer invasion and metastasis. Adv. Cancer Res. 28:149–250.

Fidler, I. J., and I. R. Hart. 1982. Biological diversity in metastatic neoplasms: Origins and implications. Science 217:998–1003.

Fidler, I. J., and G. L. Nicolson. 1981. Immunobiology of experimental metastatic melanoma. Cancer Biol. Rev. 2:171–234.

Fidler, I. J., and G. Poste. 1982. The heterogeneity of metastatic properties in malignant tumor cells and regulation of the metastatic phenotype, *in* Tumor Cell Heterogeneity: Origins and Implications, A. Owens, D. S. Coffey, and S. Baylin, eds. Raven Press, New York, pp. 111–162.

Folkman, J. 1974. Tumor angiogenesis. Adv. Cancer Res. 19:331–358.
Folkman, J. 1975. Tumor angiogenesis, *in* Cancer: A Comprehensive Treatise, Vol. 3, Biology of Tumors: Cellular Biology and Growth, F. F. Becker, ed. Plenum Press, New York, pp. 355–388.
Hanna, N. 1982. Inhibition of experimental tumor metastasis by selective activation of natural killer cells. Cancer Res. 42:1337–1342.
Hart, I. R. 1981. Mechanisms of tumor cell invasion. Cancer Biol. Rev. 2:29–58.
Hart, I. R. 1982. Seed and soil revisited. Mechanism of site specific metastasis. Cancer Metastasis Rev. 1:5–16.
Hart, I. R., and I. J. Fidler. 1981. The implications of tumor heterogeneity for studies on the biology and therapy of cancer metastasis. Biochim. Biophys. Acta 651:37–50.
Heppner, G. H. 1982. Tumor subpopulation interactions, *in* Tumor Cell Heterogeneity: Origins and Implications, A. H. Owens, Jr., D. S. Coffey, and S. B. Baylin, eds. Academic Press, New York, pp. 225–236.
Honn, K. V., and S. B. Sloane, eds. 1983. Hemostatic Mechanisms and Metastasis. Martinus Nijhoff Publishers, The Hague. (in press).
Kim, U. 1970. Metastasizing mammary carcinomas in rats: Induction and study of their immunogenicity. Science 164:72–74.
Liotta, L., and I. R. Hart, eds. 1982. Tumor Invasion and Metastasis. Martinus Nijhoff Publishers, The Hague, The Netherlands.
Liotta, L. A., U. P. Thorgeirsson, and S. Garbisa. 1982. Role of collagenases in tumor cell invasion. Cancer Metastasis Rev. 1:277–317.
Mareel, M. M. K. 1979. Is invasiveness in vitro characteristic of malignant cells? Cell. Biol. Int. Rep. 3:627–640.
Mareel, M. M. K. 1980. Recent aspects of tumor invasiveness. Int. Rev. Exp. Pathol. 22:65–129.
Nicolson, G. L. 1982a. Cancer metastasis: Organ colonization and the cell surface properties of malignant cells. Biochim. Biophys. Acta 695:113–176.
Nicolson, G. L. 1982b. Cell surface properties of metastatic tumor cells, *in* Tumor Invasion and Metastasis, L. Liotta and I. R. Hart, eds. Martinus Nijhoff Publishers, The Hague, The Netherlands, pp. 57–59.
Nicolson, G. L., and G. Poste. 1982. Tumor cell diversity and host responses in cancer metastasis. I. Properties of metastatic cells. Curr. Prob. Cancer 7(6):1–83.
Nicolson, G. L., and G. Poste. 1983a. Tumor cell diversity and host responses in cancer metastasis. II. Host immune responses and therapy of metastases. Curr. Probl. Cancer 7(7):1–43.
Nicolson, G. L., and G. Poste. 1983b. Tumor implantation and invasion at metastatic sites. Int. Rev. Exp. Pathol. 25:77–181.
Poste, G. 1982a. Experimental systems for analysis of the malignant phenotype. Cancer Metastasis Rev. 1:141–199.
Poste, G. 1982b. Methods and models for studying tumor invasion, *in* Tumor Invasion and Metastasis, L. A. Liotta and I. R. Hart, eds. Martinus Nijhoff Publishers, The Hague, pp. 148–177.
Poste, G., and I. J. Fidler. 1980. The pathogenesis of cancer metastasis. Nature 283:139–146.
Sugarbaker, E. V. 1979. Cancer metastasis: A product of tumor-host interactions. Curr. Probl. Cancer 3(7):3–59.
Sugarbaker, E. V. 1981. Patterns of metastasis in human malignancies. Cancer Biol. Rev. 2:235–278.
Sugarbaker, E. V., N. Weingrad, and J. M. Roseman. 1982. Observations on cancer metastasis in man, *in* Tumor Invasion and Metastasis, L. A. Liotta and I. R. Hart, eds. Martinus Nijhoff Publishers, The Hague, pp. 427–465.
Talmadge, J. E., and I. J. Fidler. 1982. Cancer Metastasis is selective or random depending on the parent tumour population. Nature 297:593–596.
Turner, G. A. 1982. Surface of the metastatic cell. Invasion Metastasis 2:197–216.
Varani, J. 1982. Chemotaxis of metastatic tumor cells. Cancer Metastasis Rev. 1:17–28.
Warren, B. A. 1981. Origin and fate of blood-borne tumor emboli. Cancer Biol. Rev. 2:95–169.
Weiss, L. 1977. A pathobiologic overview of metastasis. Semin. Oncol. 4:5–19.
Weiss, L. 1980. Metastasis: Differences between cancer cells in primary and secondary tumors. Pathobiol. Annu. 10:51–18.
Zeidman, I. 1981. Metastasis: An overview. Cancer Biol. Rev. 2:1–27.

Cancer Invasion and Metastasis: Biologic and Therapeutic Aspects edited by Garth L. Nicolson and Luka Milas. Raven Press, New York © 1984.

The Ernst W. Bertner Memorial Award Lecture: The Evolution of Biological Heterogeneity in Metastatic Neoplasms

Isaiah J. Fidler

Cancer Metastasis and Treatment Laboratory, NCI-Frederick Cancer Research Facility, Frederick, Maryland 21701

The propensity of malignant neoplasms to produce metastases in organs distant from the primary tumor is one of the most devastating aspects of neoplasia. With the exception of skin cancer, by the time many cancers are diagnosed, metastasis to many organs has already occurred. Despite remarkable advances in surgical treatment of primary neoplasms, in development of aggressive adjuvant therapies, and in improvement of patient care, most cancer patients die of metastatic disease. For this reason, a major goal of clinical oncology should be the prevention or eradication of metastases.

The most formidable obstacle to the treatment of established metastases may well be the heterogeneity of cells within neoplasms. This biological heterogeneity, which results from the continuing evolution of tumors, is reflected by the emergence of variants from the primary tumor and is responsible for differences in response to treatment that exist within cells populating a primary tumor, between the primary tumor and its metastases, and even among different metastatic lesions. The biological diversity of neoplasms implies that the successful treatment of the disease will require the total destruction of all tumor cells.

This concept is illustrated in Figure 1. By the time primary tumors (or metastases) are diagnosed, the lesions can well approximate 1 cm^3 in size, i.e., contain about 10^9 cells (De Vita et al. 1975). The destruction of 99.9% of the cells, a remarkable achievement indeed, still leaves 10^6 cells to proliferate and provide a large basis for the further, and more rapid, generation of biological diversity, including the emergence of treatment-resistant variants. Understanding the mechanisms responsible for the development of biological heterogeneity in neoplasms and how metastatic cells spread from primary tumors to produce secondary lesions is, therefore, an important goal of cancer research.

THE METASTATIC PROCESS

The development of new approaches to the treatment of metastasis will be forthcoming once we better understand the biology of the process. Research

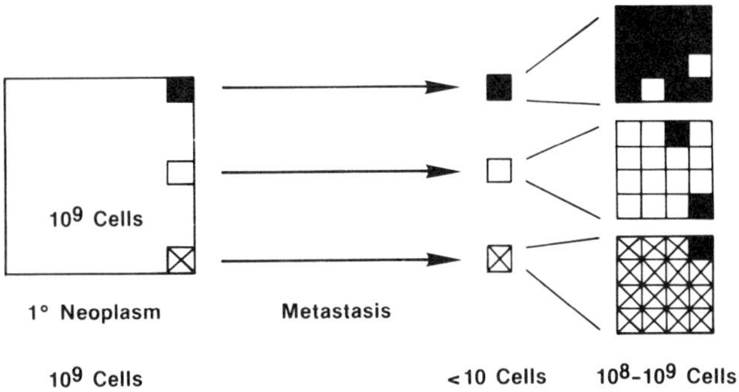

FIG. 1. The implications of tumor heterogeneity for therapy. In a tumor mass containing 10^9 cells, the destruction of 99.9% of the cells still leaves 10^6 cells that can give rise to metastases, which can originate from fewer than 10 cells.

originating from many laboratories indicates that the outcome of metastasis depends on the properties of both tumor cells and host factors and that the balance of these contributions varies among different tumor systems (Zeidman 1957, Fidler et al. 1978, Sugarbaker 1979, Hart and Fidler 1980a, Poste and Fidler 1980, Poste 1982, Nicolson 1982).

The pathogenesis of a metastasis can be divided, albeit somewhat arbitrarily, into various sequential steps as illustrated in Figure 2. Metastasis begins with the local invasion of the surrounding host stroma by either single cells or multicellular clumps of cells from the primary tumor (Hart 1981). Once the invading tumor cells have penetrated the vascular or lymphatic channels, they may grow at the site of penetration or they may detach as individual cells or small embolic aggregates. These neoplastic cells are then transported via the circulatory system, where they are more susceptible to various host immune and nonimmune defenses such as blood turbulence, lymphocytes, monocytes (Fidler 1974, Fidler et al. 1979), and natural killer cells (Hanna 1982). Surviving tumor cells are then arrested in the capillary beds of distant organs either by adhering to capillary endothelial cells (Kramer and Nicolson 1979) or by attaching at the sites of endothelial cell retraction where the underlying basement membrane is exposed (Hart and Fidler 1980a, Poste and Nicolson 1980). The next step, extravasation, probably occurs by many of the same mechanisms that determine initial invasion (Hart 1981). To grow in the organ parenchyma, the metastases must develop a vascular network and evade the host immune system (Wheelock et al. 1977). When the metastases have attained a certain size, they may give rise to additional metastases (Hart and Fidler 1980b). Thus, in a short time a small primary tumor can produce a multitude of metastases.

Few cells in the primary tumor can complete all these steps to develop into metastases. The difficulty of completing the arduous metastatic process may account, in part, for the fact that metastasis is an inefficient process (Weiss 1980, Weiss et al. 1980). Most tumor cells that enter the circulation die rapidly

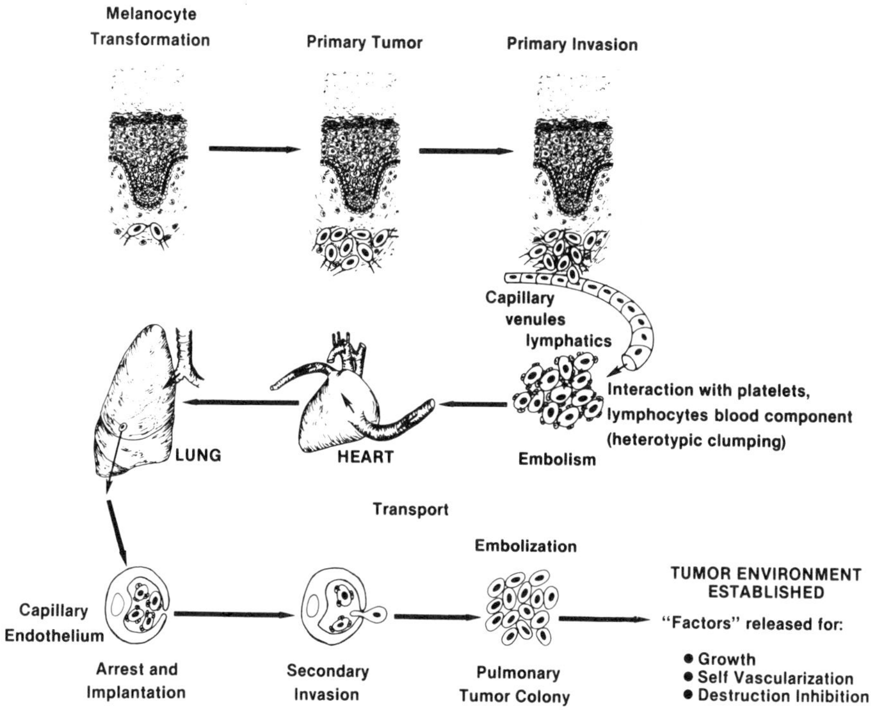

FIG. 2. The pathogenesis of cancer metastasis. At every step of the process, the rules of "survival of the fittest" apply with regard to the interplay of tumor cells with their host.

(Fidler 1970); therefore, the mere presence of tumor cells in the circulation does not predict that metastases will develop (Salsbury 1975). Several years ago we investigated the fate of circulating tumor emboli (Fidler 1970). Using tumor cells labeled with [^{125}I]5-iodo-2′-deoxyuridine, we found that by 24 h after entry into the venous circulation, less than 0.1% of the original inoculum survived to proliferate into metastases (Fidler 1970). The fact that most circulating emboli did not survive to produce metastases was not surprising, but it rasised the question of whether the pathogenesis of metastasis is a random or a selective process. That is, given the large number of tumor cells that can enter the circulation, does the development of metastases represent the fortuitous survival of a few neoplastic cells (Weiss et al. 1983) or the selection from the parent tumor of minor metastatic subpopulations of cells (Fidler and Kripke 1977)?

The Selective Nature of the Metastatic Process

Our studies, and most data reported by others, have led us to conclude that metastasis is a highly selective process regulated by a number of as yet imperfectly understood mechanisms (Fidler 1978, Fidler and Poste 1982). This belief is contrary to the once widely accepted notion that neoplastic dissemination is the ultimate expression of cellular anarchy. In fact, suggesting that cancer metastasis is a selective process is a more optimistic view in terms of cancer therapy than one that postulates that tumor dissemination is an entirely random event. Belief that certain rules govern the spread of neoplastic disease implies that elucidation and understanding of these rules will lead to better therapeutic interventions. If the event is entirely random, little more can be said about the nature of the process. Irrespective of our subjective feelings about these two interpretations, the weight of evidence supports the view that metastasis is a selective process.

PATTERNS OF METASTASIS

Clinical observations of human and domestic animals afflicted with malignant neoplasms have revealed that certain tumors have a marked predilection for metastasis to specific organs (Sugarbaker 1981) and these metastatic patterns are not determined entirely by vascular anatomy, rate of blood flow, and number of tumor cells delivered (Weiss et al. 1980, Sugarbaker 1981). Interest in factors that affect metastatic patterns is by no means new. As early as 1889, Paget analyzed 735 autopsies of patients with breast cancer to answer the question, "What is it that decides what organs shall suffer in a case of disseminated cancer?" The nonrandom pattern of metastases suggested to Paget that the process was not due to chance but rather that certain tumor cells (the "seed") had a specific affinity for the milieu provided by certain organs (the "soil"). This "seed and soil" hypothesis has received considerable support. Comparable site-specific metastasis occurs with many of the transplantable tumors used in laboratory animals (Fidler and Nicolson 1976, 1977, 1978, Brunson and Nicolson 1978, Brunson et al. 1978, Tarin and Price 1979, Raz and Hart 1980, Hart et al. 1981, Talmadge et al. 1981, Hart 1982, Tarin 1982). Indeed, this preference of certain tumors for specific organs is maintained even when the organs are transplanted into ectopic sites (Kinsey 1960, Sugarbaker et al. 1971, Hart and Fidler 1980b, Hart 1982, Nicolson 1982). The fact that patterns of metastasis are predictable for tumors of a defined histological type suggests that metastasis is not an entirely random event.

THE METASTATIC HETEROGENEITY OF MALIGNANT NEOPLASMS

At the time of diagnosis, many human and animal neoplasms are composed of numerous subpopulations of cells with distinctly different biological properties. Cells isolated from individual neoplasms have been shown to differ with respect to their morphology, karyotype, growth rate, antigenicity-immunogenicity, cell surface receptors for lectins, hormone receptors, response to therapies, and potential for invasion and metastasis (for review, see Calabresi et al. 1979; also see Hart and Fidler 1981, Fidler and Hart 1982, Fidler and Poste 1982, Heppner and Miller 1983).

Cells with different metastatic properties have been isolated from parent or primary tumors, thus supporting the hypothesis that not all the cells in a primary tumor can successfully disseminate. Two general approaches have been used to isolate populations of cells that differ from the parent neoplasm in metastatic capacity. In the first, tumor cells are selected in vivo. These cells are implanted subcutaneously or intramuscularly or injected intravenously into mice, and metastasis is allowed to occur. The metastatic lesions are harvested, and the cells that are recovered can first be expanded in culture or can be used immediately to repeat the process. The cycle is repeated several times. The behavior of the cycled cells is compared with that of the cells of the parent tumor to determine whether the selection process enriched the lines with cells of enhanced metastatic capacity. [Studies have shown that the increase in metastatic capacity of the recovered cells does not result from the adaptation of tumor cells to preferential growth in a particular organ (Brunson and Nicolson 1979, Raz et al. 1981, Fidler and Nicolson 1981, Nicolson and Custead 1982, Talmadge and Fidler 1982a,b, Nicolson 1982, Poste 1982, Kiernan and Longenecker 1983).] This procedure was originally used to obtain the B16-F10 line from the unselected B16 melanoma (Fidler 1973a, 1975) (Figure 3). It has also been successfully used to produce tumor cell lines with increased metastatic capacity from many of the experimental tumors tested (Fidler and Hart 1982, Poste 1982, Nicolson 1982, Talmadge 1983).

In the second approach, cells are selected for the enhanced expression of a phenotype believed to be of importance in one or another step of the metastatic sequence, and then they are tested in the appropriate host to determine whether concomitant metastatic potential has been increased or decreased. This method has been used to examine whether properties as diverse as resistance to T lymphocytes (Fidler et al. 1976, Frost and Kerbel 1981) (Figure 4), adhesive characteristics (Briles and Kornfeld 1978), invasive capacity (Hart 1979, Poste et al. 1980), lectin resistance (Kerbel 1979a, Reading et al. 1980a,b), resistance to natural killer cells (Hanna and Fidler 1981), and antibody-complement-dependent cytotoxicity (Kerbel et al. 1982) are important in metastasis.

One obvious criticism of these studies is that the surviving isolated tumor line may have arisen as a result of adaptive rather than selective processes. To determine whether differences between metastatic capacities of tumor cell populations are preexistent or arise as a result of adaptation to local environmental conditions, in 1977 Margaret Kripke and I applied the classical fluctuation analysis of Luria and Delbruck (1943) to our studies of the B16 melanoma (Figure 5). A culture of the B16 melanoma was established from a subcutaneous mass grown in a syngeneic C57BL/6N mouse and was divided into two portions. One portion was maintained as a mass culture; the other portion was cloned

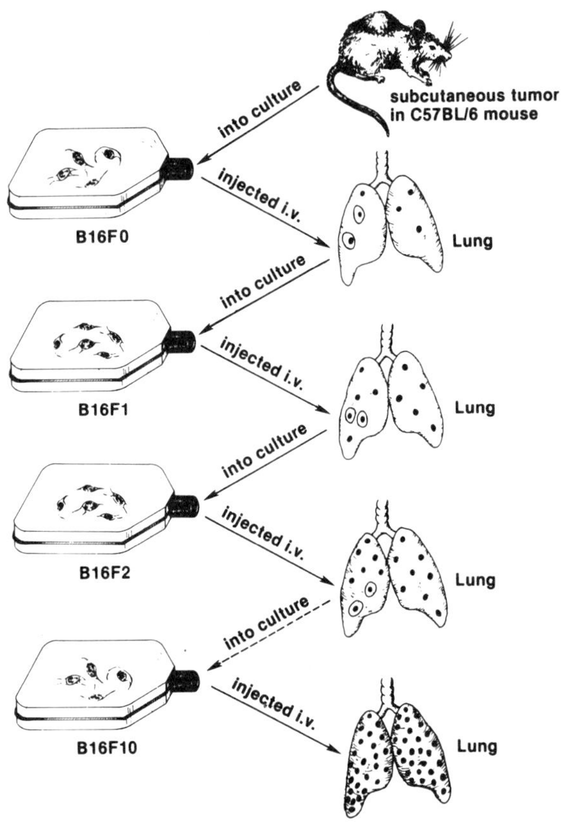

FIG. 3. The in vivo selection for cells with increased metastatic capacity. Tumor cell variants of the B16 melanoma were selected by injecting parent tumor cells intravenously into syngeneic C57BL/6 mice. Two to three weeks later, grossly visible pigmented lung tumor colonies were removed, and the tumor cells were adapted to tissue culture. The B16 cells that grew in culture after the first in vivo selection were established as a continuous line and were designated B16-F1. Cells from this line were reinjected into new syngeneic animals, and 3 weeks later a new group of lung tumor colonies was removed and cultured to yield B16-F2. With each succeeding cycle in vivo, the ability of the selected B16 lines to implant, survive, and form lung tumors increased (Fidler 1973a, 1975). After 10 such selections, the B16-F10 tumor line was obtained. This cell line forms significantly more gross lung tumors per input of cells than the B16-F1 tumor after intravenous or intracardiac injection into syngeneic C57BL/6 mice (Fidler and Nicolson 1976).

to produce 17 cell lines, each one established from an individual cell. After incubation for the same period of time, equal numbers of tumor cells in suspension from each of the cloned lines and from the parent tumor were injected into syngeneic mice. We reasoned that if the parent tumor was homogeneous, i.e., populated by cells with uniform metastatic capacity, cells from isolated clones would produce the same number of metastases as cells from the parent tumor. Alternatively, if the cloned lines gave rise to very different numbers of lung colonies, this would suggest that the tumor was heterogeneous, that cells of both low and high metastatic potential preexisted in the parent population, and that metastatic foci did not result from adaptation to local organ environment during the process of metastasis.

The study clearly demonstrated that the B16 melanoma is heterogeneous for metastasis and that a few highly metastatic tumor cell variants preexisted in the parent population. The groups of animals inoculated with the uncloned, mixed line all produced a similar number of lung metastases, whereas the cloned sublines differed markedly from the parent tumor and among themselves in the numbers of metastases produced. Control subcloning experiments showed that this variability was not introduced by the process of cloning per se.

The B16 melanoma has been repeatedly passaged in animals or culture for many times the life span of its natural host. The observed metastatic heterogeneity of this tumor could be an artifact resulting from its longevity. However, comparable data have been obtained with several other murine tumors of much more recent origin (Kripke et al. 1978, Fidler and Cifone 1979, Fidler and Kripke 1980a, Fidler et al. 1981, Nicolson 1982, Poste 1982).

In 1979, Kripke described the induction and isolation of a new melanoma syngeneic to the C3H/HeN mouse. The K-1735 melanoma arose in a C3H mouse subjected to ten 1-h exposures to UV radiation followed by weekly applica-

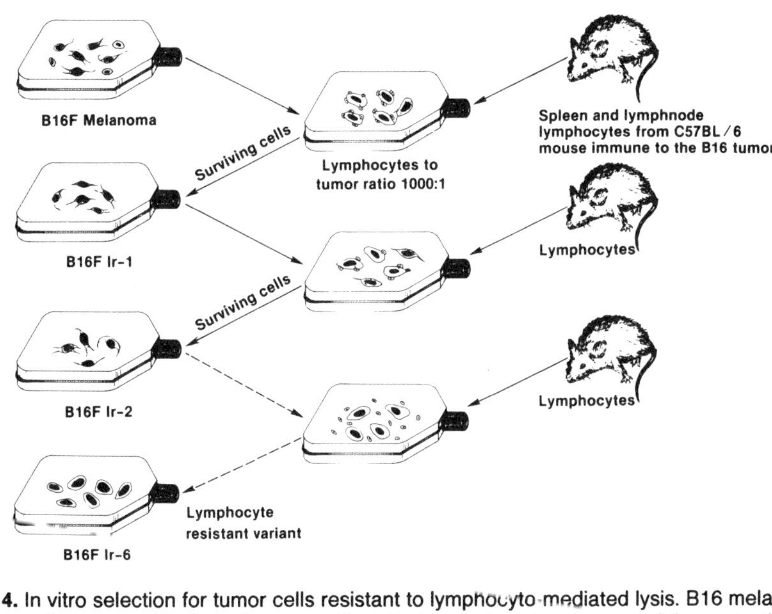

FIG. 4. In vitro selection for tumor cells resistant to lymphocyto-mediated lysis. B16 melanoma parent cells were cultivated alone or with splenic lymphocytes harvested from specifically immunized syngeneic mice. The surviving target cells were expanded and then cultured again with immune lymphocytes. The cycle was repeated six times. The resultant B16F Ir-6 line was resistant to lymphocyte-mediated lysis. Surprisingly, this variant line was also poorly metastatic (Fidler et al. 1976).

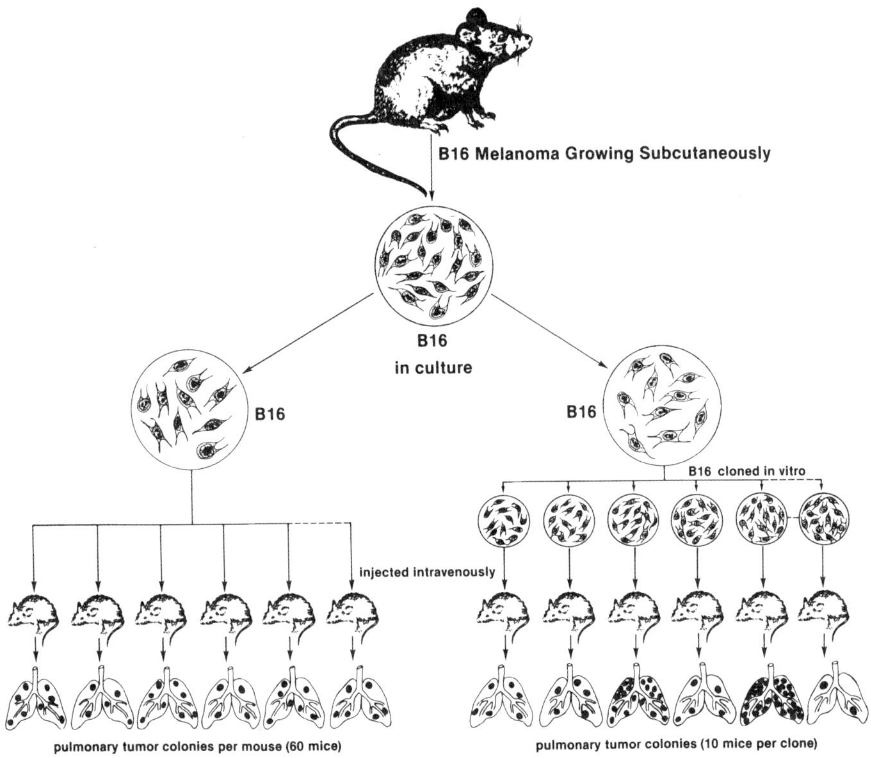

FIG. 5. Experimental design for the demonstration that metastatic variants preexist within a malignant tumor. A culture of parent B16 melanoma cells was divided into two parts. One part was maintained as a mass culture; the other part was cloned to produce 17 cell lines. After the same period of culture, equal numbers of tumor cells in suspension from each of the cloned lines and from the parent tumor were injected into syngeneic mice (Fidler and Kripke 1977).

tions of 2.5% croton oil in acetone to the skin of the scapular region for 2 years. The primary tumor was removed and fragments were transplanted into immunodeficient animals to circumvent the possibility of immune selection. Several weeks later, a tissue culture line was established, and cells from the fifth passage were used to produce clones. Clones and tumor lines were stored frozen until they were analyzed for metastatic capacity in syngeneic mice (Fidler and Kripke 1980b, Fidler et al. 1981). The clones differed dramatically from each other and from the parent line in their production of metastases in the lungs, lymph nodes, and other organs (Figure 6). Statistical analysis indicated that 20 of 22 clones differed significantly from the K-1735 parent tumor with regard to metastatic capacity (Fidler et al. 1981). In the B16 melanoma system, 15 of 17 clones were significantly different from the parent tumor (Fidler and Kripke 1977), and in a third tumor system (a recently induced fibrosarcoma), 15 of 21 clones were different from the parent tumor (Kripke et al. 1978).

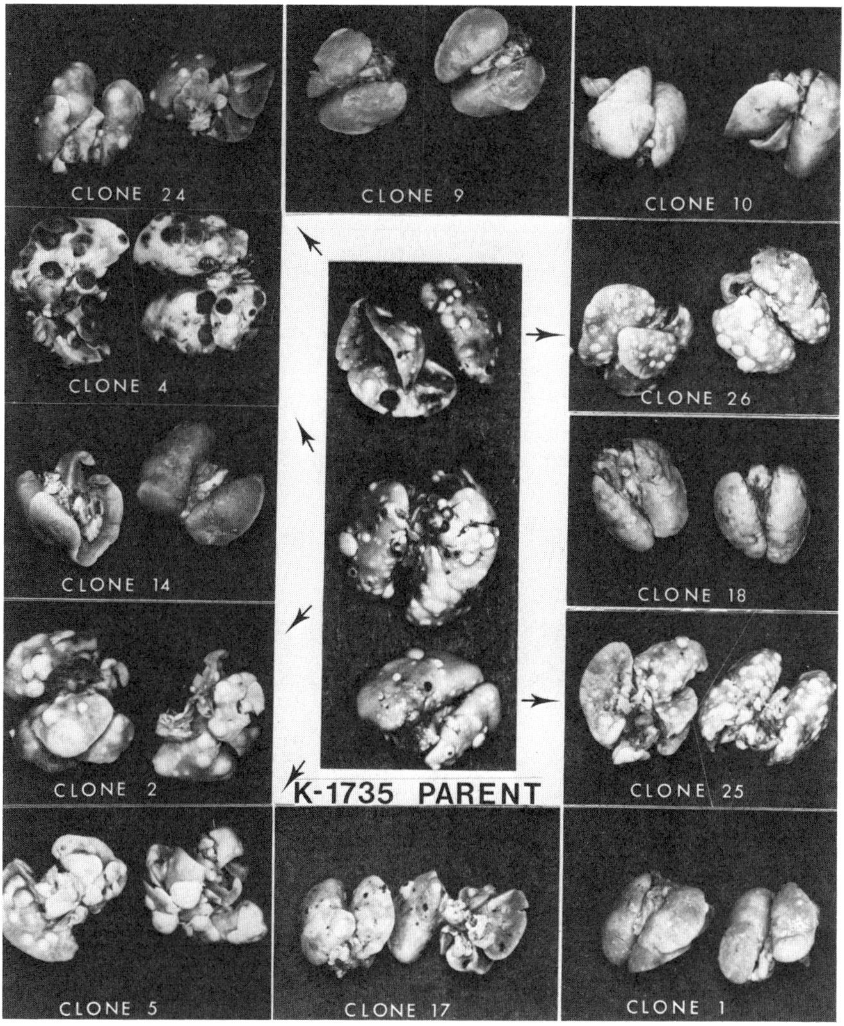

FIG. 6. Pulmonary metastases produced by cells of parent K-1735 melanoma and various cloned subpopulations. Heterogeneity in number, size, and pigmentation of metastases is readily observed (Fidler et al. 1981).

These results clearly indicate the high degree of heterogeneity of tumors and show that tumors of recent origin are no less heterogeneous with regard to metastatic capacity than the B16 melanoma. Longevity of neoplasms, therefore, is not a prerequisite for the generation of metastatic heterogeneity.

Recently, we addressed the question of whether the cells that survive to form metastases possess a greater metastatic capacity than most cells that populate the parent neoplasm (Talmadge and Fidler 1982b). As already stated, some support for this possibility comes from the initial in vivo selection experiments of the more highly metastatic B16-F10 cell line derived from the parent B16 melanoma (Fidler 1973a, 1975). Again, comparable results have been obtained with the K-1735 tumor. Cells derived from the parent tumor were injected intramuscularly into the hind footpads of syngeneic mice. The resulting "primary tumors" were allowed to grow large enough to produce spontaneous pulmonary metastases. Four cell lines, designated Met-1, Met-2, Met-3, and Met-4, were established from four individual lung nodules harvested from four different mice. The metastatic capacity of cells from these four lines was compared with that of cells from the parent tumor, using both experimental metastases (those that occur following intravenous injection of tumor cells) and spontaneous metastases (those that develop from a subcutaneously implanted tumor) as end points. All the lines derived from metastatic deposits produced significantly more metastases than the parent line ($P \leq 0.01$) in both types of assay (Figure 7). Similar data were obtained with three other tumors (Talmadge and Fidler 1982b). These results indicate that cells populating metastases have an increased metastatic capacity.

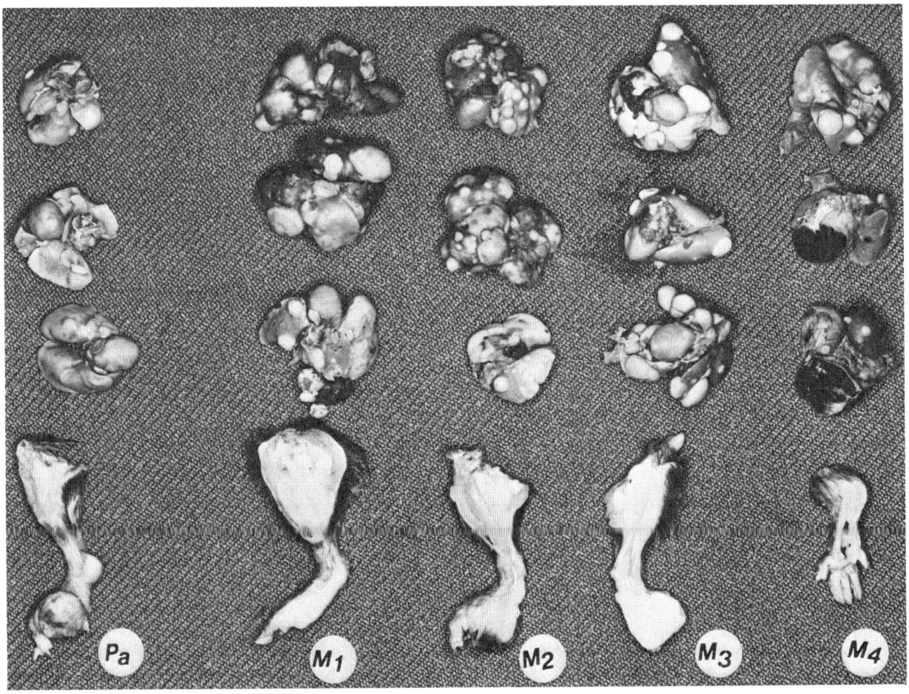

FIG. 7. Spontaneous lung metastases produced by cells from parent K-1735 cell line (Pa) or spontaneous metastases (SM1 through SM4) implanted into the footpads of syngeneic C3H/HeN mice (Talmadge and Fidler 1982b).

METASTASIS CAN APPEAR RANDOM OR SELECTIVE DEPENDING ON THE EXPERIMENTAL TUMOR SYSTEM

The question of whether metastasis is due to chance has been debated for almost a century (Paget 1889). The data discussed in the preceding section support the nonrandom nature of tumor spread. Yet there are inconsistencies among several reports that require explanation. Some investigators who used the in vivo selection procedure (Figure 3) reported results that differed from ours (Giavazzi et al. 1980, Eccles et al. 1980, Weiss et al. 1983). The discrepancies in the data may have been caused by differences in experimental conditions (Stackpole 1981) and in the heterogeneity or homogeneity of the various tumor systems used.

We attempted to minimize such variables by using three variant lines isolated from the B16 melanoma: (1) the B16-F1 variant, an unselected tumor line that is heterogeneous and poorly metastatic; (2) the B16-F10 variant, a tumor line selected in vivo for its high lung-colonizing potential (Fidler 1975); and (3) the B16-BL6 variant, a tumor line selected in vitro for its invasiveness and its high metastatic capacity (Hart 1979). All tumor lines were implanted subcutaneously in normal C57BL/6 mice and allowed to produce lung metastases, which were recovered and established in culture as individual cell lines. The metastatic abilities of cells from these new cell lines were compared with cells of the respective parent variant tumors. Metastases produced by the unselected (i.e., heterogeneous) and poorly metastatic parent B16-F1 tumor were composed of cells with increased metastatic capacity. In contrast, metastases produced by the previously selected (more homogeneous), highly metastatic B16-BL6 tumor line were not. Thus, even under controlled conditions the process of metastasis could give the appearance of being either selective or random depending on the nature of the starting population (Talmadge and Fidler 1982a). The heterogeneous nature of unselected cell lines allows selection of variants with higher metastatic capacity, whereas the homogeneous nature of already selected cell lines restricts further selection.

THE ORIGIN OF CELLULAR HETEROGENEITY IN MALIGNANT NEOPLASMS

If metastatic cells are more metastatic than most cells populating the parent tumor, why were 10 selection cycles, rather than a single passage, required to attain the biological behavior of the B16-F10 melanoma line? We believe the answer to this apparent paradox lies in understanding the origin of the exhibited heterogeneity of cells in malignant neoplasms. Two mechanisms, not necessarily mutually exclusive, can be proposed to explain the biological diversity of various neoplasms. Tumors of multicellular origin (Reddy and Fialkow 1979) may merely reflect the characteristics of the multiple progenitor cells. However, it is generally agreed that most spontaneous tumors probably originate from a single cell (Fialkow 1972, 1976, Iannaccone et al. 1978). Nonetheless, by the time of clinical presentation, most human tumors are heterogeneous with respect to various characteristics (Baylin et al. 1978, Calabresi et al. 1979, Baylin 1982). Heterogeneity in these tumors is probably generated through the process of tumor evolution and progression.

Clinical observations of neoplasms have suggested that tumors undergo a series of detectable changes during the course of the disease. For example, a tumor that was initially diagnosed as benign can, over a period of many months or even years, evolve into a malignant tumor. This neoplastic progression has been defined by Foulds (1954, 1956) as acquisition of permanent, irreversible qualitative changes of one or more characteristics in a neoplasm. The loss or acquisition of a characteristic can be independent of changes in other characteristics and is influenced by host homeostatic factors that act as selection pressures (Klein 1955, Prehn 1976, Klein and Klein 1977).

To explain the process of tumor evolution, Nowell (1976) suggested that acquired genetic variability within developing clones of tumor cells, coupled with the selection pressure exerted by host responses, leads to the emergence of new sublines with enhanced survivability manifested by increased malignancy. This hypothesis predicts that increasing progression toward malignancy would be accompanied by increasing genetic instability of the evolving cells. To test this hypothesis, we have examined the metastatic stability of several tumor lines with different capacities for spontaneous and experimental metastasis. Concomitantly, the rates of mutation to ouabain resistance or 6-thioguanine resistance of paired metastatic and nonmetastatic cloned lines isolated from four different neoplasms was determined (Cifone and Fidler 1981). Poorly metastatic and highly metastatic clones were isolated from the UV-2237 fibrosarcoma (Kripke et al. 1978) and were cultivated in vitro for 72 or 60 days, respectively. Simultaneously, both clones were also grown subcutaneously in syngeneic mice. Then, cell cultures were established from these solid tumors, and 1 week later subclones were isolated. The ability of these subclones to form experimental metastases was compared to that of subclones derived from clones grown in culture and to that of subclones isolated and frozen when parent clones were initially established.

The patterns of behavior of all the subclones derived from the poorly metastatic clone were remarkably similar to that of the parent clone, regardless of whether the subclones were derived at the time of isolation or after 72 days of continuous growth in vitro or in vivo. In contrast, after 60 days of cultivation in vitro or in vivo, the metastatic behavior of the subclones derived from the highly metastatic clone differed considerably from that of the parent clone, suggesting that the metastatic phenotype of the highly metastatic clone was unstable (Cifone and Fidler 1981). This rapid generation of diversity may have been caused in part by increased genetic instability.

The rates of spontaneous mutation resulting in resistance to 5 mM ouabain or to 6-thioguanine (4 μg/ml) were determined for cells of the two UV-2237 fibrosarcoma clones using the fluctuation assay of Luria and Delbruck (1943). In clones with high metastatic potential the rate of mutation to ouabain resistance was threefold higher and to 6-thioguanine it was 4.6-fold higher than in clones with low metastatic potential. Similar results were found when these studies were extended to three other tumor systems. Furthermore, in these studies with the UV-2237 fibrosarcoma, the K-1735 melanoma, and the SF-19 fibrosarcoma (spontaneous in origin), the increase in the rate of spontaneous mutation to ouabain resistance (6.5-, 7.0- and 5.8-fold, respectively) correlated with the degree of metastatic capacity.

These results are in accord with the hypothesis that tumor progression could occur as a result of acquired genetic alterations. However, the evolution of metastatic heterogeneity did not progress in a unidirectional manner (some subclones were less metastatic than the parent clone), and therefore the results are not incompatible with Nowell's hypothesis (1976). Perhaps the characteristic lack of selection pressure in in vitro conditions and the relatively benign milieu of the subcutis combined with the increased rate of mutation led to the emergence of both less-metastatic and more-metastatic variants. Indeed, recent experiments on mutagenesis in other murine neoplasms support this explanation. Mutagenesis of malignant cell lines has produced clones incapable of progressive growth in normal hosts (Boon and Kellerman 1976, Boon and Van Pel 1978, Van Pel et al. 1979, Boon et al. 1980) and variants with metastatic capacities more than (Fisher and Cifone 1981), less than, or equal to the parent tumor (Kerbel 1979a,b, Dennis et al. 1981a,b, Kerbel and Frost 1982, Kerbel et al. 1982). We conclude from our studies that increased metastatic capacity is frequently associated with an increased rate of spontaneous mutation, a state of affairs reflected in the relative lack of stability of the metastatic phenotype and the generation of variants of both higher and lower metastatic capacity.

THE STABILITY OF HETEROGENEOUS TUMOR POPULATIONS

Since malignant cells have higher mutation rates than benign cells, the fact that cells populating metastases so frequently exhibit greater metastatic capacity than cells of primary tumors is remarkable. Given the existence of tumor progression and lack of genetic stability, we may ask how degrees of difference can be maintained between various tumor populations. For example, the B16-F1, the B16-F10, and the B16-BL6 sublines have maintained their relative metastatic capacities for several years (Fidler and Nicolson 1981, Poste et al. 1981). What has prevented these differences from being obliterated by the bidirectional emergence of new variants?

One answer may be that subpopulations of tumor cells within the tumor mass are not autonomous units but are regulated by the proximity of other neoplastic cells. Different subpopulations of mammary tumor cells have been shown to affect the growth patterns (Miller and Heppner 1979, Miller 1982) and chemosensitivity (Miller et al. 1980, Heppner and Miller 1983) of other groups of cells. Similar regulatory control may exist for the metastatic phenotype of different cells within a mixed tumor (Poste et al. 1981). To test for this regulatory control, two poorly metastatic clones and two highly metastatic clones were isolated from the B16-F10 melanoma line. These clones were cultured in vitro or in vivo for 10, 20, or 40 passages (5, 10, or 20 weeks), and then subclones derived at each of these intervals were reassessed for their metastatic ability. After only 10 in vitro passages, many subclones that differed significantly from the parent clone were isolated. Continued cultivation introduced more variability such that by 20 and 40 passages, most clones tested differed significantly from their parent clones. In marked contrast, the metastatic phenotype of the uncloned B16 melanoma lines B16-F1 and B16-F10 remained remarkably stable over 30 in vivo passages or 60 in vitro passages. Similar stability was attained when different clones were mixed together and cocultivated as polyclonal populations; however, the subsequent removal of all but one clone led to the rapid generation of biological diversity in that remaining clone (Poste et al. 1981).

These data provide evidence that different subpopulations of tumor cells stabilize their relative proportions and thereby impose an equilibrium on the combined population. Removal of the stabilizing effect, by isolating clones or by applying a strong selection pressure such as chemotherapy, leads to rapid diversification in the resurgent populations (Figure 1). Although the nature of these stabilizing influences and their mode of action are not yet understood, their very existence argues against randomness in tumor development. Rather, the society of tumor cells imposes regulatory constraints upon its individual members to maintain cellular diversity and its concomitant benefits for tumor survival. Certainly, this phenomenon, irrespective of its underlying mechanisms, further complicates attempts to understand the process of tumor progression toward malignancy.

THE EVOLUTION OF BIOLOGICAL DIVERSITY IN METASTASES

Metastases within one host can exhibit heterogeneity with regard to many characteristics besides metastatic capacity, such as hormone receptors (Sluyser and Van Nie 1974, Brennen et al. 1979), marker enzymes (Fialkow 1976, Baylin et al. 1978), antigenicity or immunogenicity (Pimm and Baldwin 1977, Fogel et al. 1979, Kerbel 1979a, Olsson and Ebbesen 1979, McCune et al. 1981, Albino et al. 1981, Kerbel et al. 1982, Schirrmacher et al. 1982), growth rate (Fidler et al. 1981), and response to various chemotherapeutic agents (Fugmann et al. 1972, Trope 1975, 1982, Heppner et al. 1978, Tsuruo and Fidler 1981). This biological diversity may be a consequence of tumor progression, or it may result from the nature of tumor cell dissemination. Several questions remain unanswered: Do tumor emboli that survive the many steps of metastasis to form metastases consist of single cells or cell aggregates (Fidler 1973b)? How does the composition of these emboli affect the malignant process? Can embolic clumps survive in the circulatory system and give rise to homogeneous metastases of monoclonal origin (Figure 8)?

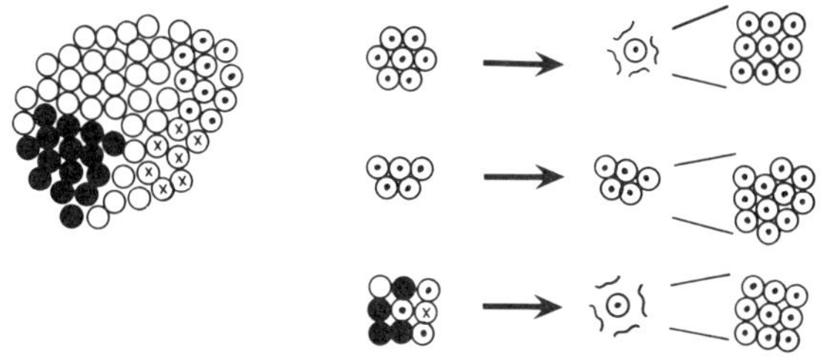

FIG. 8. The origin of metastases. Metastases may result from the proliferation of a single cell or multicellular clumps that reach distant organs. Metastatic origin notwithstanding, the process of tumor progression can generate biological diversity in metastases.

Pathologists have long recognized that primary tumors are made up of zones of morphologically distinct cells. Recent studies have demonstrated that these zonal differences are not restricted to morphology, but include many other characteristics (Henderson and Rous 1962, Prehn 1970, Fidler and Hart 1981a, Trope 1982, Raz 1982). We have shown that repeated passage of small tumor fragments can rapidly impose a uniformity on tumor cell populations that is absent when larger, more representative populations are used (Fidler and Hart 1981b). It is conceivable that embolic aggregates may arise from a single one of these zones and thus exhibit a degree of uniformity for specific characteristics. Then, irrespective of whether only the central cell or all the cells of the clump survive, the resulting metastatic growth will be analogous to a primary tumor of unicellular origin with regard to the subsequent development of heterogeneity. The same situation will arise when the embolus is derived from an area of zonal junctions, so that, though the embolus contains populations with varying phenotypes, selective cell death leads to the survival of only one cell. Alternatively, many or all of the cells forming such a mixed embolus may survive to act as the progenitors of metastatic tumors so that the generation of diversity, as in some primary tumors, is then a consequence of the multicellular origin of the neoplasm.

We performed a series of experiments to determine (a) whether individual metastases are clonal in their origin and (b) whether the metastases from one tumor originate from different progenitor cells (Talmadge et al. 1982). We examined the metastases that arose from subcutaneously growing X-irradiated cells with induced chromosomal damage. We reasoned that if a metastasis were derived from one cell, all the cells within the metastasis would exhibit the same karyotype. In contrast, a metastasis derived from more than one progenitor cell would exhibit different chromosomal arrangements. In these experiments, cells from a metastatic line of the K-1735 melanoma were exposed to 700 R X radiation to induce chromosomal breaks and rearrangements. The irradiated line was implanted into the footpads of syngeneic C3H/HeN mice. Eight to

10 weeks later, spontaneous lung metastases were isolated, grown in culture as individual lines, and karyotyped (Figure 9). In 10 of 21 lines, all the chromosomes were telocentric, and, therefore, these metastases were noninformative. In the other 11 lines, single or multiple marker chromosomes (submetacentric, metacentric, minute) were observed. In 8 of these lines, unique chromosome patterns were found in most spreads, suggesting that each metastasis originated from a single progenitor cell. In the remaining 3 lines, the pattern of markers varied, suggesting a bimodal or multimodal origin. However, G-band analysis indicated that these variations probably represented evolution within the individual metastasis. This experiment did not resolve whether metastases arose as a consequence of individual cells surviving in the blood stream or whether homogeneous clumps survived in the circulation, but it does indicate that many secondary foci can originate from the progeny of single cells. Moreover, because the metastases each exhibited a unique pattern of marker chromosomes, the data also indicate that different metastases could originate from different progenitor cells (Talmadge et al. 1982).

It is possible, therefore, to explain how diversity rapidly develops in metastases (Poste et al. 1982). Our finding that different metastases can originate from different progenitor cells (Talmadge et al. 1982) can account for the biological diversity that exists among various metastases. Moreover, even within a solitary metastasis of proved clonal origin, heterogeneity for various characteristics can develop rapidly. This may be due to the fact that clonal populations tend to

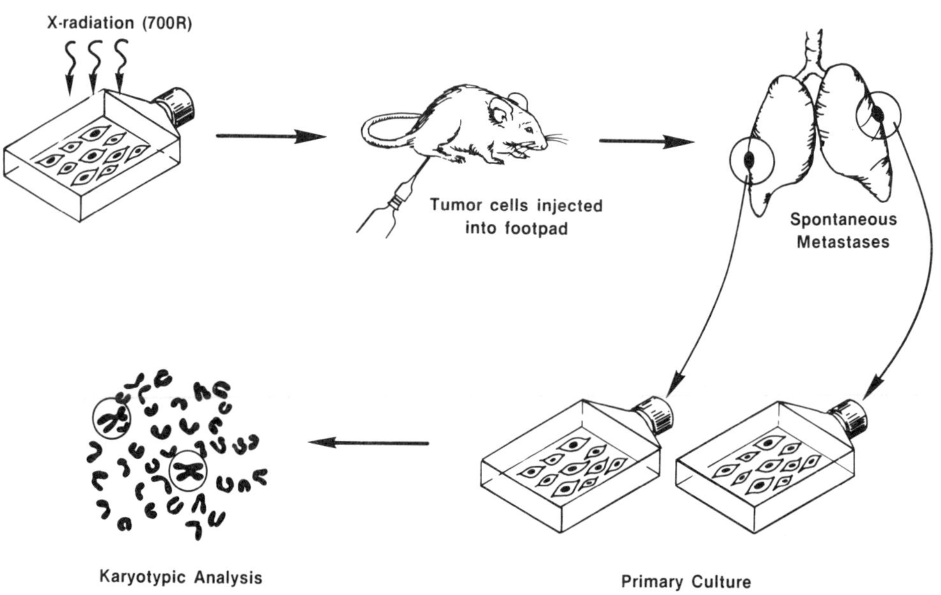

FIG. 9. Experiment designed to determine whether metastases are clonal in their origin.

be phenotypically unstable (Poste et al. 1981) and that cells populating metastases could well have a high rate of spontaneous mutation (Cifone and Fidler 1981).

SUMMARY AND CONCLUSIONS

The complexity of the processes of tumor progression and metastasis makes it difficult to provide generalized rules. Results and hypotheses that are based upon a single tumor system or a simple experimental technique are likely to be revised as more data become available. However, bearing these limitations in mind and ignoring the above warnings, I wish to conclude the following:

1. By the time of diagnosis, many malignant neoplasms are heterogeneous, i.e., they contain subpopulations of cells with different biological characteristics.
2. The process of metastasis involves a sequence of complex events whose outcome depends on tumor cell properties and host factors.
3. The metastatic process selects variants from a heterogeneous starting population.
4. The diversity for the metastatic phenotype may be a consequence of the multicellular origin of a neoplasm or it may be the result of continuous evolution and progression in tumors of unicellular origin.
5. Metastatic clones appear, in general, to be less stable than nonmetastatic clones.
6. Metastatic clones exhibit an increased rate of spontaneous mutation compared with nonmetastatic clones.
7. Some metastases may be clonal in their origin, and multiple metastases can originate from different progenitor cells.
8. Biological diversity can rapidly develop within individual metastases.
9. The acquisition of phenotypic heterogeneity by populations of tumor cells imposes a degree of stability on the tumor as a whole.
10. The generation of biological diversity in malignant neoplasms and within and among metastases has profound implications both for studies on the pathogenesis of cancer metastasis and for the design of any successful approach to the treatment of this disease.

ACKNOWLEDGMENTS

Many of my colleagues have contributed to the success of the studies I have described in this review. In particular I wish to thank Drs. Maria Cifone, Douglas Gersten, Nabil Hanna, Ian Hart, Margaret Kripke, Garth Nicolson, George Poste, Avraham Raz, James Talmadge, Sandra Wolman, and Irving Zeidman for their collaboration, encouragements, and friendship. I am also grateful to all my technical and administrative staff for their dedicated support.

Research sponsored by the National Cancer Institute, DHHS, under Contract No. NO1-CO-23909 with Litton Bionetics, Inc. The contents of this publication do not necessarily reflect the views or policies of the Department of Health and Human Services, nor does mention of trade names, commercial products, or organizations imply endorsement by the U.S. Government.

REFERENCES

Albino, A. P., K. O. Lloyd, A. N. Houghton, H. F. Oettgen, and L. J. Old. 1981. Heterogeneity in surface antigen and glycoprotein expression of cell lines derived from different melanoma metastases of the same patient. J. Exp. Med. 154:1764–1778.

Baylin, S. B. 1982. Clonal selection and heterogeneity of human solid neoplasms, *in* Design of Models for Testing Cancer Therapeutic Agents, I. J. Fidler and R. J. White, eds. Van Nostrand, New York, pp. 50–64.

Baylin, S. B., W. R. Weisburger, J. C. Eggleston, G. Mendelshon, M. A. Bearnen, M. D. Abeloff, and D. S. Ettinger. 1978. Variable content of histaminase, L-dopa decarboxylase and calcitonin in small-cell carcinoma of the lung. Biologic and clinical implications. N. Engl. J. Med. 299:105–110.

Boon, T., and O. Kellerman. 1976. Rejection by syngeneic mice of cell variants obtained by mutagenesis of a malignant teratocarcinoma cell line. Proc. Natl. Acad. Sci. USA 74:272–277.

Boon, T., and A. Van Pel. 1978. Teratocarcinoma cell variants rejected by syngeneic mice: Protection of mice immunized with these variants against other variants and against the original malignant cell line. Proc. Natl. Acad. Sci. USA 75:1519–1523.

Boon, T., J. V. Snick, A. Van Pel, C. Uyttenhove, and M. Marchand. 1980. Immunogenic variants obtained by mutagenesis of mouse mastocytoma P815. II. T lymphocyte mediated cytolysis. J. Exp. Med. 152:1184–1193.

Brennen, M. J., W. L. Donegan, and D. E. Appleby. 1979. The variability of estrogen receptors in metastatic breast cancer. Am. J. Surg. 137:260–262.

Briles, E. B., and S. Kornfeld. 1978. Isolation and metastatic properties of detachment variants of B16 melanoma cells. JNCI 60:1217–1222.

Brunson, K. W., G. Beattie, and G. L. Nicolson. 1978. Selection and altered tumour cell properties of brain-colonising metastatic melanoma. Nature 272:543–545.

Brunson, K. W., and G. L. Nicolson. 1978. Selection and biologic properties of malignant variants of a murine lymphosarcoma. JNCI 61:1499–1503.

Brunson, K. W., and G. L. Nicolson. 1979. Selection of malignant melanoma variant cell lines for ovary colonization. J. Supramol. Struct. 11:517–528.

Calabresi, P., D. L. Dexter, and G. H. Heppner. 1979. Clinical and pharmacological implications of cancer cell differentiation and heterogeneity. Biochem. Pharmacol. 28:1933–1941.

Cifone, M. A., and I. J. Fidler. 1981. Increasing metastatic potential is associated with increasing genetic instability of clones isolated from murine neoplasms. Proc. Natl. Acad. Sci. USA 78:6949–6952.

Dennis, J. W., T. P. Donaghue, D. A. Carlow, and R. S. Kerbel. 1981a. Demonstration of a correlation between tumor cell H-2 antigen content, immunogenicity, and tumorigenicity using lectin-resistant tumor variants. Cancer Res. 41:4010–4019.

Dennis, J. W., T. P. Donaghue, and R. S. Kerbel. 1981b. An examination of tumor antigen loss in spontaneous metastases. Invasion and Metastasis 1:111–125.

De Vita, V. T., R. C. Young, and G. P. Canellos. 1975. Combination versus single agent chemotherapy: A review of the basis for selection of drug treatment of cancer. Cancer 35:98–110.

Eccles, S. A., S. E. Heckford, and P. Alexander. 1980. Effect of cyclosporin A on the growth and spontaneous metastasis of syngeneic animal tumours. Br. J. Cancer 42:252–259.

Fialkow, P. J. 1972. Use of genetic markers to study cellular origin and development of tumors in human females. Adv. Cancer Res. 15:191–226.

Fialkow, P. J. 1976. Clonal origin of human tumors. Biochim. Biophys. Acta 458:283–310.

Fidler, I. J. 1970. Metastasis: Quantitative analysis of distribution and fate of tumor emboli labeled with ^{125}I-5-iodo-2′ deoxyuridine. JNCI 45:773–782.

Fidler, I. J. 1973a. Selection of successive tumor lines for metastasis. Nature (New Biol.) 242:148–149.

Fidler, I. J. 1973b. The relationship of embolic homogeneity, number, size and viability to the incidence of experimental metastasis. Eur. J. Cancer 9:223–227.
Fidler, I. J. 1974. Immunostimulation-inhibition of experimental cancer metastasis. Cancer Res. 34:491–498.
Fidler, I. J. 1975. Biological behavior of malignant melanoma cells correlated to their survival in vivo. Cancer Res. 35:218–224.
Fidler, I. J. 1978. Tumor heterogeneity and the biology of cancer invasion and metastasis. Cancer Res. 38:2651–2660.
Fidler, I. J., and M. A. Cifone. 1979. Properties of metastatic and nonmetastatic cloned subpopulations of an ultraviolet light-induced murine fibrosarcoma of recent origin. Am. J. Pathol. 97:633–648.
Fidler, I. J., D. M. Gersten, and M. B. Budmen. 1976. Characterization in vivo and in vitro of tumor cells selected for resistance to syngeneic lymphocyte-mediated cytotoxicity. Cancer Res. 36:3160–3165.
Fidler, I. J., D. M. Gersten, and I. R. Hart. 1978. The biology of cancer invasion and metastasis. Adv. Cancer Res. 28:149–250.
Fidler, I. J., D. M. Gersten, and M. L. Kripke. 1979. The influence of immune status on the metastasis of three murine fibrosarcomas of different immunogenicities. Cancer Res. 39:3816–3821.
Fidler, I. J., E. Gruys, M. A. Cifone, Z. Barnes, and C. Bucana. 1981. Demonstration of multiple phenotypic diversity in a murine melanoma of recent origin. JNCI 67:947–956.
Fidler, I. J., and I. R. Hart. 1981a. The origin of metastatic heterogeneity in tumors. Eur. J. Cancer 17:487–494.
Fidler, I. J., and I. R. Hart. 1981b. Biological and experimental consequences of the zonal composition of solid tumors. Cancer Res. 41:3266–3267.
Fidler, I. J., and I. R. Hart. 1982. Biological diversity in metastatic neoplasms: Origins and implications. Science 217:998–1003.
Fidler, I. J., and M. L. Kripke. 1977. Metastasis results from preexisting variant cells within a malignant tumor. Science 197:893–895.
Fidler, I. J., and M. L. Kripke. 1980a. Biological variability within murine neoplasms. Antibiot. Chemother. 28:123–129.
Fidler, I. J., and M. L. Kripke. 1980b. Metastatic heterogeneity of cells from the K-1735 melanoma, *in* Cancer Campaign, vol. 3, E. Grundmann, ed. Gustav Fischer Verlag, Stuttgart, pp. 71–84.
Fidler, I. J., and G. L. Nicolson. 1976. Organ selectivity for implantation survival and growth of B16 melanoma variant tumor lines. JNCI 57:1199–1202.
Fidler, I. J., and G. L. Nicolson. 1977. Fate of recirculating B16 melanoma metastatic variant cells in parabiotic syngeneic recipients: Brief communication. JNCI 58:1867–1872.
Fidler, I. J., and G. L. Nicolson. 1978. Tumor cell and host properties affecting the implantation and survival of blood-borne metastatic variants of B16 melanoma. Isr. J. Med. Sci. 14:38–50.
Fidler, I. J., and G. L. Nicolson. 1981. The immunobiology of experimental metastatic melanoma. Cancer Biol. Rev. 2:1–47.
Fidler, I. J., and G. Poste. 1982. The heterogeneity of metastatic properties in malignant tumor cells and regulation of the metastatic phenotype, *in* Tumor Cell Heterogeneity, A. H. Owens, Jr., ed. Academic Press, New York, pp. 127–145.
Fisher, M. S., and M. A. Cifone. 1981. Enhanced metastatic potential of murine fibrosarcomas treated in vitro with ultraviolet radiation. Cancer Res. 41:3018–3023.
Fogel, M., E. Gorelik, S. Segal, and M. Feldman. 1979. Differences in cell surface antigens of tumor metastases and those of the local tumor. JNCI 62:585–588.
Foulds, L. 1954. The experimental study of tumor progression: A review. Cancer Res. 14:327–339.
Foulds, L. 1956. The histologic analysis of mammary tumors of mice. I. Scope of investigations and general principles of analysis. JNCI 17:701–712.
Frost, P., and R. S. Kerbel. 1981. Immunoselection in vitro of a nonmetastatic variant from a highly metastatic tumor. Int. J. Cancer 27:381–385.
Fugmann, R. A., J. C. Anderson, R. Stoli, and D. S. Martin. 1972. Comparison of adjuvant chemotherapeutic activity against primary and metastatic spontaneous murine tumors. Cancer Res. 37:496–500.

Giavazzi, R., G. Alessandri, F. Spreafico, S. Garattini, and A. Mantovani. 1980. Metastasizing capacity of tumor cells from spontaneous metastases of transplanted murine tumors. Br. J. Cancer 42:462–472.

Hanna, N. 1982. Role of natural killer cells in control of cancer metastasis. Cancer Met. Rev. 1:45–65.

Hanna, N., and I. J. Fidler. 1981. Relationship between metastatic potential and resistance to natural killer cell-mediated cytotoxicity in three murine tumor systems. JNCI 66:1183–1190.

Hart, I. R. 1979. The selection and characterization of an invasive variant of the B16 melanoma. Am. J. Pathol. 97:587–600.

Hart, I. R. 1981. Mechanisms of tumor cell invasion, *in* Cancer Biology Reviews, vol. 2, J. J. Marchalonis, M. G. Hanna, Jr., and I. J. Fidler, eds. Marcel Dekker, Inc., New York, pp. 29–58.

Hart, I. R. 1982. "Seed and soil" revisited: Mechanisms of site specific metastasis. Cancer Met. Rev. 1:5–17.

Hart, I. R., and I. J. Fidler. 1980a. Cancer invasion and metastasis. Q. Rev. Biol. 55:121–142.

Hart, I. R., and I. J. Fidler. 1980b. Role of organ selectivity in the determination of metastatic patterns of the B16 melanoma. Cancer Res. 40:2281–2287.

Hart, I. R., and I. J. Fidler. 1981. The implications of tumor heterogeneity for studies on the biology and therapy of cancer metastasis. Biochim. Biophys. Acta 651:37–50.

Hart, I. R., J. E. Talmadge, and I. J. Fidler. 1981. Metastatic behavior of a murine reticulum cell sarcoma exhibiting organ-specific growth. Cancer Res. 41:1281–1287.

Henderson, J. S., and P. Rous. 1962. The plating of tumor components on the subcutaneous expanses of young mice. J. Exp. Med. 115:1211–1230.

Heppner, G. H., D. L. Dexter, T. DeNucci, F. R. Miller, and P. Calabresi. 1978. Heterogeneity in drug sensitivity among tumor cell subpopulations of a single mammary tumor. Cancer Res. 38:3758–3763.

Heppner, G. J., and B. E. Miller. 1983. Tumor heterogeneity: Biological implications and therapeutic consequences. Cancer Met. Rev. 2:5–23.

Iannaccone, P. M., R. L. Gardner, and H. Harris. 1978. The cellular origin of chemically-induced tumors. J. Cell Sci. 29:249–257.

Kerbel, R. S. 1979a. Immunologic studies of membrane mutants of a highly metastatic murine tumor. Am. J. Pathol. 97:609–619.

Kerbel, R. S. 1979b. Implications of immunological heterogeneity of tumours. Nature 280:358–360.

Kerbel, R. S., J. W. Dennis, A. E. Lagarde, and P. Frost. 1982. Tumor progression in metastasis: An experimental approach using lectin resistant tumor variants. Cancer Met. Rev. 1:99–141.

Kerbel, R. S., and P. Frost. 1982. Heritable alterations induced in tumor cell immunogenicity. Immunology Today 3:34–35.

Kiernan, M. W., and B. M. Longenecker. 1983. Organ specific metastasis with special reference to avian systems. Cancer Met. Rev. 2:165–183.

Kinsey, D. L. 1960. An experimental study of preferential metastasis. Cancer 13:674–676.

Klein, E. 1955. Gradual transformation of solid into ascites tumors. Evidence favoring the mutation-selection theory. Exp. Cell Res. 8:188–199.

Klein, G., and E. Klein. 1977. Immune surveillance against virus-induced tumors and nonrejectability of spontaneous tumors: Contrasting consequences of host-versus-tumor evolution. Proc. Natl. Acad. Sci. USA 74:2121–2125.

Kramer, R. H., and G. L. Nicolson. 1979. Interactions of tumor cells with vascular endothelial cell monolayers: A model for metastatic invasion. Proc. Natl. Acad. Sci. USA 76:5704–5708.

Kripke, M. L. 1979. Speculations on the role of ultraviolet radiation in the development of malignant melanoma. JNCI 63:541–548.

Kripke, M. L., E. Gruys, and I. J. Fidler. 1978. Metastatic heterogeneity of cells from an ultraviolet light-induced murine fibrosarcoma of recent origin. Cancer Res. 38:2962–2967.

Luria, S. B., and M. Delbruck. 1943. Mutation of bacteria from virus sensitivity to virus resistance. Genetics 28:491–511.

McCune, C. S., D. V. Schapira, and E. C. Henshaw. 1981. Specific immunotherapy of advanced renal carcinoma: Evidence for the polyclonality of metastases. Cancer 47:1984–1987.

Miller, F. R. 1982. Intratumor immunologic heterogeneity. Cancer Met. Rev. 1:319–335.

Miller, F. R., and G. H. Heppner. 1979. Immunologic heterogeneity of tumor cell subpopulations from a single mouse mammary tumor. JNCI 63:1457–1463.

Miller, B. E., F. R. Miller, J. Leigh, and G. H. Heppner. 1980. Growth interaction in vivo between tumor subpopulations derived from a single mouse mammary tumor. Cancer Res. 40:3977–3981.
Nicolson, G. L. 1982. Organ colonization and the cell surface properties of malignant cells. Biochim. Biophys. Acta 695:113–176.
Nicolson, G. L., and S. E. Custead. 1982. Tumor metastasis is not due to adaptation of cells to a new organ environment. Science 215:176–178.
Nowell, P. 1976. The clonal evolution of tumor cell populations. Science 194:23–28.
Olsson, L., and P. Ebbesen. 1979. Natural polyclonality of spontaneous AKR leukemia and its consequences for so-called specific immunotherapy. JNCI 62:623–627.
Paget, S. 1889. The distribution of secondary growths in cancer of the breast. Lancet 1:571–573.
Pimm, M. V., and R. W. Baldwin. 1977. Antigenic differences between primary methylcholanthrene-induced rat sarcomas and post-surgical recurrences. Int. J. Cancer 20:37–43.
Poste, G. 1982. Experimental systems for analysis of the malignant phenotype. Cancer Met. Rev. 1:141–200.
Poste, G., J. Doll, and I. J. Fidler. 1981. Interactions between clonal subpopulations affect the stability of the metastatic phenotype in polyclonal populations of B16 melanoma cells. Proc. Natl. Acad. Sci. USA 78:6226–6230.
Poste, G., J. Doll, I. R. Hart, and I. J. Fidler. 1980. In vitro selection of murine B16 melanoma variants with enhanced tissue invasive properties. Cancer Res. 40:1636–1644.
Poste, G., and I. J. Fidler. 1980. The pathogenesis of cancer metastasis. Nature 283:139–146.
Poste, G., and G. L. Nicolson. 1980. Arrest and metastasis of blood-borne tumor cells are modified by fusion of plasma membrane vesicles from highly metastatic cells. Proc. Natl. Acad. Sci. USA 77:399–403.
Poste, G., J. Tzeng, J. Doll, R. Greig, D. Reiman, and I. Zeidman. 1982. Evolution of tumor cell heterogeneity during progressive growth of individual lung metastases. Proc. Natl. Acad. Sci. USA 79:6574–6578.
Prehn, R. T. 1970. Analysis of antigenic heterogeneity within individual 3-methylcholanthrene-induced mouse sarcomas. JNCI 45:1039–1044.
Prehn, R. T. 1976. Tumor progression and homeostasis. Adv. Cancer Res. 23:203–236.
Raz, A. 1982. Regional emergence of metastatic heterogeneity in a growing tumor. Cancer Letters 17:153–160.
Raz, A., N. Hanna, and I. J. Fidler. 1981. In vivo isolation of a metastatic tumor cell variant involving selective and nonadaptive processes. JNCI 66:183–194.
Raz, A., and I. R. Hart. 1980. Murine melanoma: A model for intracranial metastasis. Br. J. Cancer 42:331–341.
Reading, C. L., D. N. Belloni, and G. L. Nicolson. 1980a. Selection and in vivo properties of lectin-attachment variants of malignant murine lymphosarcoma cell lines. JNCI 64:1241–1249.
Reading, C. L., K. W. Brunson, M. Torriani, and G. L. Nicolson. 1980b. Malignancies of metastatic murine lymphosarcoma cell lines and clones correlate with decreased cell surface display of RNA-tumor virus envelope glycoprotein gp70. Proc. Natl. Acad. Sci. USA 77:5943–5947.
Reddy, A. L., and P. J. Fialkow. 1979. Multicellular origin of fibrosarcoma in mice induced by the chemical carcinogen 3-methylcholanthrene. J. Exp. Med. 150:878–886.
Salsbury, A. J. 1975. The significance of the circulating cancer cell. Cancer Treat. Rev. 2:55–61.
Schirrmacher, V., M. Fogel, E. Russmann, K. Bosslet, P. Altevogt, and L. Beck. 1982. Antigenic variation in cancer metastasis: Immune escape versus immune control. Cancer Met. Rev. 1:241–275.
Sluyser, M., and R. Van Nie. 1974. Estrogen receptor content and hormone-responsive growth of mouse mammary tumors. Cancer Res. 34:3252–3257.
Stackpole, C. W. 1981. Distinct lung-colonizing and lung-metastasizing cell populations in B16 mouse melanoma. Nature 289:798–800.
Sugarbaker, E. V. 1979. Cancer metastasis: A product of tumor-host interactions. Current Problems in Cancer 3:3–59.
Sugarbaker, E. V. 1981. Patterns of metastasis in human malignancies. Cancer Biol. Rev. 2:235–278.
Sugarbaker, E. V., A. M. Cohen, and A. Ketcham. 1971. Do metastases metastasize? Ann. Surg. 174:161–166.
Talmadge, J. E. 1983. The selective nature of metastasis. Cancer Met. Rev. 2:25–40.
Talmadge, J. E., and I. J. Fidler. 1982a. Cancer metastasis is selective or random depending on the parent tumour population. Nature 27:593–594.

Talmadge, J. E., and I. J. Fidler. 1982b. Enhanced metastatic potential of tumor cells harvested from spontaneous metastases of heterogeneous murine tumors. JNCI 69:975–980.

Talmadge, J. E., M. Key, and I. R. Hart. 1981. In vitro characterization of a transplantable murine reticulum cell sarcoma. Cancer Res. 41:1271–1280.

Talmadge, J. E., S. R. Wolman, and I. J. Fidler. 1982. Evidence for the clonal origin of spontaneous metastases. Science 217:361–363.

Tarin, D. 1982. Investigations of the mechanisms of metastatic spread of naturally occurring neoplasms. Cancer Met. Rev. 1:215–227.

Tarin, D., and J. E. Price. 1979. Metastatic colonization potential of primary tumour cells in mice. Br. J. Cancer 39:740–754.

Trope, C. 1975. Different sensitivity to cytostatic drugs of primary tumor and metastasis of the Lewis carcinoma. Neoplasma 22:171–180.

Trope, C. 1982. Different susceptibilities of tumor cell subpopulations to cytotoxic agents, *in* Design of Models for Testing Cancer Chemotherapeutic Agents, I. J. Fidler and R. J. White, eds. D. Van Nostrand, New York, pp. 64–79.

Tsuruo, T., and I. J. Fidler. 1981. Differences in drug sensitivity among tumor cells from parental tumors, selected variants, and spontaneous metastases. Cancer Res. 41:3058–3064.

Van Pel, A., M. Georlette, and T. Boon. 1979. Tumor cell variants obtained by mutagenesis of a Lewis lung carcinoma cell line: Immune rejection by syngeneic mice. Proc. Natl. Acad. Sci. USA 76:5282–5285.

Weiss, L. 1980. Metastasis: Differences between cancer cells in primary and secondary tumors. Pathobiol. Annu. 10:51–81.

Weiss, L., K. Haydock, J. W. Pickren, and W. W. Lane. 1980. Organ vascularity and metastatic frequency. Am. J. Pathol. 101:101–114.

Weiss, L., J. C. Holmes, and P. M. Ward. 1983. Do metastases arise from pre-existing subpopulations of cancer cells? Br. J. Cancer 47:81–89.

Wheelock, E. F., L. T. Goldstein, K. J. Weinhold, W. P. Carney, and P. A. Marx. 1977. The tumor dormant state, *in* Progress in Cancer Research and Therapy: Cancer Invasion and Metastasis: Biologic Mechanisms and Therapy, vol. 5, S. P. Day, W. P. Laird Myers, P. Stansly, S. Garattini, and M. G. Lewis, eds. Raven Press, New York, pp. 105–116.

Zeidman, I. 1957. Metastasis: A review of recent advances. Cancer Res. 17:157–162.

Cancer Invasion and Metastasis: Biologic and Therapeutic Aspects edited by Garth L. Nicolson and Luka Milas. Raven Press, New York © 1984.

Keynote Address: The Interdependence of Laboratory and Clinical Research in the Study of Metastases

Bernard Fisher

Department of Surgery, University of Pittsburgh, Pittsburgh, Pennsylvania 15261

To attempt to review the subject of metastasis or any aspect of it, either factually or editorially, is redundant. That has been done over the years both by ourselves (B. Fisher and E. R. Fisher 1965a, 1965b, 1967b, 1968, E. R. Fisher and B. Fisher 1967) and by others (Clarke 1979, Cole 1973, Fidler 1978, Fidler et al. 1978, Hoover and Ketcham 1975, Marchalonis et al. 1981, Nicolson 1979, Nicolson and Poste 1982, 1983, Poste and Fidler 1980, Sugarbaker 1979, Weiss 1976, 1977). In fact, there may be as many reviews as there are articles referred to in them. Those commentaries indicate that investigators of metastasis are romanticists. Their scenarios are often fascinating. What is more picturesque than a "metastatic cascade"? Is there anything that can top watching a group of tumor cells participating in a decathlon and realizing that the winner, by performing well in all events, will have the honor of becoming a metastasis? Since the history and nature of the process is so well documented, it needs no retelling by me. Not a philosopher of science or possessing precognition, I am unable to point out what direction research on the subject should take or what models should be used. After 25 years of involvement in both laboratory and clinical research in the study of the biology of tumor metastasis, I have acquired firm impressions regarding their interdependence. It is my intent to share with you some of my thoughts and experiences indicating the importance of that relationship.

BACKGROUND

Szent-Gyorgi commented, "To fix a machine one must understand how it works and to cure cancer one must understand the disease." This supposes that complete comprehension of the process with an attendant therapeutic gain is apt to occur only as a result of knowing what constitutes its component parts, what the behavior of each is, and how they function when in combination. The gross components of the metastatic process, i.e., tumor cell invasion, dissemination, lodgement, and growth, have long been familiar. Over the last two decades in vitro investigation and animal experimentation have been directed toward dismantling the metastatic "machine" into its more basic constituents and determining how each of them may function as *independent* variables. With each new methodologic development, the "breakdown" process has proceeded at a more rapid pace. Considerable information, albeit often contradictory, has resulted, providing new insight into the basic components of the metastatic process—at least in the models employed.

Despite what appears to be progress, certain perceptions I have, if they are accurate, cause concern. The position that methodology and animal models have assumed in the study of metastasis justifies comment. There is an undeniable tendency, particularly in study sections where the fate of research direction in this country is determined, frequently to be more concerned with the nuances of methodology to be employed than with the concept that has given rise to a contemplated study. Methodologic vogue is a research distraction. Despite the most elegant methodology, the time has not yet arrived when one can assume that findings obtained from in vitro studies are indicative of what takes place in the human being. Extrapolation of the significance and universality of a finding from an in vivo animal model to a patient with cancer is equally precarious, no matter how convinced proponents of a model are that it simulates the human. How each one of those well-characterized functional components becomes modulated when present in an intact environment composed of competing forces cannot possibly be predicted. My concern is intensified by the fact that there is an increasing cadre of investigators who favor the emphasis of in vitro research at the expense of in vivo animal investigation, and there is an equal, if not more dangerous, cabal who seek to abolish human clinical trial research because they perceive it to be inefficient, nonproductive, and unjustifiably competitive for research dollars. In my opinion these attitudes are regressive and arise from a lack of appreciation of the interdependence of laboratory and clinical research in the study of cancer.

Another concern relates to the impression I have obtained from comprehensive reviews that despite all of the laboratory research carried out during the last two decades, there has been little or no testing in the human of concepts derived from animal and in vitro studies of metastasis. Perhaps no new hypotheses have been formulated. Perhaps those synthesized have not been worthy of evaluation in humans. Perhaps testing has taken place, but was not recognized as such. Often the only reference to human metastasis in reviews is either observational in nature or consists of a stirring "grant application type" last sentence such as, "Learning more about metastasis and tumor progression in animal tumor systems should lead to the design of more rational therapies for the management of cancer." Moreover, there is no indication that investigations or observations in the human have given rise to concepts that have provided impetus to laboratory investigation. Do reviews reflect the true state of affairs? Have the past two decades been so devoted to experiment-driven research that awareness of purpose has been lost? Are laboratory investigators to blame, or have clinical investigators failed to translocate findings from the laboratory into the clinical setting?

After two decades of effort, there are still facets of metastatic research that have failed to produce findings unifiable into a concept capable of being tested in the human. Tumor cell invasion and penetration exemplifies one such component. Information from a number of models indicates that ". . . there is a vast indirect (histologic) evidence, but hardly sufficient direct (cinematographic) proof for the occurrence of cell locomotion in tumor penetration in vivo" (Strauli and Weiss 1977). Others have considered that a major advance in knowledge of metastasis has been the recognition of the importance of tumor cell surface properties in influencing the invasive process. Investigations have evaluated the capabilities of tumor cells to produce enzymes that enhance their invasiveness by perturbing a normal tissue matrix, and observations from in vitro models have indicated that the cells within a tumor possess variable invasive properties. Can these and other seemingly unrelated phenomena be coordinated into a concept with therapeutic relevance? Since biological events associated with the early stages of the metastatic process have been in operation prior to the discovery of a tumor, even should an intervention be devised to abort the process it could be introduced only after the fact. Perhaps its worth might be to prevent metastases from metastasizing, if this is an event of clinical importance. By discerning properties of human tumor cells that relate to invasiveness, we could make another prognostic marker available to aid in defining a patient population at risk. It is more likely that information on the invasive properties of a tumor has greater relevance to understanding normal cell biology than to the formulation of strategies that can affect the natural history of patients with cancer. These comments are not to be construed as minimizing the importance or worth of such investigations—merely to indicate how I perceive their orientation in the scheme of things.

Redundant as it may seem, it is appropriate to put into focus the purpose of in vitro and in vivo research, which is primarily to develop concepts that can be formulated into hypotheses. It is such hypotheses—not individual experiments—that require testing in the human. Clinical benefit is the fringe benefit derived from biological hypothesis testing. The perception held by many that "clinical" trial research is "product testing," i.e., testing of drugs, operations, types of radiation, etc., needs to be changed. Clinical trial research is not only a necessary corollary of laboratory investigation but is an instigator of concept and hypotheses in its own right. Those who would eliminate the testing process provided by clinical trial research may not fully appreciate that they may be supplying an open ticket for laboratory investigators to continue their studies in tangential and repetitive fashion—limited only by urgency in developing new methodology and models and, of course, funding. Without there ever being a day of reckoning, there can be no accountability for their efforts. Sooner or later it becomes necessary to assess what has been and is being done in a field such as metastasis to ascertain whether there are threads in the results capable of being woven into a worthy hypothesis that can be tested in humans. A hypothesis is of value only if it can be evaluated so that it may be rejected, supported, or modified. Otherwise, it assumes the status of armchair philosophy.

There comes a time when hypothesis testing *must* be undertaken. To continue to look for the "perfect" experiment in the "perfect" model to resolve all doubts and to satisfy all one's peers before instituting such an undertaking is apt to result in investigative stalemate and paralysis. An appropriate hypothesis derived from biological principles tested in a proper human setting will result in information not only of clinical importance but of equal if not greater biological significance. The results will clarify directions for research in metastasis that might be productive and indicate other areas that should be abandoned. Such testing in the human cannot confirm findings obtained from individual laboratory experiments. It is unlikely that more than a few of the experiments carried out in animal model systems will or can ever be duplicated in the human to determine whether findings in the former are valid in the latter.

These remarks are not to be construed as minimizing the importance of nontargeted, non-goal-oriented or fundamental research. There must be increased and unabated support for such effort. There is no conflict between fundamental research and research that may have clinical relevance. Just as one must be circumspect about considering all clinical research mundane so must one be cautious about considering all research without a clinical application as fundamental. The term "fundamental" may be considered in a sense akin to a "promissory note."

The remainder of this discussion provides a few scenarios from our experience to exemplify how a combination of laboratory and clinical research has contributed or may in the future add to the understanding of tumor metastasis and at the same time improve the therapy of cancer. Female breast cancer was the human tumor model used exclusively in these studies. How universally applicable findings from that model are to other human tumors is equally as conjectural as is the relation of findings from in vivo and in vitro systems to all or any human tumors.

EXAMPLES OF LABORATORY AND CLINICAL RESEARCH INTERACTION

Halstedian Hypothesis

The first paradigm for cancer management synthesized slightly less than 100 years ago was based on the biology of metastasis as it was perceived at that time. Information primarily from three investigations circa 1880 resulted in the formulation of a hypothesis that provided the basis for both cancer surgery and postoperative radiation. Goldman and Schmidt demonstrated that cancer cells in blood excited thrombosis. They concluded that the thrombi destroyed or rendered such cells harmless (Handley 1922). That finding was interpreted as minimizing the importance of the blood vascular system in the metastatic process. It is remarkable how many experiments carried out in recent years bear a relation to Goldman and Schmidt's observation, but not to their conclusion. It is equally remarkable that despite those efforts, so many uncertainties still remain about the pathobiology of this aspect of the metastatic process. Innumerable investigators have attempted by various means to determine the importance of fibrin, fibrinogen, platelets, and other coagulation components in the metastatic process. Many have evaluated the capacity of a variety of anticoagulants to inhibit metastasis formation. Our own studies relative to the use of such agents go back to 1961 (B. Fisher and E. R. Fisher 1961, 1967a). Despite considerable effort, the investigations have not resulted in very great dividends; their translocation into the human setting has been almost nil.

Handley's concept that tumor cells spread along lymphatic pathways by direct extension rather than by embolization also played a role in the formulation of the halstedian hypothesis (B. Fisher 1970). It considered that there was contiguity between a primary tumor and its metastasis, even when one occurred remote from the other, e.g., a breast cancer and a metastatic lesion in the femur. Finally, studies by Virchow indicating that regional lymph nodes (RLN) were effective filters that could serve as barriers to tumor cell spread influenced the evolution of the hypothesis (B. Fisher 1970). Mainly from those three studies related to metastasis came the first hypothesis that had relevance to the therapy of cancer in humans. There arose principles of cancer surgery that were anatomic and mechanistic in concept.

Two comments regarding the halstedian hypothesis are appropriate. First, it was based upon "scientific" precepts. Theories that have been replaced are not in principle unscientific. If one designates outdated concepts as "nonscientific" or "error," then scientific knowledge of today is apt to be judged in the future as nonscience and error as well. Second, the hypothesis was accepted without test of its validity because it was not replacing an already entrenched paradigm and because there were for many years few challenges to it from the results of laboratory and clinical studies.

Alternative Hypothesis

By the mid 1950s when our laboratory investigations began, little had changed in the perception of the process of metastasis. While by then it was accepted that lymphatic spread occurred by embolization instead of by direct extension, that the bloodstream was an important pathway of tumor dissemination, and that laboratory investigations had clarified certain aspects of the process, the overall concept remained unaltered. The idea prevailed that lymph-borne tumor cells had one destination—lymph nodes, that tumor cells in blood lodged in the first capillary bed they encountered, and that there was an orderly pattern of dissemination based on temporal and mechanical considerations. The only debate related to whether patterns of distant metastases were due to specific properties of various tissues, the "seed-soil" hypothesis first promulgated by Paget in 1889, or to anatomical and mechanical factors.

Intrigued by the possibility that disseminated tumor cells produced metastases only in *some* individuals, and that the soil concept was somehow related to this occurrence, we began investigations toward obtaining a better comprehension of the biology of metastasis. No convictions or hypothesis directed our efforts; we were entirely involved with experiment-driven research—fact finding. Laboratory studies carried out by us between 1958 and 1968 influenced our own thinking relative to metastatic mechanisms. They revealed that the blood and the lymphatic vascular systems are so interrelated that it is impractical to consider them as independent routes of dissemination (B. Fisher and E. R. Fisher 1966). Within minutes, viable tumor cells gaining access to the liver via the portal vein could be identified in lymph coming from the liver. Those and other findings led us to conclude as early as 1964 (B. Fisher and E. R. Fisher 1965a) that:

> . . . it would seem obsolete to ascribe either mechanical considerations *or* soil (host) factors as responsible for tumor distribution. It would seem that patterns of tumor spread are dictated by anatomic considerations *as well as* intrinsic factors in the tumor cell per se and in the tissue that it reaches.

Using labeled cells, we first obtained *quantitative* data relative to the deposition and egress of neoplastic cells from organs following their hematogenous dissemination and subcutaneous inoculation. It was observed that the residence of a vast majority of tumor cells gaining access to an organ via the bloodstream was transient (B. Fisher and E. R. Fisher 1967c), confirming and extending the seminal observation of Zeidman (1961) and his associates that tumor cells are not trapped by the first capillary bed they encounter. Such observations permitted us to adopt the thesis that there is no orderly pattern of tumor cell dissemination that could be based on mechanical and temporal factors.

Results from another series of experiments led to the conclusion that RLN are not, as Virchow proposed, effective barriers to tumor spread. Additional studies indicated the biological importance of RLN. They were found to play a role in both initiation (B. Fisher and E. R. Fisher 1971) and maintenance of tumor immunity (B. Fisher and E. R. Fisher 1972). We also demonstrated that RLN cells are capable of destroying tumor cells, indicating that the presence of negative nodes may be a result of such a circumstance as well as because tumor cells traverse nodes rather than that a tumor had been removed prior to its dissemination (B. Fisher et al. 1974a). Axillary nodes from patients (B. Fisher et al. 1972, 1974b) continued to possess immunological capabilities despite the presence of growing tumors. Those qualities vary in nodes within a patient and between patients. The findings indicated that biological rather than anatomical factors might be the reason that certain nodes contained metastases and others did not. Recent evidence indicates that RLN cells are instigators of a cascade of events giving rise to cytotoxic effector cells of both the lymphoid and myeloid series (B. Fisher et al. 1977).

Studies begun in 1958 indicated that host factors are important in the development of metastases and that a tumor is not autonomous of its host as was believed (E. R. Fisher and B. Fisher 1967). The presence of dormant tumor cells was demonstrated (B. Fisher and E. R. Fisher 1959a), and it was shown that perturbation of the host by a variety of means could produce lethal metastases from those cells (B. Fisher and E. R. Fisher 1959b, B. Fisher et al. 1969b). Our findings led us to consider that local recurrences following operation were apt to be the result of systemically disseminated cells lodging and growing at a site of trauma rather than of inadequate surgical technique (B. Fisher et al. 1967). We proposed that a tumor is a systemic disease, probably from its inception. That premise never implied that all patients would at some time develop overt metastases; nor did it imply that only those with metastases represent the population with disseminated disease.

In the 1960s, the thesis was formulated that the RLN is an indicator of host-tumor relations. The lymph node that contains tumor cells reflects an interrelation between host and tumor that permits the development of metastases rather than that the node is an *instigator* of distant disease.

Concomitant with the laboratory investigations, we obtained information from a series of clinical trials. The results of those studies failed to coincide with expectation. Recurrence and survival were independent of the number of axillary nodes removed and examined (B. Fisher and Slack 1970). Patients having few nodes removed that were all free of tumor had the same prognosis as did those with large numbers removed and free of tumor. Conversely, patients with, for example, two of five nodes positive were at the same risk as those with two of 30 nodes positive. It was also found that despite the fact that cancers of the inner half of the breast metastasize more frequently to internal mammary nodes than do outer quadrant tumors, tumor location failed to influence prognosis (B. Fisher et al. 1969a). In patients who had radical mastectomy, an operation that does not remove internal mammary nodes, the treatment failure and survival was the same whether the tumors were in the inner or outer half of the breast.

Whether the results of all of these laboratory studies and clinical observations were interpreted correctly, were due to the methodologies and models employed rather than to biologic circumstances, could or could not be confirmed in every setting and in every detail, or were obtained from simplistic experiments that did not really provide positive proof for any of our assumptions, they all had the same characteristic. They did not conform to the concepts that provided the principles for the halstedian hypothesis. They provided a matrix on which an alternative thesis could be formulated. That hypothesis, synthesized in 1968, is biological in concept rather than anatomic and mechanistic. Its components are completely antithetical to those in the one attributed to Halsted (Table 1).

Alternative Hypothesis Testing

Opportunity to confirm or deny the tenets of the alternative hypothesis became available in 1971 via a trial involving almost 2,000 women. We fully appreciated that no answers would be obtained from that clinical test that would specifically

TABLE 1. *Two divergent hypotheses of tumor biology*

Halstedian	Alternative
Tumors spread in an orderly defined manner based upon mechanical considerations.	There is no orderly pattern of tumor cell dissemination.
Tumor cells traverse lymphatics to lymph nodes by direct extension, supporting en bloc dissection.	Tumors cells traverse lymphatics by embolization, challenging the merit of en bloc dissection.
The positive lymph node is an indicator of tumor spread and is the instigator of disease.	The positive lymph node is an indicator of a host-tumor relationship that permits development of metastases rather the instigator of distant disease.
Regional lymph nodes are barriers to the passage of tumor cells.	Regional lymph nodes are ineffective as barriers to tumor cell spread.
RLN's are of anatomic importance.	RLN's are of biological importance.
The blood stream is of little significance as a route of tumor dissemination.	The blood stream is of considerable importance in tumor dissemination.
A tumor is autonomous of its host.	Complex host-tumor interrelationships affect every facet of the disease.
Operable breast cancer is a local regional disease.	Operable breast cancer is a systemic disease.
The extent and nuances of operation are the dominant factors influencing patient outcome.	Variations in local-regional therapy are unlikely to substantially affect survival.
No consideration was given to tumor multicentricity.	Multicentric foci of tumor are not of necessity a precursor of clinically overt cancer.

indicate whether each of our laboratory findings was reproducible in humans. The aim was to test the *hypothesis* synthesized from these studies, not to test the studies themselves. After a follow-up of 10 years, the results of that trial have indicated that in patients without clinical evidence of node involvement three distinctly different treatment regimens (radical mastectomy, total mastectomy with local-regional radiation, or total mastectomy without radiation and removal of nodes only if they later became involved) yielded no significant difference in overall treatment failure, distant metastases, or survival (B. Fisher et al. 1980). In patients having clinical node involvement who were treated by radical mastectomy or total mastectomy followed by local-regional radiation, there was also no significant difference in outcome. The results provide credibility to and confirmation of many of the tenets of the alternative hypothesis. To most clinicians, the results of that study provided justification for doing a lesser operation—nothing more. The nonclinician laboratory investigator of metastasis is apt to overlook the biological relevance of those results or more likely to be totally unaware of the study.

The similarity of findings in patients with clinically negative nodes was remarkable considering that approximately 40% of women subjected to total mastectomy alone had positive nodes unremoved and untreated. Those nodes should have been expected to serve as a source of further tumor dissemination, resulting in an increase in distant treatment failure and mortality. That such was not so justifies a challenge to temporal considerations in metastatic development and tends to indicate that, even if metastases do metastasize, the consequences, at least in this setting, are clinically irrelevant. Just as not removing nodes was not deleterious, their removal did not adversely affect prognosis, refuting the concept that unremoved regional nodes may provide an immunologic advantage. When considered overall, the findings refute in the human the anatomic and mechanical precepts that have dictated thinking relative to metastases and have influenced therapy. It would thus seem that laboratory research having as its specific goal the obtaining of additional information to confirm or deny the tenets of this hypothesis (which had been evaluated in the human) may not be of high priority.

Adjuvant Chemotherapy Hypothesis

Another area of metastasis that reveals the interdependence of laboratory and clinical research is that relating to adjuvant chemotherapy. The use of such therapy provides an opportunity to obtain information regarding the biological nature of micrometastases. In the late 1950s, animal experiments indicated that chemotherapeutic agents were capable of destroying hematogenously disseminated tumor cells (Cruz et al. 1956, McDonald et al. 1956). Shapiro and Fugmann (1957) noted in an animal model that whereas surgical removal of primary tumors or the administration of 6-mercaptopurine failed to achieve cure, the combination of the two was highly effective. Those early findings provided a rationale for testing the use of adjuvant chemotherapy in patients with cancer, the aim being to destroy circulating tumor cells during and shortly after operation. There was little concern for the management of established metastases.

In the 1960s and early 1970s, a new hypothesis for the use of chemotherapy began to take form. Mendelsohn (1960), and subsequently Skipper and Schabel (Skipper 1971, Skipper and Schabel 1973), defined the concept of a growth fraction in tumor cell populations. Skipper proposed additional principles that provided a basis for the use of adjuvant chemotherapy. He (a) quantitated the effects of chemotherapy on cancer cells, (b) demonstrated that cell kill follows first-order kinetics, (c) postulated the influence of body tumor burden on the outcome of treatment, and (d) estimated the number of cells remaining in patients following operation. Concepts embodying growth kinetic principles with direct relevance for micrometastases were formulated primarily from animal models and mathematical considerations (Table 2). Those principles resulted in a hypothesis that adjuvant chemotherapy would be beneficial.

Adjuvant Chemotherapy Hypothesis Testing

There was a difference of opinion as to how the adjuvant therapy hypothesis might best be tested in humans. Since Skipper (1971) had estimated that about 75% of women with stage II breast cancers who harbor between 10^6 and 10^7

TABLE 2. *Kinetic concepts for adjuvant chemotherapy* (*c. 1970*)

1. Growth fractions and doubling times of primary tumors may differ from those in micrometastases. Consequently, responsiveness to chemotherapy may differ.
2. The magnitude of response of a primary tumor in the plateau of Gompertzian growth need not reflect the response of micrometastases in exponential growth.
3. First-order kinetics relative to cell kill by cytocidal agents apply to those cells with constant growth fractions in exponential growth, i.e., micrometastases of $\leq 10^6$ cells.
4. The degree of synchronization of cell-cycle times of a primary tumor and its micrometastases may differ. On this basis, they may respond to cyclical chemotherapy differently.
5. Ablation of a primary tumor with a resultant decrease in total tumor cell burden may alter the growth characteristics of residual micrometastases. A decrease in tumor doubling time, an increase in growth fraction, and an improved synchronization of cell-cycle times may result. Such changes may enhance the sensitivity of micrometastases to chemotherapy.
6. Micrometastases approaching exponential growth kinetics could be sensitive to single-agent chemotherapy. Consequently, there exists the rationale for first evaluating the effect of single agents as adjuvants.

residual cells following primary tumor removal could benefit from single-agent therapy, some considered that there was logic to first employing single agents and, after determining their effectiveness, proceeding to determine the results of increasing numbers of drugs in combination. Others subscribed to a concept derived from patients with advanced disease: that the simultaneous use of multiple agents would increase therapeutic response by potentiating biochemical activity against tumor cells and by destroying tumor cells resistant to one or more, but not all, of the drugs in combination. An awakening awareness of the phenomenon of tumor heterogeneity suggesting the possibility that there might be a variable response to a therapeutic regimen by different patient subsets provided a third consideration. It was decided to carry out our trials in stepwise fashion. First, a single agent was compared with no treatment and then a two-drug combination was compared with the single agent. Finally, the two drugs were evaluated against a combination of three drugs. It is now appropriate to decide whether evidence has accumulated from our trials and those of others that lends support to the hypothesis that adjuvant chemotherapy is of value and whether new data have arisen that would modify the prevailing hypothesis or any of the concepts from which it was derived.

Information from the major trials indicates that the natural history of breast cancer has, indeed, been altered (B. Fisher et al. 1983c). The original hypothesis that adjuvant chemotherapy inhibits or eliminates the growth of micrometastases has been confirmed—*but only partially so.* No "penicillin effect" has been observed. Considering the empiricism employed in all trials, any positive result is remarkable. In none was there a preliminary determination of optimal drug dose. The scheduling, length of administration, decisions concerning drug dose reduction, and escalation were arbitrary. Consequently, the results obtained may well reflect the application of less-than-optimal methodology.

Some of the findings have biological importance. It became apparent that there was a heterogeneous response to a chemotherapeutic regimen. Subsets of patients were benefited to a greater or lesser degree than others or not at all (B. Fisher 1980). Some of the findings were discordant when considered in light of the hypothesis relating cell kill to tumor burden, first-order kinetics, drug resistance, etc. Postmenopausal patients with four or more positive nodes were *more* responsive to chemotherapy than were those who had one to three positive nodes. That observation is inconsistent with the concept that increasing numbers of positive nodes reflect a greater tumor burden and that chemotherapeutic effectiveness is inversely related to tumor burden.

Another observation difficult to explain utilizing current concepts is that patients 49 years old or younger with one to three positive nodes responded to single- and double-agent chemotherapy while identically selected patients 50 years old or older with the same nodal status, and presumably the same tumor burden, were unaffected by one, two, or three drugs. To ascribe such findings to the difference in menopausal status is logical. Unfortunately, that explanation is not adequate because postmenopausal patients with four or more positive nodes responded to two-drug therapy even better than did premenopausal women with a similar number of positive nodes.

Observations derived from our own trials and those of others indicating that increasing the number of agents in a combination does not necessarily increase the effectiveness of therapy are even more discordant with popular concept. In some subsets one or two drugs have been as, or almost as, effective as three or five. In others two, three, or five agents produced almost similar results and in still others any number used in combination failed to demonstrate much of an effect. Such findings, at least at the moment, suggest that in certain subgroups a plateau may have been attained with the use of progressively more drugs in combination. Since in certain circumstances patients with putatively greater tumor burdens are better responders to chemotherapy and since increasing the number of drugs may not always improve results, current concepts in the adjuvant therapy hypothesis used to explain response require reappraisal.

The observation that *all* populations of patients fail to respond uniformly to any of the regimens of treatment caused us to consider the use of adjuvant therapy from a different perspective. A chemotherapeutic agent or a combination of agents may be considered a probe to identify subpopulations whose metastases have cells with common or differing biological properties. Such a therapeutic "probe" culls responders and nonresponders from a population of heterogeneous tumors and provides direction for further investigation to determine why there is a difference in response between and within subgroups. The therapeutic "probe" strategy employed in humans is not dissimilar in concept to that which Fidler and associates have used in the B-16 mouse melanoma model. In their elegant experiments, by successive cloning and passage of tumor cells they have identified cell lines within a tumor with different properties (Fidler 1973, 1977). Our model, instead of using the Petri dish and the inbred mouse, is employing a therapy probe to identify differences. A major contrast between the two approaches is that the laboratory studies use a model that presumably controls for all variables. Rarely do studies in animals and in vitro models evaluate more than one variable simultaneously. In our clinical studies the findings are obviously the product of a multiplicity of host-tumor interactions.

Chemohormonal Therapy Testing

An alternative approach in humans is to employ therapeutic agents that affect cells possessing a previously identified biological characteristic. Since mammary tumors contain estrogen and progesterone receptors (ER and PR) and since tamoxifen (T), an antiestrogen that competitively binds to ER, is available, there was an opportunity to employ such an approach to obtain biological information about breast cancer micrometastases and at the same time evaluate the therapeutic effect of T. It seemed logical to employ a regimen containing both chemotherapy (L-phenylalanine mustard and 5-fluorouracil—PF) and T; the former to eliminate cells sensitive to the drugs employed and the latter to interfere with the replication of cells containing ER. A clinical trial of that combination opened Pandora's box. The heterogeneous response to such therapy observed in almost 2,000 patients clearly indicates the inability to predict outcome when we design therapies (B. Fisher et al. 1983b).

The overall results indicate that the addition of T to PF benefits patients with primary breast cancer and positive nodes. That advantage, however, is limited to those 50 years old or older and is associated with both the ER and the PR content of their tumors. The greatest benefit is in those with tumors having high ER and PR. A more precise examination of age relative to outcome indicates that the survival of those 50–59 years old is poorer when the tumor PR is low, whereas in those 60–70 years old, there is a benefit regardless of receptor level. Patients 49 years old or younger who have tumors with a low ER and PR have a poorer survival than those who do not receive T. The observation of no benefit from T in younger patients when both receptor levels are high while there is a benefit in older patients with receptor-poor tumors indicates that, at least according to the conditions of the study, the differences between the two age groups cannot be explained by an association of age with tumor receptor content.

Multivariate analyses considered the effects of the number of positive nodes, age, ER, and PR. They support the conclusion that, while nodes and ER exert strong prognostic influences in treated patients, the PR content of tumors is a stronger predictor of the effectiveness of therapy than is ER. They provide evidence for a heterogeneity in response to therapy that is both age and PR dependent. The advent of the computer and the evolving sophistication of modern biostatistics has made it possible to deal effectively with multiple host and tumor variables, thereby enhancing the capability and scope of research in humans.

These complex findings are presented to indicate the heterogeneity of response by micrometastases to a therapy and to inquire what in vitro model could possibly have predicted them. The adverse effect in certain subsets may be due to the effect of T on such organs as the liver, which in turn alters the metabolism of the chemotherapeutic agents. Could this have been predicted in a single-variable model?

The investigations with T have provoked several considerations. They indicate that the expression of tumor ER is related to age and that the older the patient the higher is apt to be the content of tumor ER. Are these findings the result of all tumors having been "born" genotypically similar but variably altered as a result of host modulation so that they display differences in phenotypic expression, or are all tumors "born" genotypically unequal due to differences in the environment in which they arise? Once again, it seems impossible to consider the tumor independent of its host. Preliminary laboratory investigations by us indicate that alteration of a host may indeed result in a change in the phenotypic expression of tumor ER.

A question raised from these findings is whether the disparate levels of ER in tumors are due to changes in the proportion of cells expressing the receptor or to variation in the amount of receptor in the cell population with ER. To answer that question and others relative to ER, it is necessary to determine the receptor level in single, intact viable cells. For several years we have been incubating suspensions of mouse or human mammary tumor cells with a ligand consisting of a fluorescein moiety coupled to position 17 of estrone (17-FE) (B. Fisher et al. 1982). Cells binding ligand demonstrate fluorescence. The proportion of cells in human breast cancers varied in our series from 3% to 58%. Moreover, the location of the fluorescence was not the same in all ER-positive tumor cells, further indicating the heterogeneity of the cell population. This methodology makes it possible to evaluate host influences on tumor cell ER as well as to relate ER to other cellular activities such as DNA synthesis. It should be a goal of laboratory research to develop methodology for determining individual cellular production of, for example, markers, enzymes, and CEA in human tumors rather than estimating those values in the tumor as a whole.

Before I leave this discussion of how therapy serves as a probe that points out biological differences in patient subsets, a philosophic comment is in order. By looking at finer and finer subsets to determine population(s) that respond to a therapy, one becomes caught between Scylla and Charybdis or, in the more popular vernacular, between a rock and a hard place. As a result of subdivision, comprehension of the biology of the disease is improved but at the same time the findings have less and less clinical meaning.

The phenomenon of subset analysis is synthesized by the lack of a totally or near totally favorable therapy. The situation is akin to that which existed in pneumonia prior to penicillin's discovery. Pneumococcal typing (or subsetting) was laboriously carried out. Much was learned about the pneumococcus in the process, but not many patients were cured by the type-specific antisera employed. With the advent of penicillin, almost all patients survived, and who then cared about the biology of the disease? A better cancer therapy might well have the same effect.

Hypothesis for the Use of Perioperative Therapy

Perioperative therapy provides another example of how laboratory and clinical research interacts. Several different biological premises provide justification for considering the use of perioperative chemotherapy. One relates to the effect that removal of a primary tumor has on the growth kinetics of metastases. Our studies have demonstrated that within 24 h following removal of a primary C3H mammary tumor, there is an increase in the labeling index (LI) of a distant tumor focus that persists for between 7 and 10 days (Gunduz et al. 1979). There is also a decrease in tumor doubling time and a measurable increase in tumor size that become apparent about a week following primary tumor removal. The tumor growth is probably a result of the conversion of noncycling cells in G_0 phase into proliferating cells, cells that should be more vulnerable to cytostatic agents. The rapidity of the onset of the kinetic changes and their relatively short duration provides a suitable rationale for the use of chemotherapy as soon as possible following tumor removal. Investigations carried out by us in an animal model have indeed indicated that chemotherapy had a more favorable effect when given on the day of tumor removal than 3 days later, when the LI of metastases were at a peak, and it was least effective when given at a time when the LI had returned to the preoperative level (B. Fisher et al. 1983a). The greatest benefit occurred when the chemotherapy was given prior to operation. Use at that time completely prevented the increase in LI, more effectively suppressed tumor growth, and prolonged survival to a greater extent than was noted under any other circumstance. This suggests that for more effective control of metastases, chemotherapy had best be employed before or at the time of primary tumor removal.

Aside from the therapeutic ramifications of the findings, their biological importance requires assessment. The mechanism whereby removal of a primary tumor exerts its effect on metastases is worthy of investigation. What mediates such a phenomenon and what characterizes the cells that respond to the stimulus? It hardly needs pointing out that the kinetic changes observed by us and by others (Schiffer et al. 1978, Simpson-Herren et al. 1976) in animal models provide no assurance that a similar phenomenon takes place following the removal in the human of all or even some primary tumors of the same or different types. Moreover, there is no assurance that the temporal pattern of the kinetic changes in the animal and in the patient (should they occur) are similar.

Of interest are our laboratory investigations that show that a change in the proportion of cells containing a certain marker may be associated with a change in the proportion of cells demonstrating other markers. We have noted that the increase in [^{3}H]TdR-labeled cells is accompanied by a decrease in those demonstrating ER.

Another justification for perioperative therapy is based on the contention of Goldie and Coldman (1979) that as a tumor cell population increases there is an ever-expanding number of drug-resistant phenotypic variants that become more difficult to eradicate. In that concept every minute counts. Consequently, combinations of non-cross-resistant drugs should be administered when a tumor population contains as few cells as possible. The Goldie somatic mutation theory seems to provide an alternative and independent explanation to that evoking cell kinetic principles as the basis for drug resistance. The two are not, however, mutually exclusive. With the growth of a tumor, not only are the absolute numbers of resistant cells increased but so is the percentage of resistant cells in the total cell population. The latter is presumed to occur because resistant phenotypes not only multiply as a result of their own intrinsic growth rates but as a consequence of the addition of new mutations from the pool of nonresistant (sensitive) cells (Goldie 1982). As a consequence of the enhanced proliferation of cells following tumor removal, it becomes more likely that the number of resistant phenotypes will increase in the metastatic population. Thus, appropriate perioperative therapy should not only destroy cells made more sensitive by their kinetic alteration but also prevent cell proliferation and so prevent an increase in resistant cells.

A third justification for the use of perioperative therapy relates to repeated observations that surgical manipulations result in "showers" of circulating tumor cells (E. R. Fisher and Turnbull 1955, Moore et al. 1957, Roberts et al. 1962). It has been reported that the presence of such cells is *not* related to patient outcome (Engell 1959, Ritchie and Webster 1961, Salsbury 1975). Examination of the studies providing evidence for such a conclusion, however, reveals that they could not have determined what the consequences of finding circulating cells might be. Insufficient patients with too short a follow-up time were inappropriately analyzed. Most important, outcome was related to the presence or absence of circulating tumor cells without regard for other variables that could have influenced prognosis.

Findings from two clinical trials employing perioperative chemotherapy have provided evidence to indicate that there may be a benefit from such therapy. Our own (B. Fisher et al. 1968) employing Thio-tepa on the day of surgery and for 2 successive days thereafter demonstrated an improvement in both disease-free survival and survival in some patients—the first evidence indicating the worth of adjuvant chemotherapy. A Scandinavian trial (Nissen-Meyer et al. 1978) in which cyclophosphamide was administered for 6 consecutive days starting on the day of operation also indicated an advantage for treated patients.

Since such therapy is apt to neutralize only events that are transient, i.e., cells disseminated and kinetic alterations occurring during the perioperative period, one may conjecture how much more beneficial such treatment will be than conventional treatment given a few weeks to a month following operation. Is that lead time apt to alter significantly an outcome more likely determined by events prior to operation? In that regard, one may contemplate many of the suppositions of the Goldie hypothesis, whose basis is not, to my knowledge, findings from in vivo experimental systems but has been derived from computer modeling. How can that concept relate to breast cancer metastases if they possess a relatively small growth fraction or do not grow at a constant rate? If gene amplification is a mechanism leading to resistance, earlier use of drugs may result in the more rapid emergence of resistant cells.

Despite these speculations, a trial of perioperative therapy is likely to provide more definitive biological information relative to human neoplasms than will additional in vitro and in vivo models. If it is revealed from a study that has truly been a contest (a proper evaluation) that there is no benefit to the use of perioperative therapy, then it may be concluded that the biological consequences of primary tumor removal or of circulating tumor cells released at the time of operation are not likely to be of clinical significance and that further research in that aspect of metastasis should be diminished or redirected. Current biological concepts will then need to be modified or abandoned.

Phenomenon of Breast Cancer Multicentricity

The controversy regarding breast-conserving operations in women with mammary cancer is more than a clinical polemic. It has directed attention to the phenomenon of tumor multicentricity and to the realization that in the course of determining what constitutes optimal treatment for breast cancer there is the opportunity to obtain information that animal models and in vitro preparations are apt to provide with less certainty, if at all. There is a substantial incidence of multifocal tumors in both breasts of women with breast cancer (E. R. Fisher et al. 1975). Only rarely is there evidence of two or more overt cancers in the same breast, synchronous bilateral tumors are uncommon, and the incidence of asynchronous primary tumors in uninvolved breasts fails by far to approach the incidence of occult lesions detected by random biopsy or at autopsy. Does the presence of a primary tumor inhibit the growth of other tumor foci and will its removal be followed by stimulation of their growth? Will there be an increased incidence of second tumors? Are unremoved occult tumor foci that fail to become overt lesions a persistent source of disseminated tumor cells that increase the occurrence of distant disease and death?

Answers to these simple but fundamental questions should be obtained from a clinical trial now being conducted. At its completion, 2,000 patients will have been randomized so that each underwent an operation that either removed the breast (total mastectomy and axillary node dissection) or conserved the breast (tumorectomy and axillary node dissection). One half of those subjected to local tumor removal will have received breast irradiation with the intent of eradicating multicentric tumor foci and the other half will not have. This trial should provide information to answer the preceding questions.

Answers to other questions regarding multicentricity could be obtained from this human model if those with the expertise and appreciation of its potential had access to it. It is ironic that so much is known about the morphologic, surface, adhesive, enzymatic, invasive, and immunologic properties of cells from various B-16 melanoma lines and yet there exists no information regarding the characteristics of the multicentric lesions. What, if any, differences exist in cells within and between such tumor foci and how do they relate to the characteristics of the primary tumor? Are, for example, all foci similar to each other and to the primary tumor relative to their ER? Perhaps patients with a primary tumor containing a high proportion of ER-positive cells are better candidates for local tumor excision because multicentric foci in their breast are also ER positive and thus might be less likely to develop into a second overt primary tumor. Information might be obtained to indicate whether all multicentric foci are synchronous in origin, supporting the "multifield" concept of carcinogenesis and that the single overt cancer represents the outcome of a rare transformation in one of them. On the other hand, did the tumor foci arise over time in response to a persisting or recurring etiologic stimulus and does the clinical cancer represent seniority?

Are multicentric tumor foci in the breast avascular and consequently dormant? Just as in metastasis, perhaps they grow only when they become vascularized. Are the cells in such foci variably deficient in angiogenesis factor and is it only in those foci that have angiogenic cells that malignant progression takes place? Perhaps with the development and use of antiangiogenesis factor, the risk of new tumors occurring following removal of a primary tumor could be eliminated.

It is disappointing that so little attention has been directed toward the study of multicentricity. In this methodologic era I am confident that, albeit difficult, approaches could have been developed that would have permitted the gaining of some insight into this biological puzzle. Should our clinical trial demonstrate that local tumor excision is equivalent to removal of the breast in terms of the development of distant disease and that multicentricity is not a problem to be reckoned with, we will have provided insight into those biological questions of clinical importance and the model will become unavailable since few or no breasts will be removed. Moreover, demand for answers to the biological questions will become less urgent. This scenario indicates, once again, how clinical findings are apt to set the direction for future research.

COMMENT

I hope that as you read the other chapters in this monograph, you will consider them in light of some of the comments I have made. I have attempted to show that the interdependence of laboratory and clinical research is so firm that any attempt to promote one at the expense of the other will be tragic for both. There is no separation between the two. They represent a continuum of effort. Until a proper clinical test is carried out, no matter how promising a line of investigation seems to be, it remains just a promise. On the other hand, without a firm biological basis acquired from laboratory investigation clinical research is apt to be nothing more than product testing. There can be no disagreement that laboratory and clinical research are of different genders. Putting them into the same bed will be more productive than keeping them apart.

ACKNOWLEDGMENT

I acknowledge with gratitude the contribution of Elizabeth Saffer to many of these studies and my discussions with Dr. Norman Wolmark, which led to this presentation.

REFERENCES

Clarke, R. L. 1979. Systemic cancer and the metastatic process. Cancer 43:790–797.

Cole, W. H. 1973. The mechanisms of spread of cancer. Surg. Gynecol. Obstet. 137:853–871.

Cruz, E. P., G. O. McDonald, and W. H. Cole. 1956. Prophylactic treatment of cancer: The use of chemotherapeutic agents to prevent tumor metastasis. Surgery 40:291–296.

Engell, H. C. 1959. Cancer cells in the blood. A five to nine year follow-up study. Ann. Surg. 149:457–461.

Fidler, I. J. 1973. Selection of successive tumour lines for metastases. Nature New Biol. 242:148–149.

Fidler, I. J. 1977. Metastasis results from preexisting variant cells within a malignant tumor. Science 197:893–895.

Fidler, I. J. 1978. General considerations for studies of experimental cancer metastases. Methods in Cancer Research 15:399–439.

Fidler, I. J., D. M. Gersten, and I. R. Hart. 1978. The biology of cancer invasion and metastasis. Adv. Cancer Res. 28:149–250.

Fisher, B. 1970. The surgical dilemma in the primary therapy of invasive breast cancer: A critical appraisal. Curr. Probl. Surg. (October), pp. 1–53.

Fisher, B. 1980. Laboratory and clinical research in breast cancer—A personal adventure: The David A. Karnofsky memorial lecture. Cancer Res. 40:3863–3874.

Fisher, B., and E. R. Fisher. 1959a. Experimental evidence in support of the dormant tumor cell. Science 130:918–919.

Fisher, B., and E. R. Fisher. 1959b. Experimental studies of factors influencing hepatic metastases. III. Effect of surgical trauma with special reference to liver injury. Ann. Surg. 150:731–744.

Fisher, B., and E. R. Fisher. 1961. Experimental studies of factors which influence hepatic metastases. VIII. Effect of anticoagulants. Surgery 50:240–247.

Fisher, B., and E. R. Fisher. 1965a. Biologic aspects of cancer-cell spread, *in* Fifth National Cancer Conference Proceedings (Sponsored by the American Cancer Society and the National Cancer Institute, 1964). J. B. Lippincott Co., Philadelphia, pp. 105–122.

Fisher, B., and E. R. Fisher. 1965b. The biology of metastasis, *in* Current Concepts in Surgery, J. H. Davis, ed. McGraw Hill Book Company, Inc., New York, pp. 321–351.

Fisher, B., and E. R. Fisher. 1966. The interrelationship of hematogenous and lymphatic tumor cell dissemination. Surg. Gynecol. Obstet. 122:791–798.

Fisher, B., and E. R. Fisher. 1967a. Anticoagulants and tumor cell lodgment. Cancer Res. 27:421–425.

Fisher, B., and E. R. Fisher. 1967b. Metastases of cancer cells, *in* Methods in Cancer Research, H. Busch, ed. Academic Press, vol. I. New York, pp. 243–286.

Fisher, B., and E. R. Fisher. 1967c. The organ distribution of disseminated ^{51}Cr-labeled tumor cells. Cancer Res. 27:412–420.

Fisher, B., and E. R. Fisher. 1968. Role of the lymphatic system in dissemination of tumor, *in* Lymph and the Lymphatic System (Proceedings of the Conference on Lymph and the Lymphatic System, sponsored by Tulane University School of Medicine and Committee on Shock of the National Research Council). Charles C Thomas Publishers, Springfield, Illinois, pp. 324–347.

Fisher, B., and E. R. Fisher. 1971. Studies concerning the regional lymph node in cancer. I. Initiation of immunity. Cancer 27:1001–1004.

Fisher, B., and E. R. Fisher. 1972. Studies concerning the regional lymph node in cancer. II. Maintenance of immunity. Cancer 29:1496–1501.

Fisher B., E. R. Fisher, and N. Feduska. 1967. Trauma and the localization of tumor cells. Cancer 20:23–30.

Fisher, B., N. Gunduz, and E. A. Saffer. 1983a. Influence of the interval between primary tumor removal and chemotherapy on kinetics and growth of metastases. Cancer Res. 43:1488–1492.
Fisher, B., N. Gunduz, S. Zheng, and E. A. Saffer. 1982. Fluoresceinated estrone binding by human and mouse breast cancer cells. Cancer Res. 42:540–549.
Fisher, B., J. Hanlon, J. Linta, and E. A. Saffer (with the technical assistance of J. Coyle and C. Ruddock). 1977. Tumor specificity, serum inhibition, and influence of regional lymph nodes on cytotoxic macrophages from cultured bone marrow. Cancer Res. 37:3628–3633.
Fisher, B., R. G. Ravdin, R. K. Ausman, N. H. Slack, G. E. Moore, R. J. Noer, and Cooperating Investigators. 1968. Surgical adjuvant chemotherapy in cancer of the breast: Results of a decade of cooperative investigation. Ann. Surg. 168:337–356.
Fisher, B., and C. K. Redmond, in collaboration with N. Abramson, D. M. Bowman, T. N. Campbell, R. K. Desser, N. V. Dimitrov, R. W. Frelick, P. H. S. Geggie, A. G. Glass, D. Plotkin, D. Prager, L. Stolbach, J. M. Wolter, and other NSABP Investigators. 1983c. Topics in oncology: Advances in adjuvant chemotherapy of breast cancer, *in* Current Hematology II, V. F. Fairbanks, ed. John Wiley and Sons, Inc., New York, pp. 415–446.
Fisher, B., C. Redmond, A. Brown, D. L. Wickerham, N. Wolmark, J. Allegra, G. Escher, M. Lippman, E. Savlov, J. Wittliff, and E. R. Fisher, with the contributions of D. Plotkin, D. Bowman, J. Wolter, R. Bornstein, R. Desser, R. Frelick, and other NSABP Investigators. 1983b. The influence of tumor estrogen and progresterone receptor levels on the response to tamoxifen and chemotherapy in primary breast cancer. J. Clin. Oncol. 1:227–241.
Fisher, B., C. Redmond, E. R. Fisher, and participating NSABP investigators. 1980. The contribution of recent NSABP clinical trials of primary breast cancer therapy to an understanding of tumor biology—An overview of findings. Cancer 46:1009–1025.
Fisher, B., E. A. Saffer, and E. R. Fisher. 1972. Studies concerning the regional lymph node in cancer. III. Response of regional lymph node cells from breast and colon cancer patients to PHA stimulation. Cancer 30:1202–1215.
Fisher, B., E. Saffer, and E. R. Fisher. 1974a. Studies concerning the regional lymph node in cancer. IV. Tumor inhibition by regional lymph node cells. Cancer 33:631–636.
Fisher, B., E. A. Saffer, and E. R. Fisher. 1974b. Studies concerning the regional lymph node in cancer. VII. Thymidine uptake by cells from nodes of breast cancer patients relative to axillary location and histopathologic discriminants. Cancer 33:271–279.
Fisher, B., and N. H. Slack. 1970. Number of lymph nodes examined and the prognosis of breast carcinoma. Surg. Gynecol. Obstet. 131:79–88.
Fisher, B., N. H. Slack, R. K. Ausman, and I. D. J. Bross. 1969a. Location of breast carcinoma and prognosis. Surg. Gynecol. Obstet. 129:705–716.
Fisher, B., O. Soliman, and E. R. Fisher. 1969b. Effect of antilymphocyte serum on parameters of tumor growth in a syngeneic tumor-host system. Proc. Soc. Exp. Biol. Med. 131:16–18.
Fisher, E. R., and B. Fisher. 1967. Host-tumor relationship in the development and growth of hepatic metastases, *in* Endogenous Factors Influencing Host-Tumor Balance (International Symposium Sponsored by the Argonne Cancer Research Hospital, University of Chicago, 1966). R. W. Wissler, T. L. Dao, and S. Wood, Jr., eds. University of Chicago Press, Chicago, pp. 149–166.
Fisher, E. R., R. Gregorio, C. Redmond, F. Vellios, S. C. Sommers, and B. Fisher. 1975. Pathologic findings from the National Surgical Adjuvant Breast Project (Protocol No. 4). I. Observations concerning the multicentricity of mammary cancer. Cancer 35:247–254.
Fisher, E. R., and R. B. Turnbull, Jr. 1955. Cytologic demonstration and significance of tumor cells in the mesenteric venous blood in patients with colorectal carcinoma. Surg. Gynecol. Obstet. 100:102–108.
Goldie, J. H. 1982. Drug resistance and chemotherapeutic strategy, *in* Tumor Cell Heterogeneity: Origins and Implications, A. H. Owens, Jr., D. S. Coffey, and S. B. Baylin, eds. Academic Press, New York, pp. 115–125.
Goldie, J. H., and A. J. Coldman. 1979. A mathematic model for relating the drug sensitivity of tumors to their spontaneous mutation rate. Cancer Treat. Rep. 63:1727–1733.
Gunduz, N., B. Fisher, and E. A. Saffer. 1979. Effect of surgical removal on the growth and kinetics of residual tumor. Cancer Res. 39:3861–3865.
Handley, W. S. 1922. Cancer of the Breast and Its Operative Treatment, Ed. 2. P. B. Hoeber, New York.
Hoover, H. C., Jr., and A. S. Ketcham. 1975. Techniques for inhibiting tumor metastases. Cancer 35:5–14.

Marchalonis, J. J., M. G. Hanna, and I. J. Fidler, eds. 1981. Cancer Biology Reviews. Marcel Dekker, Inc., New York and Basel, p. 278.

McDonald, G. O., E. P. Cruz, and W. H. Cole. 1956. The effect of cancer inhibitor drugs on the "take" of Walker carcinosarcoma 256 in rats. Surg. Forum 7:486–489.

Mendelsohn, M. L. 1960. The growth fraction: A new concept applied to tumors. Science 132:1496.

Moore, G. E., A. A. Sanberg, and J. R. Schulbarg. 1957. Clinical and experimental observations of the occurrence and fate of tumor cells in the bloodstream. Ann. Surg. 146:580–587.

Nicolson, G. L. 1979. Cancer metastasis. Sci. Am. 240:66–76.

Nicolson, G. L., and G. Poste. 1982. Tumor cell diversity and host responses in cancer metastases—Part 1. Properties of metastatic cells. Curr. Probl. Cancer 7:1–83.

Nicolson, G. L., and G. Poste. 1983. Tumor cell diversity and host responses in cancer metastases—Part 2. Host immune responses and therapy of metastasis. Curr. Probl. Cancer 7:3–23.

Nissen-Meyer, R., K. Kjellgren, K. Malmio, B. Mansson, and T. Norin. 1978. Surgical adjuvant chemotherapy. Results with one short course with cyclophosphamide after mastectomy for breast cancer. Cancer 41:2088–2098.

Poste, G., and I. J. Fidler. 1980. The pathogenesis of cancer metastasis. Nature 283:139–145.

Ritchie, A. C., and D. R. Webster. 1961. Tumor cells in the blood, *in* Proceedings of the Fourth Canadian Cancer Conference, 1960. R. W. Begg, A. Ham, C. P. Leblond, R. L. Noble, and R. J. Rossiter, eds. Academic Press, New York, pp. 225–236.

Roberts, S., O. Jonasson, L. Long, E. A. McGrew, R. McGrath, and W. H. Cole. 1962. Relationship of cancer cells in the circulating blood to operation. Cancer 15:232–240.

Salsbury, A. J. 1975. The significance of the circulating cancer cell. Cancer Treat. Rev. 2:55–72.

Schiffer, L. M., P. G. Braunschweiger, and J. J. Stragand. 1978. Tumor cell population kinetics following noncurative treatment. Antibiot. Chemother. 23:148–156.

Shapiro, D. M., and R. A. Fugmann. 1957. A role of chemotherapy as an adjunct to surgery. Cancer Res. 17:1098–1101.

Simpson-Herren, L., A. H. Sanford, and J. P. Holmquist. 1976. Effects of surgery on the cell kinetics of residual tumor. Cancer Treat. Rep. 60:1749–1760.

Skipper, H. E. 1971. Kinetics of mammary tumor cell growth and implications for therapy. Cancer 28:1479–1499.

Skipper, H. E., and F. M. Schabel, Jr. 1973. Quantitative and cytokinetic studies in experimental tumor models, *in* Cancer Medicine, J. F. Holland and E. Frei, III, eds. Lea and Febiger, New York, pp. 629–650.

Strauli, P., and L. Weiss. 1977. Cell locomotion and tumor penetration: Report on a workshop of the EORTC cell surface project group. Eur. J. Cancer 13:1–12.

Sugarbaker, E. V. 1979. Cancer metastasis: A product of tumor host interactions. Curr. Probl. Cancer 3:1–59.

Weiss, L., ed. 1976. Fundamental Aspects of Metastases. North Holland, Amsterdam-Oxford, American Elsevier, New York, p. 443.

Weiss, L. 1977. A pathobiologic overview of metastases. Semin. Oncol. 4:5–17.

Zeidman, I. 1961. The fate of circulating tumor cells. I. Passage of cells through capillaries. Cancer Res. 21:38–39.

Tumor Cell Properties and Metastasis

Cancer Invasion and Metastasis: Biologic and Therapeutic Aspects edited by Garth L. Nicolson and Luka Milas. Raven Press, New York © 1984.

Relevance of Spontaneous In Vivo Tumor-Host Cell Fusion to Tumor Progression and Metastasis Evaluated Using a Series of Lectin-Resistant Mutant Tumor Sublines

Robert S. Kerbel, Alain E. Lagarde, James W. Dennis, Fred P. Nestel, Terrence P. Donaghue, Louis Siminovitch,* and Marie Claude Fulchignoni-Lataud*

*Cancer Research Division, Department of Pathology, Queen's University, Kingston, Ontario, Canada K7L 3N6 and *Department of Medical Genetics, Hospital for Sick Children, University of Toronto, Toronto, Ontario, Canada*

Malignant tumors have two special qualities that endow them with their formidable capacity for relentless growth, even when confronted with the most aggressive therapies. These qualities are the ability to spread to distant sites (metastasis) and the ability, from a cellular viewpoint, to continuously diversify and change. The lament of the surgical oncologist—"cancers could be cured with a scalpel if only they didn't spread"—while true, is only part of the story. For even if a metastasis lies beyond a surgeon's knife, it was hoped that it should not escape the physical assault of chemotherapeutic drugs. But the quality for continuous change inevitably results in the emergence, and eventual outgrowth, of variants resistant to the drugs, an event that can sometimes occur at very high frequency. Therefore, the capacity for metastasis is necessary, but not necessarily sufficient, to render a cancer lethal: metastases, even if clonally derived, must be capable of further cellular variation.

These considerations have led to the emergence of a series of important questions, the answers to which are crucial if we are to understand and successfully tackle the cancer problem: What are the forces responsible for driving tumor cell populations towards a heterogeneous state? Are the mechanisms genetic or epigenetic? And what are the special features of metastatic cancer cells that endow them with this unique characteristic?

These are the questions we have had in mind during our own experimental metastasis and tumor progression studies, studies that were initially concerned with defining the contribution of the cell membrane to the metastatic phenotype.

Membranes and Metastasis

Metastasis is a rather complicated biological process involving a series of discrete steps (Fidler 1978). Many, perhaps most, of these steps depend on cell-cell interactions, and for this reason the cell membrane is thought to play a key role in the process. The interaction of tumor cells with normal hematopoietic cells such as platelets, lymphocytes, or monocytes, or even with other tumor cells, to form blood-borne microemboli is one example. The adherence of tumor cells to the endothelial cells lining blood vessels, during extravasation or arrest in capilliary beds, is another.

A logical approach to study the contribution of the cell membrane to metastasis is to derive so-called "membrane mutants" from metastatic tumor cell populations, preferably ones having glycoprotein alterations (Tao and Burger 1977, Burger 1980). The rationale for this approach is straightforward: the major constituent of cell membranes are glycoproteins, and cell surface carbohydrates are thought to play a key role in various cell-cell interaction and recognition phenomena. Hence, a surface glycoprotein mutant may, as a result of the change, acquire an enhanced or decreased ability to metastasize. One can then study the mutant to assess what the change is and what aspect of the metastatic process it affects; in short, a classic structure-function relationship study.

Several experimental approaches can be used to isolate such mutants.

1. Any reagent whose mode of action is known to perturb the initiation, progression, or regulation of the glycosylation processes is likely to ultimately provoke a block of cell division and cell death. Rare cells (mutants) may survive if the drug is prevented from exerting its lethal action—e.g., reduction of drug access to its intracellular target molecule (which may include the loss of a surface receptor if implicated), the loss or amplification of an enzyme activity, or the loss of the drug binding site of the target molecule. Structural analogues such as 2-deoxyglucose, antibiotics such as tunicamycin, streptovirudin, tsushimycin, amphomycin, showdomycin, and alkaloids such as swainsonine have been used to alter the glycosylated moieties of membrane proteins. However, plant lectins that bind to sugar residues with a relatively high specificity have been the most useful molecules to probe the structure and function of mammalian cell membranes (Burger 1980). That lectins can indeed be used to select for tumor cell mutants having stable membrane alterations was clearly shown by Stanley et al. (1975a).

2. Antibodies, in the presence of complement directed against surface antigens, most of which are glycosylated, can also be used as a selective device to isolate antigen-loss membrane variants, through resistance to antibody-mediated lysis (Frost and Kerbel 1981). Alternatively, they can be labeled with a fluorescent dye that can be detected on the cell by flow cytometry.

3. Other methods of selection can be imagined based on the fact that the cell membrane defines the cell morphology, which itself is governed by adherence to chemically defined substratum (Liotta et al. 1982).

Derivation and Properties of Lectin-Resistant Mutants of MDAY-D2—A Highly Metastatic Murine Tumor

We decided to select a variety of membrane mutants from an extremely metastatic mouse tumor called MDAY-D2 (Kerbel 1979). This is a DBA/2 strain leukemialike tumor whose precise cellular origin is unclear (Kerbel et al. 1978, 1980). Its extremely malignant nature (Kerbel et al. 1978) made it an ideal candidate from which to select nonmetastatic mutant sublines. Not only would such mutants, because of disparity in their ability to metastasize, be useful in studies of cellular properties relevant to the metastatic phenotype, but our studies, described below, have also revealed that they can potentially be used to study tumor progression by monitoring the instability (or stability) of the nonmetastatic phenotype of mutants. In short, would the mutants remain nonmetastatic? If not, how quickly and by what mechanisms is the ability to metastasize acquired?

In our initial studies, we selected lectin-resistant (Lec^r) mutants using phytohemagglutinin (PHA), concanavalin A (Con A), or wheat germ agglutinin (WGA) as the selective lectins (Kerbel 1979). Prior mutagenesis by ethylmethane sulphonate (EMS) was used to increase the frequency of Lec^r mutants, and some mutants were selected in a single step, others in two or more steps (Kerbel 1979). More recently, spontaneous single-step mutants have been selected (Lagarde et al. 1983b). As will become apparent in the results section, the method of selection, and especially the use of prior mutagenesis, may have an effect on the frequency or nature of the mutants obtained, especially in relation to their metastatic properties.

Quantitation of metastasis is usually done by counting the number of nodules in a particular organ such as the lungs (Fidler 1978). On this basis, it appeared we were successful, using WGA, in deriving Lec^r mutants having a significantly reduced metastatic phenotype (Dennis and Kerbel 1981). Thus, whereas subcutaneous injection of MDAY-D2 cells produced many hundreds of small liver nodules, an equivalent injection of some WGA^r mutants (e.g., MDW4, a mutagen-induced, single-step WGA^r mutant, resistant to about 50 μg/ml WGA, as outlined in Kerbel 1979) gave rise to much smaller numbers (10–50) of conspicuously larger nodules. Given the fact that most spontaneous metastases are monoclonal in origin (Poste et al. 1982, Talmadge et al. 1982), the results could be taken as evidence that fewer numbers of WGA^r MDW4 cells were reaching or surviving in the liver, i.e., they are "less metastatic" (Kerbel et al. 1982). In fact, on the basis of changes in the status of Lec^r phenotype, as well as changes in other drug (genetic) markers, following an in vivo passage, we eventually concluded that the MDW4 cells were *nonmetastatic*, as amplified below.

Spontaneous In Vivo Tumor-Host Cell Fusion

If a liver tumor nodule isolated from an animal that had previously been injected with 10^5 MDW4 cells was disaggregated and the cells injected into a new host, the metastatic properties of the cells were indistinguishable from the highly metastatic MDAY-D2 parent: livers were confluent with tumor and the nodules were far too numerous to count. Thus, the attenuated metastatic phenotype of MDW4 appeared unstable in vivo. We therefore monitored metastases obtained from MDW4 injected animals for the stability of their WGA^r phenotype: in every case metastases consisted of WGA-sensitive (WGA^s) "revertant" tumor cells (Dennis et al. 1981a). Cells from late-stage primary subcutaneously growing solid tumor also consisted of WGA^s cells (Dennis et al. 1981a), the proportion of which increased progressively with time (Kerbel et al. 1982).

In order to obtain more information on the fate of the injected cells, we incorporated an additional independent genetic marker into WGA^r cells—resistance to ouabain (Oua^R), which is a well-known codominant genetic marker (Siminovitch 1976). Our initial experiments indicated that the injection of a double-marked mutant (Oua^RWGA^r) of MDAY-D2 into DBA/2 mice allowed us to recover metastases populated with WGA^SOua^R tumor cells (Dennis et al. 1981a). This result was very important in two very different respects. First, it provided us with an indication of the potential usefulness of studying tumor progression by monitoring changes in the status of stable recessive or dominant drug-resistant genetic markers introduced into tumor cell populations in vitro (Kerbel et al. 1982). Second, it was the first indication that a spontaneous tumor-host cell fusion event could be occurring in the MDW4-injected animals. Thus the fusion of a WGA^rOua^R tumor cell with any WGA^SOua^s cell (i.e., a normal host cell) would result in loss of the WGA^r marker because of its presumed recessive nature (Stanley et al. 1975b), whereas the Oua^R marker, being codominant, would be retained unless the relevant chromosome was lost through segregation from a hybrid. If in fact the cause of the $WGA^r \rightarrow WGA^s$ shift is a tumor–host cell fusion event, this would imply MDW4 cells per se are "benign" (i.e., nonmetastatic) but acquire metastatic ability through the cell-cell fusion event. As such, the process could constitute a novel pathway for tumor progression.

Over the last decade a number of investigators have reported spontaneous tumor–host cell fusion in vivo, as we reviewed in detail recently (Kerbel et al. 1982, 1983). With rare exceptions, these studies did not address the question of whether this phenomenon might have any relevance to the evolution of tumor heterogeneity and the subsequent emergence of metastatic variants during tumor progression, points first raised by Goldenberg et al. (1974) and Warner (1975).

It occurred to us that the use of certain genetically marked WGA^r mutants of MDAY-D2, such as MDW4, could be very useful devices to study aspects of spontaneous tumor-host cell fusion in vivo and its possible relevance to tumor progression and metastasis. We therefore undertook a detailed series of experiments (Kerbel et al. 1983, Lagarde et al. 1983a) to determine whether the $WGA^r \rightarrow WGA^s$ phenotypic shift was in fact a consequence of a tumor-host cell fusion event, and if so, what the nature of the host cell is and why MDW4 cells are unable to metastasize—unlike their parents and hybrid counterparts. These experiments are summarized in this paper. Regardless of the relevance of spontaneous tumor-host cell fusion to tumor progression—a highly contentious issue that is reviewed in the Discussion section—the last question highlights the considerable usefulness of Lec^r membrane mutants as tools to help dissect various aspects of the cell biology of metastasis and the tumor-host relationship.

THE EXPERIMENTAL APPROACH: SOME GENERAL COMMENTS ON MATERIALS AND METHODS

As most of the material presented in this paper has already been published elsewhere, we will not give a detailed description of materials and methods. Some general comments, however, are in order. One of the principle procedures involves the quantitation of lectin resistance, and we have used several different assays for it. Initially, we used a simple cell count assay (Kerbel 1979): 5,000 cells were plated in Petri dishes in varying concentrations of WGA or other lectins, and the cells were counted 5–7 days later. This procedure is equivalent to plating efficiency experiments (Lagarde, unpublished observations).

The second method involves a modification of the thymidine incorporation assay described by Trowbridge et al. (1978) as recently described (Kerbel et al. 1983). It involves the growth of tumor cells in varying concentrations of lectins for 24 h, followed by a 4-h pulse with [^{3}H]thymidine, which is incorporated into DNA in dividing (i.e., lectin-resistant), viable cells.

The third method used was a clonogenic assay (described in detail in Lagarde et al. 1983a), which involves an estimation of plating efficiency. This procedure was also used for establishing changes in the status of drug-resistant genetic markers, e.g., 6-Thg^r and Oua^R, as discussed in the results section.

RESULTS

Altered Metastatic Properties of Some WGA^r Mutants of the Highly Metastatic MDAY-D2 Tumor

Tao and Burger (1977) found that a WGA^r mutant of the B16 melanoma, a C57BL/6 mouse strain tumor, had a considerably reduced ability to metastasize spontaneously. The mutant, called Wa4, was selected without prior mutagenesis, using a four-step selection protocol. Our initial studies were carried out with the highly metastatic MDAY-D2 tumor, encompassed the use of PHA, Con A, and WGA, and entailed prior mutagenesis of the tumor cells with EMS to increase the frequency of Lec^r mutants. The origin and properties of MDAY-D2 have been described in detail (Kerbel et al. 1978, 1980). Its metastatic phenotype can best be described as ferocious: subcutaneous (s.c.) inoculation of 10^2–10^5 cells leads to the rapid development of overwhelming visceral metastases in which the liver and spleen are the most conspicuous sites of involvement (Kerbel et al. 1978). The lungs and kidneys are also infiltrated, although to a lesser degree.

The way the livers become progressively involved by the tumor is an important process that deserves some amplification. At about 7–10 days after a s.c. inoculation of 10^5 MDAY-D2 cells (regardless of whether the cells were derived from an established tissue culture line or from a mouse ascites donor), a number of very small, pinpoint nodules appear in the liver (data not shown). These quickly grow in number, but not so much in size, so that by day 25 much of the normal liver tissue is replaced by many hundreds of small nodules (Figure 1A). At autopsy, as shown in Figure 1B, it is impossible to estimate the number of nodules, because the nodules coalesce and the liver essentially becomes a solid internal tumor mass.

Quite a different picture emerged with some of the WGA^r mutants we initially selected (Kerbel 1979, Dennis and Kerbel 1981), an example of which is shown

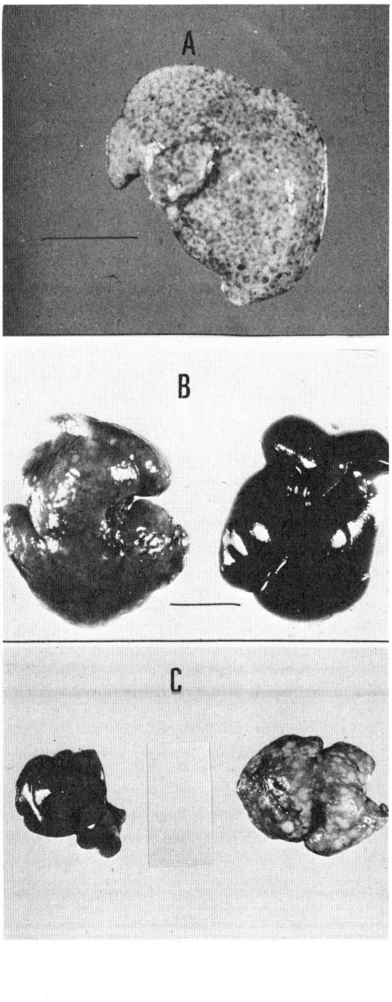

FIG. 1. Metastatic burden and pattern in the livers of mice given 10^5 MDAY-D2 cells or the WGA^r mutant MDWA. **A.** A typical picture of a liver 25 days after injection showing hundreds of very small nodules. **B.** These coalesce to form a confluent tumor mass by day 35; normal liver on *right.* **C.** Much smaller numbers of large discrete (and countable nodules) in the livers of mice injected with MDW4 cells, even at terminal stages of the disease; normal liver on *left.* Bars in **A** and **B** are 1 cm.

in Figure 1C. The number of nodules at autopsy was greatly reduced, but they tended to be much larger, often reaching several millimeters in diameter. The mutant used in the experiment shown in Figure 1C is called MDW4: it was a single-step WGA^r mutant obtained after the MDAY-D2 cells were mutagenized with EMS (Kerbel 1979). One could claim, quite justifiably, that the final "metastatic burden" in the liver is as great, if not greater, in the MDW4-injected recipients as in those mice that received MDAY-D2 cells. But if one quantitates metastasis on the basis of the number of nodules in a particular organ—the most commonly employed and accepted practice (Fidler 1978), although it does have its limitations (Stackpole 1981)—then the only conclusion that can be drawn is that the WGA^r MDW4 cells are less malignant (i.e., metastatic) than MDAY-D2.

In fact there is now sound experimental evidence for accepting tumor nodule counts as an index of relative metastatic potential. We refer to the apparent clonal origin of either artificial or most spontaneous metastases (Poste et al. 1982, Talmadge et al. 1982). Thus, it appears likely that fewer tumor cells migrate to the liver or are able to survive there and give rise to visible metastatic foci once they do migrate and establish themselves. Either way, it would be reasonable to conclude that MDW4 had a reduced metastatic phenotype.

Having satisfied ourselves that we had in fact successfully derived a mutant much less able to metastasize than the parent MDAY-D2 line, we next decided to monitor the cells for the stability of this phenotypic change. This seemed a necessary precaution in view of the fact that many laboratories have reported a rapid "phenotypic drift" among clones selected for either decreased or enhanced metastatic ability (Kerbel 1979, Chambers et al. 1981, Neri and Nicolson 1981, Poste et al. 1981). It would clearly be impractical to use such lines for certain structure-function studies in metastasis, as discussed recently by Harris et al. (1982).

Reversion of the WGA^r Genetic Marker in MDW4 Cells After Growth and Metastasis In Vivo

It was immediately clear to us that the attenuated metastatic phenotype of MDW4 was probably not stable. This was revealed through two types of in vivo growth experiments. First, if the tumor cells from a metastatic nodule (obtained from an MDW4-injected animal) were established in tissue culture and then injected s.c. (10^5 cells) into syngeneic DBA/2 mice, the resultant tumor grew in a manner virtually indistinguishable from MDAY-D2: animals died in 30–35 days and almost all the normal liver tissue of the hosts was replaced by tumor, as described above. Second, if 10^2–10^5 MDW4 cells were injected intravenously into the tail veins of DBA/2 mice, the incidence of tumor take was very low, usually about 1 in 10 mice (Dennis et al. 1981a). In contrast, intravenous (i.v.) injection of MDAY-D2 or cells from metastases obtained from MDW4-injected mice invariably gave rise to rapidly growing lethal tumors (death within 15 days, with massive involvement of liver, spleen, and lungs) (Dennis et al. 1981a).

We therefore decided to monitor the WGA^r phenotype of MDW4 tumor cells recovered from metastases or the solid subcutaneously growing solid tumor. We already knew this phenotype was stable in tissue culture: MDW4 cells, and other independent WGA^r mutants, could undergo hundreds of population doublings in vitro over several years and in the absence of selection still maintain their relative WGA^r phenotype (Kerbel 1979). Our results were quite clear: every metastasis examined, regardless of its anatomical location, possessed a WGA-sensitive (WGA^s) phenotype, i.e., the cells had fully reverted to the wild-type phenotype, as described in Table 1 (Dennis et al. 1981a). The picture that emerged from the solid tumor studies was a little more variable: sometimes the cells retained the WGA^r phenotype whereas in other cases the cells were almost all WGA^s (Dennis et al. 1981a). We subsequently found that this was

TABLE 1. *WGA^r phenotype of primary tumors and spontaneous metastatic nodules obtained from MDW4-injected DBA/2 mice*

Cell line	Source	Number of cells injected	WGA resistance	50% mortality (days)	Liver metastasis pattern, at death
MDAY-D2	Tissue culture	10^5	5	35	Confluent
MDW4	Tissue culture	10^5	50	63	Nodular
MDW4-11	Primary	10^2	2	33	Confluent
MDW4-21a	Liver metastasis		2	30	Confluent
MDW4-21b	Liver metastasis		2	35	Confluent
MDW4-21c	Liver metastasis		2	32	Confluent
MDW4-12	Primary	10^4	2	29	Confluent
MDW4-22a	Liver metastasis		2	30	Confluent
MDW4-22b	Liver metastasis		2	27	Confluent
MDW4-22c	Kidney metastasis		2	31	Confluent
MDW4-14	Primary	10^4	2	32	Confluent
MDW4-24a	Liver metastasis		2	34	Confluent
MDW4-24b	Liver metastasis		2	34	Confluent
MDW4-24c	Liver metastasis		2	35	Confluent
MDW4-13	Primary	10^5	43	30	Confluent
MDW4-23a	Liver metastasis		2	31	Confluent
MDW4-23b	Liver metastasis		2	29	Confluent
MDW4-23c	Spleen metastasis		2	33	Confluent
MDW4-23d	Gut metastasis		2	30	Confluent

MDW4 cells were injected s.c. into syngeneic DBA/2 mice. Approximately 2 months later, the "primary" tumor or liver, kidney, gut, and spleen metastases were removed and the tumor cells adapted to tissue culture. Their level of resistance to WGA was then determined as described in Dennis et al. (1981a). Samples of the cells from the various lines were also injected s.c. (10^5 cells/mouse) into DBA/2 mice and the days until death and metastatic pattern at autopsy in the livers noted. Confluent refers to many hundreds of coalescent small nodules; nodular refers to 10–50 larger discrete nodules as described in the text and shown in Figure 1. (Reproduced, with modification, from Dennis et al. 1981a, with permission of *Nature,* MacMillan Journals Ltd.)

a function of when the solid tumor was sampled, i.e., how long the tumor had been growing in the animal (Kerbel et al. 1982). During the first 4 weeks, almost all of the cells retained their WGA^r phenotype, but thereafter, an increasing proportion of the cells became WGA^s (Kerbel et al. 1982) until at terminal stages of illness more than 99.9% of the cells were WGA^s (Lagarde et al. 1983a).

Our results could be explained on the basis that the cells we injected were "nonmalignant," i.e., incapable of metastatic growth, but then gradually acquired this attribute as a result of a change in vivo, one which resulted in reversion of the WGA^r phenotype of the cells (Dennis et al. 1981a, Kerbel et al. 1982). This reasoning obviously assumes that WGA^s revertants did not arise spontaneously at high rate in tissue culture. The presence of such cells could account for the results if they possessed a strong selective advantage in vivo over their WGA^r counterparts. Prima facie, this seems unlikely because, as mentioned earlier, the original mutants are stable over many generations in vitro. In fact, WGA^s revertants do indeed arise spontaneously, at a frequency of about 2×10^{-5} per cell per generation (Lagarde 1983). Although this rate is high, it is still too low to account for some of our results; e.g., s.c. injection with as few as 10^2 MDW4 still led to the emergence of multiple WGA^s metastases (Dennis et al. 1981a). Second, the $WGA^r \rightarrow WGA^s$ reversion event still took place even if the MDW4 cells injected were grown in vitro in the presence of WGA so as to counterselect for any spontaneously arising WGA^s revertants present in the cultures (Lagarde 1983). Hence, the reversion phenomenon appeared to take place in vivo some time after injection of the MDW4 cells.

The phenomenon we have described therefore seems to involve what could be a new model of tumor progression. In the absence of selection pressures, the cells that populated distant metastases and late-stage "primary" tumors were clearly different from, and in particular more malignant than, the MDW4 cell population injected. That the change had an underlying genetic basis was implied by its stability once it occurred: WGA^s revertants virtually never regain the original WGA^r phenotype, either in vivo or in vitro (Dennis et al. 1981a).

Changes in the Status of Additional Genetic Markers After Growth of WGA^r Cells In Vivo

The next question we addressed was whether the change in MDW4 was unique to the WGA^r phenotype as opposed to the possibility of much broader changes taking place. Our initial approach was to introduce genetic markers other than one for lectin resistance into MDW4 cells, some recessive, some dominant, and assess their status in WGA^s revertants. We therefore introduced Oua^R, a codominant genetic marker (Siminovitch 1976), into WGA^r mutant cells. When metastases were recovered and analyzed from DBA/2 mice given a s.c. injection of such a mutant (MDOW2b), we found, as shown in Figure 2, that the tumor cells possessed a WGA^sOua^R phenotype. Thus, the codominant

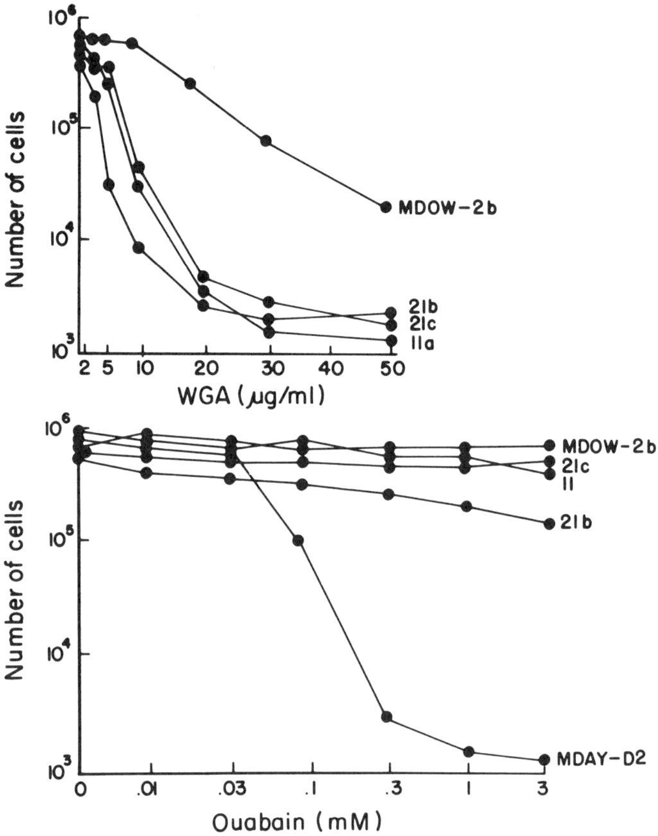

FIG. 2. WGA and ouabain sensitivity of MDAY-D2 and MDOW-2b and of cell lines established from spontaneous metastases removed from the liver of an MDOW-2b-bearing mouse. DBA/2 mice were given a s.c. injection of 10^5 MDOW-2b cells followed 60 days later by removal of tumor tissue from the site of injection (MDOW-11). Three discrete metastatic nodules were found in the liver (MDOW-21a, MDOW-21b, MDOW-21c). Tumor tissue removed from the mouse was minced and trypsin treated, and the resulting cell suspension placed in tissue culture for at least 3 weeks to allow tumor cells to outgrow host-derived cells. The established tissue culture lines were then tested for the ability to grow in the presence of either WGA (*upper panel*) or ouabain (*lower panel*). (Reproduced from Dennis et al. 1981a, with permission of *Nature,* Macmillan Journals Ltd.)

Oua^R marker was retained, whereas, once again, the WGA^r marker was lost.

Previous experiments by Stanley and Siminovitch (1977) indicated the WGA^r mutants behaved recessively in somatic cell hybrids of Chinese hamster ovary (CHO) cells, a characteristic that was also subsequently observed in WGA^r mutants of MDAY-D2 (Kerbel et al. 1983). Therefore, it was possible that our findings could be explained by a spontaneous somatic cell fusion event in vivo involving the Oua^RWGA^r tumor cells and a Oua^sWGA^s normal host cell. This would lead to extinction of recessive markers but not dominant or codominant markers—unless the chromosome containing the relevant gene for the dominant type of marker was segregated from the hybrids. In this connection, a number of laboratories had already reported that tumor cells could spontaneously fuse in vivo with normal host cells (see Discussion, and Kerbel et al. 1983, for review).

To examine this possibility more fully, a new mutant was derived that was marked with genetic markers, two of them recessive and one codominant (Lagarde et al. 1983a). A clone from MDW4 was derived, called MDW4-1. Subsequently, a clone resistant to 3 mM Ouabain was obtained after mutagenesis (MDW4-Oua^R1). The latter cells were mutagenized, and two independent clones (W4OT3 and W4OT4) were selected for 6-thioguanine resistance (6-Thg^r), an X-chromosome-linked recessive genetic marker (Siminovitch 1976). W4OT3 cells were then injected s.c. into a large group of DBA/2 mice, and a time course analysis was performed on the status of the three markers on cells obtained from the primary tumor site. Metastases obtained at autopsy were also assessed. The rationale for this experiment was that the putatively independent recessive markers (WGA^r and 6-Thg^r) would simultaneously revert, in contrast to the Oua^R marker. This reversion would be expected to occur in any hybrid formed between the drug-marked cells and normal drug/lectin-sensitive cells.

As the results in Figure 3 show this reversion in fact occurred (Lagarde et al. 1983a). Over a period of 65–70 days, the majority of the cells retained the Oua^R marker, whereas there was a gradual and virtually simultaneous decline in the proportion of cells carrying the two recessive markers (Figure 3A). At day 65, by which time the animals were dying of widespread metastases, about 40% of the cells were still Oua^R whereas only 0.05–0.1% were WGA^r or Thg^r. Twenty-six metastases obtained only at a late stage of progression (between day 55 and 70) were examined. These were found, in the main (17/26), to retain the Oua^R marker to some degree, whereas 21 did not contain any WGA^r cells and the remaining 5 had only 10^{-4}–10^{-6} WGA^r cells (Figure 3B). Similarly, there were no 6-Thg^r cells in seven metastases and only about 10^{-6} in two others.

In summary, the two recessive markers were lost, essentially simultaneously, whereas the Oua^R marker was retained in a substantial proportion of the cells. The fact that the Oua^R marker was lost in some of the cells is still consistent with the cell fusion hypothesis, since segregation of the relevant chromosome could account for the reappearance of the Oua^S phenotype. Thus, all the results obtained were consistent with—but did not prove—a tumor–normal cell fusion event. They also provided an illuminating example of how informative and useful genetic markers introduced into tumor cell populations can be in helping to delineate genetic versus epigenetic events associated with tumor progression and tumor heterogeneity.

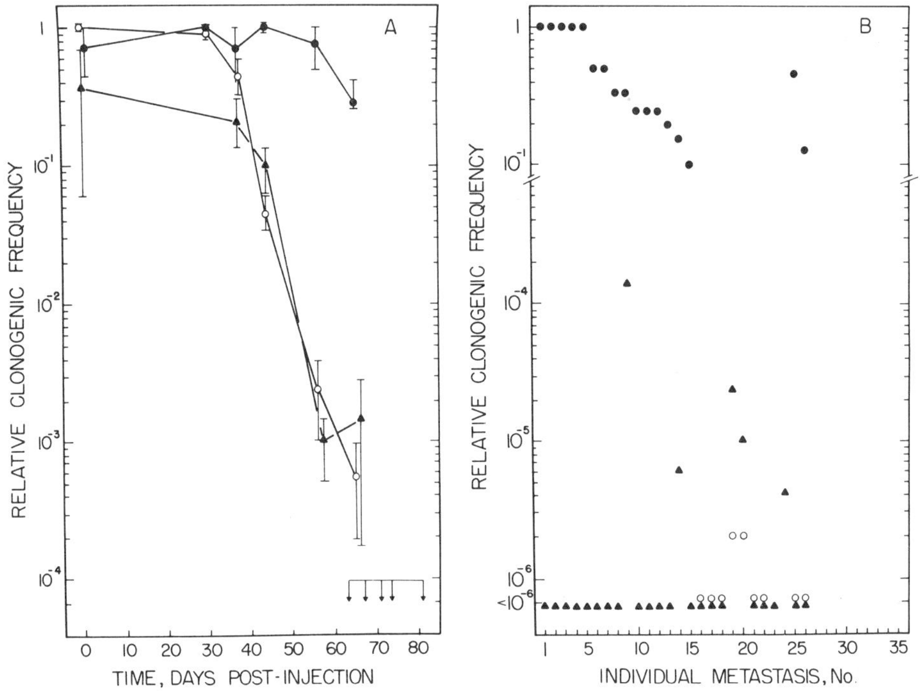

FIG. 3. Frequency of Oua^R, Thg^r, and WGA^r cells in primary tumor and metastatic sites after s.c. inoculation of MDW4 drug-resistant derivatives. **A.** 3×10^5 cells of the triply-marked W40T3 cell line were injected s.c. into a group of DBA/2 mice. At time intervals, one animal was sacrificed and the relative clonogenic frequency of Oua^R (●), Thg^r (0), and WGA^r (△) cells present in the tumor growing at the site of inoculation was measured as described in Lagarde et al. (1983a). Each point represents the mean frequency ± S.D. from two independent experiments separated by a 3-month interval. Arrows indicate times at which five animals died of metastasis. **B.** Relative clonogenic frequency of Oua^R (●), Thg^r (0), and WGA^r (△) cells was measured in 26 independent liver or spleen metastatic nodules, 60–80 days after s.c. injection of 1×10^5 cells from MDW4-Oua^{R}1 (no. 1–15), MDW4-TG^{r}2 (no. 16–22), MDW4-1 (no. 23, 24), and W40T3 (no. 25, 26) cell lines. MDW4-TG^{R}2 is a 6-thioguanine-resistant (6-Thg^r) derivative of MDW4. MDW4-Oua^{R}1 is a ouabain-resistant (Oua^R) derivative of MDW4. These lines and W40T3 are described in detail in Lagarde et al. (1983), from which the results are reproduced.

Chromosome Analysis

A further series of experiments were performed in which we examined the karyotypes of the MDW4 WGA^r mutant (or W4OT3) and the WGA^s revertants obtained in vivo after s.c. injection of these cells. One would expect to find an increase (up to 40) in the number of chromosomes of the WGA^s revertants if they were the progeny of hybrids between MDW4 cells and a normal host cell. This was found to be the case (Lagarde et al. 1983), as shown in Figure 4. Whereas MDAY-D2 had a near diploid number of chromosomes (Kerbel et al. 1978) with a modal chromosome number of 38 and 2 or 3 metacentric

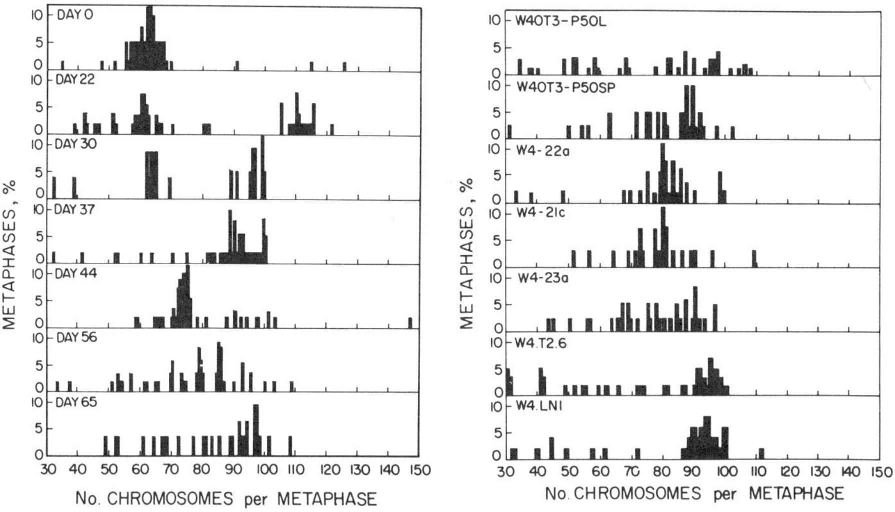

FIG. 4. Karyotype distributions of cell populations removed from the metastatic nodules after s.c. inoculation of a Oua^R and Thg^r derivative of the MDW4-1 mutant cell line, namely W40T3. **Left:** Distribution of karyotypes of tumor cells from primary tumors removed at the various times indicated after s.c. injection of 10^5 cells. Cell chromosome counts are displayed as a histogram. **Right:** Chromosome number histogram for independent uncloned populations and clones removed from the metastatic sites following the s.c. inoculation of MDW4-1 derivative cell lines designated within brackets: W40T3-P50L (W40T3, day 50, liver); W40T3-P50SP (W40T3, day 50, spleen); W4-22a (MDW4-Oua^R1, day 65, liver); W4-21c (MDW4-TG^R2, day 56, spleen); W4-23a (MDW4-TG^R2, day 70, liver); W4-T2.6 (MDW4.1, day 68, liver, cloned twice, WGA-sensitive); W4-LN1 (MDW4.1, day 68, liver, cloned once, WGA^r). Reproduced from Lagarde et al. (1983).

chromosome markers, MDW4 cells, the MDW4-1 subclone and its drug-resistant derivatives W4OT3 and W4OT4, had a hypotetraploid mode (68 $\pm$ 2) and an average of 7 metacentric chromosomes per metaphase. This latter karyotype has been designated class B and the former (MDAY-D2) class A.

In contrast, the WGA^s revertants invariably contained significantly more chromosomes than MDW4. The mode at day 22 was 110 chromosomes (range 80–110), consistent with the fusion of MDW4 cells with a normal mouse somatic cell containing 40 chromosomes. At a later (e.g., preterminal) stage, namely day 65, the mode drops to 98 (range 80–109). The results are suggestive of cell fusion followed by some chromosome loss. The karyotypes of spontaneous metastases obtained from W4OT3-injected animals were similar to the karyotypes of cells obtained from late-stage primary tumors (Lagarde et al. 1983). We refer to such cells as having a class C karyotype. The kinetic evolution of W4OT3 tumor progression, as analyzed at the population level, clearly implies that new cell subsets originate at the site of inoculation and that these cell subsets are the ones capable of forming distant metastases.

A subsequent clonal analysis by Lagarde et al. (1983) revealed that, whether derived from the primary site or metastatic foci, clones carrying the WGA^s, Thg^s, or Oua^S phenotypes are always associated with a class C karyotype and are highly malignant upon reinoculation. In contrast, cells carrying all three resistant alleles are always associated with a class B karyotype and are equivalent in malignant status to MDW4 cells. Furthermore, the number of metacentric chromosome markers in class C cells never exceeded that in class B cells.

All of the results are consistent with the possibility that the class C cells, i.e., the WGA^s revertants, originated through a spontaneous tumor–host cell fusion event followed by varying degrees of chromosome loss.

Acquisition of Identifiable Host-Related Characteristics by WGA^s Revertants After Growth in F_1 Hybrid Recipients

More direct evidence for tumor-host cell hybridization was obtained in the following way: MDW4 cells were injected s.c. into (DBA × C57BL/6)F_1 or (DBA/2 × C3H/HeJ)F_1 hybrid recipients. Somatic cells in the former hybrid strain (B6D2F1) carry the $H\text{-}2^b$ major histocompatibility antigen of the C57BL/6 mouse strain, whereas the latter hybrid (C3D2F1) carries the $H\text{-}2^k$ antigens associated with the C3H/HeJ strain. Therefore, a tumor cell hybrid formed between $H\text{-}2^d$-positive (DBA strain) MDW4 cells and a normal somatic cell from a (DBA/2 × C57BL/6)F_1 or (DBA/2 × C3H/HeJ)F_1 mouse would be expected to express $H\text{-}2^b$ or $H\text{-}2^k$ antigens, respectively (Wiener et al. 1974), since H-2 antigens are expressed in a codominant fashion. A positive result would of course depend on retention of the H-2 carrying host chromosome no. 17 in the hybrids.

Results from such an experiment, which used cytotoxic T cells for the H-2 typing, are shown in Figure 5 (adapted from Kerbel et al. 1983). They clearly reveal evidence for acquisition of opposite parental strain H-2 antigens on tumor cells recovered from all of the metastases or late-stage primary tumors sampled. The expression of this new phenotype was stable in tissue culture cell lines established from metastases over the several months they were tested. Serological analysis using anti-H-2 polyclonal or monoclonal antibodies confirmed the T-cell typing tests (Kerbel et al. 1983). All of these lines were WGA^s; i.e., they had reverted for the WGA^r phenotype in the F_1 hybrid hosts just as in normal DBA/2 animals.

Evidence for a Bone Marrow Origin of the Normal Host Cell Involved in the Tumor–Host Cell Fusion Process

Wiener et al. (1976) obtained evidence that the normal cell involved in some cases of spontaneous in vivo tumor–host cell fusion was of bone marrow origin. This was accomplished by injection of tumor cells into allogeneic bone marrow "radiation chimeras," i.e., mice that were lethally irradiated and then hemato-

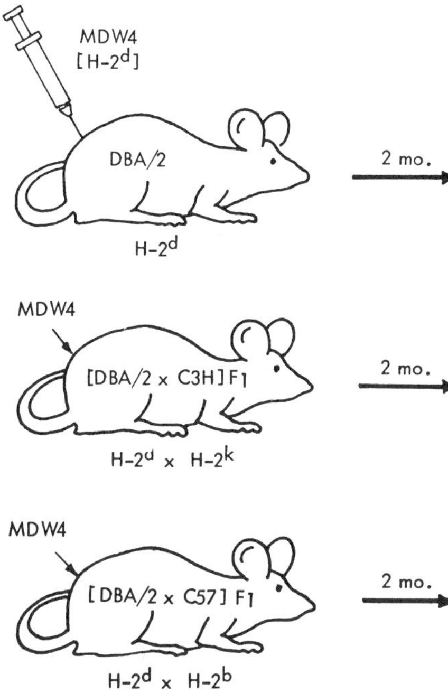

Mouse strain	Tissue	PERCENTAGE CELLS KILLED BY ANTISERUM TO: H - 2d	H - 2k	H - 2b
DBA/2 (H-2d)	primary	88.8	3.2	0
	liver met	90.3	1.6	1.2
	spleen met	83.6	0.9	0.9
	lung met	90.2	2.2	3.1
[DBA/2 x C3H] F1 (H-2d x H-2k)	primary	81.2	63.5	0
	liver met	90.9	97.4	3.8
	lung met	79.1	88.8	0
	spleen met	91.0	92.0	3.4
	kidney met	94.0	76.1	0
[DBA/2 x C57] F1 (H-2d x H-2b)	primary	88.5	1.1	78.1
	liver met	88.3	0	95.0
	lung met	89.1	3.2	13.5 *
	spleen met	69.0	0	88.7
	kidney met	87.7	0	0 *

FIG. 5. Summary of the H-2 antigen phenotypes of WGA^s revertant metastases and primary tumors recovered from various mouse strains given a prior injection of H-2^d-positive MDW4 cells (Kerbel et al. 1983). H-2 analysis was done by harvesting cytotoxic T cells (CTL) from mixed lymphocyte cultures (MLC) using H-2 congenic mouse strains such that CTL were generated against H-2^d, H-2^k, or H-2^b antigens only. 10^5 MDW4 cells were injected s.c. into the various mouse strains indicated. Approximately 2 months later metastases and late-stage primary tumors were removed, adapted to tissue culture as cell lines, and then analyzed for their WGA^r and H-2 phenotypes. All lines were found to be WGA^s. The asterisks (*) signify that the two lines found to be H-2^b-negative by serology were positive for H-2^b by CTL analysis (Kerbel et al. 1983). Met, metastasis. (Adapted from Kerbel et al. 1983 with permission of the American Society for Microbiology.)

poietically reconstituted with bone marrow cells from an H-2 incompatible donor strain.

To examine this question in our system, DBA/2 mice were lethally irradiated (850 R) and then reconstituted with 5×10^6 bone marrow cells from CBA/HT6T6 mouse donors. This latter strain possesses the H-2^k allele. MDW4 cells were injected s.c. into these so-called CBA/HT6T6 → DBA/2 radiation chimeras, spontaneous metastases isolated from several different organ sites removed from animals, and the cells established in tissue culture. Primary tumors at a late stage of growth were also analyzed. Using the thymidine incorporation assay, we found that all the lines tested had once again reverted to the WGA^0 phenotype (Kerbel et al. 1983), just as in normal DBA/2 mice. When tested for the presence of the foreign H-2^k antigens, either by CTL typing or by serological analysis, every one of these lines was positive (Table 2). These results indicate

TABLE 2. *H-2 profiles of WGA^S revertant tumor cells recovered from CBA/HT6T6 → DBA/2 bone marrow radiation chimeric recipients injected with WGA^R MDW4 cells**

	% Specific lysis‡ by CTL to				% Cells killed by antiserum (+RC) to:§			
	H-2^d		H-2^k					
Cell line†	100/1	50/1	100/1	50/1	H-2^d	H-2^k	H-2^k (m)	H-2^b
MDAY-D2	79.3	76.0	2.1	2.4	93.9	1.2	0	0
MDW4-1	82.0	79.2	2.3	3.2	?″	?	?	?
73: 1–1	63.8	59.5	69.8	57.7	91.4	79.8	27.6	0
73: 1–2b	71.3	64.6	58.6	56.5	93.4	43.3	0	0
73: 2–1	74.3	61.5	74.8	64.1	90.2	67.2	61.9	1.1
73: 2–2b	71.3	63.2	63.4	59.3	60.0	68.6	53.7	0
73: 2–2c	58.6	46.9	64.1	47.2	78.8	52.9	0	6.2
73: 2–2d	70.8	61.7	64.0	56.8	58.0	49.8	5.2	0

* CBA/HT6T6-DBA/2 bone marrow radiation chimeric recipients refer to lethally irradiated DBA/2 mice reconstituted with allogeneic CBA/HT6T6 bone marrow cells as described in Kerbel et al. (1983). (Results reproduced from Kerbel et al. (1983) with permission of the American Society for Microbiology.)

† The notation for the cell lines is described in Kerbel et al. (1983). They were established from metastases of various organs (liver, spleen, kidneys, lungs) (e.g., 73: 1–2b, 73: 2–2b, 73: 2–2c, and 73: 2–2d, respectively) or the late-stage solid tumors growing at the site of inoculation (e.g., 73: 1–1 and 73: 2–1). The cell lines were established from the radiation chimera recipients after s.c. injection of MDW4 cells.

‡ CTL (cytotoxic T lymphocytes) were obtained from mixed lymphocyte cultures (MLC) as described in Kerbel et al. (1983).

§ Antisera sources and conditions of assay as described in Kerbel et al. (1983). H-2^k (m) refers to a test using a monoclonal (m) anti-H-2^k antibody. RC refers to rabbit complement.

″ MDW4 cells are highly susceptible to the toxic effects of rabbit complement alone, without any antiserum added, as described in Kerbel et al. (1983). Hence serological analysis was not possible by performing cytotoxicity assays. The cells are (H-2^k)- and (H-2^b)-negative, however, by CTL typing.

that the host cell involved in vivo in the fusion process is derived from bone marrow cells. It is interesting to note that in the experiments of Wiener et al. (1976) similar results were obtained only when ascites tumors were tested. In the case of solid tumors, the normal cells implicated in the formation of hybrids were not of bone marrow origin; their lineage has never been identified.

Further proof for the cell fusion hypothesis and for the bone marrow origin of the normal cell partner was obtained by intentional in vitro hybridization of a Oua^R 6-Thg^r derivative of MDW4 (W4OT3) with normal bone marrow or spleen cells from DBA/2 mice. The hybrids obtained were indistinguishable from the WGA^s hybrids obtained in vivo, in terms of lectin-resistance phenotype, karyotype, and malignant phenotype (Kerbel et al. 1983), as shown in Table 3. The WGA^S phenotype of such hybrids also showed the recessive nature of this genetic marker, as was found by Stanley and Siminovitch (1977) in CHO cells. By lectin-resistance phenotype, we mean the pattern of resistance or sensitivity to several different lectins as shown in Table 3. Thus, MDW4 cells, which were selected for resistance to WGA, were also found to become "collaterally

TABLE 3. *Properties of hybrids generated in vitro between MDW4 cells and normal DBA/2 bone marrow or spleen cells*

Cell line	Origin	H2 haplotype*	Karyotype†	Lectin-resistance (D_{50} values)‡ WGA (μg/ml)	PHA (μg/ml)	Con A (μg/ml)	RIC (μg/ml)	Metastatic properties§ s.c. injection	i.v. injection
KD2-3	MDAY-D2 subclone (14)	d	A	4	3	33	0.5	5/5 (35 ± 5)	5/5 (14 ± 2)
MDW4-1	WDW3 subclone (14)	d	B	23	>80	13	1.7	6/6 (72 ± 7)	2/22 (143 ± 22)
W4OT3	Oua^R, Thg^R derivative of MDW4-1 (14)	d	B	50	>80	11	1.9	6/6 (77 ± 17)	2/5 (114 ± 50)
DBM	Normal bone marrow cells DBA/2	d	N	3	63	80	2.0	n.d.	n.d.
HWW-1	W4OT3 × MDW4-1	d	D	5	18	7	1.4	3/3 (103 ± 11)	0/3 (>150)
HWW-2	W4OT3 × MDW4-1	d	D	16	80	12	1.7	2/3 (95 ± 58)	0/3 (>150)
HWW-3	W4OT3 × MDW4-1	d	D	14	32	9	1.5	3/3 (71 ± 39)	0/3 (>150)
HWKD-1	W4OT3 × KD2–3	d	E	5	3	21	n.d.	n.d.	3/3 (35 ± 22)
HWKD-2	W4OT3 × KD2–3	d	E	3	2	20	n.d.	n.d.	3/3 (33 ± 5)
HWDSP-1	W4OT3 × DBA/2 spleen cells	d	C	2	1	16	3.3	2/3 (92 ± 50)	3/3 (29 ± 4)
HWDSP-2	W4OT3 × DBA/2 spleen cells	d	C	3	2	29	4.2	3/3 (71 ± 12)	3/3 (39 ± 5)
HWDBM-1	W4OT3 × DBA/2 bone marrow cells	d	C	3	2	18	0.9	3/3 (62 ± 19)	3/3 (35 ± 4)
HWDBM-2	W4OT3 × DBA/2 bone marrow cells	d	C	3	1	17	3.2	3/3 (57 ± 8)	3/3 (33 ± 3)
HWDBM-3	W4OT3 × DBA/2 bone marrow cells	d	C	5	2	35	3.6	3/3 (68 ± 13)	3/3 (24 ± 10)

* Determined with polyclonal and monoclonal anti-H-2 antibodies and rabbit complement using the microcytotoxicity assay, as described in Kerbel et al. (1983).

† Chromosomal mode, range, and average number of metacentric chromosomes per metaphase are: 39 ± 1, 30 to 45, 3 (class A); 68 ± 2, 50 to 75, 7 (class B); 90 ± 10, 30 to 110, 6 (class C); no mode, 38 to 142, 12 (class D); 95 ± 5, 86 to 103, 8 (class E); 40, no range, no marker (class N); as described in Kerbel et al. (1983).

‡ Determined from dose-response curves, using a [^{3}H]thymidine incorporation assay as described in Kerbel et al. (1983).

§ 1×10^5 cells inoculated per DBA/2 mouse. The ratios give the number of animals dying of metastasis before 150 days per number of animals injected. Numbers within parenthesis are mean animal survival time per group ±S.D. n.d., not done.

(Reproduced from Kerbel et al. (1983) with permission of the American Society for Microbiology.)

resistant" to PHA, while being more sensitive to Con A than the parent MDAY-D2 cells. Indeed, Stanley and Siminovitch have grouped CHO cells into several different Lec^R classes on the basis of lectin resistance profiles, and the same appears true for MDAY-D2 cells (Lagarde et al. 1983a, 1983b). In any event, the lectin-resistance phenotype of in vivo MDW4–normal cell hybrids and hybrids generated in vitro between MDW4 and normal bone marrow or spleen cells are virtually identical.

The Reason Some WGA^r Mutants of MDAY-D2, such as MDW4, Are Nonmetastatic

It now seems clear that the detection of the WGA^S hybrid revertants was made possible by what appears to be a host-mediated selection process against the WGA^r mutant cells injected. This becomes readily apparent from the results shown in Figure 3, where there was a gradual decline in the proportion of WGA^r tumor cells in the tumor growing at the site of inoculation, until they comprised less than 0.01% of the tumor cells. From these results it could even be argued that MDW4 cells are nontumorigenic, or only minimally tumorigenic, since they appear to grow only transiently and then regress, to be replaced by the WGA^S revertants. Similarly, they do not grow after i.v. inoculation (Dennis et al. 1981a, Lagarde et al. 1983). And finally, we have never seen WGA^r cells in distant metastases—clearly showing they cannot metastasize.

These results raise the obvious question of what prevents MDW4, and similar WGA^r mutants, from growing progressively and metastasizing. Answering this question could provide insights into cellular and host-related factors that govern or affect the expression of the metastatic phenotype. In this connection, we wish to stress that classic changes involving antigenic alteration of the mutants do not appear to be involved. MDW4 is no more, or less, immunogenic than the MDAY-D2 cells from which it was derived, and appears to possess the same tumor antigens (Dennis et al. 1981b, 1981c).

One would therefore predict that the cell fusion phenomenon would take place in nude mice, and this is exactly what we have found, as shown in Figure 6. MDW4 cells were injected s.c. into adult Balb/c nude mice and the resultant metastases, as well as late-stage primary tumors, were tested for the status of the WGA^r phenotype. Using the thymidine incorporation assay, we obtained evidence that the cells behaved in nude mice as they do in the normal syngeneic DBA/2 host. The inability of MDW4 cells to grow after i.v. inoculation, however, implies that other types of host defense mechanisms that are sometimes referred to as paraimmune might be a causative factor. We are referring in particular to natural killer (NK) cells: the evidence is mounting that the blood-borne phase of metastasis can be curtailed by these cells (e.g., Hanna et al. 1982).

A series of experiments were therefore undertaken to examine the relative susceptibility to NK cells of MDAY-D2, MDW4, and WGA^s revertants derived in vivo from MDW4 (Nestel and Kerbel, unpublished observations). As shown

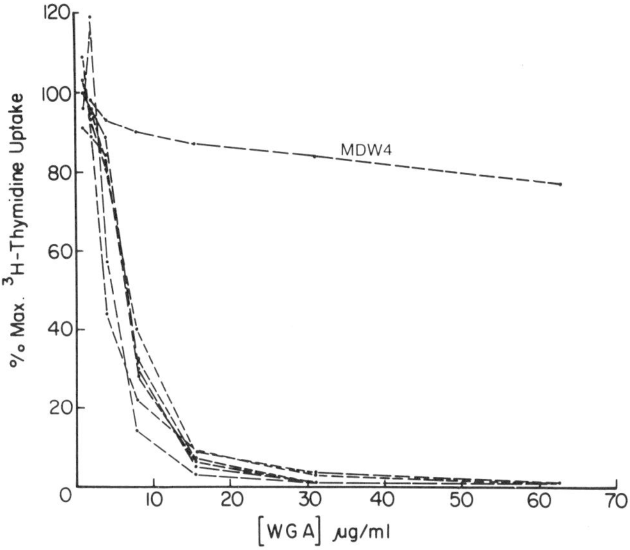

FIG. 6. Wheat germ agglutinin resistance (WGA^r) profiles of MDW4 (*upper curve*) and several metastases (or primaries) (*lower curves*) obtained from nude mice. An inoculum of 10^5 MDW4 cells was injected s.c. into 12-week-old Balb/c nude mice. Two months later several spontaneous metastases from two anatomical sites and several primaries were removed from the livers or lungs of two different nude mice and tested for their WGA^r phenotype using the [^{3}H]thymidine incorporation assay. All metastases and primaries were revertant for the WGA^r marker as shown.

in Table 4, an excellent correlation was observed. Thus, MDAY-D2 cells and WGA^s hybrid revertants of MDW4 were highly resistant to NK cells. In contrast, MDW4 cells were susceptible. Similar experiments were undertaken to examine the susceptibility of the various lines to activated tumoricidal macrophages (Nestel et al., unpublished observations). We found the converse: MDW4 cells were much more resistant to activated macrophages than any of the WGA^s revertants tested or MDAY-D2 cells. Hence, the results suggest that NK cells do indeed play some kind of role in the behavior of MDW4 cells, possibly related to their survival in the bloodstream, where NK cell levels are normally very high.

Nevertheless, it would be premature to conclude that the NK cells are the *only* host controlling element. For example, we have obtained evidence (unpublished) that i.v. inoculation of MDW4 cells into nude mice results in 100% tumor take. The tumors that arose had a WGA^S phenotype, or a mixed phenotype (WGA^S and WGA^r) (Kerbel, unpublished observations). Since nude mice have high NK cell levels, but lack T cells (see Kindred 1979), the MDW4 cells should not have grown after i.v. inoculation if the mechanism responsible for this behavior was the same as it is in DBA/2 mice and is related solely to NK cells.

TABLE 4. *NK-cell-mediated cytotoxicity of WGA^r MDW4 cells versus MDAY-D2 and WGA^s hybrid revertants generated in vivo after s.c. injection of MDW4 cells*

Cell line*	NK% specific lysis ± S.E.M.†, mediated by: Crude spleen cells	Nylon wool–passaged cells‡	Tumor growth§ in vivo
KD2-3	n.d.	11.6 ± 1.4	5/5 (14 ± 2)
MDW4	30.9 ± 1.4 (3)	52.5 ± 11.4	0/5 (>150)
MDW4-110c1	33.4 ± 7.9 (3)	42.5 ± 4.9	9/9 (53 ± 12)
MDW4-110c2	4.5 ± 2.0 (3)″	16.6 ± 5.1	5/5 (17 ± 1)
MDW4-14	4.2 ± 0.1 (2) #	15.5 ± 1.3	n.d.
MDW4-24a	5.0 ± 0.6 (3) #	18.6 ± 0.8	5/5 (11 ± 2)
MDW4-24b	n.d.	21.9 ± 1.5	5/5 (15 ± 2)
MDW4-23a	5.7 ± 1.1 (2)	11.3 ± 2.0	4/4 (15 ± 1)

* MDW4-24a, 24b, and 25c are cell lines established from WGA^s revertant metastases obtained from MDW4-injected animals (Dennis et al. 1981c). MDW4-110c1 is a clone from a primary tumor obtained from an MDW4-injected DBA/2 host in which the cells retained the WGA^r marker, whereas MDW4-110c2 is a clone from the same tumor in which the cells lost the WGA^r marker. MDW4-14 is an uncloned line established from a primary tumor obtained from an MDW4 marker (Dennis et al. 1981a).

† NK (natural killer) cell assays were carried out using an 18-h ^{111}In radioisotope release assay at a 100:1 effector:target ratio. Effector cells were from poly I:C boosted CBA mice. A total of 5×10^3 target cells were added to each well. Number of experiments performed in parentheses.

‡ % Specific lysis of YAC-1 lymphoma cells in 2 separate experiments equalled 64.4 ± 0.6. All results are expressed as % specific lysis ± S.E.M. of 2 experiments.

§ DBA/2 mice were injected i.v. with 10^5 tumor cells. Numerator indicates number of animals dying of metastases. Numbers in brackets are mean survival time in days ± S.D.

″ $P < 0.02$ level of significance as compared to MDW4.

\# $P < 0.01$ level of significance as compared to MDW4.

Membrane Structural Change and the Change in Malignant Phenotype of MDW4 Cells

It appears that a membrane structural change explains the alteration in malignant phenotype of MDW4 cells. Dennis et al. (1982) found significant reductions in the total amount of cell surface sialic acid in MDW4 cells compared with the WGA^s revertants of MDAY-D2 cells (Table 5). This result is of considerable interest since a direct relationship between levels of cell surface siliac acid and metastatic ability has been reported by several investigators (Yogeeswaran et al. 1978, Yogeeswaran and Salk 1981, Finne et al. 1980, Dobrossy et al. 1981, Burger et al. 1982). Conversely, an inverse relationship between cell surface sialic acid levels and NK cell susceptibility has been noted (Yogeeswaran et al. 1981). These results are not unexpected since sialic acid is the only charged sugar and therefore could (and should) affect many membrane-related functions, not just NK susceptibility. Indeed, Dennis et al. (1982) found that reduced sialic acid levels increased the ability of MDW4 cells to adhere to collagen type IV and fibronectin but not to laminin or other types of collagens. Such alterations could obviously affect the metastatic capability of cells.

TABLE 5. *Comparison of neuraminidase-accessible sialic acid on WGA^r mutant and wild-type MDAY-D2 cells**

Tumor cell lines	Phenotype†	Release of counts from ^{3}H-N-acetylmannosamine-labeled cells‡	Thiobarbituric acid assay (nM sialic acid per mg cell protein)§
MDAY-D2	met$^+$ WGA^S Oua^S	16.7 ± 5.1	1.91 ± 0.35 (5)
MDW4	met$^-$ WGA^r Oua^R	4.1 ± 1.8	0.59 ± 0.13 (4)
W40M1	met$^+$ WGA^S Oua^R	22.2 ± 9.5	1.89 ± 0.06 (2)
W40M4	met$^+$ WGA^S Oua^R	16.0 ± 5.7	1.69 ± 0.12 (3)

* Met$^+$ = metastatic; met$^-$ = nonmetastatic; WGA^r = wheat germ agglutinin-resistant. (Results reproduced from Dennis et al. (1982) with permission of *Nature*, MacMillan Journals Ltd.)

† WGA (2-5 μg ml^{-1}) and ouabain (0.1 mM) added to MDAY-D2 in tissue culture reduced cell growth by 90% (D_{10}) (WGA^s,Oua^s). MDW40 is an Oua^R mutant (D_{10} = 3 mM) and WGA^r mutant (D_{10} = 50 μg ml^{-1}) of MDW4. MDW40 cells have been shown to grow only locally at the site of a s.c. inoculation, and when 10^5 cells are injected i.v. less than 5% of the mice die of tumor takes. W40M1 and W40M4 are WGA^s, Oua^R resistant tumor cell lines isolated from the liver and spleen, respectively, of two DBA/2 mice injected s.c. with 10^5 MDW40 cells 90 days earlier, i.e. the cells were WGA^s tumor cell–host cell hybrid revertants.

‡ Tumor cells, 5 × 10^5 per ml, were cultured in RPMI plus 10% fetal calf serum and 2 μCi ml^{-1} [6-^{3}H]N-acetylmannosamine. After 48 h, the cells were washed three times in Dulbecco's phosphate-buffered saline (PBS) and samples of 10^6 cells in 100 μl of PBS, 5 mM $CaCl_2$, pH 6.1, were incubated alone (C) or with 0.02 U of neuraminidase (N) for 60 min at 37°C. The cells were washed twice in PBS and solubilized, and radioactivity was measured. The formula (C-N/C) × 100 was used to calculate the percentage of neuraminidase-accessible sialic acid. The results are the mean ± s.e. of three experiments.

§ Tumor cells were incubated with 2 U of neuraminidase for 60 min at 37 ° C. The cells were pelleted, and sialic acid in the supernatant was measured using the thiobarbituric acid assay. The results represent the mean ± s.e. of the number of experiments indicated in parentheses.

Preliminary results have been obtained on the cause of the reduced amounts of cell surface sialic acid and on what structures are actually affected. MDW4 cells seem to lack terminal galactose and sialic acid residues in the N-linked oligosaccharides of cell surface glycoproteins (Dennis, Schacter and Carver, unpublished observations). This lack may be related to a missing glycosyltransferase enzyme, and as such, the cells may be representative of a certain class of "transferase-deficient" mutant. Elucidating the nature of these biochemical changes and what their effects on certain cell properties are will clearly be an informative way of establishing cellular structure-function relationships relevant to the metastatic phenotype.

The Possible Role of Prior Mutagenesis in the Growth Properties of MDW4 and Related Mutants In Vivo

There are basically four ways in which WGA^r mutants can be selected: (1) spontaneously in a single step, (2) spontaneously in two or more steps, (3) after mutagenesis in a single step, or (4) after mutagenesis in two or more steps. The method of selection appears to have a significant impact on the nature of mutants obtained. Thus, Lagarde et al. (1983, and unpublished observations) found that most WGA^r mutants selected without prior mutagenesis (spontaneous WGA^r mutants) behave in a fashion similar to MDAY-D2; none has yet been found that spontaneously fuse in vivo. An independent series of selections by M.-C. Fulchignoni-Lataud (manuscript in preparation) revealed that a significant proportion of WGA^r mutants of MDAY-D2 selected in a single step after mutagenesis (which is how MDW4 was isolated) behaved similarly (but not identically) to MDW4 in vivo insofar as reversion of the WGA^r phenotype was concerned. An example of this is shown in Figure 7. The WGA^r mutant tested was designated 310.5A, and s.c. injection of DBA/2 mice with 310.5A WGA^r cells led to the emergence of WGA^s revertants, but not in all cases. This result is an interesting departure from MDW4, whose every metastasis was WGA^s.

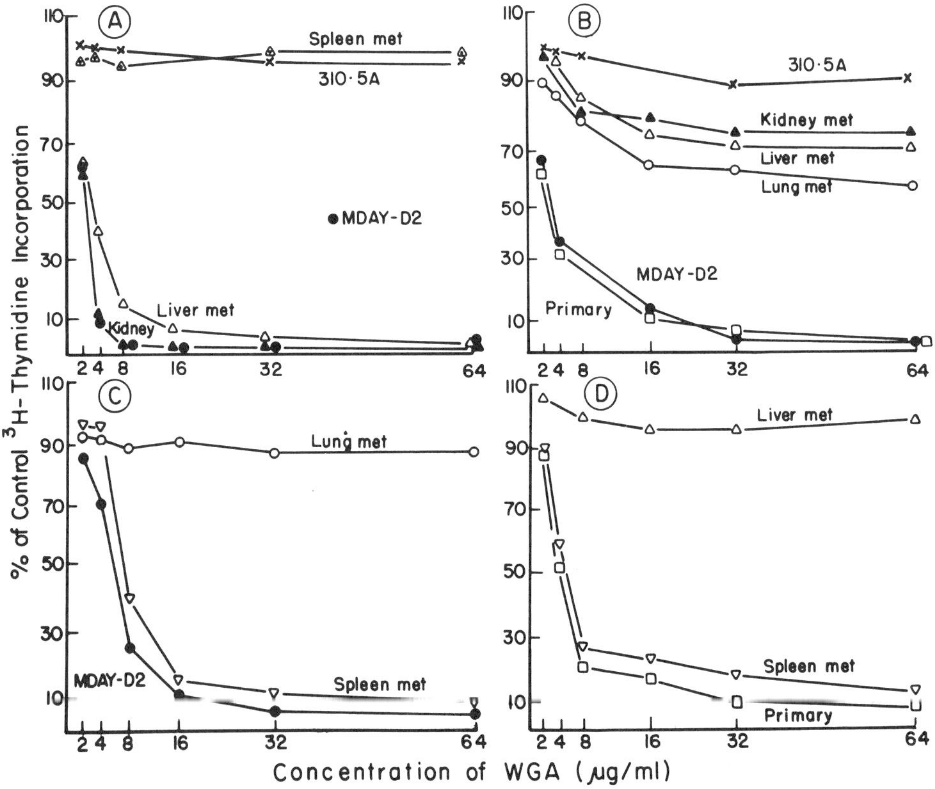

FIG. 7. WGA^r phenotypes of MDAY-D2, a WGA^r mutant called 310.5A, or spontaneous metastases and primary tumors obtained from DBA/2 mice given a s.c. inoculation of 310.5A mutant cells 50–70 days earlier. WGA resistance was assessed using a [^{3}H]thymidine incorporation assay as described previously (Lagarde et al. 1983a, Kerbel et al. 1983). Each panel represents a different experiment performed over a 3-month period, using individual mice. The 310.5A mutant, like MDW4, was obtained in a single-step selection after mutagenesis of MDAY-D2 cells (Fulchignoni-Lataud et al. unpublished observations). Met, metastasis.

A somatic cell genetic analysis on a large series of independently derived WGA^r mutants of MDAY-D2 cells by Fulchignoni-Lataud et al. (manuscript in preparation) revealed that there are a number of genotypic classes involved, as was found for CHO cells by Stanley (1981). Genetic complementation analysis has revealed that cell hybrids made in vitro between the MDW4 and 310.5A WGA^r mutants have a WGA^s phenotype that would imply they may belong to different complementation groups. This conclusion is strengthened by the finding that the PHA^r, Con A^r, and RIC^r profiles (i.e., the overall lectin-resistant phenotype) of the two mutants is quite different. Thus, 310.5A cells are RIC^R whereas MDW4 cells are RIC^S and 310.5A cells are much less PHA^r than MDW4 cells are (Fulchignoni-Lataud et al. manuscript in preparation).

Thus it seems that there is more than one type of WGA^r mutant (genotype) that can spontaneously fuse in vivo with a normal host cell; moreover, it is possible that the underlying mechanisms may be different. This could explain the differences between MDW4 and 310.5A cells in terms of the consistency with which they revert (i.e., fuse) in vivo, as discussed above and shown in Figure 7. Comparative characterization of the mutants should therefore be useful in gaining a better understanding of the unique in vivo properties of mutants such as MDW4.

An important issue these results raise is the contribution of the prior mutagenesis treatment to the outcome of the results. Arguments can be made both for and against the view that the derivation and properties of WGA^r mutants such as MDW4 and 310.5A are dependent on the mutagen treatment. This issue is addressed in detail in the Discussion section. To summarize, it is possible to derive a number of independent WGA^r mutants from MDAY-D2 in a single-step selection that completely or substantially lose the ability to grow progressively and metastasize, but acquire metastatic growth potential by cell fusion in vivo. Prior mutagenesis may be necessary to obtain these types of mutants, and their individual behavior suggests that they are not identical, but instead belong to different classes of WGA^r mutants.

DISCUSSION

Using a series of lectin-resistant membrane mutant tumor sublines, we have performed experiments that demonstrate a clear case of tumor progression occurring as a consequence of spontaneous in vivo tumor–host cell fusion, followed by chromosome segregation. Our results raise several issues with implications for many aspects of tumor biology.

Because of the progression of both clinical and experimental solid tumors and the evolution of tumor heterogeneity and progression is often accompanied by an increase in ploidy levels, it would seem reasonable to propose that spontaneous tumor–host cell fusion is one of many ways by which this could occur (Goldenberg et al. 1974, Warner 1975, Kerbel et al. 1982, 1983). However, there are several questions raised about the relevance of our experimental model and overall approach. These must be addressed before it can be said with assurance that the model is indeed appropriate. These are addressed in the discussion that follows.

Is the Spontaneous "Fusogenicity" of the WGA^r Mutants Unique to the Mutants or a General Property of the MDAY-D2 Tumor?

If one accepts the possibility that spontaneous tumor–normal host cell fusion is a mechanism by which tumor cell heterogeneity and the emergence of metastatic subpopulations can be generated, then our experimental approach may be an informative method to study the phenomenon. At first glance, it may appear that those WGA^r mutants of MDAY-D2 that spontaneously fuse in vivo do so at a very high frequency. Because these mutants were intentionally selected on the basis of having membrane alterations, it would not be surprising to isolate mutants that are far more spontaneously fusogenic than the wild-type cells from which they were derived. This could be taken as a criticism of the model, since it could be argued that such types of mutants would rarely, if ever, arise during the normal course of events of tumor growth in vivo.

In this regard, two considerations are pertinent. First, one reason the hybrids were so easy to detect in our experimental model was that the WGA^r mutant cells injected were unable to grow indefinitely and progressively at the site of inoculation. Nor were they able to metastasize. In other words, they were at a marked selective disadvantage compared to the WGA^s hybrids. Thus, it is quite possible that the cell fusion event is *not* frequent. Rather, the few WGA^s hybrids that arose early were quickly able to displace the WGA^r tumor cell population at the site of inoculation and then to metastasize. If so, the spontaneous fusion process may be a general property of the MDAY-D2 tumor line itself, but it is not readily detected (in the case of MDAY-D2 tumor growth) because the hybrids generated have no selective advantage over the highly malignant MDAY-D2 cells.

Second, it is probable that it is not so much a question of whether spontaneous tumor-host cell fusion events occur (or even how often they do so), but rather, whether such hybrids—or their segregating progeny—have a strong selective growth advantage over their tumor cell "parents." For if they do not, their numbers would always remain negligible, and they could never have any influence on the course of tumor progression. In this connection it should be noted that a number of reports over the last decade have described spontaneous tumor–host cell fusion in vivo (for reviews see Kerbel et al. 1982, 1983). As pointed out by Fenyo et al. (1973), such fusions with a large variety of tumors occur in a number of different experimental circumstances. However, the malignant phenotype of the hybrids was not assessed except by Goldenberg et al. (1974). A summary of some of these results is given in Table 6. Thus it cannot be argued that the ability of mutants like MDW4 or 310.5A to spontaneously fuse in vivo is either unusual or unique.

TABLE 6. *A summary of the literature documenting spontaneous in vivo cell fusion between tumor cells and normal host cells*

Tumor*	Method of detecting tumor-host cell hybrids	Tumorigenic and malignant properties of hybrids	Reference
SEWA sarcoma; SEYF fibrosarcoma; MSWB sarcoma	Chromosome and H-2 antigen markers	Tumorigenicity of hybrids and parent tumor comparable; metastatic properties not assessed	Fenyo et al. (1973)
TA3 mammary tumor; SEWA sarcoma; A9HT fibrosarcoma	Chromosome, H-2 antigen, and drug-resistance genetic markers	Not assessed	Wiener et al. (1974) Wiener et al. (1972) Ber et al. (1978)
Human astrocytic glioma transplanted to cheek pouch of hamsters	Isoenzyme and chromosome analysis	Hybrids metastatic but human tumor cell nonmetastatic in hamster hosts	Goldenberg et al. (1974)
PAZG melanoma	Chromosome and drug-resistance genetic markers	Tumorigenicity of hybrids suppressed relative to parent tumor; metastatic properties not assessed	Hu and Pasztor (1975)
C1.1D fibrosarcoma	Chromosome and drug-resistance genetic markers	All hybrids were tumorigenic; relative changes and metastatic phenotype not assessed	Aviles et al. (1977) Jami and Ritz (1975) Aviles et al. (1980)
A9HT (L cell) fibrosarcoma	Chromosome and drug-resistance genetic markers	Hybrids were 200-fold less tumorigenic than A9HT cells; metastatic properties not assessed	Kao and Hartz (1977)
Cloudman melanoma	Chromosome and drug-resistance genetic markers; isoenzyme analysis	Tumorigenic properties of hybrids and parent tumor comparable; metastatic properties not assessed	Halaban et al. (1980)
Ehrlich ascites tumor	Chromosome and H-2 antigen markers	Not assessed	Lala et al. (1980)

* All tumors listed are of mouse origin (and injected into mice for the in vivo experiments), with the exception of the human glioma.

Malignant Status of Somatic Cell Hybrids Between Normal Cells and Tumor Cells

Given the distinct possibility that spontaneous tumor–host cell fusions do occur in a more general way, the key question then shifts to the malignant status of such hybrids. Based on the somatic cell genetics literature in this field, one might justifiably claim that hybrids of this nature should *not* acquire an increased malignant phenotype. To begin with, it is now generally accepted that the trait of malignancy is suppressed in tumor–normal cell hybrids made in vitro and then grown in vivo; i.e., it behaves as a recessive characteristic (Harris 1971). Malignancy, if it reappears, does so only after chromosome segregation in vivo from the hybrids, and it appears that the balance of chromosomes No. 4 (derived from both the tumor and normal cells) is critical to the outcome of the expression of the malignant phenotype in mouse-mouse hybrids (Evans et al. 1982). It is then appropriate to ask whether there is any evidence that some of the malignant segregants might be significantly *more* malignant than the tumor cell parents once they arise.

The answer to this question is far from clear for the simple reason that almost all previous investigations on the malignant status of cell hybrids, and their segregants, utilized growth at the site of inoculation as the sole criterion of "malignancy." This test therefore measures the "tumorigenic" (as distinct from the malignant) potential of a cell population. Many authors (e.g., Poste and Fidler 1980) have stressed that a malignant tumor is defined as one that is invasive or metastatic. Hence it could be said that many experimental animal tumors are in fact nonmalignant, or very poorly so, even though they may be capable of killing their hosts by relentless growth at the site of inoculation. Thus, the use of a dose-response curve to compare the growth properties of tumor cells and cell hybrids derived from them could be quite misleading in respect to malignancy. Put another way, a slow-growing, poorly tumorigenic tumor may ultimately be more malignant than a faster growing, more-tumorigenic line because of its greater propensity for metastasis.

The recent findings of Stackpole (1981) and more recently of Sweeney et al. (1982) are of interest in this connection. They showed that it is possible to derive tumor clones that give rise to large numbers of "artificial" lung nodules after i.v. inoculation, but that are nonmetastatic after s.c. inoculation. Conversely, other clones can be derived that are highly metastatic after s.c. injection (spontaneous metastases) but are completely incapable of lung colonization after i.v. growth. Which type of clone is more malignant? Most would argue that it is the latter. Whatever the conclusion, the results illustrate the caution one must use before comparing the relative malignant status of tumor cell lines.

One additional point is of interest. The nature of the normal cell partner in a tumor–normal cell hybrid may be critical to the expression of its relative malignant phenotype. A good example was shown by De Baetselier et al. (1981), who found that a nonmetastatic murine plastocytome acquired extremely strong metastatic properties after it was intentionally hybridized in vitro with normal spleen B lymphocytes. The resultant hybridomas spontaneously metastasized to the liver, or spleen, or both. Although control experiments with other types of normal cells (e.g., fibroblasts) were not performed, the results show that hybrids can indeed be more malignant than their tumor cell parent; this may depend on fusion with normal cells that possess a "quasi-metastatic" phenotype, a characteristic, incidentally, of virtually all types of bone marrow–derived hematopoietic cells. Such cells are obviously programmed for survival in the bloodstream, migration, and the ability to extravasate. Therefore, some of these biological characteristics could be conferred by cell fusion to tumor cells that ordinarily lack them, thereby producing metastatic hybrids.

Chromosome Segregation in Human-Human Cell Hybrids

Since chromosome segregation must take place in tumor–normal cell hybrids in order for them to express the tumorigenic phenotype (Harris 1971, Stanbridge et al. 1982), one could argue that this phenomenon would be of dubious relevance in clinical cancer for the simple reason that chromosome segregation from human–human cell hybrids is far more limited and occurs much less readily than in mouse-mouse or mouse-human hybrids (Stanbridge et al 1982). Thus, studies like ours utilizing a mouse tumor model may yield results that exaggerate the role of spontaneous cell fusion in the progression of human cancers.

Another possible criticism of the relevance of the fusion phenomenon to the progression of clinical cancers comes from biochemical genetic studies on the clonality of cancers, using the isoenzyme glucose-6-phosphate dehydrogenase (G-6-PD) as a marker (Fialkow 1979). Tumors with a clonal origin have a type A or type B G-6-PD phenotype, whereas tumors with a multicellular origin could have both types. By exploiting this cellular mosaicism, most studies have shown that virtually all tumor samples thus far analyzed have a single enzyme phenotype (and are therefore of probable clonal origin). However, one would anticipate that in vivo hybridization between tumor cells and host cells should lead to tumors of metastases having a double (A + B) G-6-PD enzyme phenotype (Warner 1975).

Close examination of the literature in this area, however, reveals that the vast majority of tumors examined in such G-6-PD phenotyping studies have been leukemias (Fialkow 1979). Relatively few samples of carcinomas (and especially metastases) have been tested. Furthermore, it is interesting to note that of the few reports of human tumors with double enzyme phenotypes, almost all have been carcinomas: e.g., metastatic carcinoma of the colon, invasive carcinomas of the cervix, and breast carcinoma (reviewed by Kerbel et al. 1983). Clearly, more analyses of tissue culture cell lines established from metastatic carcinomas might reveal evidence for the possibility of tumor–host cell fusions occurring during clinical tumor progression.

The Contribution of Prior Mutagenesis to the Properties of WGA^r Mutants That Behave Like MDW4 and 310.5A

We alluded to the fact that Lagarde et al. (unpublished observations) have not detected any spontaneous WGA^r mutants that possess the properties of mutants such as MDW4 or 310.5A—i.e., those that cannot metastasize but acquire the ability to do so after spontaneous cell fusion in vivo. Thus far, about 20 spontaneous WGA^r mutants of MDAY-D2 have been isolated and tested by Lagarde. MDW4 and similar mutants were all isolated independently by a single-step selection following conventional mutagenesis with EMS. Most of the mutants that acquired properties similar to MDW4 had a subtetraploid chromosome mode (68), whereas the spontaneous WGA^r mutants retained the near-diploid number of chromosomes normally seen in MDAY-D2 cells. This difference clearly raised the possibilities that the polyploid state might somehow be a cause of the in vivo behavior of mutants like MDW4 and that the change in ploidy was induced by prior mutagenesis treatment. However, the 310.5A WGA^r mutant has a near-diploid (A) karyotype and it behaves similarly to the MDW4 mutant. Nonetheless, both mutants were derived after mutagenesis.

One could still argue both for and against the proposal that the mutagenesis procedure is instrumental in our system. As far as the arguments against, we draw attention to some recent results of Stanley (1981) that are quite pertinent. Using CHO cells she found numerous WGA^r phenotypes or classes (based on unique patterns of collateral resistance or sensitivity to other lectins such as PHA, Con A, and RIC, as well as lectin-binding characteristics) and that each phenotype occurs "at a similar frequency" in an unmutagenized population of CHO cells (Stanley 1981). In an unmutagenized population of cells, she found that out of 25 WGA^r isolates tested, 6 belonged to class I, 14 to class II, and 1 to class III, and 4 to class VIII. However, if the cells were mutagenized with EMS, the relative proportion of the various classes subsequently isolated changed considerably: evidence suggested that class III WGA^r mutants comprised all, or most, of the WGA^r mutants isolated after EMS treatment. Thus, a class of mutant that existed in the minority before mutagenesis could become the dominant mutant after mutagen treatment.

These results are perhaps not surprising in view of recent work showing that different gene loci are differentially susceptible to different mutagens (Siciliano et al. 1983). There is evidence for hypermutable DNA base sequences similar to the so-called hot spots in prokaryotes (e.g., see Tischfield et al. 1982). Because each WGA^r phenotype is associated with a different genotype (Stanley 1981), it could be argued that the gene responsible for the emergence of MDW4-related WGA^r phenotypes are hypersensitive to EMS. One can see from Stanley's results that the approximately 20 spontaneous WGA^r mutants so far isolated may be insufficient to pick up what could be a rare WGA^r class (e.g., 1/25–1/50) in an unmutagenized population of cells. Additional spontaneous WGA^r mutants may need to be isolated and tested to resolve this problem. Finally we point out, as we have before (Kerbel et al. 1982), that reduction or loss of metastatic or tumorigenic phenotypes in WGA[r] tumor mutants obtained *without* prior mutagenesis has been noted by other investigators using a variety of tumors (Tao and Burger 1977, Reading et al. 1980, Bramwell and Harris 1978).

In support of the view that mutagenesis may be a relevant factor is an argument that stems from recent findings on the induction of "mutationlike" epigenetic changes in cells by mutagens or carcinogens—the result of changes in demethylation patterns of DNA (Kasten et al. 1982, Wilson and Jones 1983). It is now known that a small portion of the cytosine residues of DNA are methylated and that the resulting 5-methylcytosine residues occur in specific sequences in the DNA, most often adjacent to guanine residues (Razin and Riggs 1980, Ehrlich and Wang 1981). It appears that gene transcription can be profoundly affected by the degree of methylation of cytosine residues: demethylation leads to gene activation (e.g., Taylor and Jones 1979, Jones and Taylor 1980, Niwa and Sugahara 1981, Harris 1982). Because the methylation pattern in the parental DNA strand is semiconservatively copied after replication, it can be passed on as a heritable trait to the daughter cells after cell division. A disturbance in methylation patterns, e.g., a reduction, can therefore erase the normal pattern that previously existed and in turn lead to activation of certain genes and a heritable change in the phenotypic properties of a cell so affected.

Hence, mutagens such as EMS, because they damage DNA—a process that itself leads to hypomethylation of the "repair patches" of DNA—must now be viewed as agents that can cause genetic *and* epigenetic changes, both of which would be heritable. How such epigenetic changes may influence the isolation and behavior of mutants, such as MDW4, is something we can only speculate about at this time. But because an effect is possible, it is clear that the selection of drug- or lectin-resistant mutants using prior mutagen treatment could itself influence how these amounts behave in vivo. We have stressed this possibility before in relation to possible immunologic alterations of tumor cells by prior mutagen treatment (Kerbel et al. 1982, Kerbel and Frost 1982, Frost and Kerbel 1984).

Tumor Cell Membrane Mutants, Tumor Progression, and Metastasis: A Summary

From this discussion, it can be seen that there are problems in trying to assess the relevance of spontaneous in vivo tumor–host cell fusion to tumor progression, tumor heterogeneity, and metastasis using membrane mutants selected through such procedures as lectin resistance in vitro. It is not yet clear whether they amplify what is normally a rare and physiologically trivial phenomenon. Nevertheless, on the basis of the results we have obtained, we think it is reasonable to hypothesize that tumor progression and the emergence of metastatic subpopulations can occasionally occur through spontaneous cell fusion between tumor cells and normal bone marrow–derived cells, followed by chromo-

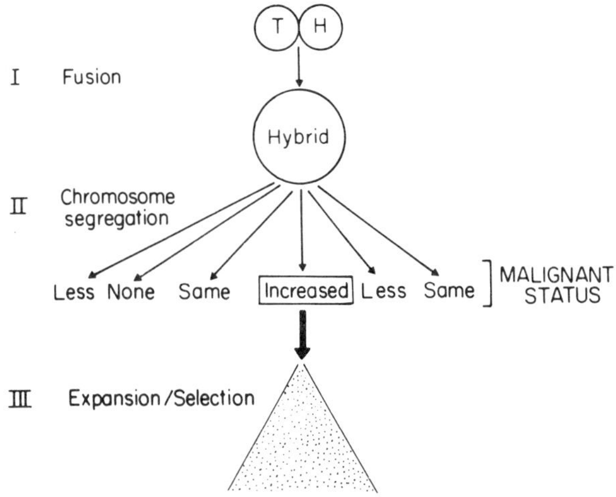

FIG. 8. Summary of the hypothesis that spontaneous tumor cell–normal host cell fusion in vivo followed by chromosome segregation is a possible mechanism for the generation of tumor progression and the emergence of more-malignant variants. The chromosome segregation phase would result in the emergence of variants less malignant, equally malignant, or more malignant than the parent tumor cell population. Even if the more-malignant variants were rare, they could, by selection, eventually overgrow the existing population.

some segregation. This is summarized in Figure 8. The chromosome segregation process would be a mechanism to promote karyotypic heterogeneity and thereby the emergence (and subsequent selection) of the "fittest" cells. As such, the hypothesis is a restatement of Nowell's hypothesis (1976) of tumor progression; but here the genetic changes leading to the generation of more-malignant variants arise as a consequence of the fusion/segregation phenomena rather than mutational events. However, we stress that we are proposing this as a *possible additional* mechanism, not an alternative to mutational or epigenetic mechanisms of tumor progression.

Even if tumor–host cell fusion proves not to be a valid mechanism of tumor progression, such mutants will nonetheless be very useful tools for studying the contribution of specific membrane-related structures to various steps of the metastatic process. Furthermore, the use of tumor cell populations having well-defined genetic markers introduced into the cells in vitro appears to be promising for studying aspects of tumor progression in vivo—provided the investigator is aware of some of the pitfalls that the introduction (or the process of their introduction) of these markers can have on the functional and physiological properties of the cells in vivo.

ACKNOWLEDGMENTS

The persevering and excellent secretarial help of Mrs. Beverley Fluhrer and Mrs. Beverley Muller is gratefully appreciated. Miss M. S. Man, Miss Dorothy

Vriezen, and Mrs. Majka Florian provided excellent technical assistance. This work was supported by grants from the National Cancer Institute of Canada and the Medical Research Council of Canada. R. S. Kerbel is a Research Associate of the National Cancer Institute of Canada.

REFERENCES

Aviles, D., J. Jami, J.-P. Rousset, and E. Ritz. 1977. Tumor x host cell hybrids in the mouse: Chromosomes from the normal cell parent maintained in malignant hybrid tumors. Proc. Natl. Acad. Sci. USA 58:1391–1397.

Aviles, D., E. Ritz, and J. Jami. 1980. Chromosomes in tumors derived from mouse tumor x diploid cell hybrids obtained in vitro. Somatic Cell Genet. 6:171–186.

Ber, R., F. Wiener, and E.-M. Fenyo. 1978. Proof of in vivo fusion of murine tumor cells with host cells by universal fusers. JNCI 60:931–933.

Bramwell, M. E., and H. H. Harris. 1978. An abnormal glycoprotein associated with malignancy in a wide range of different tumors. Proc. R. Soc. London Ser. B 201:87–106.

Burger, M. M. 1980. The cell surface and metastasis, *in* Biology of the Cancer Cell, K. Letnansky, ed. Amsterdam, Kugler Publications, pp. 193–208.

Burger, M. M., T. W. Tao, J. Finne, and J.-P. Prieels. 1982. The influence of membrane mutations on metastasis. Bioscience Reports 2:597–599.

DeBaetselier, P., E. Gorelik, Z. Eshhar, Y. Ron, S. Katzav, M. Feldman, and S. Segal. 1981. Metastatic properties conferred on nonmetastatic tumors by hybridization of spleen B-lymphocytes with plasmacytoma cells. JNCI 67:1079–1087.

Dennis, J. W., T. P. Donaghue, D. A. Carlow, and R. S. Kerbel. 1981a. Demonstration of a correlation between tumor cell H-2 antigen content, immunogenicity, and tumorigenicity using lectin-resistant tumor variants. Cancer Res. 41:4010–4019.

Dennis, J., T. Donaghue, M. Florian, and R. S. Kerbel. 1981b. Apparent reversion of stable in vitro genetic markers detected in tumour cells from spontaneous metastases. Nature 292:242–245.

Dennis, J. W., T. P. Donaghue, and R. S. Kerbel. 1981c. An examination of tumor antigen loss in spontaneous metastases. Inv. Metastasis 1:111–125.

Dennis, J. W., and R. S. Kerbel. 1981. Characterization of a deficiency in fucose metabolism in lectin-resistant variants of a murine tumor showing altered tumorigenic and metastatic capacities in vivo. Cancer Res. 41:98–104.

Dennis, J., C. Waller, R. Timpl, and V. Schirrmacher. 1982. Surface sialic acid reduces attachment of metastatic tumour cells to collagen type IV and fibronectin. Nature 30:274–276.

Dobrossy, L., Z. P. Pavelic, and R. J. Bernacki. 1981. A correlation between cell surface sialyltransferase, sialic acid, and glycosidase activities and the implantability of B16 murine melanoma. Cancer Res. 41:2262–2266.

Ehrlich, M., and Y. H. Wang. 1981. 5-Methylcytosine in eukaryotic DNA. Science 212:1350–1357.

Evans, E. P., M. D. Burtenshaw, B. B. Brown, R. Hennion, and H. Harris. 1982. The analysis of malignancy by cell fusion. IX. Re-examination and clarification of the problem. J. Cell Sci. 56:113–130.

Fenyo, E. M., F. Wiener, G. Klein, and H. Harris. 1973. Selection of tumor-host cell hybrids from polyoma virus- and methylcholanthrene-induced sarcomas. JNCI 51:1865–1875.

Fialkow, P. J. 1979. Clonal origin of human tumors. Ann. Rev. Med. 30:135–176.

Fidler, I. J. 1978. General considerations for studies of experimental cancer metastasis. Methods Cancer Res. 15:399–439.

Finne, J., T.-W. Tao, and M. M. Burger. 1980. Carbohydrate changes in glycoproteins of a poorly metastasizing wheat germ agglutinin-resistant melanoma clone. Cancer Res. 40:2580–2587.

Frost, P., and R. S. Kerbel. 1981. Immunoselection in vitro of a nonmetastatic variant from a highly metastatic tumor. Int. J. Cancer 27:381–385.

Frost, P., and R. S. Kerbel. 1984. On the possible epigenetic origins of tumor cell heterogeneity. Cancer Metastasis Rev. (in press).

Goldenberg, D. M., R. A. Pavia, and M. C. Tsao. 1974. In vivo hybridization of human tumour and normal hamster cells. Nature 250:649–651.

Halaban, R., J. Nordlund, U. Francke, G. Moellmann, and J. M. Eisenstadt. 1980. Supermelanotic hybrids derived from mouse melanomas and normal mouse cells. Somatic Cell Genet. 6:29–44.
Hanna, N., T. W. Davis, and I. J. Fidler. 1982. Environmental and genetic factors determine the level of NK activity of nude mice and affect their suitability as models for experimental metastasis. Int. J. Cancer 30:371–376.
Harris, H. 1971. Cell fusion and the analysis of malignancy. Proc. R. Soc. Lond. B 179:1–20.
Harris, J. F., A. F. Chambers, R. P. Hill, and V. Ling. 1982. Metastatic variants are generated spontaneously at a high rate in mouse KHT tumor. Proc. Natl. Acad. Sci. USA 79:5547–5551.
Harris, M. 1982. Induction of thymidine kinase in enzyme-deficient Chinese hamster cells. Cell 29:483–492.
Hu, F., and L. M. Pasztor. 1975. In vivo hybridisation of cultured melanoma cells and isogenic normal mouse cells. Differentiation 4:93–97.
Jami, J., and E. Ritz. 1975. Nonmalignancy of hybrids derived from two mouse malignant cells. II. Analysis of malignancy of LM (TK^-) Cl 1D parental cells. JNCI 54:117–122.
Jones, P. A., and S. M. Taylor. 1980. Cellular differentiation, cytidine analogs and DNA methylation. Cell 20:85–93.
Kao, F.-T., and J. A. Hartz. 1977. Genetic and tumorigenic characteristics of cell hybrids formed in vivo between injected tumor cells and host cells. JNCI 59:409–413.
Kastan, M. B., B. J. Gowans, and M. W. Lieberman. 1982. Methylation of deoxycytidine incorporated by excision-repair synthesis of DNA. Cell 30:509–516.
Kerbel, R. S. 1979. Immunologic studies of membrane mutants of a highly metastatic murine tumor. Am. J. Pathol. 97:609–622.
Kerbel, R. S., J. W. Dennis, A. E. Lagarde, and P. Frost. 1982. Tumor progression in metastasis: An experimental approach using lectin resistant tumor variants. Cancer Metastasis Reviews 1:99–140.
Kerbel, R. S., M. Florian, M. S. Man, J. W. Dennis, and I. F. C. McKenzie. 1980. Carcinogenicity of tumor cell populations: Origin of a putative H-2 isoantigenic loss variant tumor. JNCI 64:1221–1230.
Kerbel, R. S., and P. Frost. 1982. Heritable alterations induced in tumor cell immunogenicity. Immunology Today 3:34–35.
Kerbel, R. S., A. E. Lagarde, J. W. Dennis, and T. P. Donaghue. 1983. Spontaneous fusion in vivo between normal host cells and tumor cells: Possible contribution to tumor progression and metastasis studied with a lectin resistant mutant tumor. Mol. Cell. Biol. 3:523–538.
Kerbel, R. S., R. R. Twiddy, and D. M. Robertson. 1978. Induction of a tumor with greatly increased metastatic growth potential by injection of cells from a low-metastatic H-2 heterozygous tumor cell line into an H-2 incompatible parental strain. Int. J. Cancer 22:583–594.
Kindred, B. 1979. The nude mouse in immunology. Prog. Allergy 26:137–238.
Lagarde, A. 1983. A fluctuation analysis of the rate of re-expression of the metastatic potential in a non-metastatic mutant of the MDAY-D2 murine tumor. Inv. Metastasis 3:52–64.
Lagarde, A., T. P. Donaghue, J. W. Dennis, and R. S. Kerbel. 1983. Genotypic and phenotypic evolution of a murine tumor during its progression in vivo towards metastasis. JNCI 71:183–191.
Lala, P. K., V. Santer, and K. S. Rahil. 1980. Spontaneous fusion between Ehrlich ascites tumor cells and host cells in vivo: Kinetics of hybridization and concurrent changes in the histocompatibility profile of the tumor after propagation in different host strains. Eur. J. Cancer 16:487–510.
Liotta, L. A., U. P. Thorgeirsson, and S. Garbisa. 1982. Role of collagenases in tumor cell invasion. Cancer Metastasis Reviews 1:277–288.
Neri, A., and G. L. Nicolson. 1981. Phenotypic drift of metastatic and cell surface properties of mammary adenocarcinoma cell clones during growth in vitro. Int. J. Cancer 28:731–738.
Niwa, O., and T. Sugahara. 1981. 5-Azacytidine induction of mouse endogenous type C virus and suppression of DNA methylation. Proc. Natl. Acad. Sci. USA 78:6290–6294.
Nowell, P. 1976. The clonal evolution of tumor cell populations. Science 194:23–28.
Poste, G., J. Doll, A. E. Brown, J. Tzeng, and I. Zeidman. 1982. Comparison of the metastatic properties of B16 melanoma clones isolated from cultured cell lines, subcutaneous tumors, and individual lung metastases. Cancer Res. 42:2770–2778.
Poste, G., J. Doll, and I. J. Fidler. 1981. Interactions between clonal subpopulations affect stability of the metastatic phenotype in polyclonal populations of B16 melanoma cells. Proc. Natl. Acad. Sci. USA 78:6226–6230.

Poste, G., and I. J. Fidler. 1980. The pathogenesis of cancer metastasis. Nature 283:139–146.
Razin, A., and A. D. Riggs. 1980. DNA methylation and gene function. Science 210:604–610.
Reading, C. L., P. N. Belloni, and G. L. Nicolson. 1980. Selection and in vivo properties of lectin-attachment variants of malignant murine lymphosarcoma cell lines. JNCI 64:1241–1249.
Siciliano, M. J., B. F. White, and R. M. Humphrey. 1983. Electrophoretically detectable mutations induced in CHO cells by varying doses of ultraviolet radiation. Mutat. Res. 107:167–176.
Siminovitch, L. 1976. On the nature of heritable variation in cultured somatic cells. Cell 7:1–11.
Stackpole, C. W. 1981. Distinct lung colonizing and lung metastasizing cell populations in B16 mouse melanoma. Nature 289:798–800.
Stanley, P. 1981. Selection of specific wheat germ agglutinin-resistant (WGA^R) phenotypes from Chinese hamster ovary cell populations containing numerous Lec^R genotypes. Mol. Cell. Biol. 1:687–696.
Stanley, P., V. Caillibot, and L. Siminovitch. 1975a. Stable alterations at the cell membrane of Chinese hamster ovary cells resistant to the cytotoxicity of phytohemagglutinin. Somatic Cell Genet. 1:3–26.
Stanley, P., V. Caillibot, and L. Siminovitch. 1975b. Selection and characterization of eight phenotypically distinct lines of lectin-resistant Chinese hamster ovary cells. Cell 6:121–128.
Stanley, P., and L. Siminovitch. 1977. Complementation between mutants of CHO cells resistant to a variety of plant lectins. Somatic Cell Genet. 3:391–405.
Stanbridge, E. J., C. J. Der, C.-J. Doersen, R. Y. Nishimi, D. M. Peehl, B. E. Weissman, and J. E. Wilkinson. 1982. Human cell hybrids: Analysis of transformation and tumorigenicity. Science 215:252–259.
Sweeney, F. L., J. Pot-Deprun, M.-F. Poupon, and I. Chouroulinkov. 1982. Heterogeneity of the growth and metastatic behavior of cloned cell lines derived from a primary rhabdomyosarcoma. Cancer Res. 42:3776–3782.
Tao, T. W., and M. M. Burger. 1977. Non-metastasizing variants selected from metastasizing melanoma cells. Nature 270:437–438.
Talmadge, J. E., S. R. Wolman, and I. J. Fidler. 1982. Evidence for the clonal origin of spontaneous metastases. Science 217:361–363.
Taylor, S. M., and P. A. Jones. 1979. Multiple new phenotypes induced in $10T^{1/2}$ and 3TC cells treated with 5-azacytidine. Cell 17:771–779.
Tischfield, J. A., J. J. Trill, Y. I. Lee, K. Coy, and M. W. Taylor. 1982. Genetic instability at the adenine phosphoribosyltransferase locus in mouse L cells. Mol. Cell. Biol. 2:250–257.
Trowbridge, I. S., and R. Hyman. 1978. Expression of Thy-1 glycoprotein on lectin-resistant lymphoma cell lines. Eur. J. Immunol. 8:716–723.
Warner, T. F. C. S. 1975. Cell hybridization: An explanation for the phenotypic diversity of certain tumours. Medical Hypothesis 1:51–56.
Wiener, F., E. M. Fenyo, and G. Klein. 1974. Tumor-host cell hybrids in radiochimeras. Proc. Natl. Acad. Sci. USA 71:148–152.
Wiener, F., E. M. Fenyo, G. Klein, and A. J. S. Davies. 1976. Tumor-host cell hybrids in radiochimeras reconstituted with bone marrow and thymus grafts. Somatic Cell Genet. 2:81–92.
Wiener, F., E. M. Fenyo, and G. Klein. 1972. Fusion of tumour cells with host cells. Nature 238:155–159.
Wilson, V. L., and P. A. Jones. 1983. Inhibition of DNA methylation by chemical carcinogens in vitro. Cell 32:239–246.
Yogeeswaran, G., A. Gronberg, M. Hansson, T. Dalianis, R. Kiessling, and R. M. Welsh. 1981. Correlation of glycosphingolipids and sialic acid in YAC-1 lymphoma variants with their sensitivity to natural killer-cell-mediated lysis. Int. J. Cancer 28:517–526.
Yogeeswaran, G., B. S. Stein, and H. Sebastian. 1978. Altered cell surface organization of gangliosides and sialylglycoproteins of mouse metastatic melanoma variant lines selected in vivo for enhanced lung implantation. Cancer Res. 38:1336–1344.
Yogeeswaran, G., and P. L. Salk. 1981. Metastatic potential is positively correlated with cell surface sialylation of cultured murine tumor cell lines. Science 212:1514–1516.

Cancer Invasion and Metastasis: Biologic and Therapeutic Aspects edited by Garth L. Nicolson and Luka Milas. Raven Press, New York © 1984.

Phenotypic and Genotypic Differences Between High- and Low-Metastatic Related Tumor Lines and the Problem of Tumor Progression and Variant Generation

Volker Schirrmacher, Rule Dzarlieva,* Peter Altevogt, Mina Fogel, Catherine A. Waller, James W. Dennis, Georg F. Springer,† Israel Vlodavsky,‡ Michael Kramer, and Rachanee Cheingsong-Popov

*Institut für Immunologie und Genetik and *Institut für Biochemie, Deutsches Krebsforschungszentrum, D-6900 Heidelberg, West Germany, †Evanston Hospital, Northwestern University, Evanston, Illinois, and ‡Department of Radiation and Clinical Oncology, The Hebrew University, Hadassah School of Medicine, Jerusalem, Israel.*

The first contact of a cell with its microenvironment is exerted at the external plasma membrane. In malignant transformed cells, the plasma membrane is involved in physiological changes that are linked to the malignant state and lead to changes in growth, cell division, cell-cell communication, and cell motility. Contacts of tumor cells with cells of the host's immune defense system also take place at the plasma membrane. Tumor cells that can grow in spite of an immunological attack seem to have plasma membranes that are altered in such a way as to allow escape from immune destruction. The tumor cell's plasma membrane is thus an important object of tumor biology and also a promising target in cancer therapy.

Research in cancer metastasis has provided ample evidence for heterogeneity in metastatic capacity of individual cells of a tumor (for review, see Fidler et al. 1978). This evidence was made possible by isolating single cells, growing them up to clones, transplanting them into appropriate hosts, and testing them for tumorigenicity and ability to metastasize. High-metastatic cells have been described as subpopulations of a growing tumor that differ from low-metastatic cells of the same tumor in particular cell surface properties (Nicolson 1982). Relatively little is known, however, about which changes might have general importance for acquisition of malignant potential and what is the molecular and genetic basis for such changes (Schirrmacher 1980).

In this report, we summarize our results on cell surface differences between high- and low-metastatic tumor cell lines from one particular animal tumor system. These phenotypic differences are complemented by genotypic differences that were also observed within these cells. The data are discussed in the context of their possible relevance for mechanisms of cancer metastasis.

Most experimental studies in cancer metastasis compare particular tumor cells and their different variants. Tumor variants have been isolated, for instance, by cloning in vitro (Kripke et al. 1978), by selecting for organ specificity (Nicolson and Winkelhake 1975), for resistance to plant lectins (Burger 1980, Kerbel et al. 1982), or for immunoresistance (Fidler et al. 1976). More recently, other procedures such as the fusion of vesicles (Poste and Nicolson 1980) or of complete normal cells (De Baetselier et al. 1981) have also been used to analyze cell surface properties important in metastasis.

Our approach was to study variants that arose naturally from cells that had not been mutagenized or otherwise interfered with. For these studies we selected the Eb/ESb tumor lines because they fulfill certain prerequisites of a model system for cancer metastasis (Schirrmacher et al. 1979b). The two transplantable tumor lines are sublines from a murine T-cell lymphoma that was induced originally by methylcholanthrene A in a DBA/2 mouse (Parr 1972). Eb is the original low-metastatic parental line and ESb a spontaneous variant thereof that is highly metastatic. Fewer than 10 cells of the metastatic variant transplanted s.c. into a normal DBA/2 mouse can grow, metastasize, and kill the host within a few weeks (Schirrmacher et al. 1979b). The tumor system thus is syngeneic, can be studied in the inbred strain of origin, and allows comparison of closely related cell lines that differ greatly in metastatic capacity. In several respects the tumor lines show similarities to extranodal lymphoma in human beings (Johnson et al. 1975).

SPONTANEOUS TUMOR CELL VARIANTS IN THE EB/ESB SYSTEM

The chronological history of the Eb/ESb tumor system is depicted in Figure 1. A number of differences were observed in general properties between Eb/

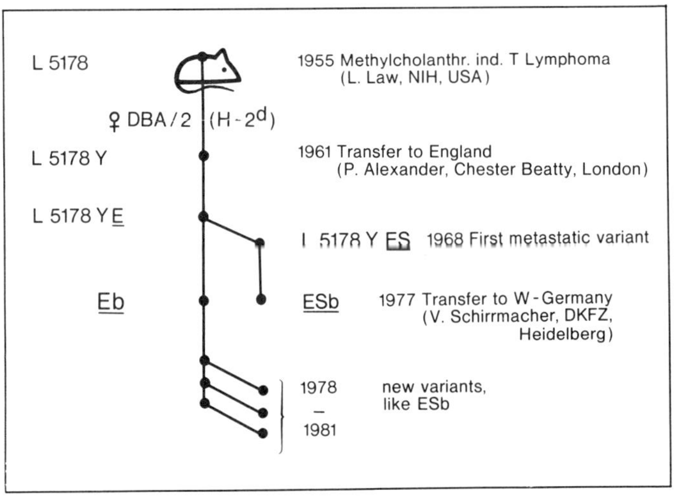

FIG. 1. Chronological history of the Eb/ESb tumor system.

ESb tumor cells, some of which will be discussed below. Before considering them, however, we want to discuss the important question of the genetic relationship between these two lines, because it could be argued that after so many years of separation the tumor lines could have diverged to such an extent that they could no longer be considered related. Apart from the history, we have other indications for the close relationship between Eb and ESb type cells: (1) the transition from Eb to ESb that was first observed in 1968 in England (Parr 1972) could be reproduced under similar conditions (successive i.p. transplantation) or by immunoselection experiments in our laboratory (Schirrmacher and Bosslet 1980). Eb/ESb mixing experiments revealed that the standard Eb cell line did not contain ESb type cells, at least not at a detectable level, which was less than one in 10^5 (Schirrmacher and Bosslet 1980). (2) Further support for a relationship between Eb and ESb came from a karyotype analysis employing the G-banding technique (Dzarlieva et al. 1982). It revealed that particular chromosomal abnormalities were constantly maintained in all metaphases from either Eb or ESb type cells. We could conclude from the cytogenetic analysis that the two tumor lines were genetically related, with the metastatic variant ESb representing a later form of tumor progression.

Figure 2 lists the different selection procedures employed. The first procedure—successive transfer of Eb cells in ascites form, which selected for eventual outgrowth of metastatic ESb type variant cells—has already been mentioned.

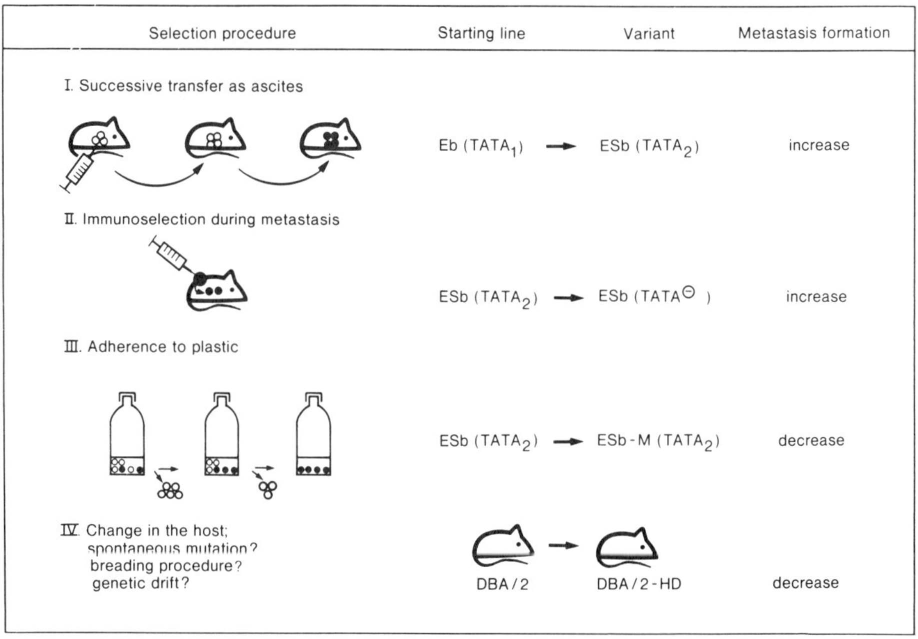

FIG. 2. Origin of spontaneous variants from the tumor and the host.

The second selection procedure—immunoselection during metastasis from a s.c. site—resulted in the appearance of high-metastatic immune escape variants from ESb. The third procedure—in vitro selection for increased adhesiveness to plastic—led to the isolation of a plastic-adherent ESb variant (ESb-M) with greatly decreased metastatic capacity (Fogel et al. 1983).

Metastasis formation was influenced not only by changes in the properties of the tumor cells but also by changes in properties of the host. Among DBA/2 strains from many different sources one was found that showed increased resistance to ESb metastases (Schirrmacher et al. 1982, Schirrmacher 1981).

Phenotypic Differences

Cell Surface Antigens

Tumor-associated transplantation antigens

The expression of tumor-associated transplantation antigens (TATA) by the different tumor variants is also indicated in Figure 2. Three phenotypes could be distinguished, namely $TATA_1$ for Eb cells, $TATA_2$ for ESb cells, and $TATA^-$ for the immunoresistant variant. These tumor antigens could be distinguished by in vivo immunization/protection experiments (Bosslet et al. 1979) and by typing with tumor-specific cytolytic T lymphocytes (CTL) (Schirrmacher et al. 1979a).

Anti-TATA CTL were used as typing reagents to investigate the stability or variability of TATA expression by cloned tumor cell lines. A clone-dependent variation in the sensitivity to anti-TATA CTL lysis was seen upon prolonged growth of individual clones in tissue culture (Schirrmacher and Bosslet 1982). Furthermore, TATA expression was highly variable in vivo during the process of metastasis formation from a s.c. site. Under these conditions, $TATA^+$ clones regularly gave rise to $TATA^-$ immune escape variants (Schirrmacher et al. 1979a).

Figure 3 illustrates the experimental protocol and overall results for the generation of immunoresistant variants during metastasis in vivo. The figure also shows the experimental evidence against the preexistence of these variants (Bosslet and Schirrmacher 1982), which was derived from an immunoselection experiment in vitro. In this part of the experiment, the twice-cloned ESb-Cl 18.1 cells were coincubated twice with a 500-fold excess of specific anti-ESb CTL for 4 h. A small number of surviving cells turned out to be still immunosensitive. When these cells were subcloned, all 17 subclones isolated were immunosensitive. In contrast, when the spleen-derived tumor variants from the same tumor line were subcloned, all 28 subclones tested were immunoresistant (Bosslet and Schirrmacher 1982). The implications of these findings are discussed in more detail elsewhere (Bosslet and Schirrmacher 1982).

The relative inefficiency of specific immunization procedures against ESb tu-

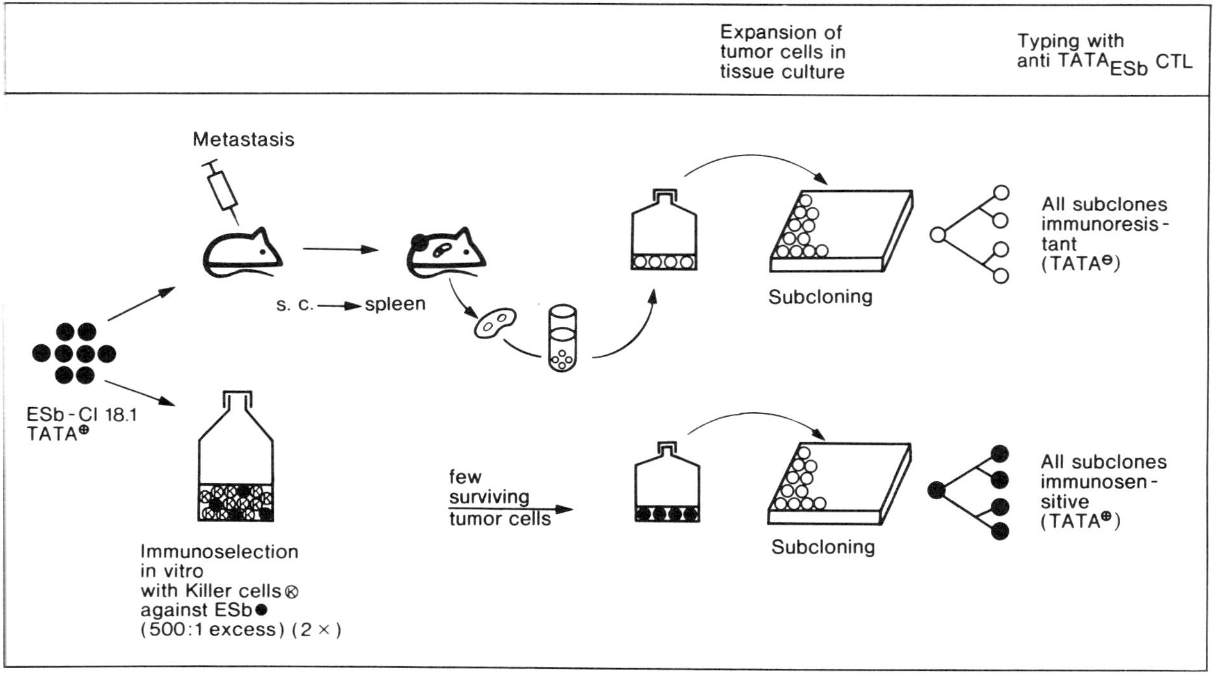

FIG. 3. Generation of immunoresistant $TATA^-$ variants during metastasis and evidence against preexistence of these variants. ●, ESb $TATA^+$ cells (immunosensitive); ○, ESb $TATA^-$ cells (immunoresistant).

mor cells (Bosslet et al. 1979, Bosslet and Schirrmacher 1981, 1982) was found to be due to the effective generation of TATA$^-$ variants by this highly malignant tumor. The possible genetic basis of the generation of such specifically immunoresistant variants will be discussed below.

C-type viral antigens (VA)

In spite of the evidence presented for the existence of TATA from in vivo immunization and in vitro CTL studies, we still do not know the physicochemical nature of these structures. The analysis of these structures would be facilitated if we were successful in our present efforts at raising monoclonal antibodies.

It has been suggested that tumor antigens from murine tumors may be virally related because murine tumor cells are notorious for harboring C-type viruses. Membrane-budding C-type particles were seen only very occasionally when we screened a great number of Eb and ESb cells on transmission electron micrographs. A cytoplasmic A-type virus was, however, found to be quite abundant, especially but not exclusively in ESb type cells (Schirrmacher et al. 1982). We do not believe that the A-type viruses, which are not expressed on the cell surface, or the occasionally found C-type viruses have anything to do with the TATA on the Eb/ESb tumor cells, because of the uniqueness of these TATA. Both the TATA$^+$ and the TATA$^-$ tumor target cells stained to a similar extent with a polyspecific antiserum against GP70 of C-type viruses and contained biochemically similar GP70 molecules.

Histocompatibility antigens (HA)

Both types of lymphoma cells, Eb and ESb, expressed H-2K^d and H-2D^d molecules on the cell surface. Quantitative absorption experiments and indirect immunofluorescence tests revealed that ESb type cells expressed more of the H-2 antigens than the Eb cells. Qualitative differences of the class 1 H-2 glycoproteins of Eb and ESb cells were seen after immune precipitation and analysis by two-dimensional gel electrophoresis. ESb H-2D^d antigens were found to be similar to those found on DBA/2 splenic ConA blasts and appeared to be more acidic than those of Eb cells. Pulse chase experiments revealed that the unglycosylated H-2D^d chains of Eb and ESb cells possessed very similar characteristics in sodium dodecyl sulfate–polyacrylamide gel electrophoresis (SDS-PAGE), while the processed forms differed (Altevogt et al. 1982b). This is direct evidence that prominent cell surface molecules of Eb and ESb cells are glycosylated in different ways (Schirrmacher et al. 1983).

Differentiation antigens

Further differences between Eb and ESb cells were found in the expression of Lyt differentiation antigens and of certain T-lymphoid cell surface glycoproteins. Thus, Eb cells typed as Thy 1^+, Lyt 1^-, Lyt $2{,}3^+$, Ly 6^+, whereas the highly metastasizing variant ESb typed as Thy 1^-, Lyt 1^+, Lyt $2{,}3^-$, Ly 6^- (Altevogt et al. 1982a). The plastic-adherent variant ESb-M, which lost its metastatic potential while maintaining its tumorigenicity (Fogel et al. 1983), had the same profile of differentiation antigens and tumor antigens as the ESb type cells.

Phenotypic differences between low- and high-metastatic tumor lines have also been observed in other tumor systems. The new observation from our studies, however, is that the changes seen in membrane glycoproteins could be identified and associated with changes in the expression of normal cell surface differentiation antigens. This finding was made possible because we investigated a tumor system of lymphoid origin, which allowed the use of well-defined typing reagents such as monoclonal antibodies against lymphoid differentiation antigens. Our results suggest that tumor progression involves changes in the cell's differentiation state.

Blood group–related antigens (T, Tn, M, N, and S-active substances)

The Thomsen-Friedenreich antigens T and Tn, which are derived from the MN blood group antigens, are clinically important structures because transformation of normal epithelium to carcinoma in man is linked in about 95% of the cases with exposure of these normally masked antigens on the outer surface of the cell membrane. T and Tn antigens also occur on human T-cell lymphomas and have been found to be conserved in all metastases (Springer et al. 1979). Furthermore, these structures are known to evoke both humoral and cell-mediated immune responses (Springer et al. 1980).

Tissue culture–derived tumor cells of both the Eb and ESb cell lines were found to absorb antibodies to M,N,T, and Tn blood group antigens (Springer et al. 1983b). Live ESb cells absorbed 25 to 55% more of a given antibody than did live Eb cells.

We previously showed that the high-metastatic ESb cells formed spontaneous rosettes with isolated syngeneic hepatocytes in vitro, while the low-metastatic parental line Eb cells did not (Schirrmacher et al. 1980). We attempted to inhibit competitively the adhesion of ESb cells to syngeneic hepatocytes with T antigen from healthy human red blood cells. T antigen and some of its carbohydrate-rich cleavage products were the most highly active inhibitors of rosette formation among several glycoproteins tested (Springer et al. 1983a). These results suggest a supportive role of T- and Tn-related structures in the malignant process.

Cell Surface Receptors

Receptors for hepatocyte lectins

Rosette formation between ESb cells and syngeneic hepatocytes was found to be mediated by a lectinlike receptor of the hepatocytes with specificity for galactosyl and N-acetylgalactosyl groups. Hepatic-binding proteins could be absorbed to and eluted from ESb cells but not from Eb cells. The immunosorbent purified hepatic-binding proteins consisted of polypeptides of molecular weights in the range of 55,000 and 110,000 (Cheingsong-Popov et al. 1983). About 10 different glycoproteins of ESb cells served as cell surface receptors for these proteins. On Eb cells, these receptors were blocked by sialic acid and could be exposed only after neuraminidase treatment (Cheingsong-Popov et al. 1983).

Receptors for plant lectins

Cell surface carbohydrate composition was studied by staining the cells with FITC-conjugated lectins and analysis by flow cytofluorography. The low-metastatic tumor lines (Eb and ESb-M) expressed receptor sites for lectins with GalNAc-Gal specificity (soybean agglutinin and *Vicia villosa* (VV)). In contrast, the high-metastatic lines (ESb) and organ-derived revertants from ESb-M, called ESb-MR, did not express such receptor sites unless the cells were pretreated with neuraminidase. The metastatic lines thus had their GalNAc-specific lectin-binding sites blocked by sialic acid (Altevogt et al., in press). Similar and even more striking differences were seen with the same lectins in a different tumor system, MDAY-D2/MDW40, consisting also of high- and low-metastatic, related tumor lines (Kerbel et al. 1982). High-metastatic ESb cells showed a better expression of receptor sites for peanut agglutinin, which recognizes terminal

TABLE 1. *Changes in metastatic capacity associated with changes in expression of specific lectin-binding sites*

Tumor line*	Metastatic capacity	Binding of lectins			
		SBA†	VV†	PNA‡	HBP‡
Eb	Low	+	+	−	−
ESb	High	↓	↓	↑	↑
ESb-M	Low	↑	↑	ND	ND
ESb-MR§	High	↓	ND	ND	ND
MDAY-D2	High	−	−	ND	+
MDW4O	Low	↑↑	↑↑	ND	ND
MDW4OM1‖	High	↓↓	↓↓	ND	ND

* For further details see Schirrmacher et al. 1983.
† Carbohydrate specificity: D-GalNAc- α 1–3 D Gal →.
‡ Carbohydrate specificity: D-Gal-β1-3-D GalNAc →.
§ Organ-derived revertants from the plastic-adherent ESb-M.
‖ Organ-derived revertant from the wheat germ agglutinin–resistant variant MDW4O.
+ and − indicate positive or negative staining; ND = not done; arrows indicate direction of change (↑ increase, ↓ decrease).
SBA, soybean agglutinin; VV, *Vicia villosa;* PNA, peanut agglutinin; HBP, hepatic-binding protein.

galactosyl groups and has a specificity similar to the T antigen (D-Gal-1-3-D-GalNAc). Peanut agglutinin receptor sites were again blocked by sialic acid on the surface of the low-metastatic cells. Similar structures were recognized on ESb cells by the hepatic-binding protein. These findings are summarized in Table 1 and Figure 4.

Cell surface sialic acid

Since cell surface receptors for syngeneic hepatocytes or for plant lectins depended on the presence of sialic acid, we investigated the total amount of neuraminidase-accessible sialic acid on the cell surface of Eb, ESb, and ESb-M cells. All cell lines had about the same amount on the cell surface (Schirrmacher et al. 1983). Since the total amount of neuraminidase-accessible sialic acid was similar and yet specific lectin-binding sites were differently sialylated, we suggested that the effects of sialic acid are cell surface site specific (Schirr-

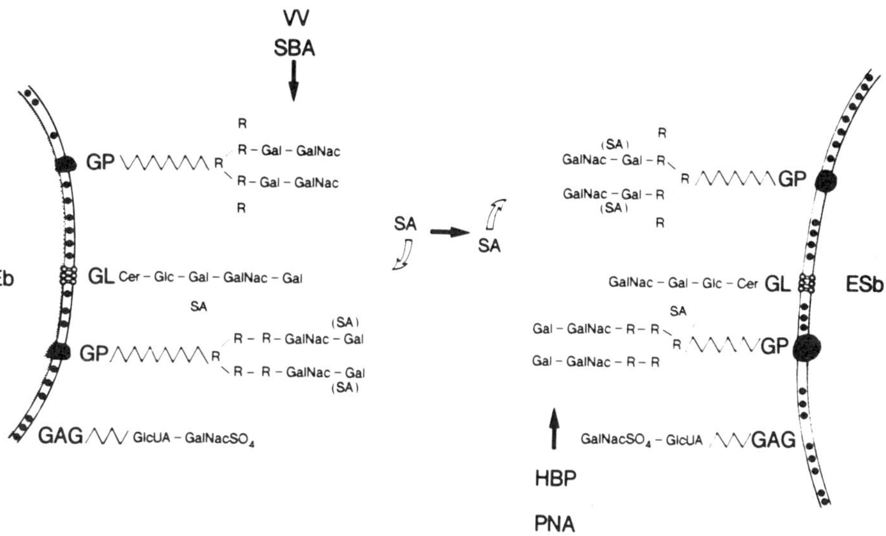

FIG. 4. Model showing the expression of terminal carbohydrates on cell surface glycoconjugates of a low-metastatic (left, Eb) and a high-metastatic (right, ESb) tumor line. Binding sites for the lectins *Vicia villosa* (VV), soybean agglutinin (SBA), and peanut agglutinin (PNA) and for the hepatic-binding protein (HBP) are indicated. These binding sites are suggested to be located on carbohydrate side chains of glycoproteins whose exact identity is not known. The respective side chains may contain other arbitrary sugar residues (R). The low-metastatic cells express receptor sites for SBA and VV that are sialylated on the high-metastatic cells. Conversely, the latter express receptor sites for HBP and PNA that are sialylated on the low-metastatic cells. The exact positioning (terminal or subterminal) or sialic acid (SA) on these receptor sites is not known. The preferential specificity of the cells' sialyl transferases is indicated by the open arrow. GP = glycoproteins; GL = glycolipids (only gangliosides are shown; Eb cells express predominantly GM1 and ESb cells GM2); GAG = glycosaminoglycans (only one type (chondroitin sulfate) is shown); Cer = ceramid; Gal = galactose; GalNAc = N-acetylgalactosamine; Glc = glucose; GlcUA = glucuronic acid.

macher et al. 1983, Altevogt et al., in press). This new concept, which we discussed in more detail in a recent review (Schirrmacher et al. 1983), is illustrated in Figure 4. It suggests: (1) Low- and high-metastatic cells show different profiles of specific lectin receptor sites and thus of terminal carbohydrates. (2) A change in the specificity or in the relative activities of sialyl transferases could have a dual effect on the expression of such receptor sites, masking some sites while exposing others. (3) The expression of receptor sites for specific cell adhesion are likely to be strictly regulated. In this concept we underline the importance of the site-specific positioning of sialic acid and give less weight to the cell's total amount of sialic acid or its overall net charge, factors previously given the greater weight.

Receptors for fibronectin, collagen type IV, and laminin

Attachment of cells to substrate containing fibronectin, laminin, or collagens has been shown to influence cell proliferation, differentiation, and migration, aspects of cellular behavior known to be altered by malignant transformation. In two tumor systems studied, we observed that high-metastatic cells showed a reduced attachment to collagen type IV and fibronectin when compared with related low-metastatic lines, while their attachment capability to laminin appeared unchanged. Furthermore, neuraminidase treatment of the metastatic tumor cells enhanced their attachment to collagen type IV and fibronectin, but not to laminin (Dennis et al. 1982). These results are consistent with the proposal that cell attachment to certain substrates such as fibronectin and collagen type IV requires expression of carbohydrate-binding sites, which can be regulated and blocked by sialic acid.

Receptors for Semliki Forest virus

We previously reported that major histocompatibility antigens of the mouse (H-2K and D molecules) and of man (HLA-A, HLA-B) could directly interact with viruses such as Semliki Forest virus (SFV) (Helenius et al. 1978). This virus has a wide host cell range and has probably adapted to the recognition of class 1 major histocompatibility antigens as a very ubiquitous cell surface glycoprotein. In this context it was surprising to find that metastatic tumor cell variants showed an increased resistance to infection by this particular virus. SFV much less easily infected and destroyed the metastatic tumor line ESb than the closely related parental line Eb. Similar results were obtained with a clonal phenotypic shift variant (Eb → ESb) and with the unrelated high-metastatic DBA/2 tumor line MDAY-D2 (Barz et al. 1981).

A cocapping experiment performed with the parental tumor line Eb clearly demonstrated selectivity of the binding of SFV to H-2 molecules, in particular to H-2D^d. Since we showed before that the glycosylated form of this molecule was different for Eb and ESb cells, it is possible that the difference in susceptibility to SFV is due to a difference in the carbohydrate side chains of the H-2 molecules of the high- and low-metastatic tumor lines.

Receptors for IgG immunoglobulin (Fcγ receptors)

The high-metastatic tumor lines from both model systems studied, ESb and MDAY-D2, contained a high percentage of Fcγ receptor-positive cells as detected in a rosette assay with IgG antibody-coated erythrocytes (EA). In contrast, the low-metastatic parental line Eb contained only a low percentage of EA rosette-forming cells.

"Soluble" Fc receptors were detectable by their ability to bind to EA and to block rosette formation. They were present in fluids from tumor-bearing animals such as serum and cell-free ascites (Schirrmacher and Jacobs 1979). This suggests that these receptors are not only expressed on the cell surface but are shed into the microenvironment.

In connection with metastasis, the acquisition of Fc receptors by tumor cells might have selective advantage for one of several reasons: (1) It would enable the cells to bind immune complexes; these could stimulate tumor growth, mask tumor-specific antigens, or lead to changes in the tumor cell traffic and enhanced sequestration in the liver. (2) A release of "soluble" Fc receptors into body fluids might have important implications in the regulation of immune responsiveness. For instance, a suppressive activity of Fc receptors produced by L5178Y tumor cells on the humoral immune response in vitro has been demonstrated (Neauport-Sautes and Fridman 1977).

Enzymatic Activities

Membrane-bound enzymes

Plasma membranes were prepared from ascites tumor cells by nitrogen cavitation, differential centrifugation to remove nuclei, mitochondria, and lysosomes, and equilibrium centrifugation in a 35% sucrose gradient. The contamination of this purified plasma membrane preparation by cytoplasmic components was low as assessed by marker enzyme analysis (Barz et al., submitted for publication).

Table 2 displays the assessed activities of membrane-bound enzymes from Eb and ESb plasma membrane preparations. As can be seen, the individual enzyme activities varied considerably. The enzyme activities of the two tumor lines were, however, quite similar. This was surprising in view of the many differences between Eb and ESb cells reported before.

Glycosyl transferases

Sialyl transferase activities were tested using asialofetuin as acceptor glycoprotein (Table 3). They turned out to be only half as active in ESb cells as in Eb

TABLE 2. *Plasma membrane-bound enzymes in Eb/ESb tumor cells*

Enzyme	Enzyme activity* Eb	ESb
5′Nucleotidase, EC 3.1.3.5.	535	555
Alkaline phosphatase, EC 3.1.3.1.	1079	1077
γ-Glutamyltransferase, EC 2.3.2.2.	8.1	10.8
ATPase (total), EC 3.6.1.3.	139	114
Lysolecithinacyl		
-transferase: EC 2.3.1.2.3.		
-arachidonoyl	2.9	2.8
-oleyl	1.2	0.9

* nmol per mg protein per min.

TABLE 3. *Glycosyl transferase activities of Eb/ESb tumor cells*

Enzyme	Acceptor	Relative activity* ESb:Eb
Sialyl transferase	Asialofetuin	0.54
Galactosyl transferase	Asialoagalactofetuin	1.44
Fucosyl transferase A	Asialofetuin	0.80
Fucosyl transferase B	Asialoagalactofetuin	0.74
N-Ac-glucosaminyl transferase 1	Ovalbumin	0.20
N-Ac-glucosamyl transferase 2	Ribonuclease A	0.23

* For details see Schirrmacher et al. 1983.

cells. Conversely, galactosyl transferases tested in a similar way were nearly twice as active in ESb cells as in Eb cells. Asialofetuin expresses numerous terminal Gal residues and thus can be assumed to test selectively for galactosyl-specific sialyl transferases. The findings of higher galactosyl-specific sialyl transferase activity in Eb cells and of a higher galactosyl transferase activity in ESb type cells could account for the better expression on these cells of determinants recognized by peanut agglutinin or by the hepatocytes (see Figure 4).

Fucosyl transferases A and B were only slightly less active in ESb than in Eb cells. ESb cells, however, had strongly reduced activities of N-acetylglucosaminyl transferases 1 and 2. Since N-acetylglucosaminyl transferase 1 controls the whole carbohydrate side-chain elongation process, these results might indicate a less complete biosynthesis of carbohydrate side chains in ESb than in Eb cells.

In conclusion, the analysis of glycosyl transferase activities of Eb and ESb cells has revealed a number of differences (Altevogt et al., in press). Although much more has to be learned about these enzymes—their fine specificity, localization, and regulation—these results point toward an important role for cell surface carbohydrates in cancer metastasis (Schirrmacher et al. 1983).

Enzymes degrading the basal lamina of blood vessels

A common and most important route for the dissemination of neoplastic cells within the body involves invasion and penetration of tumor cells into blood vessels and lymphatics. The interaction of metastatic and nonmetastatic tumor cells with the vascular endothelium and its underlying basal lamina has been studied in vitro. Two different types of degradative enzymes were detected and investigated biochemically, namely a trypsinlike serine protease with plasminogen activator activity and an endoglycosidase. The protease of ESb type cells was found to be shed from these cells in serum-free medium and has been partially purified. In contrast to most lysosomal enzymes, which are most effective in acidic conditions, this enzyme has a pH optimum of 8.0. The enzyme degrades ^{125}I-labeled extracellular matrix produced by blood vessel endothelial cells in vitro (Kramer et al. 1983).

The endoglycosidaselike activity was detected when the extracellular matrix was metabolically labeled with $Na_2\,[^{35}S]O_4$, which is incorporated into sulfated glycosaminoglycans. After coincubation with the tumor cells, the released labeled degradation products were analyzed by gel filtration. More than 90% of the labeled material released upon incubation of ESb cells with the ECM was in the form of low-molecular-weight, heparin sulphate–containing fragments. In contrast, coincubation with the low-metastatic Eb cells led to a release of only high molecular weight glycosaminoglycan components. The same high- and low-molecular-weight degradation products were obtained by incubation of the extracellular matrix with a serum-free medium conditioned by the low (Eb) and high (ESb) metastatic sublines, respectively, indicating that the enzyme activities were released by the tumor cells into the culture supernatants (Vlodavsky et al., submitted for publication).

While the protease activity was expressed by both Eb and ESb cells, the endoglycosidaselike activity was expressed only by the metastatic variant ESb. Further experiments suggested a sequential degradation of the subendothelial extracellular matrix by attack of the protease followed by the endoglycosidaselike enzyme. The significance of these two enzymes for the whole process of cancer invasion and extravasation of blood vessels is not known yet and requires further experimentation.

Plasma Membrane Proteins

An important issue of tumor variant generation is the distinction between phenotypic and genotypic variants. Whereas the former can arise as a result of epigenetic changes, the latter must involve changes in gene expression. All the phenotypic differences that we have described so far do not allow a distinction between genetic or epigenetic phenomena. Many of the differences seen could be due to differences in the glycosylation of cell surface glycoproteins, glycolipids, or glycosaminoglycans. Glycosylation differences have in fact been identified on these tumor variants. For instance, defined lymphoid differentiation antigens such as the T200 antigen and the H-2 histocompatibility antigens of Eb and ESb cells were found to differ in their glycosylation (Altevogt et al. 1982b).

In order to find out whether or not genetic changes have occurred during progression in our tumor system, we analyzed the composition of total plasma membrane proteins. For this purpose a procedure was worked out that allowed the purification of mouse plasma membrane proteins from biosynthetically labeled cells. When [^{35}S]methionine-labeled proteins of such plasma membrane preparations from cloned Eb and ESb cells were compared by two-dimensional gel electrophoresis, it was found that the highly metastatic variant ESb had acquired about 50 new protein spots, which were not found on the two-dimensional gel maps of the parental Eb cells. A major proportion of these spots were also found on maps derived from syngeneic splenic ConA blasts. This indicated that many of the newly expressed membrane proteins were possibly differentiation related and not tumor cell specific (Altevogt and Schirrmacher, submitted for publication).

Although the carbohydrate moieties of a given membrane protein can have a strong influence on its molecular weight and electrophoretic mobility, we consider it unlikely that the noted differences in gel spots between Eb and ESb were the result of altered glycosylation of otherwise similar membrane proteins. We rather suggest that the differences in the composition of total membrane proteins represent changes in the gene activation state between the two cell types. The possible relationships between the gene activation state of these cell lines and their differentiation state has been discussed in more detail elsewhere (Schirrmacher 1981).

Genotypic Differences

While the 50 new plasma membrane proteins on ESb cells as compared to Eb cells suggest that new genes are activated or derepressed in the metastatic variant, we sought direct evidence for genetic changes within these cells. We therefore recently performed a detailed cytogenetic comparison between the parental line Eb, its spontaneous TATA$^+$ metastatic variant ESb, and the TATA$^-$ immunoresistant variant. These studies demonstrated chromosomal relationships between the cell lines as well as individual characteristics and elucidated cytogenetic changes associated with the formation of tumor variants during tumor progression (Dzarlieva et al. 1982).

All three cell lines were characterized by a near-diploid chromosome count and by some common chromosomal markers derived from chromosomes no. 6, 13, and 16. Large-scale chromosomal rearrangements resulted in the formation of 8 marker chromosomes in Eb cells, 16 in ESb TATA$^+$ cells, and 18 in ESb TATA$^-$ cells. Table 4 shows the distribution of these marker chromosomes in the three cell lines. Nine marker chromosomes were identical in the two ESb sublines. In spite of their chromosomal relationships, each line had some distinct

TABLE 4. *Cytogenetic characteristics of Eb, ESb TATA⁺ and ESb TATA⁻ tumor lines*

		Marker chromosomes†			
Cell type	Modal chromosome number (range)*	Total number/ metaphase	Common in 1+3	Common in 2+3	Distinct
Eb	41(40–43)	8	M:3,7,16[d]		M:1,2,4,5,8
ESb $TATA^+$	40(39–42)	16	M′:4,8,16[d]	M′:1,3,5–8,10–13	M′:2,9
ESb $TATA^-$	39(37–40)	18	M″:4,9,16[d]	M″:1,3,6–9,10–13	M″:2,5,14

* Analysis performed from 20 to 25 G-banded metaphases.

† Present in 100% of the metaphases; marker chromosomes of Eb cells are designated as M1-M8; of ESb $TATA^+$ cells as M′1-M′16 and of ESb $TATA^-$ cells as M″1-M″18.

For characteristics and details see Dzarlieva et al. 1982.

characteristics. The cytogenetic characteristics were sufficient to delineate the evolutionary relationship between the lines as Eb → ESb $TATA^+$ → ESb $TATA^-$.

Chromosome 15 was trisomic in Eb cells, monosomic in ESb $TATA^+$ cells, and hardly detectable in ESb $TATA^-$ cells. Chromosome no. 15 seems to be particularly prominent in tumorigenesis and has recently been shown to carry the myconcogene. In view of this, it was rather surprising to see that progression in the Eb/ESb system seemed to be associated with a decrease rather than with an increase in chromosomal material derived from chromosome no. 15.

The Ig heavy chain gene–carrying region of both no. 12 chromosomes was found in translocation with a number of other chromosomes. These were nos. 5, 13, and 14 in Eb cells and nos. 1 and 17 in ESb cells. These results could indicate the translocation of strong promoter sequences from the Ig heavy chain genes to other chromosomes, thus leading to the activation of other previously silent genes. This change could be an important factor in tumor progression.

An illustrative example of genotypic and phenotypic differences arising during tumor progression is the generation of immunoresistant $TATA^-$ tumor variants. As mentioned before, these variants arose at a high frequency and reproducibility in tumor bearing or tumor immune mice (Bosslet and Schirrmacher 1982). Such variants arose even from carefully cloned ESb $TATA^+$ cell lines during metastasis from a local s.c. inoculation site to the spleen. ESb $TATA^+$ and $TATA^-$ cells were found to carry the same chromosomal abnormalities involving the two homologous no. 12 chromosomes. There were, however, several cytogenetic differences between these lines consisting of amplifications and deletions.

Recent observations indicated that highly metastatic tumor cells have an increased ability to generate tumor cell variants (Cifone and Fidler 1981, Dennis et al. 1981). This could explain the phenomenon of recurrence of tumor growth and metastasis in patients who underwent radio- or chemotherapy. Such growing cells are likely to represent variants resistant to the drug or the radiation used.

Our cytogenetic studies support and extend previous findings about the significance of certain chromosomes in murine malignancies, in particular nos. 15

Characteristic	Eb —Tumor Progression→ ESb	Comments
A. Chromosomes 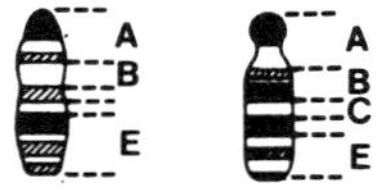	Increase of degeneration Breakage, translocations, losses or duplications in certain chromosomes	Support of Nowell's hypoth.
B. Cell surface carbohydrates 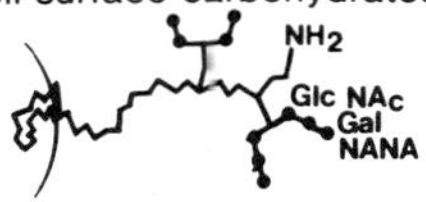	Changes in lectin binding characteristics Increase in binding to hepatocytes Increase in resistance to infection by Semliki-Forest-Virus, which binds to H-2 molecules	
C. Cell surface differentiation antigens 	Phenotypic change from: Thy 1^+, Ly 1^-, Ly $2,3^+$ to Thy 1^-, Ly 1^+, Ly $2,3^-$	Change in differentiation state
D. Microvilli and Motility 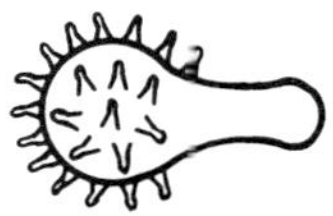	Increase in microvilli and shedding Increase in cell motility	
E. Invasive capacity 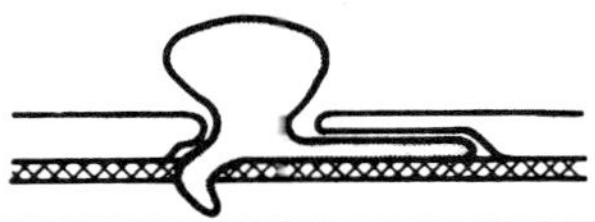	Increased binding and invasion into lung tissue Increased invasion into embryonic brain aggregates Increased ability to penetrate endothelial cell monolayer Increased ability to degrade endothelial extracellular matrix	

FIG. 5. Differences between the parental line Eb and its high-metastatic variant ESb.

and 12. Of relevance for tumor progression in general may be the following observations from this system: (1) numerical and structural chromosomal aberrations seem to be a basis and possibly a prerequisite for the generation of cellular variants; (2) in vivo tumor growth and metastasis possibly selects from these variants only those that have the proper malignant phenotype; (3) variants with the metastatic phenotype show involvement of some distinct chromosomes and not of others; (4) the more malignant cells show a higher number of chromosome breakages and reunions (translocations) resulting in new marker chromosomes; (5) tumor progression has a tendency to monosomies (full or partial) involving an ever-increasing proportion of the cells (Dzarlieva et al. 1982).

SUMMARY AND CONCLUSIONS

We have described a number of phenotypic and genotypic differences between defined tumor sublines from the Eb/ESb model system that differ greatly in metastatic capacity. Some of these differences are summarized in Figure 5. It can be seen that the differences are both structural and functional. They include differences in the glycosylation of membrane glycoproteins as well as differences in total membrane protein composition. The functional differences refer particularly to enzymatic activities, cell motility, and invasive capacity. In addition, a change in membrane fluidity and membrane dynamics was seen when we investigated membrane vesicles shed spontaneously from these tumor lines. ESb type cells were found to shed about three times as much membrane material as the low-metastatic, Eb cells. Since such vesicles carried degradative enzyme activity, they could play a role in the invasion process. The vesicles also carried TATA and thus could also play a role in preventing immunological attack against these tumor cells.

Another immunological escape mechanism was found to be based on the ability of the high-metastatic cells to generate immunoresistant variants that no longer expressed the respective TATA. A cytogenetic comparison of such immunoresistant variants with the TATA^{+} line revealed several chromosomal changes. The contribution of chromosomal rearrangements to the ability of malignant cells to generate variants was discussed.

REFERENCES

Altevogt, P., M. Fogel, R. Cheingsong-Popov, J. Dennis, and V. Schirrmacher. Related high and low metastatic tumor lines show different patterns of lectin binding and cell surface sialylation. Cancer Res. (in press).

Altevogt, P., J. T. Kurnick, A. K. Kimura, K. Bosslet, and V. Schirrmacher. 1982a. Different expression of Lyt differentiation antigens and cell surface glycoproteins by a murine T lymphoma line and its high metastatic variant. Eur. J. Immunol. 18:300–307.

Altevogt, P., P. Robinson, K. Bosslet, R. Cheingsong-Popov, and V. Schirrmacher. 1982b. Phenotypic differences between primary and metastasizing tumor cells in a T lymphoma model system of DBA/2 mice, *in* Tumour Progression and Markers, Proceedings of the VI Meeting of EACR, 1981. Kugler, Amsterdam, pp. 171–181.

Barz, D., K. Bosslet, and V. Schirrmacher. 1981. Metastatic tumor cell variants with increased resistance to infection by Semliki-Forest-virus. J. Immunol. 127:951–954.

Bosslet, K., and V. Schirrmacher. 1981. Escape of metastasizing clonal tumor cell variants from tumor-specific cytolytic T lymphocytes. J. Exp. Med. 154:557–562.

Bosslet, K., and V. Schirrmacher. 1982. High-frequency generation of new immunoresistant tumor variants during metastasis of a cloned murine tumor line (ESb). Int. J. Cancer 29:195–202.

Bosslet, K., V. Schirrmacher, and G. Shantz. 1979. Tumor metastases and cell-mediated immunity in a model system in DBA/2 mice. VI. Similar specificity patterns of protective anti-tumor immunity in vivo and of cytolytic T cells in vitro. Int. J. Cancer 24:303–313.

Burger, M. M. 1980. The cell surface and metastasis, *in* Biology of the Cancer Cell. Kugler, Amsterdam, pp. 193–208.

Cheinsong-Popov, R., P. Robinson, P. Altevogt, V. Schirrmacher. 1983. A mouse hepatocyte carbohydrate-specific receptor and its interaction with liver-metastasizing tumor cells. Int. J. Cancer 32:359–366.

Cifone, M., and I. J. Fidler. 1981. Increasing metastatic potential is associated with increasing genetic instability of clones isolated from murine neoplasms. Proc. Natl. Acad. Sci. USA 78:6949–6952.

De Baetselier, P., E. Gorelik, Z. Eshhar, Y. Ron, S. Katzav, M. Feldman, and S. Segal. 1981. Hybridization between plasmacytoma cells and B lymphocytes confers metastatic properties on a nonmetastatic tumor. JNCI 67:1079–1087.

Dennis, J., T. Donaghue, M. Florian, and R. S. Kerbel. 1981. Apparent reversion of stable in vitro genetic markers detected in tumor cells from spontaneous metastases. Nature 292:242–245.

Dennis, J., C. Waller, R. Timpl, and V. Schirrmacher. 1982. Surface sialic acid reduces attachment of metastatic tumour cells to collagen and fibronectin. Nature 300:274–276.

Dzarlieva, S., V. Schirrmacher, and N. Fusenig. 1982. Cytogenetic changes during tumor progression towards invasion, metastasis and immune escape in the Eb/ESb model system. Int. J. Cancer 30:633–642.

Fidler, I. J., D. M. Gersten, and M. B. Budmen. 1976. Characterization in vivo and in vitro of tumor cells selected for resistance to syngeneic lymphocyte-mediated cytotoxicity. Cancer Res. 36:3160.

Fidler, I. J., D. M. Gersten, and I. R. Hart. 1978. The biology of cancer invasion and metastasis. Adv. Cancer Res. 28:149–250.

Fogel, M., P. Altevogt, and V. Schirrmacher. 1983. Metastatic potential severely altered by changes in tumor cell adhesiveness and cell surface sialylation. J. Exp. Med. 157:371–376.

Helenius, A., B. Morein, E. Fries, K. Simons, P. Robinson, V. Schirrmacher, C. Terhorst, and J. L. Strominger. 1978. Human (HLA-A and HLA-B) and murine (H-2K and H-2D) histocompatibility antigens are cell surface receptors for Semliki Forest virus. Proc. Natl. Acad. Sci. USA 75:3846–3850.

Johnson, R. E., V. T. De Vita, B. R. Chabner, P. B. Chretien, C. D. Berard, and S. K. Johnson. 1975. Patterns of involvement with malignant lymphoma and implications for treatment decision making. Br. J. Cancer 31 (Suppl. II): 237–241.

Kerbel, R. S., J. W. Dennis, A. E. Lagarde, and P. Frost. 1982. Tumor progression in metastasis: an experimental approach using lectin resistant tumor variants. Cancer Metastasis Rev. 1:99–140.

Kramer, M., I. Vlodavsky, D. Barz, P. Robinson, and V. Schirrmacher. 1983. Degradation of endothelial extracellular matrix by tumor cell derived proteolytic activity. J. Cancer Res. Clin. Oncol. (in press).

Kripke, M. L., E. Gruys, and I. J. Fidler. 1978. Metastatic heterogeneity of cells from an ultraviolet light-induced murine fibrosarcoma of recent origin. Cancer Res. 38:2962–2967.

Neauport-Sautes, C., and W. H. Fridman. 1977. Characterization of suppressive immunoglobulin-binding factor (IBF). II. Purification and molecular weight determination of IBF produced by L-5178-Y θ-positive lymphoma. J. Immunol. 119:1269–1274.

Nicolson, G. L., 1982. Cancer metastasis: Organ colonization and the cell surface properties of malignant cells. Biochim. Biophys. Acta 695:113–176.

Nicolson, G. L., and J. L. Winkelhake. 1975. Organ specificity of blood-borne metastasis determined by cell adhesion. Nature 255:230.

Parr, I. 1972. Response of syngeneic murine lymphomata to immunotherapy in relation to the antigenicity of the tumour. Br. J. Cancer 26:174–182.

Poste, G. and G. L. Nicolson. 1980. Arrest and metastasis of blood-borne tumor cells are modified by fusion of plasma membrane vesicles from highly malignant cells. Proc. Natl. Acad. Sci. USA 77:399–403.
Schirrmacher, V. 1980. Shifts in tumor cell phenotypes induced by signals from the microenvironment: Relevance for the immunobiology of cancer metastasis. Immunobiology 157:89–98.
Schirrmacher, V. 1981. Immunogenetic studies on the resistance of mice against highly metastatic DBA/2 tumor cell variants. I. Effect of incompatibilities at H-2 or non-H-2 genes in normal and nude (nu/nu) mice. Invasion and Metastasis 1:4–21.
Schirrmacher, V., P. Altevogt, M. Fogel, J. Dennis, C. A. Waller, D. Barz, R. Schwartz, R. Cheingsong-Popov, G. Springer, P. J. Robinson, T. Nebe, W. Brossmer, I. Vlodavsky, N. Paweletz, H.-P. Zimmermann, and G. Uhlenbruck. 1982. Importance of cell surface carbohydrates in cancer cell adhesion, invasion and metastasis. Does sialic acid direct metastatic behavior? Invasion and Metastasis 2:313–360.
Schirrmacher, V., and K. Bosslet. 1980. Tumor metastases and cell-mediated immunity in a model system in DBA/2 mice. X. Immunoselection of tumor variants differing in tumor antigen expression and metastatic capacity. Int. J. Cancer 25:781–788.
Schirrmacher, V., and K. Bosslet. 1982. Clonal analysis of expression of tumor-associated transplantation antigens and of metastatic capacity. Cancer Immunol. Immunother. 13:62–68.
Schirrmacher, V., K. Bosslet, G. Shantz, K. Clauer, and D. Hübsch. 1979a. Tumor metastases and cell-mediated immunity in a model system in DBA/2 mice. IV. Antigenic differences between the parental tumor line and its metastasizing variant. Int. J. Cancer 23:245–252.
Schirrmacher, V., R. Cheingsong-Popov, and H. Arnheiter. 1980. Hepatocyte tumor cell interaction in vitro. I. Conditions for rosette formation and inhibition by anti H-2 antibodies. J. Exp. Med. 151:984–989.
Schirrmacher, V., M. Fogel, E. Russmann, K. Bosslet, P. Altevogt, and L. Beck. 1982. Antigenic variation in cancer metastasis: Immune escape versus immune control. Cancer Met. Rev. 1:241–274.
Schirrmacher, V., and W. Jacobs. 1979. Tumor metastases and cell-mediated immunity in a model system in DBA/2 mice. VIII. Expression and shedding of Fcγ receptors on metastatic tumor cell variants. J. Supramol. Struct. 11:105–111.
Schirrmacher, V., G. Shantz, K. Clauer, D. Komitowski, H. P. Zimmermann, and M. L. Lohmann-Matthes. 1979b. Tumor metastases and cell-mediated immunity in a model system in DBA/2 mice. I. Tumor invasiveness in vitro and metastasis formation in vivo. Int. J. Cancer 23:233–244.
Springer, G. F., R. Cheingsong-Popov, V. Schirrmacher, P. Desai, and H. Tegtmeyer. 1983a. Proposed molecular basis of murine tumor cell-hepatocyte interaction. J. Biol. Chem. 258:5702–5706.
Springer, G. F., P. R. Desai, M. S. Murthy, H. Tegtmeyer, and E. F. Scanlon. 1979. Human carcinoma-associated precursor antigens of the blood group MN system and the host's immune responses to them. Progr. Allergy 26:42–96.
Springer, G. F., P. R. Desai, H. Tegtmeyer, V. Schirrmacher, and R. Cheingsong-Popov. 1983b. Murine lymphoma cells possess blood group Tn-, T-, N-, M-, and S-active substances. Naturwissenschaften 70:98–99.
Springer, G. F., M. S. Murthy, P. R. Desai, and E. F. Scanlon. 1980. Breast cancer patient's cell mediated immune response to Thomsen-Friedenreich (T) antigen. Cancer 45:2949–2954.
Vlodavsky, I., Z. Fuks, M. Bar-Nev, Y. Ariav, P. Altevogt, and V. Schirrmacher. 1983. Lymphoma cell mediated degradation of sulfated proteoglycans in the subendothelial extracellular matrix: relationship to tumor cell metastasis. Cancer Res. 43:2704–2777.

Cancer Invasion and Metastasis: Biologic and Therapeutic Aspects edited by Garth L. Nicolson and Luka Milas. Raven Press, New York © 1984.

Immunogenetic Control of Metastatic Competence of Cloned Tumor Cell Populations

Lea Eisenbach, Patrick De Baetselier,* Shulamit Katzav, Shraga Segal,† and Michael Feldman

*Department of Cell Biology, The Weizmann Institute of Science, Rehovot, Israel 76100, *Service of General Biology, Free University of Brussels, Belgium, and †Department of Microbiology, Ben-Gurion University of the Negev, Beer-Sheva, Israel*

Tumor cells capable of metastasizing seem to be equipped with enzymatic activities for degrading matrices and penetrating basement membranes and with the capacity to survive host-defense mechanisms, to recognize cells of the target organs for metastatic growth, and to induce angiogenesis for metastatic growth. The survival of disseminating tumor cells while circulating in the organism is obviously a determining step for metastasis formation. In view of the diversity of tumor cells with respect to metastatic competence, we tested individual clones of the 3LL Lewis lung carcinoma, a tumor that originated spontaneously in a C57BL animal and that, following transplantation, generates massive metastases in the lungs.

We found that different clones had different metastatic potentials. Metastatic clones of the 3LL tumor were significantly more resistant to natural killer (NK) cells than nonmetastatic clones (Segal et al. 1982). The capacity to resist NK cells seems to be causally related to metastatic competence because a nonmetastasizing, NK-susceptible clone did produce spontaneous metastases when grown in NK-depleted Bg/Bg mice (Segal et al. 1982). The host's immune system might control the generation of tumor metastases by specific immune responses. Furthermore, it appears that spontaneous metastases are significantly more susceptible to T cell–mediated allogeneic immune responses than the local tumor. Thus, when transplated into allogeneic hosts, the local 3LL tumor grows across any allogeneic barriers tested, and yet metastases developed only in syngeneic recipients (Isakov et al. 1982). If T cell–mediated immune responses against some tumor-associated antigens were generated in syngeneic hosts, metastases would be more susceptible to such responses than the local tumor. To generate metastases, disseminating tumor cells should then be deficient in their capacity to either generate or be susceptible to cellular immunity.

Since such T cell–mediated responses are likely to be major histocompatibility complex (MHC)-restricted, we wanted to elucidate the following main questions: (1) Do MHC gene products on the tumor cell surface participate in controlling the tumor's malignant (i.e., metastatic) properties? (2) Is tumor progression, in particular the acquisition of metastatic potential by nonmetastatic neoplastic cells, associated with alterations in the expression of MHC gene products? (3) Is the differential expression of the different haplotypes in heterozygous tumors, as distinct from the differential expression of subregions of the same haplotypes, relevant to the acquisition of metastatic potential by nonmetastatic tumors? (4) Can somatic cell hybridization result in the acquisition of metastatic potential by nonmetastatic tumors?

In the initial phase of our studies, the 3LL Lewis lung carcinoma constituted our main tumor model. Since this tumor grows locally both in syngeneic and allogeneic mice, but spontaneous lung metastases develop only in syngeneic recipients, we studied the minimal requirements of genetic identity between the tumor and the host that are needed for metastasis formation. We found that lung metastases are formed only when the 3LL tumor grows in mice that share the tumor's strain of origin, the D-end of the $H\text{-}2^b$ haplotype, and the genetic background (Isakov et al. 1982). Serological analysis demonstrated that, in fact, the tumor cells had lost cell surface expression of $H\text{-}2K^b$, while retaining expression of $H\text{-}2D^b$ (Isakov et al. 1983). Is this imbalance between the H-2D and H-2K phenotypes relevant to the malignant properties of the 3LL tumor?

3LL CLONES THAT DIFFER IN METASTATIC COMPETENCE ALSO DIFFER IN THE CELL SURFACE EXPRESSION OF THE H-2 SUBREGIONS

We cloned 3LL tumor cells in soft agar (Pluznik and Sachs 1965). Individual colonies were isolated after seeding and were expanded in liquid medium. We selected two clones, clone D122 and clone A9. Testing their metastatic competence following transplantation, we found that D122 did generate lung metastases, whereas A9 did not. We then tested the expression of the $H\text{-}2^b$ molecules on cell surfaces of the two clones, by staining cells with monoclonal antibodies to the $H\text{-}2K^b$ and the $H\text{-}2D^b$ and analysis on the fluorescence activated cell sorter and by a direct radioimmunoassay using ^{125}I-labeled monoclonal antibodies. We found that both the uncloned 3LL and the metastatic clone D122 expressed only a marginal density of $H\text{-}2K^b$ and a high density of $H\text{-}2D^b$, whereas the nonmetastatic clone A9 expressed both the $H\text{-}2D^b$ and the $H\text{-}2K^b$ gene products (Table 1).

We subsequently tested the cell surface versus the cytoplasmic H-2 molecules. Cells externally labeled with iodine-125 were subjected to radioimmunoprecipitation and sodium dodecyl sulfate–polyacrylamide gel electrophoretic (SDS-PAGE) analysis with anti-$H\text{-}2^b$ antisera, and the results indicated that molecules of 45 kd were associated with beta-2 microglobulins. Monoclonal anti-$H\text{-}2K^b$ antibodies precipitated a 45-kd molecule from A9 cells but not from D122 cells (Figure 1). Extracts of ^{35}S-methionine metabolically labeled cells separated on lentil lectin sepharose 4B (Freed et al. 1979) and immunoprecipitation of

TABLE 1. *Expression of MHC antigens and metastasis formation of 3LL tissue culture lines*

Clone	% K^b expression (gain 8)*	% D^b expression (gain 8)*	Lung weight (mg)†
A9	35 ± 7	73 ± 7	239 ± 35
D122	9 ± 3	81 ± 10	536 ± 176
3LL	13 ± 3	70 ± 14	404 ± 180

* 2–3 × 10^6 tumor cells were incubated at 4°C for 30 min in purified (28–13–3) anti-K^b monoclonal antibody or anti-D^b (28–14–8) antibody, washed twice in phosphate-buffered saline, 1% bovine serum albumin, 0.2% sodium azide, and reincubated in fluoroscein isothiocyanate-labeled rabbit anti-mouse Ig. Fluorescence-activated cell sorter II analysis was performed with photomultiplier tube set at 550 V.

† In 10 C57Bl/6J male mice, 10^5 cells were inoculated intrafootpad. When the primary tumor reached a diameter of 8 mm, tumor-bearing legs were amputated. Metastatic load was determined 30 days postamputation.

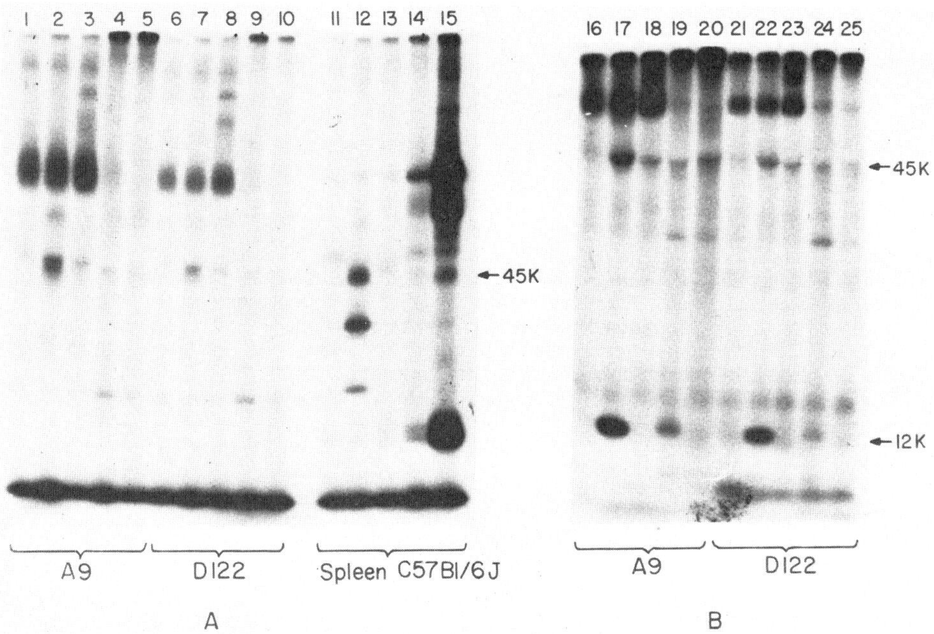

FIG. 1. Radioimmunoprecipitation of ^{125}I cell surface–labeled 3LL clones. In the presence of IODO-GEN, 10^7 living cells were labeled with 1 mCi Na ^{125}I. Cells were lysed in 0.01 M sodium phosphate pH 7.5, 0.15 M NaCl-1% Triton X-100–0.5% sodium deoxycholate-0.1% SDS. Extract equivalent to 10^6–2 × 10^6 cells was immunoprecipitated with antibody and SacI. **A.** 10% acrylamide; **B.** 15% acrylamide. Normal mouse serum (1,6,11,16,21); C3H.DiSn anti-C3H.SW (anti-H-2^b) (2,7,12,17,22); C3H.SW anti-C3H.DiSn (anti-H-2^k) (3,8,13,18,23). Rabbit anti-rat beta$_2$-microglobulin (4,9,14,19,24); monoclonal anti-H-$2K^b$ 28–13–3 plus purified anti-μ (5,10, 15,20,25).

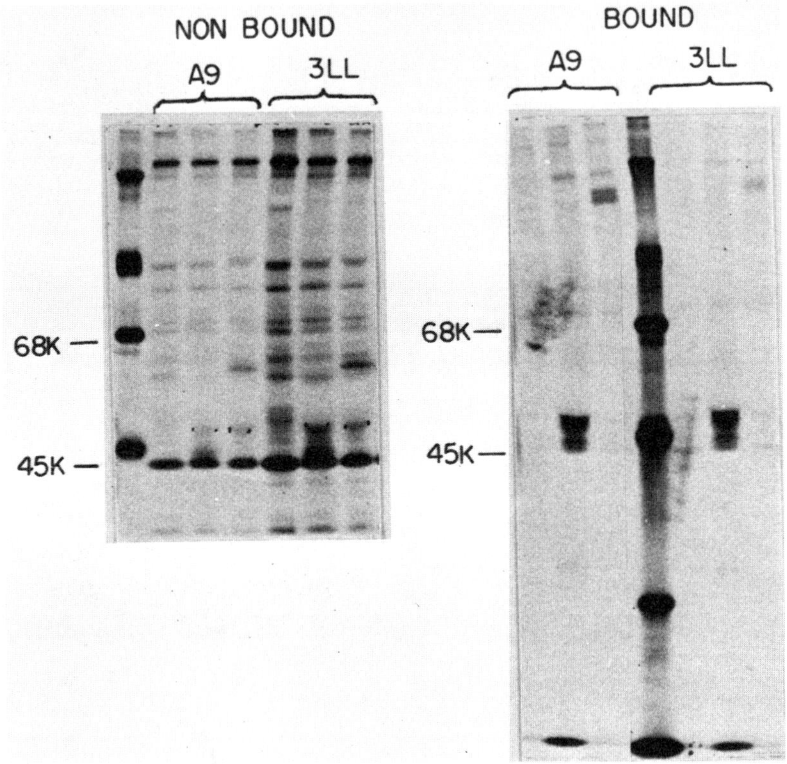

FIG. 2. Immunoprecipitation of glycosylated and nonglycosylated H-2^b molecules from [^{35}S]-methionine-labeled A9 and 3LL. *From left to right:* Lentil lectin Sepharose nonbound fraction: A9 extract (4×10^6 cpm) plus normal serum; A9 extract plus anti-H-2^b; A9 extract plus anti-H-2^k; 3LL (8×10^6 cpm) extract plus normal serum; 3LL extract plus anti-H-2^b; 3LL extract plus anti-H-2^k. Lentil lectin Sepharose bound fraction: A9 (2×10^5 cpm) plus normal serum; A9 plus anti-H-2^b; A9 plus anti-H-2^k; marker; 3LL (2×10^5 cpm) plus normal serum; 3LL plus anti-H-2^b; 3LL plus anti-H-2^k.

bound and unbound fractions showed that a substantial part of the 45-kd protein was in the glycosylated form (Figure 2).

SUBCLONING OF 3LL CELLS GENERATES VARIANTS MANIFESTING DIFFERENT METASTATIC POTENTIALS CORRELATING WITH THEIR H-2K^b/H-2D^b RATIOS

The metastatic potentials and MHC phenotypes of 3LL and the cloned A9 cells remained unchanged during 70 passages in culture. We then recloned the A9 line and cloned the in vitro passaged 3LL cells. Fourteen days following seeding of the cells in soft agar, we isolated 93 colonies of A9 and 28 colonies of 3LL cells. We intently screened a larger number of A9 clones, since one of our aims was to study the generation of phenotypic diversities within the progeny of a clonal tumor cell population by testing the cloned cells recloned in culture. Each clone was stained for H-$2K^b$ determinants using monoclonal antibody 28–13–3, which identifies the H-2.39 specificity. We used the monoclonal 28–14–8 anti-H-$2D^b$ antibody (and also an anti-K^b, D^b antibody) to detect H-$2D^b$ (Ozato and Sachs 1981). The distribution of H-$2K^b$ is presented in Figure 3. Table 2 presents the result of testing individual clones both for metastatic competence and for the expression of the D and K subregions of the H-2^b haplotypes. Lung metastases were assayed following intrafootpad inoculation of 10^5 viable cells to 10 mice per group. When the tumors reached a diameter of 8 mm, they were amputated. The animals were assayed for lung metastases 30 days after tumor excision, either by lung weight or by incorporation of 5-(^{125}I)iodo 2′ deoxyuridine (1 μCi per mouse) in the lung 30 min after injection of 5-fluorodeoxyuridine. The incorporation into lungs was measured 24 h later.

We found differences in the growth rate of the local tumor among the different 3LL-originated or A9-originated clones, yet there were no significant differences in local growth rates between clones manifesting high, low, or no metastatic competence (Table 3). We did find differences in the metastatic potential of the different clones; these differences correlated with the relative cell surface expression of the H-$2K^b$/H-$2D^b$ (Figure 4 and Table 2).

The results indicated that the smaller the ratio of H-$2K^b$ to H-$2D^b$, irrespective of the absolute density of each of these determinants, the greater the metastatic potential of the cloned population (Table 2). This relation was evident when we tested the frequencies of cells at fluorescent gains 8 and 4 (using a photomultiplier at 550 V). Furthermore, we found that shifts from a low metastatic potential

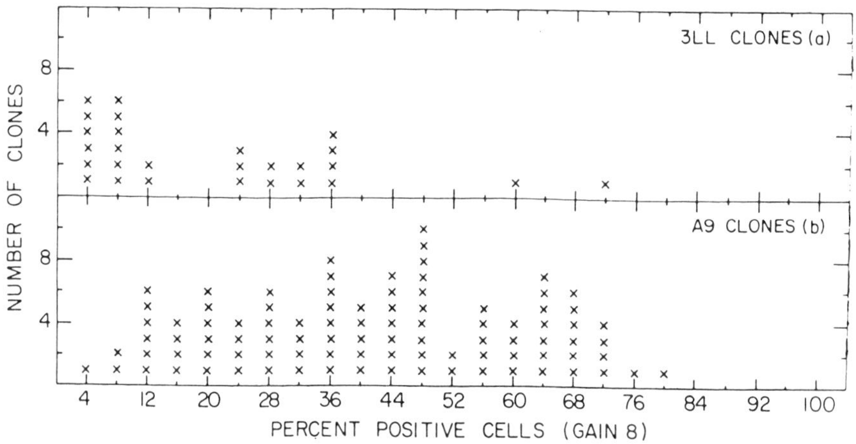

FIG. 3. Distribution of H-$2K^b$ expression on A9 and 3LL subclones. **a.** 27 clones of 3LL tissue culture line; **b.** 93 subclones of A9.

TABLE 2. *Growth rate, metastases, and H-2 expression of 3LL and A9 subclones*

Clone	Percent positive cells*				Ratio K^b/D^b		Lung weight (mg)†		50% amputation day‡
	Gain 4		Gain 8						
	K^b	D^b	K^b	D^b	Gain 4	Gain 8	Mean	Range	
A9A5	1	1	5	5	1	1	243 ± 58	126–361	30
A9FH5	2 ± 2	2 ± 3	6 ± 4	8 ± 3	1	0.75	217 ± 35	163–271	28
A9FJ1	3 ± 1	4 ± 1	13 ± 2	15 ± 2	0.75	0.87	230 ± 62	187–378	25
A9C3	11 ± 3	25 ± 6	33 ± 6	60 ± 15	0.44	0.55	233 ± 25	195–273	31
A9E2	13 ± 6	28 ± 8	43 ± 9	55 ± 18	0.46	0.78	220 ± 41	172–278	43
A9G3	10 ± 6	31 ± 10	35 ± 10	54 ± 16	0.32	0.65	229 ± 27	180–263	36
A9H3	14 ± 4	26 ± 11	30 ± 4	42 ± 9	0.54	0.71	224 ± 21	178–237	46
A9H6	16 ± 5	53 ± 15	40 ± 13	67 ± 14	0.30	0.60	236 ± 91	172–478	28
A9J2	16 ± 6	37 ± 9	53 ± 10	73 ± 14	0.43	0.73	218 ± 28	185–264	38
A9FA1	22 ± 6	37 ± 10	45 ± 2	55 ± 12	0.59	0.82	192 ± 28	145–227	27
A9FA6	16 ± 4	37 ± 0	43 ± 8	70 ± 4	0.43	0.61	208 ± 14	182–224	21
A9FI1	9 ± 3	21 ± 8	35 ± 9	47 ± 12	0.43	0.74	201 ± 18	180–239	27
A9FJ2	14	65	47	87	0.22	0.54	236 ± 30	193–273	36
A9FJ3	18 ± 7	50 ± 10	44 ± 16	75 ± 18	0.36	0.59	214 ± 31	183–278	30
3LLFI6	23 ± 5	30 ± 3	61 ± 11	61 ± 6	0.70	1	219 ± 39	173–290	43

A9E6	11 ± 6	47 ± 2	34 ± 9	84 ± 8	0.24	0.40	259 ± 73	215–458	33
A9L2	14	69	42	89	0.20	0.47	284 ± 23	252–320	33
A9FE2	5 ± 2	23 ± 16	14 ± 6	45 ± 16	0.22	0.31	367 ± 300	233–1159	36
3LLFA5	9 ± 9	51 ± 20	25 ± 9	63 ± 13	0.18	0.40	310 ± 188	204–767	35
3LLFL1	14 ± 8	35 ± 10	30 ± 41	57 ± 13	0.40	0.53	294 ± 159	185–588	27
A9FG6	7 ± 3	43 ± 17	15 ± 7	71 ± 23	0.16	0.21	429 ± 395	205–1311	35
A9FJ4	7 ± 3	29 ± 9	14 ± 7	56 ± 19	0.24	0.25	451 ± 361	168–1355	32
3LLFA3	2 ± 0	41 ± 10	11 ± 6	56 ± 18	0.05	0.20	437 ± 347	175–1226	27
3LLFB4	8 ± 7	45 ± 10	15 ± 7	61 ± 10	0.18	0.25	947 ± 243	662–1409	26
3LLFC1	6	87	22	96	0.07	0.23	641 ± 220	486–1073	24
3LLFC6	7 ± 2	32 ± 15	11 ± 8	47 ± 17	0.13	0.23	492 ± 224	336–1226	40
3LLFL5	2 ± 3	42 ± 13	9 ± 6	62 ± 12	0.05	0.15	567 ± 387	193–1290	26
3LLFC6	4 ± 4	26 ± 6	6 ± 5	52 ± 13	0.15	0.12	662 ± 367	233–1158	39
3LLFM2	4 ± 3	28 ± 7	19 ± 8	72 ± 8	0.14	0.26	518 ± 191	236–735	26

* As in Table 1.

† As in Table 1.

‡ 10^5 cells inoculated intrafootpad; 11–19 days later, tumors became palpable. Tumor diameter was measured every second day; when tumor reached 8 mm, leg was amputated. The numbers listed are the days when 50% of the group (5 mice or more) reached amputation stage.

TABLE 3. *Mean of growth rates and H-2 expression of low-, moderate-, and high-metastatic-potential groups**

	n	Percent positive cells (gain 8)				50% amputation day (mean)
		K^b mean	K^b range	D^b mean	K^b range	
Low metastatic I	3	8.0 ± 4.4	5–13	9.3 ± 5.1	5–15	27.7 ± 2.5
Low metastatic II	12	42.4 ± 8.8	30–61	62.2 ± 12.8	42–87	33.8 ± 7.7
Low combined	15	—	—	—	—	32.6 ± 7.4
Moderate metastatic	5	29.0 ± 10.4	14–42	67.6 ± 18.5	45–89	32.8 ± 3.5
High metastatic	9	13.6 ± 5.0	6–22	63.7 ± 14.6	47–96	29.4 ± 5.3

* Means and ranges of the groups described in Table 2.

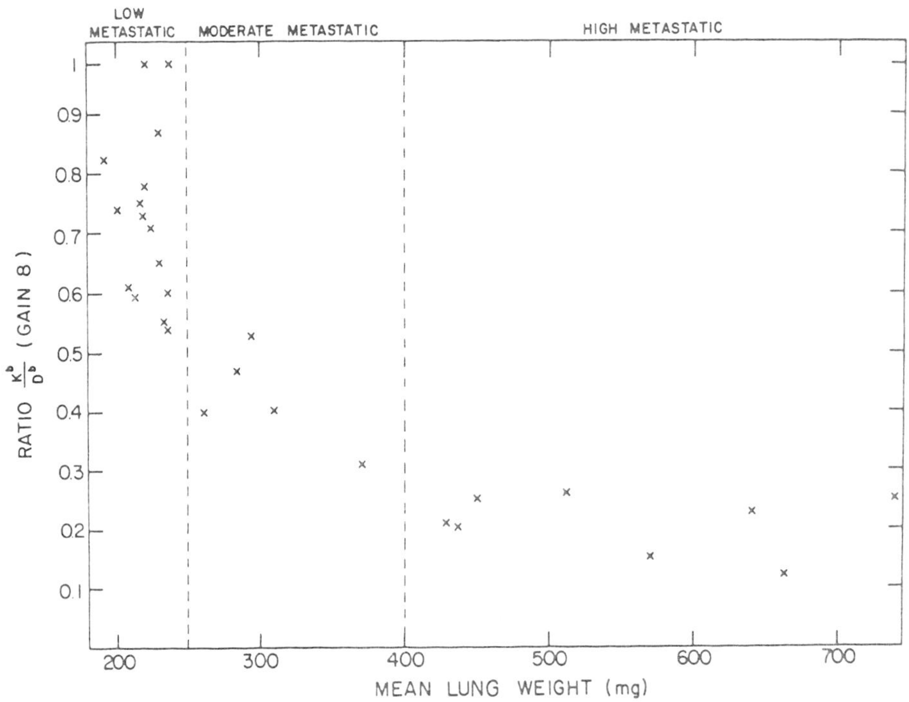

FIG. 4. Relationship between K^b/D^b ratio at gain 8 and metastatic expression of 3LL subclones.

to a medium or high metastatic competence did take place. Some of the subclones of A9, namely A9FE2 and A9L2, were categorized as medium metastatic (generating lung weights of 250–400 mg), whereas A9FG6 and A9FJ4 were highly metastatic (generating lung weights exceeding 400 mg). These properties correlated with shifts from large to small $H\text{-}2K^b/H\text{-}2D^b$ ratios.

EXPERIMENTAL MODULATION OF MHC EXPRESSION IS CORRELATED WITH SHIFTS IN METASTATIC PROPERTIES

The previous set of experiments indicated that the progeny of a low-metastatic-potential clone (A9) of the 3LL tumor yielded some clones of significant metastatic potency. These clones also manifested low $H\text{-}2K^b/H\text{-}2D^b$ ratios. We subsequently tested whether the in vitro treatment of tumor cells with interferon (which was shown to increase the synthesis of H-2 molecules (Fellous et al. 1982)) and with retinoic acid would induce alterations in the cell-surface expression of MHC determinants and whether such changes would correlate with alterations in the metastatic properties of the tumor cells. We tested two clones: the low-metastatic-potential A9 and the metastatic D122. The most dramatic effect was obtained with retinoic acid. The expression of the $H\text{-}2K^b$ was not changed on either of the two clones. Yet the expression of $H\text{-}2D^b$ was significantly increased on cells of clone A9, thus decreasing the $H\text{-}2K^b/H\text{-}2D^b$ ratio (Figure 5). Concomitantly, this low metastatic clone gains a very significant metastatic competence (Table 4). Interferon induced an increase in the cell surface expression of both the $H\text{-}2K^b$ and $H\text{-}2D^b$ on the two clones. Yet the effect on the expression of $H\text{-}2D^b$ was higher, thus again decreasing the $H\text{-}2K^b/H\text{-}2D^b$ ratio (Figure 5). This alteration of the relative expression of the two subregions was again associated with some increase in metastatic potential.

The correlation between the H-2K/H-2D ratio and the metastatic competence of the cloned 3LL tumor cell populations might be attributable to the notion that although these two subregions of the MHC developed evolutionarily by gene duplication, they differ in their immune functions. Thus, it appears from studies of various systems that, of the two class I antigens, the H-2K exerts an immunogenic effect with respect to its linked antigens distinct from that of the H-2D, which, in many antigenic systems, seems to induce a suppressive effect (Wernet and Lilly 1975, Miller et al. 1978, Hasek and Chutna 1979).

TABLE 4. *Mean lung weight* of low- and high-metastatic-potential clones treated with interferon and retinoic acid*

	Control	Interferon†	Retinoic acid†
A9	249 ± 66	410 ± 205	519 ± 270
D122	536 ± 176	794 ± 236	620 ± 178

* Spontaneous metastasis formation. For conditions see legend to Table 1.

† 10^5 tissue culture propagated cells were transferred to 100-mm Petri dishes, in 10 ml Dulbecco's modified Eagle's medium supplemented with 10% fetal calf serum, 1% glutamine, 1% sodium pyruvate, 1% nonessential amino acids, and 1% antibiotics, in the presence of 100 units/ml interferon (alpha plus beta, 10^7 units/mg) or 10^{-6} M retinoic acid (all trans). The cells were grown to confluency (1 week) with biweekly changes of growth medium.

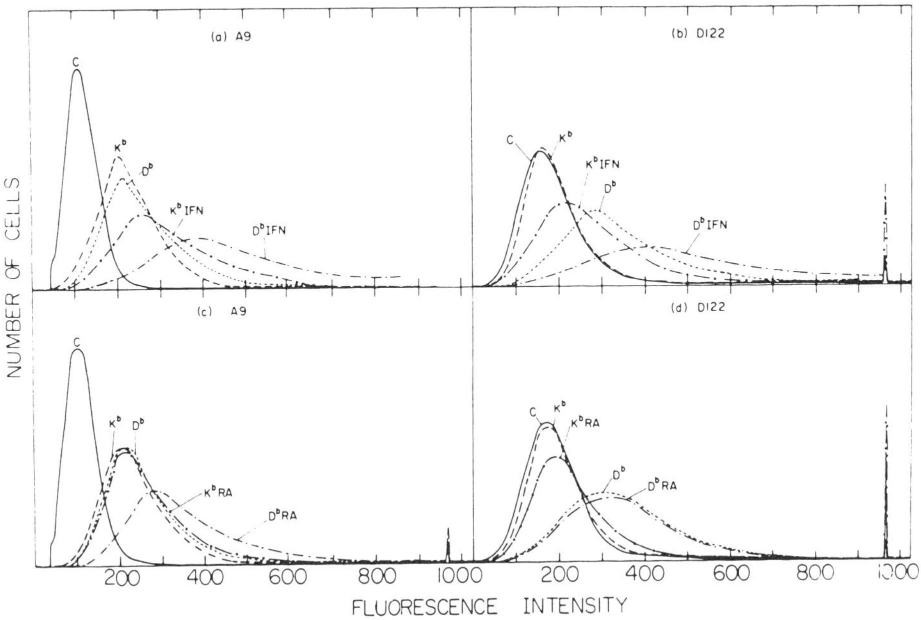

FIG. 5. Effect of interferon (IFN) and retinoic acid (RA) treatment on cell surface expression of H-2D^b and H-2K^b alloantigens of clones A9 and D122. For conditions of treatment see legend to Table 4, FACS II analyses.

That these observations are relevant to tumor-host relations gained support from Schmidt and Festenstein (1982), who reported that clones of AKR lymphomas that lost the cell surface expression of H-2K could neither elicit the production of syngeneic cytotoxic T cells directed against the Gross MuLV/H-2K^k nor serve as targets for such cells. Thus, the loss of the H-2K determinants from neoplastic cells rendered them nonimmunogenic and unsusceptible to effector cells. Since metastatic 3LL cells in allogeneic animals are significantly more susceptible to immune responses than cells of the local tumor, the relative loss in H-2K^b might determine their metastatic progression in compatible, syngeneic, yet potentially reactive, tumor-bearing organisms (Gorelik et al. 1980).

How general is the association between the "imbalance" in H-2K/H-2D expression and metastatic properties of neoplastic cells?

DIVERSITY OF THE METASTATIC T10 SARCOMA

To study further whether immunogenetic properties of tumor cells are causally related to their metastatic properties, we selected a tumor of heterozygous origin, the T10 sarcoma, induced by methylcholanthrene in a C3H/eb × C57BL/6

F1 mouse and then serially transplanted in syngeneic recipients. Comparing the phenotypes of cells of the local tumor (L-T10) grown in syngeneic mice and cells of lung metastases, we found that whereas cells from metastatic lung nodules expressed on the cell surface both the H-2^k and H-2^b haplotypes, cells from the local tumor expressed only the H-2^b haplotype (De Baetselier et al. 1980).

To test whether the expression of the H-2^k in the metastatic population of the lung is a response to a lung-modulating signal or whether it represents a selection of phenotypically heterozygous cells programmed to generate metastases, we cloned the T10 tumor in culture. Out of 10 clones, eight expressed only the H-2^b phenotype and two expressed both parental haplotypes. The inoculation of cells from each of these clones indicated that only the two clones that expressed the two haplotypes (clones IE7 and IB9) were highly metastatic (De Baetselier et al. 1980, Katzav et al. 1982). We then further examined the differential expression of the H-2 subregions by the various clones to test whether the H-2K/H-2D phenotype is also related to the metastatic potential of the cells in this tumor system. We studied clones IC9, D6, IE7, and IB9 and lines T10(8) (eight generations in vivo of the parental T10 tumor, adapted to tissue culture) and T10(40). In Figure 6 the results of a direct radioimmunoassay indicate that expression of H-$2K^b$ is completely suppressed in all clones, as is the cell surface expression of the H-$2K^k$ in metastatic and nonmetastatic clones. The clones of low metastatic potential in the T10 system (D6) express only low H-$2D^b$ densities, whereas the clones of high metastatic potential express higher densities of H-$2D^b$ and H-$2D^k$ molecules. The nonmetastatic IC9 clone does not express H-$2D^b$. Immunoprecipitation and SDS-PAGE of [^{35}S]methionine-labeled extracts show that the highly metastatic clones (IE7, IB9) and T10(40) synthesize H-$2K^k$ molecules (Figure 7), but these molecules do not bind to the beta-2 microglobulin and are not inserted into the membrane (Figure 8). On the other hand, the synthesis of H-2^b and H-2^k-encoded molecules in the nonmetastatic clone IC9 is blocked (Figure 7). Clone D6, which is of low metastatic potential, is blocked in the synthesis of only the H-2^k molecules.

These variants present an interesting sequence of MHC repression: one at the translational (or transcriptional) level of both haplotypes in IC9 and one haplotype in D6, and the second on a posttranslational level, as is the case with IE7 and IB9, in which K^k region molecules are synthesized but are not expressed. Thus, with regard to the cell surface expression of the H-2 class I antigens, the T10 clones manifest the same principle of correlation between metastatic competence and the H-2K/H-2D ratio as do the 3LL clones. The highly metastatic clones IE7 and IB9 manifest the lowest H-2K/H-2D ratio of both parental haplotypes. The low-metastatic-potential clone D6 shows a higher ratio—owing to a lower H-2D expression—confined to the H-2^b, which is the only haplotype expressed on this clone. The nonmetastatic IC9 has the highest ratio, in that the two subregions of H-2^b are hardly expressed.

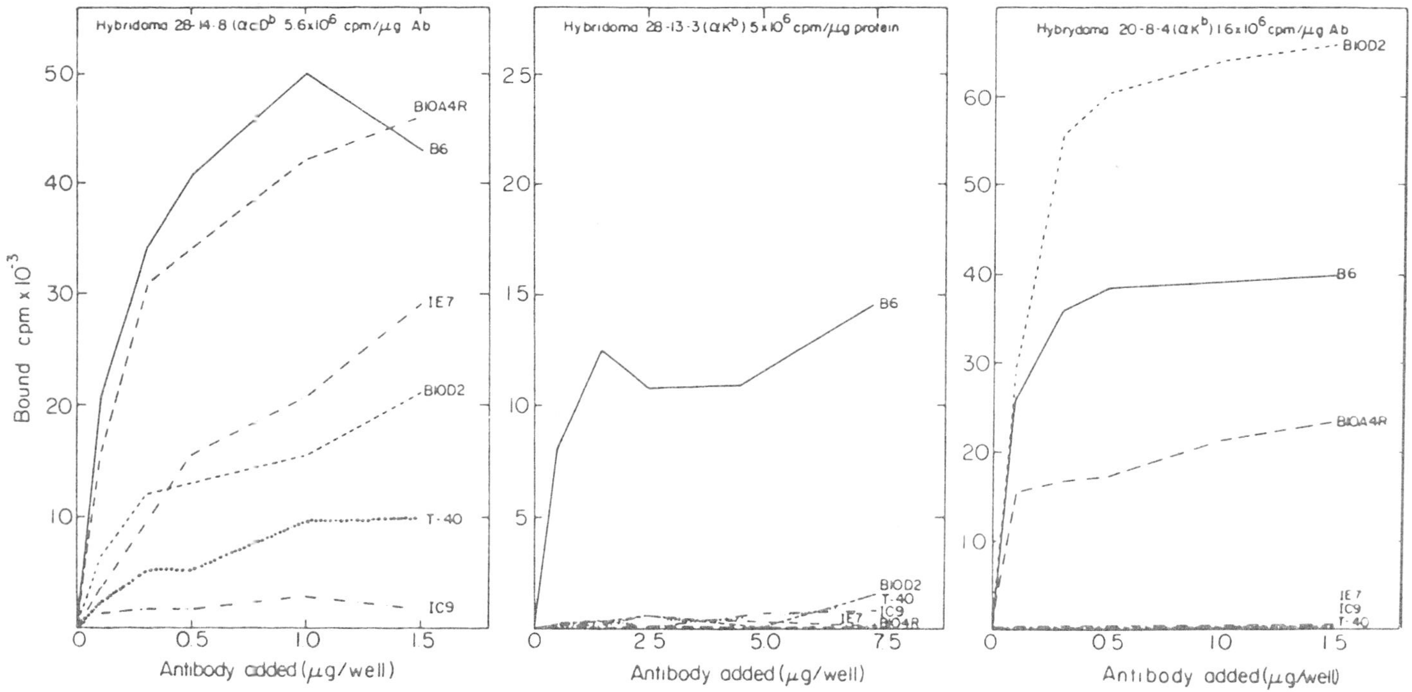

FIG. 6. Cell surface expression of H-2K^b and H-2D^b on clones of T10 sarcoma, determined by direct radioimmunoassay. 10^6 living cells were incubated with 50 μl ^{125}I-labeled antibody, 0.1 μg-1.5μg of protein A-Sepharose purified antibody (28–14–8 and 20–8–4) or 0.5–7.5 μg semipurified antibody (28–13–3). Binding was done for 1 h at 4°C, plates (24 wells) were washed four times in PBS-FCS, and cells were collected into tubes and monitored in a gamma-counter.

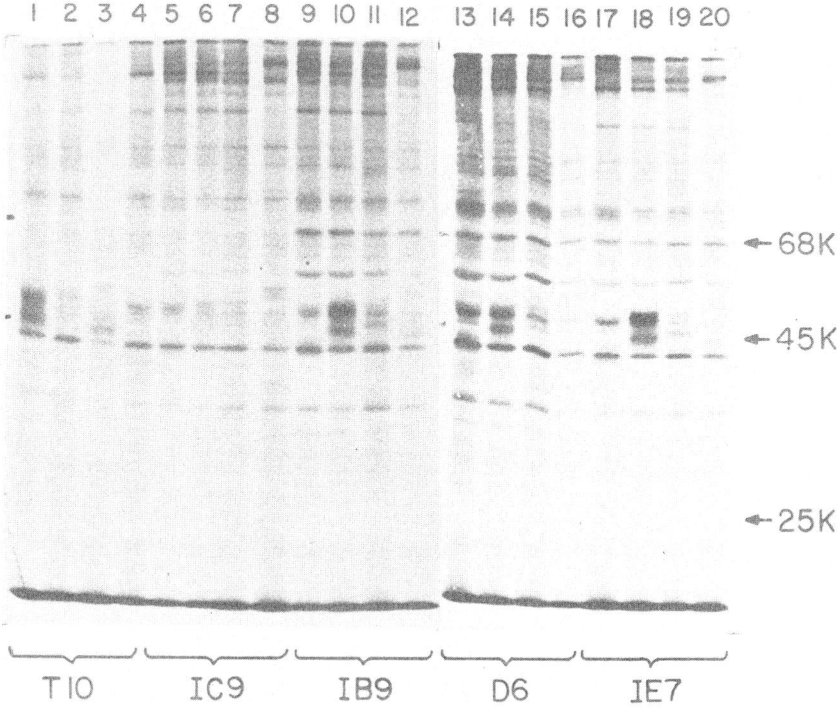

FIG. 7. Immunoprecipitation of $[^{35}S]$methionine-labeled T10 clones. 5×10^6 cells in 2 ml methionine-free Dulbecco's modified Eagle's medium supplemented with 5% dialyzed FCS were labeled for 4 h with 250 μCi $[^{35}S]$methionine. Immunoprecipitation was done as in Figure 1. Ten percent acrylamide: Normal mouse serum (4,5,9,13,17); anti-H-2^b (1,6,10,14,18); anti-H-2^k (2,7,11,15,19); monoclonal anti-H-$2K^k$ (3,8,12,16,20).

THE PROGENY OF NONMETASTATIC CLONES ACQUIRE METASTATIC CAPACITY FOLLOWING SERIAL TRANSPLANTATIONS IN SYNGENEIC F1 HYBRID MICE

The MHC phenotype of T10 clones remained unchanged for 2 years. Yet, in studying the phenotypes of T10 clones grown in vivo, we serially transplanted cells of individual clones in syngeneic F1 hybrid mice and tested at every fifth transfer both the expression of the two parental haplotypes and the generation of metastases by the cells of the cloned lines. The clones that were metastatic to begin with and expressed the two haplotypes retained these properties and, in fact, increased the density of cell surface MHC determinants and their metastatic potential (Katzav et al. 1982). On the other hand, clones that were nonmetastatic and phenotypically H-2^b-positive, H-2^k-negative acquired, following 15–35 transfers, the expression of the H-2^k haplotypes and, concomitantly, metastatic competence (Katzav et al. 1982).

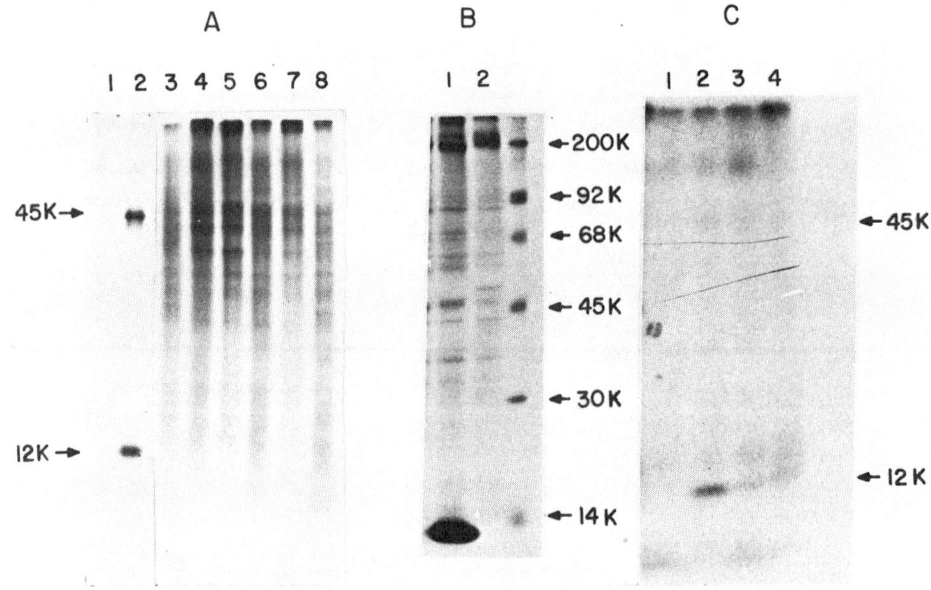

FIG. 8. Immunoprecipitation of T10 clones. **(A)** [^{35}S]methionine-labeled extracts, analysis on 15% acrylamide: spleen eb/Bl plus normal mouse serum (1); spleen eb/Bl plus anti-H-2K^k monoclonal antibody (2); T40 plus normal serum (3); IE7 plus anti-H-2K^k (4); IB9 plus anti-H-2K^k (5); IC9 plus anti-H-2K^k (6); T40 plus anti-H-2K^k (7); D6 plus anti-H-2K^k (8). **(B)** [^{35}S]methionine-labeled IE7 extract analyzed on 10–15% acrylamide gradient: Rabbit anti-mouse beta$_2$-microglobulin (1); anti-H-2K^k (2). **(C)** ^{125}I-labeled IE7 extract analyzed on 15% acrylamide: Normal serum (1); anti-H-2^b (2); anti-H-2^k (3); anti-beta$_2$-microglobulin (4).

In one particular case in the third transfer of clone IC9, which was H-2^b-positive and H-2^k-negative, H-2^b surface expression was lost and the cells of that clone remained nonmetastatic. However, upon repeated transplantation, the two parental haplotypes became expressed and the cells concomitantly metastatic. Thus, the loss of H-2 expression did not render the tumor cells metastatic. Rather, the expression of H-2^k and H-2^b seemed to be associated with the acquisition of metastatic competence. How did H-2^k-negative, H-2^b-positive cells acquire the phenotypic pattern of the original parental H-2^k-positive, H-2^b-positive cells? The "conservative" interpretation would attribute this to the selection of tumor cells in which the H-2^b haplotype had been randomly "de-repressed," and thus expressed phenotypically. An alternative possibility is based mainly on the fact that such conversions took place only in vivo, during transfers in F1 hybrid recipients, and never in vitro. This conversion could be attributed to somatic hybridization between cells of the nonmetastatic H-2^b-positive, H-2^k-negative T10 clones and normal heterozygous (H-2^b × H-2^k) F1 cells of the tumor-bearing mice.

SOMATIC CELL FUSION OF NONMETASTATIC PLASMACYTOMAS AND B CELLS PRODUCES HYBRIDOMAS MANIFESTING ORGAN-SPECIFIC METASTATIC PROPERTIES

In subsequent experiments, we studied whether somatic hybridization between a nonmetastatic cancer cell and a normal cell would result in a metastatic hybrid. Early studies of somatic cell hybrids obtained by fusing cells of highly malignant lines with cells of lines of low malignancy suggested that malignancy was a dominant property (Barski et al. 1961, Barski and Cornefert 1962). Later studies of somatic cell hybrids demonstrated, however, that the malignant trait could behave as a recessive property (Harris et al. 1969, Klein et al. 1971).

Since the properties of hybrids are likely to be determined by the characteristics of the hybrid partners, we chose to test first whether fusing cells of a nonmetastatic plasmacytoma with a normal cell capable of circulating would result in a hybrid cell manifesting metastatic properties. We therefore hybridized cells of the BALB/c-originated NSI plasmacytoma with normal B lymphocytes from C57BL/6 donors that had been immunized for marker purposes against either dinitrophenol-keyhole limpet hemocyanin (DNP-KLH) or micrococci (Katzav et al. 1982, De Baetselier et al. 1981, 1982). We randomly selected 10 hybridomas (Hy1-Hy10) and tested their capacity to generate spontaneous metastases when grown subcutaneously in (C57BL/6 × BALB/c) F1 recipients. We found that all hybridomas, irrespective of their Ig class and whether they were secreting antibody and irrespective of the antigenic specificity of their immunoglobulin (DNP-KLH versus micrococci), did generate metastases following subcutaneous growth (De Baetselier et al. 1981). In fact, at the first transplant generation, not all animals bearing tumors of a single hybridoma developed metastases. Yet, when tumor cells from the metastatic nodules were removed and retransplanted to normal F1 hybrid animals, 100% of these secondary recipients produced metastases.

Two types of metastatic patterns were observed. Eight hybridomas (Hy1,2,3,5,6,7,9,10) generated metastases in the spleen and liver, whereas two hybridomas, Hy4 and Hy8, generated metastases in the liver only (De Baetselier et al. 1981, 1982). To test how strict the organ specificity was, we tested the generation of "artificial" metastases by the different hybridomas following intravenous (i.v.) injection of the cells, i.e., under conditions of maximum probability of metastatic growth. We found that even following i.v. inoculation and even when relatively high doses of cells were injected (5×10^6 per recipient), cells of Hy4 and Hy8 generated metastases only in the liver, whereas the others metastasized to the spleen and liver. Upon retransplantation of cells from metastatic foci, the original target organ specificity was preserved; i.e., cells from liver metastases of Hy4 and Hy8, when regrafted to syngeneic mice, generated just liver metastases, whereas cells from metastases of either spleen or liver from the other hybridomas produced, following transplantation, both spleen and liver metastatic foci (De Baetselier et al. 1981, 1982). It thus appears that the two hybridoma categories follow two distinct patterns of target organ recognition. Furthermore, we found that the generation of liver metastases by hybridomas that metastasize to the liver only (Hy4 and Hy8) is under the control of a different mechanism from the generation of liver metastases by the other hybridomas. Whereas the latter hybrids do not generate liver metastases when injected into splenectomized recipients, hybridomas Hy4 and Hy8 did produce liver metastases even in animals from which the spleen had been surgically removed (De Baetselier et al. 1981, Katzav et al. 1982). It appears that the generation of liver metastases by the spleen- and liver-seeking hybridomas requires an inductive signal emitted by spleen cells. This may, in fact, be a differentiation signal, in accordance with the observation of the spleen's effect on the murine B cell leukemia BCL1 (Slavin et al. 1980).

THE NORMAL PARENTAL CELL DETERMINES THE ORGAN SPECIFICITY OF THE METASTATIC HYBRIDOMA

We subsequently aimed at studying whether a plasmacytoma other than the NSI, when similarly hybridized to B lymphocytes, would generate hybridomas of metastatic competence and, if so, whether the target organ specificity was similar to that observed following crossing of the NSI cells and B lymphocytes. Furthermore, since in the previous set of experiments the neoplastic (NSI) cells and the normal B cell partners were of two distinct H-2 phenotypes, we tested whether fusing two parental cells of identical H-2 phenotype similarly results in cells with metastatic potential.

For this purpose, we selected the BALB/c-originated nonmetastatic SP2/0 plasmacytoma and somatically hybridized it with BALB/c B lymphocytes from mice that had been immunized against micrococci. The hybridoma thus produced (Hy11H11) was inoculated i.v. into syngeneic BALB/c recipients. The inoculation generated multiple metastatic foci in the liver and scattered nodules in

TABLE 5. *Experimental metastasis in BALB/c mice, following i.v. inoculation of plasmacytoma (SP2/0) or hybridoma (Hy11H11) cells*

		Metastatic pattern					
		Spleen			Liver		
Tumor	Days*	Incidence	Growth†	Weight (mg)	Incidence	Growth	Weight (mg)
SP2/0	36	0/5	−	112	0/5	−	1380
Hy11H11	30	2/5	+	130	4/5	++	1800

* Day after inoculation at which mice were killed.

† Growth refers to tumor development. Scale: −, no metastases; +, limited involvement (scattered nodules); ++, moderate involvement (multiple nodules); +++, extensive involvement (numerous, confluent nodules).

the spleen (Table 5). It thus appeared that somatic hybridization between either NSI or SP2/0 plasmacytoma cells and normal B lymphocytes resulted in somatic hybrids with similar metastatic growth patterns.

To test whether the tumor cells that metastasized to the spleen and those that produced liver metastases constitute two subpopulations with distinct "homing" patterns, or whether the segregation to spleen and liver tumors is a random process, cells from spleen and liver nodules were analyzed for capacity to develop experimental metastases. The results (Table 6) were that cells from both spleen and liver resegregated to produce both spleen and liver metastases upon subsequent i.v. inoculation. Yet cells from spleen metastases seemed to be more malignant than cells from liver metastases, since they were significantly more effective in re-forming both spleen and liver tumors. Furthermore, cells from liver metastases, upon retransplantation, generated predominantly liver foci. It thus appears that, like the Hy hybrids, the spleen seems to induce a level of differentiation in the Hy11H11 cells inversely correlated with malignancy.

Thus far, we have reviewed the metastatic properties acquired by somatic cell hybridization of plasmacytomas and B cells. To what extent does the normal partner determine the metastatic pattern of the hybrid cell? Following fusion of the NSI plasmacytoma and C57BL/6 spleen cells, we obtained a hybridoma, the Hy38, with morphological properties different from those of the Hy1-10 B cell hybridomas. Further analysis demonstrated that it is composed of adherent cells and does not secrete antibodies. It has, in fact, none of the typical T or B cell markers. Thus, it may have resulted from fusion with a spleen macrophage or dendritic cell. Functional tests indicated that the Hy38 hybridoma exerts accessory cell properties: it can present antigen to T cells, it secretes a colony-stimulating factor, and it secretes lymphocyte-activating factor. Tested for its capacity to generate metastases in syngeneic animals following i.v. inoculation, we found that it was metastatic, yet manifested a pattern of organ-specific tumor growth different from that of the B cell hybridomas. Metastases were formed

TABLE 6. *Experimental metastasis in BALB/c mice following i.v. inoculation of spleen- or liver-derived hybridoma cells (Hy11H11)*

		Metastatic pattern					
		Spleen			Liver		
Tumor	Days	Incidence	Growth	Weight (mg)	Incidence	Growth	Weight (mg)
Experiment No. 1							
11H11 (LI)	30	2/5	+	175	5/5	++	2290
11H11 (SP)	32	3/3	+++	533	3/3	+++	4366
Experiment No. 2							
11H11 (LI)	24	1/3	−	86	3/3	+	1233
11H11 (SP)	24	4/4	++	262	4/4	++	1725

See legend to Table 5.

by the Hy38 cells only in the lungs (Katzav et al. 1982, De Baetselier et al. 1982). No metastatic nodules were formed in the spleen or liver. Thus, a splenic non-B-lymphocyte parental cell, when somatically hybridized to an NSI hybridoma, generates a hybrid manifesting metastatic competence yet possessing different organ specificity from the B cell hybrids.

SOMATIC CELL FUSION OF AN AKR LYMPHOMA WITH A NONSPLEEN B CELL

The previous experiment suggested that in a somatic hybrid of nonmetastatic neoplastic and normal cells, the normal cell controls the organ specificity of the acquired metastatic property. To test the participation of the neoplastic cell in determining the organ specificity of metastases, we studied a hybridoma produced via somatic fusion between the BW5145 lymphoma and a putative CBA macrophage or dendritic cell. These hybridomas (DCH10) were a gift from Dr. J. Peters (Institute for Biological Research in Cologne, FRG). Following i.v. inoculation into CBA animals, the parental BW lymphoma did not generate metastases. The DCH10 hybridoma cells, however, did produce metastases in the liver (Table 7). Following retransplantation of these metastatic cells from the liver, they generated heavy metastatic masses in the spleen, liver, and kidneys (Table 7). Liver metastases produced by the DCH10 hybridoma cells were morphologically different from the liver metastases produced by the B-cell plasmacytoma hybrids: they followed a diffuse pattern of tumor growth in the liver, distinct from compact nodular growth.

ALTERING CELL SURFACE COMPONENTS ALTERS THE METASTATIC SPREAD OF HYBRIDOMA CELLS

Cell surface molecules seem to be implicated in controlling the metastatic spread, survival, and target organ recognition of neoplastic cells. Studying the Hy hybridomas, in which the lymphocyte partner seemed to have determined the metastatic potential and its target-organ specificity, we attempted to apply

TABLE 7. *Experimental metastases in animals inoculated with macrophage-derived hybridomas DCH10 and DCH-Li*

	Metastatic pattern					
	Spleen		Liver		Kidney	
Tumor	Growth	Weight	Growth	Weight	Growth	Weight
DCH10	−	90	+	1683	−	208
DCH10-Li	+	233	+++	5300	++	350

See legend to Table 5.

agents known to affect lymphocyte traffic and homing properties. We therefore selected for these experiments the Hy2 hybridoma, which produces spleen and liver metastases, and the Hy8 hybridoma, which metastasizes to the liver only.

Cells of these hybridomas were treated with neuraminidase, concanavalin A (Con A), and antibodies directed against the lymphocyte parental H-2 and were subsequently injected into syngeneic recipients. The results (Table 8) indicated that each of the two hybridomas manifesting different organ specificity of metastases was affected differently by the cell surface treatments. Thus, treatment with anti $H\text{-}2^b$ antibodies abolished completely the generation of spleen metastases by the Hy2 hybridomas and severely reduced liver metastases. Neuraminidase and Con A significantly decreased spleen and liver metastases. The latter metastases were affected more markedly by neuraminidase than by Con A. On the other hand, Hy8 cells, metastasizing to the liver only, were not affected by these agents. In fact, anti-$H\text{-}2^b$ antibodies and neuraminidase seemed to increase growth of liver metastases. It thus appears that the homing ability of hybridomas generating spleen and spleen-dependent liver metastases is affected by antibodies directed against the parental lymphocyte H-2, by neuraminidase and Con A, agents that diminish homing of lymphocytes, whereas the homing ability of hybridomas generating liver metastases is affected to a lesser extent.

To what extent does somatic hybridization take place in vivo? Can it determine the acquisition of metastatic properties by nonmetastatic neoplastic cells? Somatic hybridization between tumor and host cells has been reported (Hu and Pasztor 1975), and yet the alterations that occur in such neoplastic cells as a result of the hybridization remain unspecified. An intriguing observation relevant to the problem of metastases was made by Goldenberg et al. (1974), who performed studies on xenotransplantation of human malignant tumors. Generally,

TABLE 8. *Influence of traffic-modulating agents on the organ-specific growth of B cell hybridomas*

		Metastatic pattern			
		Spleen		Liver	
Tumor	Treatment*	Growth†	Weight (mg)	Growth	Weight (mg)
Hy2	None	+++	899	+++	5954
	Concanavalin A	+++	581	+++	3830
	Neuraminidase	+++	524	++	2179
	Anti-$H\text{-}2^b$	–	241	+	1939
Hy8	None	–	131	+	1419
	Concanavalin A	–	192	+	1349
	Neuraminidase		138	++	2038
	Anti-$H\text{-}2^b$	–	248	++	2232

* Cells were pretreated for 30 min. with different reagents, washed, and inoculated i.v.
† Growth = tumor development. See legend to Table 5.

when such tumors are grafted into immune-deficient mouse recipients (nudes), they may grow locally but do not produce metastases. A case in which metastases were generated by a human tumor was reported when hamsters received transplants of the latter cells. The metastatic cells contained hamster chromosomes, thus suggesting that in vivo somatic hybridization had taken place. More recently, Kerbel and his co-workers (1983 and see pages 47 to 79, this volume) reported observations of in vivo somatic hybridization between neoplastic and normal host cells resulting in metastatic tumor cell variants.

ACKNOWLEDGMENTS

This investigation was supported by Grant No. 28139, awarded by the National Cancer Institute, Department of Health and Human Services of the United States, the Hermann and Lilly Schilling Foundation, Essen, FRG, and the Leukemia Research Foundation, Inc., Chicago, Illinois.

REFERENCES

Barski, G., and F. Cornefert. 1962. Characteristics of "hybrid" type clonal cell lines obtained from mixed cultures in vitro. JNCI 28:801–821.

Barski, G., S. Sorieul, and F. Cornefert. 1961. Hybrid type cells in combined cultures of two different mammalian cell strains. JNCI 26:1269–1291.

De Baetselier, P., E. Gorelik, Z. Eshhar, S. Katzav, M. Feldman, and S. Segal. 1981. Metastatic properties conferred on nonmetastatic tumors by hybridization of spleen B lymphocytes with plasmacytoma cells. JNCI 67:1079–1087.

De Baetselier, P., E. Gorelik, Z. Eshhar, Y. Ron, S. Katzav, M. Feldman, and S. Segal. 1982. Organ specific homing of B cell hybridomas, *in* In Vivo Immunology, Nieuwenhuis, van den Broek and Hanna, eds. Plenum Publishing Corp, New York, pp. 179–185.

De Baetselier, P., S. Katzav, E. Gorelik, M. Feldman, and S. Segal. 1980. Differential expression of H-2 gene products in tumor cells is associated with their metastatic properties. Nature 288:179–181.

Fellous, M., U. Nir, D. Wallach, G. Merlin, M. Rubinstein, and M. Revel. 1982. Interferon dependent induction of mRNA for the major histocompatibility antigens in human fibroblasts and lymphoblastoid cells. Proc. Natl. Acad. Sci. USA 79:3082–3086.

Freed, J. H., D. W. Sears, J. L. Brown, and S. G. Nathenson. 1979. Biochemical purification of detergent solubilized H-2 alloantigens. Mol. Immunol. 16:9–21.

Goldenberg, D. M., R. A. Pavia, and M. C. Tsao. 1974. In vivo hybridization of human tumor and normal hamster cells. Nature 250:649–651.

Gorelik, E., S. Segal, and M. Feldman. 1980. Control of lung metastasis progression in mice: Role of growth kinetics of 3LL Lewis lung carcinoma and host immune reactivity. JNCI 65:1217–1264.

Harris, H., O. J. Mimmer, G. Klein, P. Worst, and T. Tachibana. 1969. Suppression of malignancy by cell fusion. Nature 223:363–368.

Hasek, M. and J. Chutna. 1979. Complexity of the state of immunological tolerance. Immunol. Rev. 46:3–26.

Hu, F. and L. M. Pasztor. 1975. In vivo hybridization of cultured melanoma cells and isogenic mouse cells. Differentiation 4:92–97.

Isakov, N., M. Feldman, and S. Segal. 1982. An immune response against the alloantigens of the 3LL Lewis lung carcinoma prevents the growth of lung metastases but not of local allografts. Invasion Metastasis 2:12–32.

Isakov, N., M. Feldman, and S. Segal. 1983. Lewis lung carcinoma cells possess immunogenic $H\text{-}2D^b$ region gene products but lack $H\text{-}2K^b$ region products. JNCI 71:139–147.

Katzav, S., P. De Baetselier, B. Tartakovsky, S. Segal, and M. Feldman. 1982. Immunogenic properties of tumor metastases, *in* B and T Cell Tumors, E. S. Vitetta, ed. Academic Press, New York, pp. 233–245.

Kerbel, R. S., E. A. Lagarde, J. W. Dennis, and T. P. Donaghue. 1983. Spontaneous host cell × tumor cell hybridization in vivo: Contribution to the emergence of metastatic cell variants. Mol. Cell. Biol. 3:523–538.

Klein, G., U. Bregula, F. Wiener, and H. Harris. 1971. The analysis of malignancy by cell fusion. I. Hybrids between tumor cells and L-cell derivatives. J. Cell Sci. 8:659–672.

Miller, S. D., M. S. Sy, and H. N. Claman. 1978. Genetic restriction for the induction of suppressor T cells by hapten-modified lymphoid cells in tolerance to DNFB contact sensitivity. J. Exp. Med. 147:788–799.

Ozato, K, and D. H. Sachs. 1981. Monoclonal antibodies to MHC antigens. Hybridoma antibodies reacting to antigens of $H\text{-}2^b$ haplotype reveal genetic control of isotype expression. J. Immunol. 126:317–321.

Pluznik, D. H. and L. Sachs. 1965. The cloning of normal "mast" cells in tissue culture. J. Cell. Comp. Physiol. 66:319–324.

Schmidt, W., and H. Festenstein. 1982. Resistance to cell mediated cytotoxicity is correlated with reduction of H-2K gene products in AKR leukemia. Immunogenetics 16:257–264.

Segal, S., S. Kingsmore, E. Gorelik, and M. Feldman. 1982. Control by NK cells of the generation of lung metastases by the Lewis lung carcinoma, *in* Current Concepts in Human Immunology and Cancer Immunomodulation, B. Serrou et al., eds. Elsevier Biomedical Press, Amsterdam, pp. 227–234.

Slavin, S., S. Morecki, and L. Weiss. 1980. The role of the spleen in tumor growth kinetics of the murine B cell leukemia (BCL1). J. Immunol. 124:586–589.

Wernet, D., and F. Lilly. 1975. Genetic regulation of the antibody response to $H\text{-}2D^b$ alloantigens in mice. I. Differences in activation of helper T cells in C57BL/10 and BALB/c congenic strains. J. Exp. Med. 141:573–583.

Cancer Invasion and Metastasis: Biologic and Therapeutic Aspects edited by Garth L. Nicolson and Luka Milas. Raven Press, New York © 1984.

Prostaglandins and Metastasis

Dale A. Stringfellow

Cancer Research, Pharmaceutical Research and Development, Bristol Myers Company, Syracuse, New York 13201

Although progress has been made on a variety of fronts in the chemotherapy of human neoplastic diseases, one of the major problems still confronting cancer therapy is the phenomenon of metastasis. Cells are released from a primary tumor site and are distributed to form secondary tumors at distal sites. Once disseminated, the disease is much more difficult to treat. Over the past several years, it has been suggested that prostaglandins may play a role in this metastatic process. One of the first demonstrations was reported by Fitzpatrick and Stringfellow (Fitzpatrick and Stringfellow 1979, Stringfellow and Fitzpatrick 1979). They suggested that prostaglandins released by murine B16 malignant melanoma cells might help modulate metastatic potential.

Prostaglandins are fatty acid metabolites of arachidonic acid (AA) produced by cells (Figure 1). Membrane-bound phospholipids are enzymatically converted by phospholipase to AA. AA can in turn be enzymatically converted by 5- or 12-lipoxygenase to a series of leukotriene or lipoxygenase products or by cyclo-oxygenase to an endoperoxide intermediate. Our discussion in this paper will center on cyclo-oxygenase rather than lipoxygenase products, although the latter may also play a significant role in modulation of cellular function. At any rate, AA is converted enzymatically by cyclo-oxygenase to an endoperoxide intermediate that is in turn enzymatically converted to prostacyclin, thromboxane, or the classic prostaglandins such as PGA, E, F, and Ds. Treatment of cells with a nonsteroidal antiinflammatory agent such as indomethacin or aspirin will block cyclo-oxygenase conversion of AA to endoperoxide and as a result block prostaglandin synthesis in the treated cell.

PROSTAGLANDIN D_2 AND METASTASIS

The initial publications (Fitzpatrick and Stringfellow 1979, Stringfellow and Fitzpatrick 1979) reported an inverse correlation between the ability of murine F_1 and F_{10} malignant melanoma cells (obtained from Isaiah Fidler, National Cancer Institute) to metastasize and their ability to produce prostaglandin D_2 (Figure 2). Stringfellow and Fitzpatrick were surprised with the finding, since most cells studied had not produced prostaglandin D_2 as a major AA metabolite.

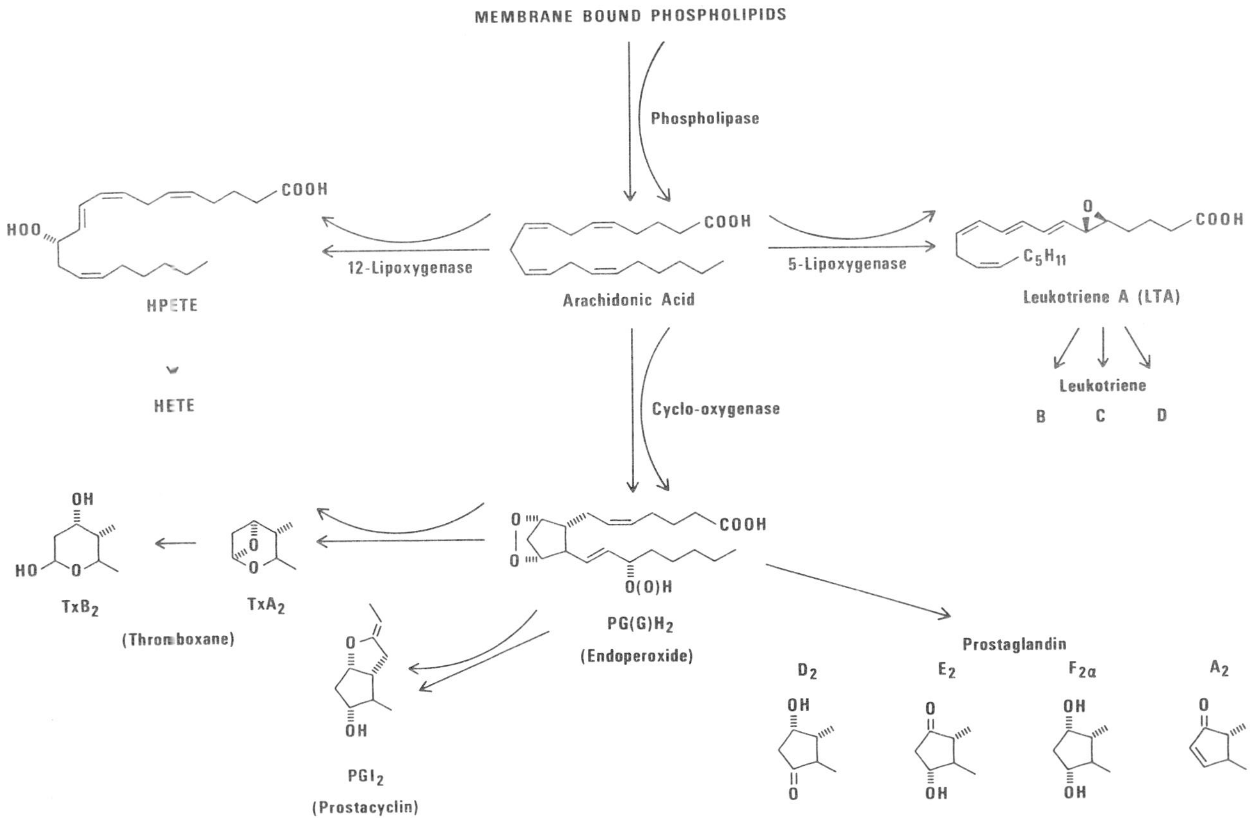

FIG. 1. Arachidonic acid cascade.

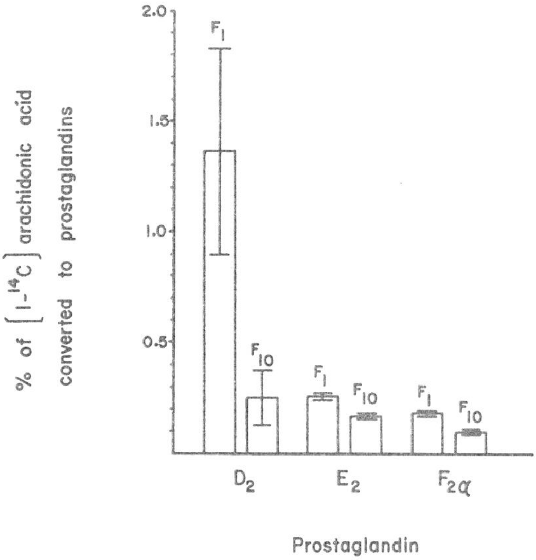

FIG. 2. Quantitative results by radiometric thin-layer chromatography. Under identical conditions, B16 F_1 cells produced significantly more ($P < 0.001$) prostaglandin D_2 than did B16 F_{10} cells. (Reproduced from Fitzpatrick and Stringfellow 1979 with permission.)

Interestingly, the F_1 cell that was less metastatic produced six times more prostaglandin D_2 than did the more metastatic F_{10} cell. Since platelet adhesion to tumor cells had been implicated in the metastatic process and since prostaglandin D_2 can inhibit the aggregation of platelets, Stringfellow and Fitzpatrick (1979) postulated that the prostaglandin D_2 being released by the F_1 cells might inhibit the adhesion of platelets to the surface of the tumor cell, thereby reducing its metastatic potential.

To investigate this possibility, Stringfellow and Fitzpatrick cultured both F_1 and F_{10} malignant melanoma cells to 70% confluency and treated these cells in vitro with indomethacin at a concentration of 5 μg/ml (which was not cytotoxic to the cell but did block cyclo-oxygenase activity, thereby inhibiting the release of prostaglandins by the melanoma cell). After a 2-h in vitro treatment with indomethacin, the cells were rinsed thoroughly to remove any extracellular indomethacin, suspended as a single-cell suspension, and promptly injected i.v. into C57 black mice. Stringfellow and Fitzpatrick (1979) reported that in vitro treatment of the F_1 cells with indomethacin strikingly enhanced the metastatic rate of the F_1 cells but did not have a significant effect on the metastatic rate of the F_{10} cells (Table 1). This again suggested that the prostaglandin D_2 being produced by F_1 cells might be involved in controlling metastasis.

To further explore this possibility, the F_1 and F_{10} cells were again treated in vitro with indomethacin, the indomethacin was rinsed from the cells, and

TABLE 1. *Prostaglandin D_2 and indomethacin treatment of B16 cells*

	F_{10} control	F_{10} + INDO	F_{10} + INDO + D_2	F_1 control	F_1 + INDO	F_1 + INDO + D_2
	10*	11	2	0	12	1
	11	12	1	0	10	2
	18	9	0	0	16	0
	7	10	2	0	9	4
	11	13	1	0	6	0
	8	7	0	3	2	2
	7	12	1	1	15	7
	16	6	1	0	13	4
	12	3	0	1	8	12
	10	5	2	1	6	5
Mean ± SEM	11.0 ± 1.15	8.8 ± 1.07	1.0 ± 0.26	0.6 ± 0.31	9.7 ± 1.39	3.7 ± 1.16

F_1 and F_{10} cells incubated at 37°C for 2 h with 5 μg/ml indomethacin (INDO). These were thoroughly rinsed, suspended as single-cell suspensions, and injected i.v. at ~2×10^4 cells. Prostaglandin D_2 (D_2) (2 mg/kg) was injected either i.p. or i.v. at time of cell injection.
* Number of metastatic nodules/lung.

these cells were injected i.v. into mice with and without added prostaglandin D_2 (2 mg/kg i.v.). The enhanced metastatic rate of F_1 cells that had been treated with indomethacin reverted to the more normal control F_1 rate, and the metastatic rate of F_{10} cells that did not normally produce as much prostaglandin D_2 was decreased by coadministration of prostaglandin D_2. These results suggest that prostaglandin D_2 normally produced by the F_1 but not the F_{10} cells played a role in their rate of metastasis. Soon after the report of Stringfellow and Fitzpatrick, Honn et al. (1981) demonstrated that other prostaglandins that reduce platelet aggregation, such as prostacyclin, also reduced the metastatic rate of malignant melanoma cells, further implicating platelet aggregation in the metastatic process.

OTHER HOST DEFENSES

There are other potential explanations for the results of Stringfellow and Fitzpatrick (1979) and Honn et al. (1981), including the modulation of host defenses or regulatory mechanisms that control metastasis, which might also be affected by prostaglandins. For example, Schultz (1980) has reported that prostaglandins can reverse the tumoricidal activity of activated macrophages. This suggests that prostaglandins produced by tumor cells may enable tumor cells to evade host defense mechanisms such as macrophages. Likewise, a number of other researchers (Brunda et al. 1980, Muscoplat et al. 1979, Taffett and Russell 1961, DiRosa and Parente 1980, Ferreira and Vane 1974) have reported that prostaglandins released by tumor cells may act as immunosuppressants and inhibit the ability of the host to mount a cellular or humoral immune response against the invading cell.

These reports led us to explore what effect the prostaglandins released by the F_1 and F_{10} tumor cells might have on host defense mechanisms. We initially turned our attention to an in vitro assay of the ability of peritoneal macrophages harvested from animals to kill F_1 and F_{10} target cells in vitro. The data are summarized in Table 2. In these studies macrophages were harvested from *Corynebacterium parvum*-treated animals and control animals that had not previously been treated. *C. parvum* was injected seven days before macrophage harvest. The macrophages harvested from *C. parvum*-treated mice had previously been demonstrated to be more cytotoxic for tumor cells than macrophages harvested from control animals (Stringfellow et al. 1978), as summarized in Table 2. However, the F_{10} target cells were more sensitive to the cytotoxicity of the macrophages than were the F_1 cells. Since prostaglandins have been reported to block macrophage or NK cell killing of tumor cells, then the prostaglandin D_2 being produced by the F_1 cells may have reduced macrophage cytotoxicity, thus explaining the difference in sensitivity.

To explore this possibility, we treated F_1 and F_{10} target cells with aspirin and indomethacin for 2 h in vitro, rinsed the cyclo-oxygenase inhibitors from the cells, and used the cells as targets in the in vitro tumoricidal assay. Treatment with aspirin or indomethacin enhanced F_1 but not F_{10} cell susceptibility to macrophage cytotoxicity, suggesting that indeed prostaglandins being released by the F_1 cells might have reduced macrophage killing. This suggestion was further strengthened by results from studies in which exogenously added prostaglandin D_2 significantly reduced the ability of macrophages to kill both F_1 and F_{10} target cells.

The preceding results led to a series of studies aimed at determining if naturally occurring mediators of host defense mechanisms such as interferons or interleukins would play a regulatory role in cellular metastasis and whether the metastasis rate might actually be controlled by them. As summarized in Table 3, murine interferon did significantly reduce the metastasis rate of F_{10} malignant melanoma cells but had relatively little effect on F_1 melanoma cells. Prostaglandin D_2

TABLE 2. *Percent cytotoxicity of murine peritoneal macrophages for F_1 and F_{10} B16 target cells in vitro*

	F_1		F_{10}	
Treatment	C. parvum	Controls	C. parvum	Controls
Control	28	10	58	21
INDO	40	11	60	5
ASP	57	7	49	13
PGD_2	11	11	23	10

Percent cytotoxicity (at 72 h) of peritoneal macrophages for F_1 and F_{10} target cells treated with minimum essential medium (control), indomethacin (INDO) (2 μg/ml) or aspirin (ASP) (20 μg/ml). Prostaglandin D_2 (PGD_2) (1 μg/ml) added at time of macrophage addition.

TABLE 3. *Interferons and regulation of cellular metastasis through endogenous regulation of arachidonic acid cascade*

	Murine interferon*		Control	
	F_{10}	F_1	F_{10}	F_1
	8†	1	10	1
	6	0	23	0
	0	0	18	0
	11	0	22	1
	3	1	17	2
	0	0	21	0
	1	2	6	2
	3	0	12	0
	0	1	19	1
	5	0	13	1
Mean	3.7	0.5	16.1	0.8

* 100 u/ml.

† Number of metastatic nodules/lung.

Interferon treatment increased the levels of prostaglandin D_2 produced by F_{10} cells from 0.2 ng/10^6 cells to 1.3 ng/10^6 cells.

F_1 cells were increased from 0.8 ng/10^6 cells to 1.2 ng/10^6 cells.

production was significantly enhanced in F_{10} cells that had been exposed to interferon. Control F_{10} cells that made 0.2 ng prostaglandin D_2 per 10^6 cells produced 1.3 ng of prostaglandin D_2 per 10^6 cells after being exposed to interferon. The enhancement of prostaglandin D_2 production by F_1 cells was not as great, it's being a twofold increase (from 1.0 to 1.8 ng/10^6 cells).

These findings were similar to those reported by Fitzpatrick and Stringfellow (1980); they demonstrated that the increased prostaglandin production by cells in response to interferon was nearly ubiquitous. To determine if the enhanced levels of prostaglandin D_2 being produced by the F_{10} cell was responsible for the antimetastatic effect of interferon treatment, F_{10} cells were cultured in vitro and treated with indomethacin (2 h at 37°C, 2 μg/ml), interferon (100 u/ml), and interferon with indomethacin together. The theory was that if interferon's antimetastatic effect was mediated by increased prostaglandin D_2 production, then indomethacin blockage of that prostaglandin D_2 production would reduce interferon's antimetastatic effect. Results from these studies are presented in Table 4. Treatment of cells in vitro with indomethacin did block the antimetastatic activity of interferon, further suggesting that it was an AA metabolite (prostaglandin D_2) produced by the F_{10} cells after exposure to interferon that mediated the antimetastatic effect.

To determine whether the in vitro effect on F_{10} cells could be produced by in vivo treatment, animals were injected i.v. with 2×10^4 F_{10} B16 cells and were immediately begun on twice-daily treatment with interferons (5×10^5

TABLE 4. *In vitro effect of indomethacin on interferon-decreased metastasis*

	Control	INDO	INF	INF + INDO
	12*	15	1	12
	15	8	5	8
	23	11	0	11
	7	13	3	17
	20	10	2	8
	19	12	0	17
	8	19	1	21
	12	26	0	12
	29	17	2	8
	11	19	1	13
Mean	15.6	15.0	1.5	12.7

F_{10} cells incubated with indomethacin (INDO) (2 μg/ml) or placebo for 2 h prior to exposure to interferon (INF) (murine, specific activity of 5 × 10^7 units/mg protein) for 2 h just prior to i.v. injection of F_{10} cells.

* Number of metastatic nodules/lung.

u/day) and indomethacin (1 mg/kg/day). In these studies, animals were treated with indomethacin alone, interferon alone, or interferon and indomethacin (Table 5). Again, in vivo treatment of mice with interferon significantly reduced the metastatic activity of the F_{10} cells. However, indomethacin did not have as dramatic an effect in vivo as it had in vitro on blocking the antimetastatic activity of interferons. This may be due to the other effects of interferon on host defense mechanisms such as activation of macrophages and T-cell cytotoxicity, which would reduce metastasis rather than increase it.

Stringfellow and Brideau (1983) previously demonstrated that in vivo and

TABLE 5. *In vivo evaluation of the antimetastatic activity of interferon and indomethacin*

	Control	INDO	INF	INF + INDO
	23*	20	11	20
	36	42	7	17
	27	38	5	13
	13	17	21	11
	21	12	7	17
	15	11	3	16
	29	15	12	7
	11	21	8	12
	17	12	15	5
	18	28	0	9
Mean	21.0	21.6	8.9	12.7

Animals treated twice daily with interferon (INF) (5 × 10^5 units/mouse/day) and indomethacin (INDO) (1 mg/kg/day) beginning immediately after F_{10} injection.

* Number of metastatic nodules/lung.

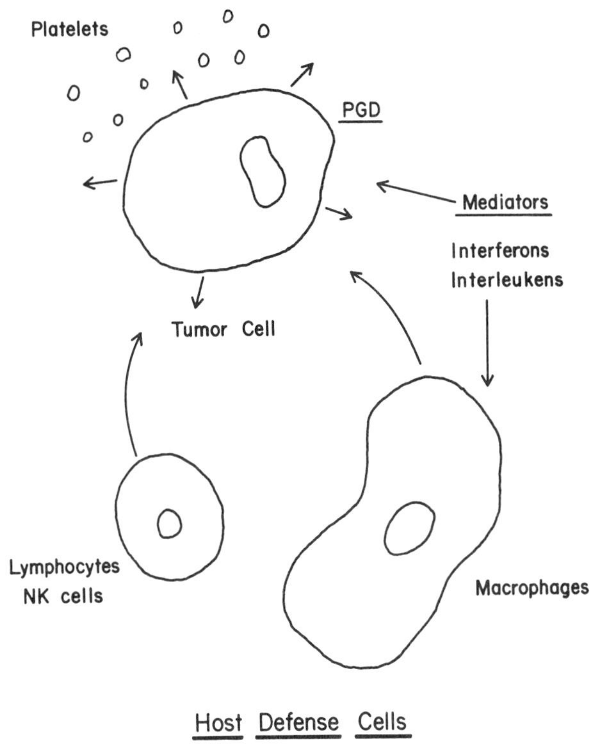

FIG. 3. Prostaglandins produced by metastasizing tumor cells. (1) Affect platelet adhesion to tumor cells and probably modulate adhesion of tumor cells to endothelial lining. (2) Host defense cells which would normally clear invading tumor cells may be counter-regulated by PGs produced by tumor cells, allowing the tumor cells to be sequestered and establish metastatic foci. (3) Other natural modulators of cell function such as interferons and interleukins may not only activate host defense mechanisms such as NK cell and macrophage tumoricidal activity but also appear to enforce the PG production by B16 tumor cells, which may counter-regulate or turn off host defenses and may affect cellular adhesion and platelet aggregation.

in vitro macrophage activation by interferon is not blocked by indomethacin. Therefore, the inability of indomethacin to block the interferon response may not be due to an effect on the tumor cell but may be more of a reflection of the other effects of interferon on host defense mechanisms, including elimination of tumor cells at the metastatic site by cells of the reticuloendothelial system such as macrophages. This suggests that reducing or controlling metastasis in the animal is not a simple phenomenon. It is a complex interplay, apparently between platelets and other host defense mechanisms, including macrophages, NK cells, and lymphocytes (Figure 3).

SUMMARY

The data presented suggest that F_1 and F_{10} cells display an inverse relationship between their levels of metastasis and prostaglandin D_2 production. Prostaglandin D_2 was able to reduce in vitro aggregation of platelets from C57 black mice. Other prostaglandins that decreased platelet aggregation such as prostacyclin also reduced the metastatic rate. Prostaglandin D_2 also reduced macrophage cytotoxicity for B16 target cells in vitro. Interferons stimulated prostaglandin D_2 synthesis in F_{10} cells and reduced lung metastasis.

F_{10} metastasis was not blocked by interferon to the same extent by in vivo treatment as it had been in vitro, suggesting that interferons and other modulators of cell function have broader activity in vivo than simply increasing the level of prostaglandins being produced by metastatic cells. Metastasis can therefore be viewed as being modulated in vivo by several mechanisms that may include platelet aggregation and elimination of metastasized cells by host defenses such as macrophages. Prostaglandins and other naturally occurring modulators of host resistance, such as interferons, appear to affect the metastatic rate of tumor cells. Although prostaglandin D_2 is not a common major AA product of most cells and therefore may not operate in all cell systems, the B16 cells may provide a system to address the importance of these mediators and mechanisms in the metastatic process.

REFERENCES

Brunda, M. J., R. B. Herberman, and H. T. Holden. 1980. Inhibition of murine natural killer cell activity by prostaglandins. J. Immunol. 124:2682–2687.

DiRosa, M., and L. Parente. 1980. Prostaglandins and inflammation. Mater. Medica Polona 3:187–194.

Ferreira, S. H., and J. R. Vane. 1974. New aspects of the mode of action of non-steroidal anti-inflammatory drugs. Annu. Rev. Pharmacol. 14:57–73.

Fitzpatrick, F. A., and D. A. Stringfellow. 1979. Prostaglandin D_2 formation by malignant melanoma cells correlates with their metastatic potential. Proc. Natl. Acad. Sci. USA 76:1765–1769.

Fitzpatrick, F. A., and D. A. Stringfellow. 1980. Virus and interferon effects on cellular prostaglandin biosynthesis. J. Immunol. 125:431–437.

Honn, K. V., B. Cicone, and A. Skoff. 1981. Prostacycline: a potent antimetastatic agent. Science 212:1270–1272.

Muscoplat, C. C., D. J. Klausner, C. J. Brunner, E. D. Sloane, and D. W. Johnson. 1979. Regulation of mitogen and antigen stimulated lymphocyte blastogenesis by prostaglandins. Infec. Immun. 26:311–315.

Schultz, R. M. 1980. E-type prostaglandins and interferons: Yen-yang modulation of macrophage tumoricidal activity. Med. Hypotheses 6:831–843.

Stringfellow, D. A., and R. Brideau. 1983. Prostaglandins and interferons in inflammation, *in* Interferons, N. Finter, ed. North Holland Publications, Amsterdam, (in press).

Stringfellow, D. A., and F. A. Fitzpatrick. 1979. Prostaglandin D_2 controls pulmonary metastasis of malignant melanoma cells. Nature 282:76–78.

Stringfellow, D. A., F. A. Fitzpatrick, F. F. Sun, and J. C. McGuire. 1978. Prostacyclin and thromboxane biosynthesis in activated, stimulated, and normal peritoneal cell populations. Prostaglandins 16:901–910.

Taffett, S. M., and S. W. Russell. 1981. Macrophage mediated tumor cell killing: Regulation of expression of cytolytic activity by prostaglandin E. J. Immunol. 127:121–124.

Cancer Invasion and Metastasis: Biologic and Therapeutic Aspects edited by Garth L. Nicolson and Luka Milas. Raven Press, New York © 1984.

Tumor Cell Hybridization and Neoplastic Progression

Ian R. Hart

Cancer Metastasis and Treatment Laboratory, NCI-Frederick Cancer Research Facility, Frederick, Maryland 21701

Neoplasms are not collections of identical cells, nor are they static entities in which the qualities and characteristics of later growth periods are indistinguishable from those exhibited during initial development. Rather, it might be said that a universal characteristic of tumors is a quite remarkable degree of diversity. This diversity is both a consequence of and a controlling factor in the other general characteristic of tumors, which is their dynamic evolution. Foulds (1969) termed this acquisition of different behavioral characteristics tumor progression and defined it as "the development of a tumor by way of permanent irreversible qualitative change in one or more of the characters of its cells."

Tumor progression is said to be subject to six general principles: (1) Multiple tumors progress independently; thus, no two tumors, whether in the same or different hosts, evolve at the same rate. (2) Different characteristics progress independently. (3) Progression is independent of growth, so even small, slow-growing neoplasms can show considerable evolution and change. (4) Progression can be either continuous or discontinuous (meaning that it could be due to discrete steps). (5) Progression follows one of the alternative paths of development. (6) Progression does not always reach an end point within the lifetime of the host.

This scenario of tumor development and evolution has become widely accepted, and Nowell (1976) has suggested that such tumor progression is caused by the inherent genetic instability of neoplastic cells coupled with the selection pressures exerted by the host. Thus, mutant subpopulations are continually being produced by the genetically unstable tumor cells. Most of these subpopulations are eliminated, possibly because of immunologic or metabolic disadvantage, whereas those cells that survive host selection pressure manifest their increased survival capacity by displaying increasingly malignant (metastatic) behavior. The unpredictable nature of these mutational events, coupled with the vagaries of host and intralesional selection pressures, ensures that rates of tumor progression are unique for individual tumors (Dexter and Calabresi 1982). It should be stressed that such a mechanism also allows for tumor progression to a less, as well as a more, malignant state. While paraphrasing Peyton Rous and indicating that generally tumors do "go from bad to worse," Foulds (1969) stressed that overemphasis had been placed on the progression of tumors from "benign" to "malignant" and indicated that "relentless progressive growth to a fatal ending is by no means an invariable characteristic of malignant neoplasia." Thus, any mechanism of tumor progression must be capable of generating less-malignant neoplasms, as well as more-malignant ones.

Recent interest, as can be gathered from many of the other chapters in this volume, has centered on the diversity of the metastatic phenotype in cells of clonal origin (Fidler and Kripke 1977) and on the role that such clonal populations may play in regulating one another (Poste et al. 1981). There is a tendency to think of neoplastic growth as being an expression of chaos or anarchy at the cellular level; this is not so. Many tumors, even highly malignant ones, retain a high degree of differentiation and specialized function, and there is now increasing evidence to suggest that the clonal populations of such tumors do not behave in completely autonomous fashion but are capable of exerting an effect on each other to modify their metastatic behavior (Poste et al. 1981), their tumor-forming capacities and growth rates (Woodruff et al. 1982), and their responses to antineoplastic drugs (Miller et al. 1981). Thus, interactions between various clones of tumor cells closely, or even distantly, apposed within the developing tumor mass may serve to modulate the degree and rate of tumor progression. What role does this polyclonality play in neoplastic progression and how might it modify tumor development? One proposed mechanism by which tumors evolve is somatic cell hybridization (Goldenberg et al. 1974), a process that can be affected drastically by the nature of the cell types involved in the fusion.

SOMATIC CELL HYBRIDIZATION AND TUMOR PROGRESSION

A considerable body of literature shows that fusion between cells does occur in experimentally transplanted tumors; furthermore, there is some strong circumstantial evidence to suggest that such a phenomenon also takes place in naturally occurring human neoplasms (Atkin 1979). Goldenberg and his colleagues (Goldenberg et al. 1971, 1974), using chromosomes and isoenzymes as markers, unequivocally showed that implantation of a human tumor into hamster cheek pouches resulted in hybridization of human tumor and normal hamster cells. These workers proposed that such in vivo hybridization in xenogeneic, and possibly isogeneic, systems was a possible mechanism by which tumor cells could progress to more-advanced states of malignancy as manifested by increased invasive and metastatic capacities (Goldenberg et al. 1974).

Such a phenomenon is not unique to this system, as shown by studies in which biochemically marked murine tumor cells were implanted into mice (Wiener et al. 1972, Ber et al. 1978). Fusion of mouse tumor cells with host cells was shown to be a common event that might be responsible for increasing the genetic variation in the growing cell population (Wiener et al. 1972). Later studies, in which radiation-induced chimeras were used as tumor bearers, showed that the presumptive host cell involved in the fusion was of bone marrow origin and probably was a macrophage (Wiener et al. 1974a, 1976). Unfortunately, these hybrids were not recovered and subsequently tested for their tumorigenic and metastatic behavior, and so there is no way to evaluate the direction in which tumor progression had evolved as a result of hybridization. However, the major emphasis in these studies and in many others (see for example Kerbel et al. 1983, pages 47–79, this volume) has been on fusion between neoplastic cells and the normal infiltrating host cells that may comprise a large portion of tumor mass.

Somatic hybridization of normal host cells with neoplastic cells has been used in numerous studies to try to identify chromosomes or genes involved in the suppression or expression of neoplastic capacity. Conflicting results have been obtained from this type of experiment. The neoplastic trait originally appeared to be dominant (Barski et al. 1961, Barski and Belehradek 1979), but now most experimental results seem to indicate that in hybrids between normal and neoplastic cells, the tumor-forming capacity of the latter are suppressed (Harris et al. 1969, Wiener et al. 1974b, Evans et al. 1982, Stanbridge 1976, Stanbridge et al. 1981). Tumorigenic hybrid lines, when they arise, are thought to do so by chromosomal segregation and the loss of specific suppressor chromosomes (Harris 1971, Stanbridge et al. 1981). This suppression of the in vivo growth capacity of tumorigenic lines has often been referred to as "suppression of malignancy" (Wiener et al. 1971, 1974b, Harris 1971, Evans et al. 1982), but, as has been pointed out recently, the observed effects correlate poorly with malignancy as defined by invasion and metastasis (Watkins et al. 1982).

More recently, the metastatic capacity of hybrids between malignant and normal cells has been assessed in a few model systems, and it has been proposed that fusion of neoplastic cells with certain types of host cells may actually enhance the metastatic capacity of resultant hybrids by conferring the normal cell's special properties on these fusions (De Baetselier et al. 1981, Kerbel et al. 1982). This outcome presumably is more compatible with the mechanisms and direction of tumor progression as originally envisaged and proposed by Goldenberg et al. (1974).

Compared with the relatively large body of literature on hybridization between tumor cells and host cells, there is little information on fusions between tumor cells and tumor cells. Somatic cell hybrids composed of different-parent neoplastic cells have been shown to retain their tumorigenic capacity (Wiener et al. 1973) and even to increase their malignant behavior (Watkins et al. 1982). There is evidence to suggest that such an event can occur in vivo within artificially mixed populations of tumor cells (Janzen et al. 1971) or even in naturally occurring human cancers (Neville and Symington 1966). These considerations have prompted me to attempt to determine whether such an event occurs in the experimental models used in our laboratory. Furthermore, given the polyclonal composition of tumors alluded to in the introduction to this chapter, I was interested to learn the outcome of fusions between tumor cells of different metastatic capacity and how such occurrences might relate to the phenomenon of tumor progression.

IN VIVO TUMOR CELL–TUMOR CELL HYBRIDIZATION IN B16 MELANOMA

The ability of B16 melanoma cells to fuse in vivo was analyzed by using wild-type B16-F10 cells (Fidler 1973) and the so-called universal fuser B16-F10 line bearing a dominant and a recessive marker. This line, designated B16-F10^{RR}, was mutagenized with ethylmethanesulfonate (EMS) and subsequently selected for resistance to ouabain (3 mM) and 6-thioguanine (10 μg/ml). The experimental metastatic capacity of these tumor cells was determined by counting the number of lung nodules that formed 3 weeks after the i.v. injection of 5×10^4 viable cells into syngeneic C57BL/6 mice. Results showed that the B16-F10^{RR} cells were metastatic, producing a median number of 96 lung tumor nodules (range, 14–178).

Groups of mice were then injected i.v., i.p., and s.c. with different numbers of B16-F10^{RR} cells. At various times thereafter, recipient animals were killed, tumors were recovered and dissociated with collagenase, and aliquots of 5×10^4 cells were plated into replicate 100-mm Petri dishes containing medium with 3 mM of ouabain plus 10 μg 6-thioguanine per milliliter or into dishes containing 3 mM of ouabain plus HAT (hypoxanthine, aminopterin, thymidine) medium. Because the B16-F10^{RR} cells bear both a dominant (ouabain) and recessive [6-thioguanine resistance because of lack of hypoxanthine phosphoribosyl transferase (HPRT) activity] marker, any fusions between tumor cells and normal cells should be recovered in the 3 mM ouabain plus HAT medium (Ber et al. 1978). I screened more than 7×10^6 tumor cells in several experiments and was unable to detect any tumor cell–host cell hybrids in this tumor system, regardless of whether the tumor was growing s.c. in the flank, in the abdominal cavity, or in the lung. Plating behavior of the B16-F10^{RR} cells clearly showed that in vivo growth under nonselective conditions for up to 12 weeks failed to alter the phenotypes of these cells, which retained their resistance to 3 mM ouabain and 10 μg/ml 6-thioguanine. I concluded from these results that the rate of in vivo hybridization between tumor and host cells was almost negligible in this B16 melanoma tumor.

Very different results were obtained when B16-F10^{RR} cells were admixed with B16-F10 cells in a 1:9 ratio and the mixed tumor cell population was injected s.c. into the flanks of C57BL/6 mice. Each mouse received a final tumor cell inoculum of 1×10^4 BL6-F10^{RR} cells and 9×10^4 B16-F10 cells. The tumor was allowed to grow until it achieved an approximate size of 1×1 cm (5–6 weeks postinjection). It was then removed and subjected to collagenase dissociation, and 5×10^4 viable cells were plated into replicate culture dishes containing

3 mM of ouabain plus HAT medium. Control animals were injected with an inoculum of either 1×10^5 B16-F10 cells alone or B16-F10^{RR} cells alone, and the resultant tumors were then treated in exactly the same fashion.

The results obtained in this experiment are presented in Table 1. Whereas no tumor cell colonies were obtained in the selective medium when both of the unmixed cell populations were analyzed, a mean number of resistant colonies varying from 2.5 to 24 per dish were obtained from the three mice bearing growths established from the mixed populations of tumor cells (Table 1). The frequency of presumptive fusions was less than 6×10^{-5} cells for the unmixed populations, but it ranged from 2.1×10^{-3} to 2×10^{-4} cells for the mixed populations. Cells growing in replicate dishes from mice 7 and 8 were prepared for karyotype analysis; the mean number of chromosomes counted in 20 individual metaphase spreads are presented in Table 2. As can be seen, the mean number of chromosomes obtained in the presumptive fusions was very close to the sum of the mean chromosomal content of the two separate tumor cell lines. The apparent infrequency (less than 7×10^{-6} cells detected) of fusions between host cells and tumor cells in this model system and the chromosomal content of the resistant colonies provide preliminary evidence that fusion between tumor cells does occur at a low but detectable level.

To determine the likely outcome of hybridization in terms of general tumor evolution and progression, I conducted studies with the B16-F10^{RR} line and a

TABLE 1. *Plating behavior of neoplastic cells recovered from subcutaneous tumors*

Cell line	Mouse	No. colonies* (3 mM ouabain + HAT)	Mean no. colonies
B16-F10	1	0, 0, 0, 0	0
	2	0, 0, 0, 0	0
	3	0, 0, 0, 0	0
B16-F10^{RR}	4	0, 0, 0, 0	0
	5	0, 0, 0, 0	0
	6	0, 0, 0, 0	0
B16-F10 + B16-F10^{RR}	7	6, 6, 0, 0, 1, 2	2.5
	8	1, 5, 5, 8, 8, 12	6.5
	9	9, 22, 26, 27, 31, 31	24

* 5×10^4 viable tumor cells were plated into each dish.

TABLE 2. *Karyotypes of recovered cell lines*

Cell line	Mean no. chromosomes* (± SD)
B16-F10	69 ± 4
B16-F10^{RR}	64 ± 5
B16-F10 + B16-F10^{RR}	127 ± 15

* Counts on minimum of 20 metaphase spreads.

UV-2237RR universal fuser line that is also resistant to ouabain and 6-thioguanine. These two universal fuser lines were fused with a variety of other murine cell lines syngeneic to C57BL/6 or C3H/HeN$^-$ mice, and the resulting hybrids were selected in 3 mM ouabain plus HAT medium. The hybrid nature of the recovered colonies was confirmed by karyotype analysis, and the tumorigenic and metastatic behavior of independently derived hybrids and their parent lines was assessed by the s.c. and i.v. injection of viable cells into (C57BL/6 × C3H/HeN)F_1 hybrid mice (B6C3F1) or 3-week-old nude mice.

The behavior of the parent cell types is summarized in Table 3. The B16-F10, B16-F10RR, and UV-2237 lines are known to be metastatic because they all form s.c. tumors within 6 weeks after the injection of 1×10^5 viable cells and because they give rise to grossly apparent and quantifiable lung nodules 3 weeks after i.v. injection. Clone 16 of the K-1735 melanoma is a benign tumor that forms s.c. tumors after s.c. implantation but does not give rise to pulmonary nodules after i.v. injection. The C3H embryo fibroblasts are normal and do not give rise to tumors at either the subcutaneous or lung site. The UV-2237RR cells were not metastatic or even tumorigenic when injected into immunocompetent B6C3F1 mice, but were highly malignant by both criteria when injected into immunodeficient animals such as nude mice and ATX (adult thymectomized, X-irradiated) mice. The behavior of this cell line, which had been mutagenized with EMS prior to selection, seems analogous to that of the so-called tum$^-$ variants of Boon (Boon and Kellerman 1976, Boon and Van Pel 1978, Van Pel et al. 1979), which were also obtained following mutagenesis and cloning; the UV-2237RR line may have major immunologic alterations that make it strongly immunogenic.

The in vivo behavior of a number of independently derived hybrids is summarized in Tables 4 and 5. There appears to be a distinct pattern of behavior of

TABLE 3. *In vivo behavior of tumor cell lines*

Cell line	Median no. chromosomes	Nude mice*: Median no. lung nodules (range)†	Nude mice*: Tumor (s.c.)	B6C3F1 mice: Median no. lung nodules (range)†	B6C3F1 mice: Tumor (s.c.)
B16-F10	09	> 300	5/5	> 300	5/5
B16-F10RR	64	238 (2–316)	5/5	201 (100–> 300)	5/5
UV-2237	42	64 (1–123)	5/5	4 (0–12)	4/5
UV-2237RR	37	60 (1–158)	5/5	0	0/5
K-1735-clone 16	40	0	5/5	0	4/5
C3H fibroblasts	69	0	0/5	0	0/5

* 1×10^5 viable tumor cells in 0.2 ml of phosphate-buffered saline injected i.v. or s.c. Tumor nodules in lungs were counted 3 weeks later.

† Lung nodules reported are medians from ten mice per group.

TABLE 4. *In vivo behavior of hybrid cell lines*

Cell line	Median no. chromosomes	Nude mice: Median no. lung nodules (range)	Nude mice: Tumor (s.c.)	B6C3F1 mice: Median no. lung nodules (range)	B6C3F1 mice: Tumor (s.c.)
B16-F10^{RR} × B16-F10-1	126	> 400	5/5	282 (35–> 400)	5/5
B16-F10^{RR} × B16-F10-2	105	372 (5–>400)	5/5	159 (17–378)	5/5
B16-F10^{RR} × Cl 16–1	128	46 (9–300)	5/5	109 (9–294)	5/5
B16-F10^{RR} × Cl 16–2	97	> 300	5/5	224 (12–> 300)	5/5
B16-F10^{RR} × Cl 16–3	96	300 (41–> 300)	4/4	259 (22–> 300)	4/4
B16-F10^{RR} × UV-2237-1	N.D.	259 (146–> 400)	5/5	18 (0–31)	5/5
B16-F10^{RR} × UV-2237-2	N.D.	84 (20–187)	N.D.	N.D.	N.D.
B16-F10^{RR} × C3H-1	97	2 (0–72)	4/5	3 (0–11)	6/10
B16-F10^{RR} × C3H-2	90	0 (0–1)	4/5	0	5/5

N.D. = no data.

the hybrids that is independent of the histologic nature of the tumors involved. Fusion between metastatic tumor cells results in hybrids that, not unexpectedly, are comparably metastatic. Thus, hybrids between B16-F10^{RR} and B16-F10, between UV-2237^{RR} and B16-F10, and between UV-2237^{RR} and UV-2237 are all tumorigenic and show metastatic capacity as evaluated by the lung-colony-forming assay. This expression of metastatic capacity is dominant in both immunocompetent and immunodeficient nude mice, even when the presumptively highly immunogenic UV-2237^{RR} line is one of the parent cell types involved in hybrid formation (Table 5). Hybridization between metastatic cells and nonmetastatic, tumorigenic cells results in progression in the malignant behavior of the hybrid cells since metastatic capacity is fully expressed. Three independently derived clones of hybrids resulting from the fusion of B16-F10^{RR} and K-1735-clone 16 cells are all tumorigenic in the s.c. site and highly metastatic as assayed by the ability to form metastases in the lung after their i.v. injection (Table 4). Fusion between two tumorigenic, but nonmetastatic, lines appears to be capable of generating more-malignant cells, as shown by the behavior of the cells derived from the hybridization of UV-2237^{RR} and K-1735-clone 16

TABLE 5. *In vivo behavior of hybrid cell lines*

		Nude mice		B6C3F1 mice	
Cell line	Median no. chromosomes	Median no. lung nodules (range)	Tumor (s.c.)	Median no. lung nodules (range)	Tumor (s.c.)
UV-2237^{RR} × B16-F10	98	149 (0–>400)	5/5	>400	5/5
UV-2237^{RR} × UV-2237-1	73	23 (0–85)	4/4	34 (1–79)	3/4
UV-2237^{RR} × UV-2237-2	75	94 (41–132)	5/5	3 (0–9)	3/5
UV-2237^{RR} × C1-16	97	98 (0–>300)	5/5	33 (4–86)	2/5
UV-2237^{RR} × C3H-1	96	0	2/5	0	0/5
UV-2237^{RR} × C3H-2	97	0	3/5	0	0/5

in immunocompetent B6C3F1 mice. Although neither of the parent cell types is able to produce lung nodules in these animals (Table 3), the progeny of the fusion between them is quite metastatic: 1×10^5 cells injected i.v. give rise to a median of 33 lung nodules 3 weeks later (Table 5). Finally, the cells derived from the fusion of metastatic and normal cells show a suppression of metastatic capacity (B16-F10^{RR} × C3H fibroblasts in B6C3F1 and nude mice; UV-2237^{RR} × C3H fibroblasts in nude mice) but not tumorigenic capacity, as determined by their ability to form progressively growing tumors in the s.c. site.

SUMMARY AND CONCLUSIONS

In the experiments reported here, I was unable to detect any fusion between host cells and transplanted tumor cells; however, spontaneous hybridization between tumor cells appears to occur in the B16 melanoma. This hybridization was demonstrated by mixing together B16-F10^{RR} cells (universal fusers) and B16-F10 cells, allowing them to grow in close juxtaposition, and recovering putative hybrids in the appropriate selection media. The tumor cell–tumor cell composition of the resultant hybrids is inferred from the relative frequency of fusions, compared with the infrequency of tumor cell–host cell fusion when single populations of B16-F10^{RR} cells were used, and by the chromosomal content of the hybrids. Definitive proof that hybridization occurs between both types of tumor cell rather than between a tumor cell and some other type of cell would require the use of a third biochemical marker on the unmarked tumor cells. I am now repeating these experiments using B16-F10 cells that exhibit resistance to the neomycinlike antibiotic G418. Nonetheless, it is not surprising to find that such closely related tumor cells fuse with one another. The efficiency of in vitro hybridization mediated by polyethylene glycol is increased when the hybridizing cells are histologically or developmentally related, so that B16 melanoma cells fuse more readily with one another than they do with unrelated cells such as UV-2237 cells (I. Hart, unpublished observations). Moreover, early hybridization protocols did not call for the use of fusogens, but merely the cocultivation of participating cells in the two-dimensional constraints of a tissue culture dish (e.g., Barski et al. 1961, Silagi 1967). Presumably, the increased contact between cells within a growing tumor mass would increase the likelihood of such spontaneous fusion.

In vivo hybridization could play a significant role in neoplastic progression and variation in metastatic efficiency by at least two separate, but not necessarily mutually exclusive, mechanisms. First, fusion of two contiguous tumor cells would increase the chromosome content of the resultant single cell; this increase in ploidy could facilitiate and heighten the apparent inherent genetic instability of neoplastic cells (Nowell 1976). Although segregation and chromosome loss may or may not be random or preferential in nature (Campbell and Worton 1981), the mere occurrence of such a phenomenon could also cause chromosomal disjunction and the possible extinction and reexpression of specific genes, which would lead to the independent variation and progression of different tumor cell characteristics in the manner cited by Foulds (1969). Second, tumors are not uniform in nature. Instead they can have zones of cloned cells (Fidler and Hart 1981) that vary in metastatic capacity (Fidler and Kripke 1977, Poste et al. 1982). If two tumor cells of different metastatic capacities are fused together, the progeny resulting from this fusion tend to be more metastatic than the starting cells; thus, in vivo hybridization could play a role in tumor progression from the benign to the malignant state. In accord with Foulds' (1969) contention that progression need not always proceed in a unidirectional fashion from benign to malignant, we found that in vivo hybridization has the potential for bidirectional progression because fusion of metastatic cells with normal cells led to suppression of the metastatic, but not the tumorigenic, state. However, this type of hybridization appears to be the less common mode of cell fusion, at least in this B16 melanoma system; therefore, in vivo hybridization is likely to be a mechanism by which neoplastic cells can progress to more advanced states of malignancy.

REFERENCES

Atkin, N. B. 1979. Premature chromosome condensation in carcinoma of the bladder: Presumptive evidence for fusion of normal and malignant cells. Cytogenet. Cell Genet. 23:217–219.

Barski, G., and J. Belehradek. 1979. Inheritance of malignancy in somatic cell hybrids. Somatic Cell Genet. 5:897–908.

Barski, G., S. Sorieul, and F. Cornefert. 1961. "Hybrid" type cells in combined cultures of two different mammalian cell strains. JNCI 26:1269–1277.

Ber, R., F. Wiener, and E.-M. Fenyo. 1978. Proof of in vivo fusion of murine tumor cells with host cells by universal fusers. JNCI 60:931–933.

Boon, T., and O. Kellerman. 1976. Rejection by syngeneic mice of cell variants obtained by mutagenesis of a malignant teratocarcinoma cell line. Proc. Natl. Acad. Sci. USA 74:272–276.

Boon, T., and A. Van Pel. 1978. Teratocarcinoma cell variants rejected by syngeneic mice: Protection of mice immunized with these variants against other variants and against the original malignant cell line. Proc. Natl. Acad. Sci. USA 75:1519–1523.

Campbell, C. E., and R. G. Worton. 1981. Segregation of recessive phenotypes in somatic cell

hybrids: Role of mitotic recombination, gene inactivation and chromosome nondisjunction. Mol. Cell Biol. 1:336–346.
De Baetselier, P., E. Gorelik, Z. Eshhar, Y. Ron, S. Katzav, M. Feldman, and S. Segal. 1981. Metastatic properties conferred on nonmetastatic tumors by hybridization of spleen B-lymphocytes with plasmacytoma cells. JNCI 67:1079–1087.
Dexter, D. L., and P. Calabresi. 1982. Intraneoplastic diversity. Biochim. Biophys. Acta 695:97–112.
Evans, E. P., M. D. Burtenshaw, B. B. Brown, R. Hennion, and H. Harris. 1982. The analysis of malignancy by cell fusion. IX. Re-examination and clarification of the cytogenetic problem. J. Cell Sci. 56:113–130.
Fidler, I. J. 1973. Selection of successive tumour lines for metastasis. Nature New Biol. 242:148–149.
Fidler, I. J., and I. R. Hart. 1981. Biological and experimental consequences of the zonal composition of solid tumors. Cancer Res. 41:3266–3267.
Fidler, I. J., and M. L. Kripke. 1977. Metastasis results from preexisting variant cells within a malignant tumor. Science 197:893–895.
Foulds, L. 1969. Neoplastic Development. Vol. 1. New York, Academic Press.
Goldenberg, D. M., R. D. Bhan, and R. A. Pavia. 1971. In vivo human-hamster somatic cell fusion indicated by glucose 6-phosphate dehydrogenase and lactate dehydrogenase profiles. Cancer Res. 31:1148–1152.
Goldenberg, D. M., R. A. Pavia, and M. C. Tsao. 1974. In vivo hybridization of human tumour and normal hamster cells. Nature 250:649–651.
Harris, H. 1971. Cell fusion and the analysis of malignancy. Proc. R. Soc. Lond. B 179:1–20.
Harris, H., O. J. Miller, G. Klein, P. Worst, and T. Tachibana. 1969. Suppression of malignancy by cell fusion. Nature (London) 223:363–368.
Janzen, H. W., P. A. Millman, and O. G. Thurston. 1971. Hybrid cells in solid tumors. Cancer 27:455–459.
Kerbel, R. S., J. W. Dennis, A. E. Lagarde, and P. Frost. 1982. Tumor progression in metastasis: An experimental approach using lectin resistant tumor variants. Cancer Metastasis Rev. 1:99–140.
Miller, B. E., F. R. Miller, and G. H. Heppner. 1981. Interactions between tumor subpopulations affecting their sensitivity to the antineoplastic agents cyclophosphamide and methotrexate. Cancer Res. 41:4378–4381.
Neville, A. M., and T. Symington. 1966. Pathology of primary aldosteronism. Cancer 19:1954–1968.
Nowell, P. 1976. The clonal evolution of tumor cell populations. Science 194:23–28.
Poste, G., J. Doll, and I. J. Fidler. 1981. Interactions between clonal subpopulations affect the stability of the metastatic phenotype in polyclonal populations of B16 melanoma cells. Proc. Natl. Acad. Sci. USA 78:6226–6230.
Poste, G., J. Tzeng, J. Doll, R. Greig, D. Rieman, and I. Zeidman. 1982. Evolution of tumor cell heterogeneity during progressive growth of individual lung metastases. Proc. Natl. Acad. Sci. USA 79:6574–6578.
Silagi, S. 1967. Hybridization of a malignant melanoma cell line with L cells in vitro. Cancer Res. 27:1953–1960.
Stanbridge, E. J. 1976. Suppression of malignancy in human cells. Nature 260:17–20.
Stanbridge, E. J., C. J. Der, C.-J. Doersen, R. Y. Nishimi, D. M. Peehl, Weissman, B. E., and J. E. Wilkinson. 1982. Human cell hybrids: Genetic analysis of transformation and tumorigenicity. Science 215:252–259.
Stanbridge, E. J., R. R. Flandermeyer, D. W. Daniels, and W. A. Nelson-Rees. 1981. Specific chromosome loss associated with the expression of tumorigenicity in human cell hybrids. Somatic Cell Genet. 7:699–712.
Van Pel, A., M. Georlette, and T. Boon. 1979. Tumor cell variants obtained by mutagenesis of a Lewis lung carcinoma cell line: Immune rejection by syngeneic mice. Proc. Natl. Acad. Sci. USA 76:5282–5286.
Watkins, J. F., G. B. Burns, and Z. Steplewski. 1982. Studies on a human melanoma × hamster hybrid line selected by metastasis. Exp. Cell Biol. 50:18–26.
Wiener, F., E. M. Fenyo, and G. Klein. 1974a. Tumor-host cell hybrids in radiochimeras. Proc. Natl. Acad. Sci. USA 71:148–152.
Wiener, F., E. M. Fenyo, and G. Klein. 1976. Tumor-host cell hybrids in radiochimeras reconstituted with bone marrow and thymus grafts. Somatic Cell Genet. 2:81–92.

Wiener, F., E. M. Fenyo, G. Klein, and H. Harris. 1972. Fusion of tumour cells with host cells. Nature (New Biol.) 238:155–159.

Wiener, F., G. Klein, and H. Harris. 1971. The analysis of malignancy by cell fusion. III. Hybrids between diploid fibroblasts and other tumour cells. J. Cell Sci. 8:681–692.

Wiener, F., G. Klein, and H. Harris. 1973. The analysis of malignancy by cell fusion. IV. Hybrids between tumour cells and a malignant L cell derivative. J. Cell Sci. 12:253–261.

Wiener, F., G. Klein, and H. Harris. 1974b. The analysis of malignancy by cell fusion. V. Further evidence of the ability of normal diploid cells to suppress malignancy. J. Cell Sci. 15:177–183.

Woodruff, M. F. A., J. D. Ansell, G. M. Forbes, J. C. Gordon, D. I. Burton, and H. S. Micklem. 1982. Clonal interaction in tumours. Nature 299:822–824.

Tumor Invasion

Cancer Invasion and Metastasis: Biologic and Therapeutic Aspects edited by Garth L. Nicolson and Luka Milas. Raven Press, New York © 1984.

Metastatic Cell Attachment to and Invasion of Vascular Endothelium and its Underlying Basal Lamina Using Endothelial Cell Monolayers

Garth L. Nicolson, Tatsuro Irimura, Motowo Nakajima, and Jaime Estrada*

*Departments of Tumor Biology and *Pediatrics, The University of Texas M. D. Anderson Hospital and Tumor Institute at Houston, Houston, Texas 77030*

Distant hematogenous metastasis occurs via a complex cascade of events whereby malignant cells undergo invasion of adjacent normal tissues, penetration of blood vessels, detachment, and passive transport to distant sites, where they then implant, invade the blood vessel wall, survive, and finally proliferate to form a metastatic colony (see reviews by Fidler et al. 1978, Poste and Fidler 1980, Fidler and Nicolson 1981, Sugarbaker 1981, Nicolson 1982a, Poste 1982a, Nicolson and Poste 1982, 1983a, 1983b). This sequence is discussed in the reviews cited above; our discussion here will be limited to the events that occur when blood-borne malignant cells arrest in the microcirculation at distant sites and invade blood vessel walls.

In clinical cancer as well as in animal tumor models, blood-borne tumor metastasis often favors particular secondary sites (Sugarbaker 1979, 1981, Nicolson 1982a, Sugarbaker et al. 1982). Although the locations of most regional metastases can be explained strictly on anatomical or mechanical grounds, such as the pattern of efferent venous and lymphatic drainage, distant blood-borne organ colonization by malignant cells does not always follow this pattern. In man and other animals, there are numerous examples of malignant tumors that tend to metastasize to particular secondary locations. For example, prostatic carcinoma metastasizes at high rates to bone, small cell carcinoma of the lung to brain, and neuroblastoma to liver and adrenal glands (reviewed in Nicolson 1982a, Sugarbaker 1981). It is well known that the initial organ distributions of malignant cells do not yield similar metastatic distributions (Fidler 1976, Hart and Fidler 1981); therefore, events occurring after blood-borne dissemination must be important in determining the distributions of metastases.

The formation of hematogenous metastases requires that blood-borne tumor cells implant within the microcirculation by adhesion to blood vessel walls, usually in capillaries or postcapillary venules. Subsequently, malignant cells must penetrate the vessel wall to reach the extravascular tissues, where they proliferate to generate visible metastases. This suggests that hematogenous metastasis formation requires recognition of target organ cells or stroma by the circulating malignant cells, selective survival or growth at specific distant sites, or combinations of these processes in order to form clinically important metastatic lesions (Nicolson 1982a, Hart 1982).

The entry of malignant cells into the circulation does not necessarily determine that implantation, invasion, and metastatic colonization will occur. There are numerous examples in which the presence of malignant cells or their emboli in the blood does not correlate with metastatic disease (Salsbury 1975). This failure is due to the rapid death of most malignant cells in the circulation; only a small fraction of the circulating tumor cells survive each subsequent step of metastasis formation (Fidler 1976, Fidler et al. 1978, Fidler and Nicolson 1981, Nicolson and Poste 1983b). The distribution of tumor cells in the blood has been followed by the injection of radiolabeled malignant cells via intravenous or intracardiac routes. These studies have demonstrated that tumor cells initially arrest in the microvascular system of the first organ encountered, but they then often recirculate to other organs where they rearrest, invade, and colonize these sites (Zeidman and Buss 1952, Fidler and Nicolson 1976, 1977).

The abilities of metastatic cells to home to, survive, and grow at particular organ sites such as the lung have been shown by implanting lung tissue into the thighs of syngeneic mice and examining whether lung-colonizing tumor cells can recirculate to and form metastatic colonies in these ectopic organs (Kinsey 1960, Sugarbaker et al. 1971, Hart and Fidler 1980). When Hart and Fidler (1980) examined the kinetic distribution of radiolabeled, lung-colonizing B16 melanoma cells in animals bearing ectopic lung implants, they did not find differences in the kinetic distribution patterns of the B16 melanoma cells between animals without organ implants and those bearing ectopically implanted lung or kidney tissues. These results suggest that events subsequent to implantation, such as invasion, survival, vascularization, and growth, are important in determining tumor colonization of the ectopic lung implants. Nonetheless, other explanations are possible. For example, it is likely that a substantial portion of the vascular system in the ectopic implants is derived from surrounding tissues. In addition, the localization of radiolabeled tumor cells at the ectopic implant site does not indicate their exact location. Many of the melanoma cells that Hart and Fidler (1980) found associated with the ectopic lung implants in mice would not be expected to extravasate and survive to form detectable tumor lesions. In such experiments, similar numbers of lung-colonizing B16 melanoma cells were found in ectopically implanted lung or kidney tissues, although gross tumors were not subsequently found in the kidney implants.

It is now well established that malignant neoplasms are populated by cells with differing phenotypic properties and that only certain subpopulations of tumor cells within primary tumors are capable of metastasizing to distant sites (Hart and Fidler 1981, Nicolson 1982a, Poste 1982a). From the work of several laboratories it is now thought that as malignant tumors grow progressively, variant cell subpopulations arise that are subject to host selection pressures. These pressures result in malignant tumors that are composed of various cell subpopulations. This process has been described by Foulds (1956a, 1956b) as neoplastic evolution. Neoplastic evolution, or tumor progression, is the phenomenon in which a tumor gradually changes, acquiring or losing certain characteristics under the influence of host selection pressures. As a result of tumor progression, neoplasms can become more malignant. Several different experimental approaches using in vivo or in vitro selection techniques or tumor cell cloning procedures have provided strong evidence for the phenotypic variability of tumor cell subpopulations in malignant neoplasms and also for the gradual evolution of certain cell subpopulations within malignant tumors (see Poste and Fidler 1980, Fidler and Poste 1982, Fidler and Nicolson 1981, Nicolson 1982a, Poste 1982a, Nicolson and Poste 1982).

The use of in vitro or in vivo selection procedures and in vitro cloning techniques to obtain subpopulations of malignant cells is particularly advantageous for studies of the role of tumor and host properties in metastasis formation. The success of such procedures in certain tumor systems, however, does not guarantee that in every tumor system dramatic differences in cell phenotypic properties will be found, nor do they guarantee that cell phenotypes will remain stable during propagation in vivo or in vitro. In fact, several studies have shown that great care must be taken in growing tumor cell subpopulations in order to avoid changing their metastatic properties and other phenotypes (Nicolson 1982a, Fidler and Hart 1982, Poste 1982a, Nicolson and Poste 1982, Hart and Fidler 1981). Using tumor cells of known metastatic potentials derived from the same neoplasm allows tumor cell properties essential in certain steps of the metastatic process to be identified and eventually studied in detail. With the reservations that such malignant cells are potentially unstable in their phenotypic properties, certain comparisons are likely to yield important data on metastasis formation.

The interactions of malignant cells with their environment, and particularly their interactions with host cells, are mediated by constituents present at the cell surface (Nicolson 1982a, 1982b, Nicolson and Poste 1982, 1983a, 1983b). Several lines of evidence have illustrated the involvement of cell surface components in certain aspects of metastasis formation, such as blood-borne tumor cell implantation. One of the earliest series of such experiments demonstrated that enzymatic modification of cell surface glycoproteins can alter tumor cell implantation properties in the microcirculation without modifying tumor cell viability (Fidler 1978, Hagmar and Norrby 1973). In addition, specific biosynthetic modifications of cell surface glycoproteins have been shown to inhibit blood-borne implantation and experimental metastasis formation (Irimura et al. 1981, Irimura and Nicolson 1981a). Finally, the role of the plasma membrane in blood-borne arrest and organ colonization have been demonstrated by the transfer of portions of these membranes from highly metastatic B16 melanoma cells to B16 cells of lower metastatic potential (Poste and Nicolson 1980). In these studies, Poste and Nicolson (1980) took advantage of the fact that B16 melanoma cells spontaneously shed closed plasma membrane vesicles in vivo as well as in vitro. These vesicles were harvested, purified, and subsequently fused with the plasma membranes of homologous or heterologous cells to introduce membrane components into the surface membranes of recipient cells. When vesicles from the high lung-colonizing line B16-F10 were fused into the cell surfaces of the low lung-colonizing subline B16-F1, the ability of these F10 vesicle-modified B16-F1 cells to localize in lung and form experimental pulmonary metastases was increased significantly. These vesicle-induced changes were reversible and correlated with the natural turnover of cell membrane components. There are now numerous examples (reviewed in Nicolson 1982a, 1982b) in which differences in the display, dynamics, amounts, or structures of cell surface proteins, glycolipids, and glycoproteins may be involved in various steps of the metastatic process.

THE INTERACTIONS OF METASTATIC TUMOR CELLS DURING BLOOD-BORNE TRANSPORT

During their dissemination in the blood, malignant cells are involved in several types of interactions, including homotypic or self-interactions and interactions with other host cells or blood components. Such interactions can result in the formation of multicell tumor emboli, which implant in the microcirculation at greater efficiencies than single tumor cells (Fidler 1973, Liotta et al. 1976). These results suggest that mechanical factors, such as the size and deformability of the circulating tumor cells and tumor cell emboli, as well as host capillary deformability, can modify the lodgment properties of blood-borne malignant cells (Zeidman and Buss 1952, Sato and Suzuki 1976). The cellular interactions during blood transport are certainly not the only determinants of successful arrest and metastasis formation, because tumor cell emboli of large size often pass through the first capillaries encountered and recirculate to other sites (Zeidman and Buss 1952, Fidler and Nicolson 1976, 1977, Fisher and Fisher 1967).

The interactions of malignant cells with themselves or with platelets or lymphoid cells to form multicell emboli have been examined in different tumor model systems. B16 melanoma sublines selected in vivo for increased abilities to colonize lung (Fidler 1973), ovary (Brunson and Nicolson 1979), or brain (Miner et al. 1982) or in vitro for increased tissue invasive properties (Poste et al. 1980) or resistance to lymphocyte-mediated cytolysis (Fidler et al. 1976) have been useful for such studies. Using selected B16 melanoma sublines, Nicolson et al. (1983) have shown that the B16 cells of highest lung implantation and colonization potentials possess the highest rates of homotypic adhesion measured in aggregation-type experiments. Similar results have been obtained using murine sarcoma variants selected for enhanced lung colonization (Nicolson 1978). These data are consistent with previous findings in which multicell aggregates were found to be more effective in blood-borne arrest and experimental metastasis formation. Although the actual mechanisms of homotypic aggregation have not been elucidated in the B16 melanoma system, Raz and Lotan (1981) have found that human and murine tumor cells, including B16 melanoma cells, contain cell surface lectins capable of binding galactosyl-containing glycoconjugates, suggesting that cell surface lectins or similar types of components may be responsible for mediating at least some of the intercellular interactions of tumor cells in the blood.

During their dissemination in the circulation, malignant cells can interact with blood platelets. For example, the interactions of B16 melanoma cells with platelets is thought to be important in facilitating blood-borne implantation through the formation of platelet–tumor cell emboli, which can adhere better to blood vessel walls. Gasic et al. (1973) found the B16 melanoma sublines of high lung-colonization potentials aggregated with platelets in vitro at higher rates than sublines of low lung-colonization potential. Tumor cell lines of various origins and metastatic potentials have been found to aggregate platelets (Gasic et al. 1978, Pearlstein et al. 1980). Indeed, experimental metastasis can be inhibited in certain systems by inducing thrombocytopenia or by administering antiplatelet agents (Gasic et al. 1972, Fisher and Fisher 1961, Gastpar 1977, Brown 1973). However, not all tumor cells appear to be associated with platelets during blood-borne transport and after implantation (Warren 1981), and in some metastatic systems correlations have not been found between platelet aggregation and the potentials of malignant cells to metastasize spontaneously or experimentally. We have used a spontaneously metastasizing rat mammary adenocarcinoma tumor system (Neri et al. 1982) to test the universality of malignant cell–platelet interactions and have found no correlation between platelet aggregation abilities and the incidence of spontaneous or experimental lung metastasis. In these experiments, cloned tumor cell lines of various metastatic potentials (obtained from locally growing tumors or spontaneous lung metastases) were incubated with rat platelet-rich plasma, and aggregation was monitored with an aggregometer. Mammary tumor lines such as MTLn3 of high spontaneous metastatic potential had the lowest rates of platelet aggregation (Figure 1) and caused the least amount of thrombocytopenia after intravenous administration into syngeneic animals.

Malignant cells in the blood can also undergo homotypic adhesion with host lymphocytes. Fidler (1975) noted that B16 melanoma cells of high lung-colonization potential bound to syngeneic lymphocytes to form heterotypic cell aggregates. The rates of lymphocyte-B16 cell aggregate formation correlated with lung-colonization potentials (Fidler and Bucana 1977). Further evidence for the involvement of lymphocyte tumor cell heterotypic interactions in enhancing B16 melanoma arrest was obtained by Fidler et al. (1976), who sequentially selected B16 sublines in vitro for resistance to lymphocyte-mediated cytolysis. The lymphocyte-resistant B16 sublines thus obtained were less adhesive to lymphocytes and showed lower rates of blood-borne implantation and experimental metastasis formation than the parental B16 lines (Fidler and Bucana 1977).

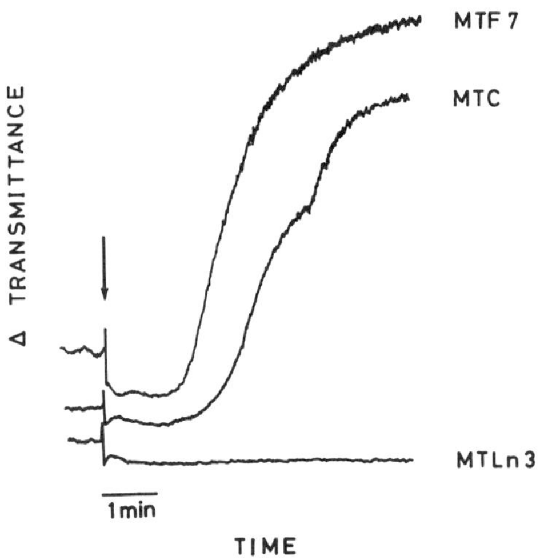

FIG. 1. Typical platelet aggregation curves induced by the addition of 5×10^5 rat mammary adenocarcinoma clones MTC, MTF7 or MTLn3, of low, intermediate, and high metastatic potential, respectively, in 0.05 ml DPBS free of calcium and magnesium, to 0.45 ml of heparinized rat platelet-rich plasma (4×10^6 platelets/ml) in a dual sample aggregometer (Sienco, Inc.). The temperature was maintained at 37°C and the platelet–tumor cell suspension was stirred at 1000 rpm with a small, siliconized bar.

Of course, there are examples of malignant cells of high metastatic potential that do not undergo these types of cellular interactions to greater extents than cells of lower metastatic potential. Thus, cellular interactions leading to the formation of multicell emboli are not required for metastasis formation, but they may enhance the potential of blood-borne tumor cells to implant and survive in the microcirculation.

Another aspect of tumor cell interaction during malignant cell dissemination in the blood involves natural host defense mechanisms against circulating tumor cells. These host defense systems involve, among others, natural antibody and natural killer (NK) cell systems, which can be important in surveillance mechanisms (Vaage and Agrawal 1976, Gorelik et al. 1979, Hanna 1982). Although natural antibody- and NK cell-mediated destruction of malignant cells during blood-borne transport may be two of the more important host defense mechanisms, these processes cannot explain the extremely rapid death rates of tumor cells in the circulation. Among others, the inability of tumor cells to withstand the excessive shear forces and deformation in the microcirculation are thought to be responsible for the death of most blood-borne tumor cells.

Host defense mechanisms such as those mediated by NK cells have been shown to be important in metastasis formation. Gorelik et al. (1979) have found that metastatic 3LL carcinoma cells can be inhibited in their spontaneous metastasis formation by mixing them with normal spleen cells before subcutaneous inoculation. However, metastasis inhibition was reduced when the authors selected NK-resistant sublines from the 3LL tumor (Gorelik et al. 1982). After eight sequential selections for resistance to NK cell-mediated cytolysis, there was a dramatic increase in the abilities of the selected 3LL cells to metastasize spontaneously to lung and to resist NK cell–mediated lysis in vitro. Similar results have been obtained by Hanna and Fidler (1981) using B16 melanoma cells. These authors utilized mature nude mice as the source of NK effector cells and sequentially selected B16 melanoma cells in vitro for their resistance to NK cell-mediated cytolysis. The NK-resistant B16 sublines possessed enhanced lung-colonization potentials and gained the capacity to metastasize in adult nude mice, in contrast to the parental B16 line, which was unable to form experimental metastases in adult nude mice.

Blood-borne malignant cells can interact with blood clotting components during their dissemination. Many types of tumor cells are thromboplastic and elicit fibrin formation in vitro and in vivo, either during blood-borne transport or soon after implantation in the microcirculation (Warren 1981, Chew et al. 1976). Sequential ultrastructural observations of malignant cells during arrest have revealed the formation of fibrin clots at the sites of tumor cell implantation in some tumor systems (Warren 1981). Alternatively, the arrest of multicell tumor emboli can result from damage to the endothelium and accumulation of platelets and fibrin clots at that spot. The evidence for and against a role for fibrin and clot formation in blood-borne metastasis has been reviewed by Warren (1981), and he has concluded that fibrin formation is not essential for blood-borne implantation or metastatic spread of tumor cells. In some experimental metastatic systems, correlations between tumor thromboplastin levels, fibrin formation, and metastatic potentials have not been found (Kinjo et al. 1979).

After blood-borne tumor cells have successfully implanted in the microcirculation, they usually extravasate or escape from the vascular compartment by invading blood vessel walls rather than by growing at the site of arrest until the endothelial vessels rupture (Dingemans 1974, Nakamura et al. 1977). The normal route of extravasation involves tumor cell invasion between adjacent endothelial cells (Sindelar et al. 1975, Kramer and Nicolson 1979, 1981, Nicolson 1982a) or direct penetration of endothelial cell cytoplasm (Dingemans 1974, Roos and Dingemans 1979). Penetration of the vessel wall endothelial cell layer is followed by adhesion to and subsequent destruction of the underlying endothelial basal lamina or basement membrane. (This process will be considered in more detail in the next section.)

Once malignant cells have undergone extravasation, they can interact with parenchymal cells and extracellular tissue stroma. Interactions of malignant cells with parenchymal cells have been measured using in vitro procedures. For example, we have measured the abilities of B16 melanoma cells to heterotypically adhere to suspended organ cells as a model for tumor cell–parenchymal cell interactions. In this experiment we found that B16 cells of high lung-colonization potentials adhered at faster rates to suspended lung cells than did B16 cells of low lung-colonization potentials. We also found that substitution of other organ cells for lung cells abolished these differences (Nicolson and Winkelhake 1975). This experiment has now been repeated using small pieces of intact organ tissue, and we have found that various organ-colonizing variants of B16 melanoma possess differing abilities to attach to and invade tissues such as lung, ovary, and heart (Nicolson 1982a). Phondke et al. (1981) have noted similar organ cell–tumor cell interactions using leukemia cells that show high spleen-colonization potentials. Phondke et al. (1981) found that their leukemia cells adhered at high rates to spleen cells, but not to suspended lung cells. In other experiments, Shirrmacher et al. (1980) noted that mouse lymphoma cells of high liver-colonization potential adhered to mouse hepatocytes at higher rates than to a parental line of low liver-colonization potential.

The biochemical mechanisms involved in the heterotypic cell interactions described above have, for the most part, not been determined; however, evidence exists that these interactions may be mediated by cell surface glycoproteins and lectins. In the studies of Schlepper-Schafer et al. (1981), various metastatic cells were found to bind to rat hepatocytes through asialogalactosaminyl- or galactosyl-binding lectins on the hepatocyte cell surface. Other experiments, such as those of Shirrmacher et al. (1980), also suggest that cell surface lectins may be involved in mediating tumor cell–host cell interactions.

Efforts to relate specific malignant cell properties with blood-borne implantation and metastasis formation have been impeded until recently by the lack of suitable animal tumor systems. Studies on the kinetics of blood-borne tumor cell implantation and clearance of radiolabeled tumor cells injected in the circulation have been useful in monitoring differences in average tumor cell distributions in different organs, in screening potential therapeutic procedures for inhibiting tumor cell implantation, and in determining differences in tumor cell survival at different sites (Nicolson and Poste 1982, 1983b, Poste 1982b, Giraldi and Sava 1981). Unfortunately, such methods have provided little insight into the cellular and molecular mechanisms underlying these phenomena. Progress in elucidating the mechanisms involved in malignant cell implantation have depended to a large degree upon the development of suitable in vitro models permitting detailed studies on malignant cell interactions with vascular endothelium and the endothelial basal lamina. These approaches would be extremely difficult, if not impossible, to employ in vivo. Our work, as well as those of other laboratories, has focused on the interactions between tumor cells and vascular endothelial cells grown on cellular (Jones 1979) or stromal (Kramer and Nicolson 1979, Zamora et al. 1980, Nicolson 1982c) matrices.

MALIGNANT CELL INTERACTIONS WITH VASCULAR ENDOTHELIAL CELLS AND THEIR BASAL LAMINA-LIKE MATRIX

To develop into distant metastatic colonies, blood-borne malignant cells must successfully implant in the microcirculation. The first cell type encountered by malignant cells at sites where they initiate organ colonization are the endothelial cells lining the microcirculation. Thus, the interactions of circulating malignant cells with endothelial cells may (under certain circumstances) be specific, because endothelial cells at different locations appear to possess unique characteristics that may determine their tissue origin. For example, antigenic differences have been found between endothelial cells established from different organs (Joseph et al. 1983), and our own experiments have shown that brain-colonizing

B16 melanoma cells attach at higher rates to brain endothelial cells than to lung endothelial cells (Nicolson 1982c). Therefore, each organ may have its own recognition system based on unique endothelial cell determinants, or alternatively, malignant cells may recognize target organs by interacting with organ-specific subendothelial basal lamina.

When malignant cells interact with endothelial cells, either in vivo or in vitro, they are often found adherent to the junctional regions between adjacent endothelial cells. When examined ultrastructurally, these malignant cells are often found bound to exposed subendothelial basal lamina between endothelial cells (Warren 1973, 1981, Chew et al. 1976, Sindelar et al. 1975, Carr et al. 1976). We have obtained similar results in vitro utilizing monolayers of vascular endothelial cells (Kramer and Nicolson 1979, 1981, Nicolson 1982c).

After malignant cells attach to the apical surfaces of endothelial cells in vitro, they induce endothelial cell junction breakage and cell retraction (Figure 2A,B).

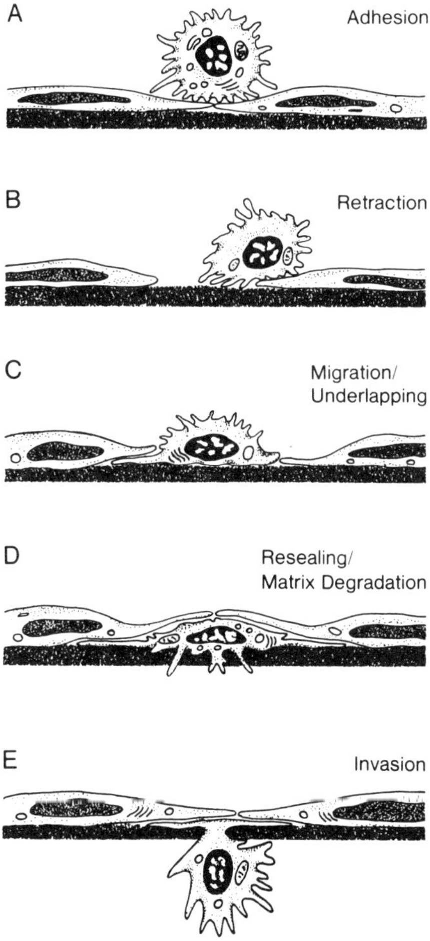

FIG. 2. The sequence of events during blood-borne metastatic cell attachment and invasion of vascular endothelium and underlying basal lamina-like matrix. **A.** Malignant cell attachment to endothelial cells. **B.** Endothelial cell retraction. **C.** Tumor cell migration and attachment to the underlying matrix. **D.** Local destruction of the endothelial basal lamina-like matrix. **E.** Invasion of the malignant cell into surrounding tissue. (Reproduced from Nicolson 1982a with permission of Elsevier Biomedical Press.)

Once the endothelial cells retract, the motile malignant cells migrate to, and adhere and spread on, the underlying basal lamina-like matrix (Figure 2B,C). A wide range of neoplastic and nonneoplastic cells have been examined for their abilities to adhere to monolayer cultures of endothelial cells and stimulate endothelial cell retraction (Kramer and Nicolson 1979, Nicolson 1982c). Apart from lymphocytes, platelets, and monocytes, which do not adhere to undamaged endothelium, qualitiative differences were not found in the adhesive behaviors of metastatic, nonmetastatic, and nonneoplastic cell lines. We found that many of the cells that bound to endothelial cell monolayers stimulated retraction. Some of the cells that attached to vascular endothelial cell monolayers remained rounded and failed to migrate to the subendothelial matrix. In our in vitro assays, most tumor cell adhesion occurred at the junctional regions between adjacent endothelial cells, suggesting that this region may contain a specialized domain of the endothelial cell surface or that microexposure of the underlying matrix occurs more readily in this region.

What distinguishes metastatic from nonmetastatic cells in their interactions with endothelial cells? The distinguishing characteristic appears to be in the abilities of basal lamina–bound metastatic cells to underlap adjacent endothelial cells, solubilize regions of the basal lamina-like matrix, and migrate through this structure (Figure 2). Events similar to these have been documented to occur in vivo (Warren 1981, Sindelar et al. 1975, Ludatsher et al. 1967). Infiltration of malignant cells through the endothelial cell layer does not result in loss of endothelial cell viability (Kramer and Nicolson 1979). After invasion of malignant cells through the endothelial cell layer, the endothelial cells quickly reconstruct their disrupted junctions to re-form an intact cell monolayer (Figure 2).

Considerable variation exists in the times required for individual tumor cells to attach to and invade endothelial cell monolayers (Kramer and Nicolson 1979, 1981, Nicolson 1982c). This is consistent with the differences reported in the speed with which different tumor cells extravasate from blood vessels in vivo (Ludatsher et al. 1967, Wood 1964) and is also consistent with the extensive tumor cell heterogeneity that exists in most, if not all, malignant tumor systems.

The endothelial cell layer possesses dramatic asymmetry in the display of components on its apical and basolateral surfaces (Birdwell et al. 1978). For example, components in the basal lamina-like matrix synthesized by endothelial cells do not appear on the apical endothelial cell surface, and this asymmetry is probably important in the preferential adhesion and movement of metastatic cells to the basal lamina-like matrix. Indeed, metastatic tumor cells exhibit greater rates of adhesion to the basal lamina-like matrix synthesized by endothelial cells than to the endothelial cells themselves (Figure 3) (Kramer et al. 1980, Nicolson et al. 1981); this same observation has been made on intact veins (Poste and Fidler 1980).

The cell matrix synthesized by vascular endothelial cells contains glycoproteins such as fibronectin (Kramer et al. 1980, Nicolson et al. 1981) and laminin

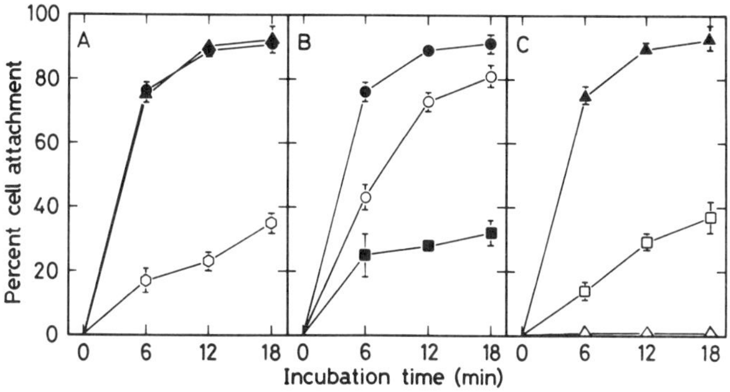

FIG. 3. Rates of attachment of radiolabeled murine B16-F10 melanoma cells to endothelial cell monolayers, basal lamina-like extracellular matrix produced by endothelial cells, or immobilized fibronectin in vitro. **A.** Adhesion of untreated B16-F10 cells to untreated endothelial cell monolayers (○), endothelial matrix (●), or immobilized fibronectin (▲). **B.** Adhesion of untreated (○,●) or tunicamycin-treated (0.5 μg/ml for 24 h) (■) B16-F10 cells to endothelial extracellular matrix or matrix pretreated with 400 μg/ml purified antifibronectin antibody (○). **C.** Adhesion of untreated (△,▲) or tunicamycin-treated (0.5 μg/ml for 24 h) (□) B16-F10 cells to immobilized fibronectin untreated or pretreated with 400 μg/ml antifibronectin (△). (Reproduced from Irimura et al. 1983b with permission of Japan Scientific Societies Press.)

(Terranova et al. 1980, Gospodarowicz et al. 1981, Vlodovsky and Gospodarowicz 1981), collagens (Murray et al. 1980, Liotta et al. 1980, Howard et al. 1976) and sulfated proteoglycans (Kramer et al. 1982, Nakajima et al. 1983, Irimura et al. 1983a, 1983b). It is likely that metastatic cells adhere to the endothelial basal lamina via these types of components, and we have proposed that different metastatic cells may utilize different adhesive mechanisms to adhere to the basal lamina structure (Nicolson et al. 1981). Evidence comes from assays in which the binding of tumor cells to specific matrix components can be blocked by affinity-purified antibodies (Figure 3) (Nicolson et al. 1981) and tumor cell adhesion assays in which purified, immobilized basal lamina components are utilized (Figure 3) (Murray et al. 1980, Liotta et al. 1980, Nicolson et al. 1981). Such assays have been conducted in parallel on a selected series of metastatic variants or on the same tumor line but with several immobilized basal lamina components. For example, metastatic B16 melanoma cells adhere with similar, rapid kinetics to immobilized fibronectin and subendothelial basal lamina-like matrix synthesized by endothelial cells (Figure 3). Whereas adhesion to immobilized fibronectin can be completely blocked by an affinity-purified antibody to fibronectin, adhesion to basal lamina-like matrix can only be partially inhibited by the same preparation (Figure 3) (Nicolson et al. 1981). These results indicate that metastatic cells probably use a variety of adhesive mechanisms, in concert, to attach to endothelial basal lamina. In addition, different metastatic cells may use different mechanisms to attach to endothelial cells or their basal lamina-like matrix, and in most cases multiple adhesive interactions probably occur. We have therefore proposed that multiple classes of adhesive interactions are important in determining organ-specific malignant cell–endothelial cell and malignant cell–basal lamina interactions (Nicolson 1982a, Nicolson et al. 1981).

Evidence supporting the hypothesis that metastatic tumor cells may use multiple adhesive mechanisms to attach to endothelial basal lamina has been obtained by several investigators. Murray et al. (1980) noted that malignant cells attach to type IV collagen, the major collagen type of endothelial basal lamina, but not to other collagens, in correlation with their metastatic potentials. In other experiments, collagen-laminin complexes were used to demonstrate differences in binding of malignant cells to basal lamina components (Terranova et al. 1982).

Metastatic cell attachment to the apical surfaces of endothelial cells and basal lamina may also occur through tumor cell surface glycoproteins. As mentioned previously, enzymatic modifications of cell surface glycoproteins modify in vivo implantation and in vitro adhesion to endothelial cells and their subendothelial matrices. The role of glycoconjugates in this process has been studied by Irimura et al. (1981) using tunicamycin, an inhibitor of cellular glycoprotein biosynthesis. Tunicamycin treatment effectively blocks tumor cell–endothelial cell adhesion and tumor cell–subendothelial matrix adhesion (Figure 3) (Irimura et al. 1981, Irimura and Nicolson 1981a, Nicolson et al. 1981). Tunicamycin modified B16 melanoma cell surface glycoproteins without altering the major cell surface proteins accessible to lactoperoxidase-catalyzed iodination (Irimura et al. 1981). Since the effects of tunicamycin were reversible within one day after drug was removed from cultures of B16 melanoma cells, these results were not due to modifications in cell viabilities. Examination of the loss of metastatic properties during tunicamycin treatment of B16 melanoma cells established the relationship between metastatic properties and the disappearance of a specific class of cell surface glycoproteins. Irimura et al. (1981) were able to implicate the cell surface sialogalactoproteins on B16 cells in endothelial cell and subendothelial matrix interactions. They also found that the treatment of B16 melanoma cells with tunicamycin effectively blocked blood-borne implantation and experimental metastasis (Irimura et al. 1981, Irimura and Nicolson 1981a).

Irimura and Nicolson (1981b) purified B16 melanoma cell surface sialogalactoproteins by affinity chromatography and then examined their binding to endothelial basal lamina-like matrix. In contrast to intact B16 melanoma cells, isolated B16 sialogalactoproteins exhibited low binding affinities to subendothelial matrix. These results suggest that B16 cell adhesion to endothelial basal lamina is the result of multiple adhesive interactions that cannot be duplicated with any isolated, single adhesion component (Nicolson 1982a, Nicolson et al. 1981).

MALIGNANT CELL DEGRADATION OF ENDOTHELIAL BASAL LAMINA-LIKE MATRIX

We have shown that the net movement of metastatic cells after attachment to endothelial cell monolayers is to the subendothelial matrix and eventually through this structure. Although mechanical destruction and enzymatic degradation have both been postulated as important in penetration of basal lamina by metastatic cells, most investigators have concentrated on the role of tumor cell degradative enzymes. Proposals for an enzymatic mechanism of basal lamina penetration are based on direct measurements of various tumor cell enzymes that can act on basal lamina components, whereas mechanical disruption of basal lamina by metastatic tumor cells has been postulated strictly on morphological observations. In the former proposal, several enzymes have been considered; among them, the enzymes involved in degrading collagens (especially those specific for type IV and other prominent basal lamina collagens), proteases capable of degrading matrix glycoproteins such as fibronectin and laminin, and endoglycosidases, which can cleave glycosaminoglycan side chains from matrix proteoglycans (Figure 4) (reviewed in Nicolson 1982a, Irimura et al. 1983b, Liotta et al. 1982). Since metastatic tumor cells can undergo extravasation of intact blood vessels in vitro and can easily penetrate endothelial cell monolayers and their underlying basal lamina-like matrix under conditions of minimal mechanical pressure, it is unlikely that simple mechanical disruption can explain extravasation. Thus, such circumstances as excessive tumor pressure due to

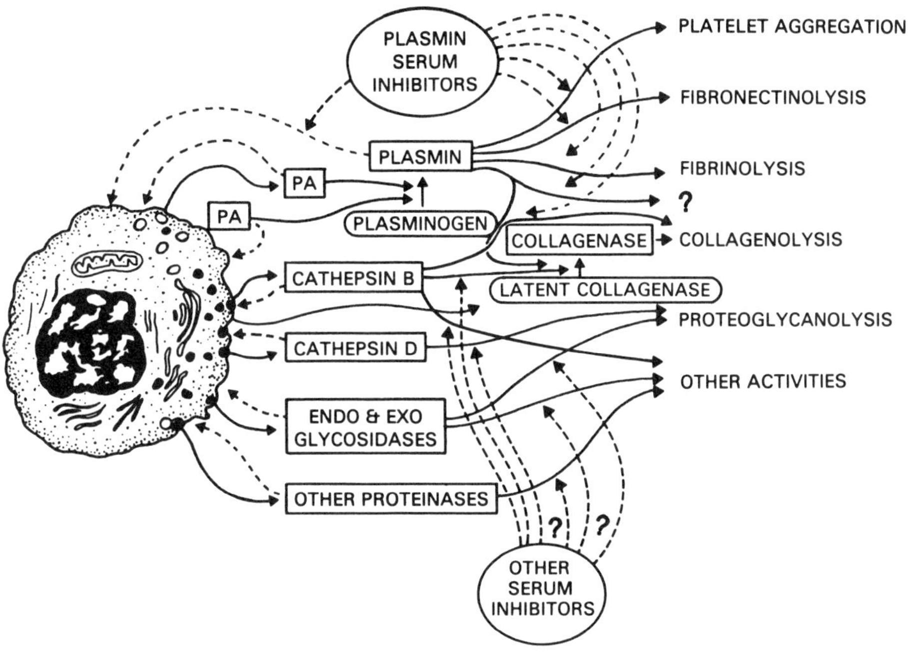

FIG. 4. Release or cell surface display of tumor-associated degradative enzymes and their possible roles in metastatic processes. The solid lines represent the possible direct or indirect effects of tumor-associated enzymes on biologic substrates that form part of the barriers to malignant cell invasion. The broken lines represent possible feedback inhibitory or autolysis mechanisms. (Modified from Nicolson 1982a.)

cell proliferation are not required in order for malignant cells to penetrate the endothelial and basal lamina layers.

Additional support for enzymatic mechanisms in endothelial cell layer and basal lamina penetration have come from the studies of Liotta et al. (1980), who have shown that highly metastatic B16 melanoma cells possess higher collagenase activities than cells of lower metastatic potential. In addition, these differences were only found when B16 sublines were tested against type IV collagen, the major collagen of the basal lamina. Measurements of B16 collagenase activities against type I or type II collagen yielded similar results with low or highly metastatic cells, indicating that highly metastatic cells possess enzymes that can degrade selectively the major collagen class of the basal lamina.

Lysosomal proteases and glycosidases may also be important in basal lamina penetration by malignant cells. Recently, Sloane et al. (1981,1982) have correlated the levels of lysosomal cathepsin B with the metastatic potentials of two B16 melanoma sublines. Although they did not find differences between low and high lung-colonizing B16 sublines when they examined several lysosomal enzymes such as cathepsin D, β-N-acetylglucosaminidase, β-glucuronidase, and acid phosphatase, they did note that cathepsin B activities were three times higher in the dispersed cells from tumors formed from the high lung-colonizing B16-F10 variant and four times higher in lysosomal preparation made from these same tumors than in tumors formed from the low lung-colonizing B16-F1 cells. The higher cathepsin B activities in tumors formed from B16-F10 cells were not due to host cell contamination. Poole et al. (1978) found that malignant breast cancer lesions secreted up to 11 times the amount of cathepsin B that benign breast lesions or surrounding normal tissues released. Cathepsin B, in contrast to other cathepsins, also possesses the ability to activate procollagenases or latent collagenases (Barrett and McDonald 1980). Thus, certain proteolytic enzymes that are released or displayed at the cell surface may also function to activate other enzymes essential in the extravasation process.

When the degradative enzymes of metastatic tumor cells are examined in detail, it is apparent that the malignant cells have all of the enzymatic machinery necessary to degrade the major components of basal lamina (Figure 4). This has been demonstrated in vitro by examining the abilities of metastatic cells to solubilize and degrade basal lamina-like matrix synthesized by endothelial cells. Metabolic labeling of subendothelial matrix with the appropriate precursors can monitor the release of major molecules or fragments upon exposure of the matrix to malignant cells. Using such assays, it is possible to determine the susceptibility of different matrix components to enzymatic degradation by tumor cells and to identify the enzymatic activities involved in such a degradative process. For example, we have placed B16 melanoma cells on [^{3}H]leucine-labeled, cell-free subendothelial matrix and have examined the release of ^{3}H into the medium in the form of solubilized macromolecules. The more metastatic B16 melanoma sublines in such assays released acid-precipitable, [^{3}H]leucine-labeled molecules and their degradative fragments from subendothelial matrix at higher rates than B16 cells of lower metastatic potential (Nicolson 1982c). In the subendothelial matrix, the predominant glycoproteins (fibronectin and laminin) are both solubilized by B16 melanoma cells. One of two fibronectin subunits released into the medium has a slightly lower (by $M_r \sim 10{,}000$) molecular weight than the other. Polyacrylamide gel electrophoresis analysis of untreated subendothelial matrix fibronectin indicated that matrix fibronectin subunits are normally equivalent in molecular weight ($M_r \sim 230{,}000$) (Kramer et al. 1982). Thus, it appears that one of the two glycopeptide chains of fibronectin is proteolytically or glycolytically fragmented while the other is unmodified by B16 cells.

In addition to their abilities to solubilize basal lamina proteins and glycoproteins, metastatic tumor cells also have the capacity to solubilize basal lamina proteoglycans. This capacity can be measured kinetically through the solubilization of [^{35}S]sulfate-labeled proteoglycans from subendothelial matrix. We have shown that the major glycosaminoglycan side chains of these matrix proteoglycans are molecules of $M_r \sim 25{,}000$–$30{,}000$. When metastatic tumor cells are added to subendothelial matrix, they solubilize glycosaminoglycan side chains of the proteoglycans by cleaving these glycans at intrachain sites and releasing fragments that are approximately one-third the original size of glycosaminoglycan chains. Analysis of these glycosaminoglycan fragments indicates that >95% of the released molecules are heparan sulfate (Kramer et al. 1982). The composition of metastatic cell–solubilized glycosaminoglycan fragments indicates that B16 cells possess endoglycosidases active against heparan sulfate molecules. More recently, we have found that the release of heparan sulfate fragments from subendothelial matrix occurs at higher rates in B16 melanoma sublines of high invasive or metastatic potential than in similar lines of low invasive potentials (Nicolson 1983c, Nakajima et al. 1983).

The heparan sulfate–specific endoglycosidase activities of metastatic B16 melanoma cells and their abilities to degrade various glycosaminoglycans have been studied in vitro using purified lung heparan sulfate and other tissue glycosaminoglycans. In our assay, we measured the appearance of glycosaminoglycan degradation products using polyacrylamide gel electrophoresis in 1,3-diaminopropane-acetate buffer according to Nakajima et al. (1983). The rates of heparan sulfate degradation by various intact B16 melanoma cells and the rates of appearance of degradation products of decreased molecular weights (Figure 5) indicated that high-molecular-weight heparan sulfate was degraded preferentially to large fragments rather than to monosaccharides by the malignant cells. This result is consistent with our previous data suggesting that metastatic cells have an endoglycosidase capable of cleaving heparan sulfate (Kramer et al. 1982). When we compared various B16 melanoma sublines for their abilities to degrade a series of different glycosaminoglycan substrates, we found that B16 melanoma cells preferentially degraded heparan sulfate (Figure 6). It is interesting that heparan sulfate is the predominant glycosaminoglycan among the basal lamina-like matrix proteoglycans.

We have recently determined the size distributions of a variety of glycosamino-

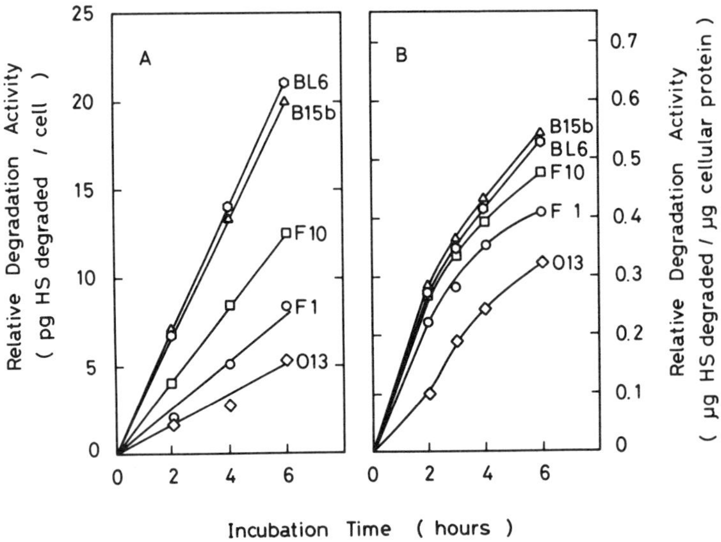

FIG. 5. Time course of lung heparan sulfate (HS) degradation by intact, viable cells and cell-free homogenates of B16 melanoma metastatic variants. **A.** B16 cells (1×10^5) were incubated with 50 μg purified HS in Dulbecco-modified Eagle's and HAM's F12 medium (1:1) containing 20 mM Tricine (pH 7.3) at 37°C for various times. **B.** B16 cell extracts (40 μg protein) were incubated with 50 μg HS in 0.1 M sodium phosphate buffer (pH 6.0) containing 0.15 M NaCl and 0.2% Triton X-100, at 37°C. Upon termination of the incubations, HS and its degradation products were analyzed by polyacrylamide gel electrophoresis in 1,3-diaminopropane-acetate buffer (pH 9.0). Toluidine blue–stained spots on polyacrylamide gels were scanned at 525 nm, and the relative degradation activities were calculated from the decreases in the high molecular weight half of the HS peak. (Reproduced from Nakajima et al. 1983 with permission. Copyright 1983, American Association for the Advancement of Science.)

glycans and their fragments produced by metastatic cell interactions using high performance liquid chromatography (Irimura et al. 1983a, 1983b). With this analytical system we have found that glycosaminoglycans such as heparan sulfate are degraded to large molecular weight fragments by endoglycosidases derived from metastatic cells. In the example shown in Figure 7, heparan sulfate of approximately 11,000 M_r synthesized by PYS-2 embryonic carcinoma cells is fragmented into molecules averaging ~6,000 M_r in the presence of the exo-β-glucuronidase inhibitor D-saccharic acid 1,4-lactone. This result confirms our previous findings that B16 melanoma cells have an endoglycosidase that recognizes a sequence in the heparan sulfate chain and cleaves this molecule at specific intrachain sites.

The heparan sulfate cleavage produced by its interaction with B16 melanoma endoglycosidase has been examined after isolation of the degradation fragments. Bovine lung heparan sulfate molecules previously reduced with $NaBH_4$ at their reducing terminal ends were incubated with B16 melanoma cell extract in the presence of D-saccharic acid 1,4-lactone, and their fragments were isolated and

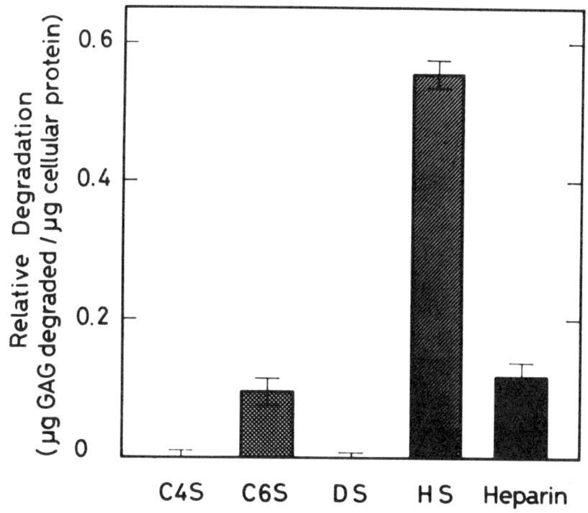

FIG. 6. Degradation of various sulfated glycosaminoglycans by B16 melanoma cell extracts. Sulfated glycosaminolglycans (50 μg) were incubated with B16-F10 cell extracts (40 μg protein) in 0.1 M sodium phosphate buffer (pH 6.0) containing 0.15 M NaCl, 0.2% Triton ×100, and 0.05% NaN_3 at 37°C for 12 h, and then glycosaminoglycans were analyzed by polyacrylamide gel electrophoresis. Relative degradation was calculated from the decrease in the high molecular weight half of the GAG peak as described in Figure 5. C4S, chondroitin 4-sulfate; C6S, chondroitin 6-sulfate; DS, dermatan sulfate; HS, heparan sulfate.

labeled at the newly formed reducing termini with $NaB[^3H]_4$. After further cleavage of heparan sulfate into monosaccharides by nitrous acid deamination and acid hydrolysis, the labeled reducing terminal sugars were analyzed by descending paper chromatography and high voltage paper electrophoresis. We found that >90% of the reducing terminal sugars of the heparan sulfate fragments were glucuronic acid, indicating that the heparan sulfate–degrading enzymes of B16 melanoma cells are endoglucuronidases specific for heparan sulfate.

Endoglycosidases specific for heparan sulfate have been described in various tissues such as skin fibroblasts (Klein et al. 1976), rat liver cells (Höök et al. 1975), human platelets (Wasteson et al. 1977), and placenta (Klein and von Figura 1976). Murine mastocytoma cells have been found to possess a heparin-specific endoglucuronidase that is capable of cleaving macromolecular heparin into physiologically active, intermediate molecular weight fragments (Ögren and Lindhal 1975), and normal human platelets have a heparan sulfate–degrading endoglucuronidase, which has been recently purified (Oosta et al. 1982). The heparan sulfate endoglycosidases of tumor and nontumor cells may be important in restructuring the basal lamina during angiogenesis, blood vessel damage, leukocyte extravasation, and blood-borne tumor cell invasion.

SUMMARY

Cellular interactions during blood-borne transport of malignant cells, including the interactions of tumor cells with themselves, platelets, lymphocytes, blood

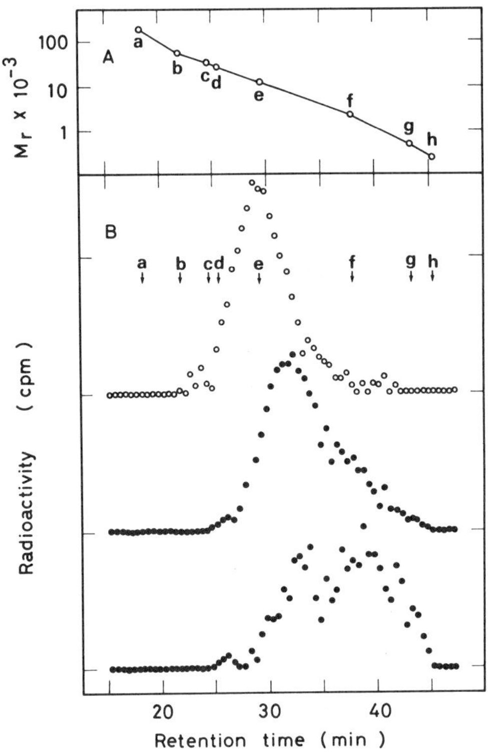

FIG. 7. High-performance liquid chromatographic analysis of ^{35}S-labeled heparan sulfate from PYS-2 embryonic carcinoma cells and its fragments produced by B16 melanoma cell heparanase. **A.** Logarithmic plot of the molecular weights versus the retention times of standard glycans separated on two sequential 0.7 × 75 cm columns of Fractogel-TSK (Toyopearl) HW-55(S). Elution was performed with 0.2 M sodium chloride at a flow rate of 1.0 ml/min at 55°C. Standard glycans used are: *a,* HA from human umbilical cord (M_r ~ 230,000); *b,* chondroitin-6-sulfate from shark cartilage (M_r ~ 60,000); *c,* heparan sulfate (HS) from bovine lung (M_r ~ 34,000); *d,* dermatan sulfate from hog mucosal tissue (M_r ~ 27,000); *e,* heparin from hog mucosal tissue (M_r ~ 11,000); *f,* monosyalosyl-biantennary complex-type glycopeptide from porcine thyroglobulin (M_r ~ 2190); *g,* tri-N-acetylchitotriose (M_r ~ 627); *h,* N-acetylglucosamine (M_r ~ 221). **B.** Elution profiles of cellular HS produced by PYS-2 embryonic carcinoma (*upper tracing*) and its fragments after incubation with B16 melanoma cell extracts in the presence (*middle tracing*) or absence (*lower tracing*) of D-saccharic acid 1,4-lactone. 2,500 cpm of [^{35}S]HS (4 μg glucuronolactone) was incubated at 37°C for 1.5 h with B16 melanoma cell extract (30 μg cellular protein) in 100 μl of 0.1 M sodium phosphate buffer, pH 6.0, containing 0.2% Triton X-100, 0.15 N sodium chloride and 0.05% sodium azide. D-Saccharic acid 1,4-lactone was added at a final concentration of 20 mM (*middle tracing*). The reaction was stopped by chilling to 4°C and the addition of one tenth volume of cold 50% trichloroacetic acid. After centrifugation at 9,000 × g the supernatant was delivered directly into the injection port. Fractions corresponding to 30S were collected and counted; a-f indicate the elution positions of the standard glycans. HA, hyaluronic acid.

components, and the vascular endothelium, can play important roles in metastasis formation. Since blood-borne metastasis often occurs to specific organ sites in vivo, recognition must occur between the circulating malignant cells and the vascular endothelium. We have used vascular endothelial cells and their underlying basal lamina-like matrix as targets for tumor cell interactions. Our findings indicate that highly metastatic tumor cells attach more rapidly and avidly to the endothelial basal lamina-like matrix than to the apical surfaces of the endothelial cells. Since the former contains cell adhesive molecules such as fibronectin and laminin, these molecules, as well as collagens and proteoglycans, may be collectively responsible for the higher rates of malignant cell binding to the basal lamina. Glycoproteins present on malignant cell surfaces are also important in these interactions, because inhibiting their biosynthesis with tunicamycin blocks blood-borne implantation and experimental metastasis formation and prevents malignant cell binding to endothelial cells or their basal lamina-like matrix.

Invasion of blood vessel walls requires that malignant cells penetrate the endothelial cell layer and underlying basal lamina. Metastatic cells appear to perform these activities using degradative enzymes such as proteases and glycosidases that solubilize the major basal lamina components: glycoproteins, collagens, and proteoglycans. We have examined the degradation of basal lamina proteoglycan side chain glycosaminoglycans using purified tissue glycosaminoglycans as substrates. B16 melanoma cells of high organ colonization capacities possess higher levels of endoglycosidase activity against heparan sulfate than B16 cells of lower organ colonization potentials. The highly malignant B16 cells were capable of cleaving the heparan sulfate molecules at specific intrachain glucuronoside sites, producing intermediate molecular weight products.

REFERENCES

Barrett, A. J., and J. D. McDonald. 1980. A glossary and bibliography, *in* Mammalian Proteases, A. J. Barrett, and J. D. McDonald, eds. Academic Press, New York, pp. 338–350.

Birdwell, C. R., D. Gospodarowicz, and G. L. Nicolson. 1978. Identification, localization and the role of fibronectin in cultured bovine endothelial cells. Proc. Natl. Acad. Sci. USA 75:3273–3277.

Brown, J. M. 1973. A study of the mechanism by which anticoagulation with Warfarin inhibits blood-borne metastasis. Cancer Res. 33:1217–1224.

Brunson, K. W., and G. L. Nicolson. 1979. Selection of malignant melanoma variant cell lines for ovary colonization. J. Supramol. Struct. 11:517–528.

Carr, I., G. McGinty, and P. Norris. 1976. The fine structure of neoplastic invasion: Invasion of liver, skeletal muscle and lymphatic vessels by the Rd/3 tumour. J. Pathol. 118:91–99.

Chew, E. C., R. K. Josephson, and A. C. Wallace. 1976. Morphologic aspects of the arrest of circulating cancer cells, *in* Fundamental Aspects of Metastasis, L. Weiss, ed. North-Holland Publishing, Amsterdam, pp. 121–150.

Dingemans, K. P. 1974. Invasion of liver tissue by blood-borne mammary carcinoma cells. JNCI 53:1813–1819.

Fidler, I. J. 1973. The relationship of embolic homogeneity, number, size and viability to the incidence of experimental metastasis. Eur. J. Cancer 9:223–227.

Fidler, I. J. 1975. Biological behavior of malignant melanoma cells correlated to their survival in vivo. Cancer Res. 35:218–224.

Fidler, I. J. 1976. Patterns of tumor cell arrest and development, *in* Fundamental Aspects of Metastasis, L. Weiss, ed. North-Holland, Amsterdam, pp. 275–289.

Fidler, I. J. 1978. General considerations for studies of experimental cancer metastasis. Methods Cancer Res. 15:399–439.

Fidler, I. J., and C. Bucana. 1977. Resistance of tumor cells to lysis by syngeneic lymphocytes: A possible mechanism. Cancer Res. 37:3945–3956.

Fidler, I. J., D. M. Gersten, and M. B. Budmen. 1976. Characterization in vivo and in vitro of tumor cells selected for resistance to syngeneic lymphocyte-mediated cytotoxicity. Cancer Res. 36:3160–3165.

Fidler, I. J., D. M. Gersten, and I. R. Hart. 1978. The biology of cancer invasion and metastasis. Adv. Cancer Res. 28:149–250.

Fidler, I. J., and G. L. Nicolson. 1976. Organ selectivity for implantation, survival and growth of B16 melanoma variant tumor lines. JNCI 57:1199–1202.

Fidler, I. J., and G. L. Nicolson. 1977. Fate of recirculating B16 melanoma metastatic variant cells in parabiotic syngeneic recipients. JNCI 58:1867–1872.

Fidler, I. J., and G. L. Nicolson. 1981. Immunobiology of experimental metastatic melanoma. Cancer Biol. Rev. 2:171–234.
Fidler, I. J., and G. Poste. 1982. The heterogeneity of metastatic properties in malignant tumor cells and regulation of the metastatic phenotype, *in* Tumor Cell Heterogeneity, A. Owens, and S. Baylin, eds. Raven Press, New York, pp. 111–162.
Fisher, B., and E. R. Fisher. 1961. Experimental studies of factors which influence hepatic metastases. VIII. Effect of anticoagulants. Surgery 50:240–247.
Fisher, B., and E. R. Fisher. 1967. Barrier function of lymph node to tumor cells and erythrocytes. I. Normal nodes. Cancer 20:1907–1918.
Foulds, L. 1956a. The histologic analysis of mammary tumors of mice. I. Scope of investigations and general principles of analysis. JNCI 17:701–712.
Foulds, L. 1956b. The histologic analysis of mammary tumors of mice. II. The histology of responsiveness and progression. The origin of tumors. JNCI 17:713–754.
Gasic, G. J., D. Boettiger, J. L. Catalfamo, T. B. Gasic, and G. J. Stewart. 1978. Aggregation of platelets and cell membrane vesiculation by rat cells transformed in vitro by Rous sarcoma virus. Cancer Res. 38:2950–2955.
Gasic, G. J., T. B. Gasic, and S. Murphy. 1972. Antimetastatic effects of aspirin. Lancet 2:932–933.
Gasic, G. J., T. B. Gasic, N. Galanti, T. Johnson, and S. Murphy. 1973. Platelet-tumor cell interaction in mice. The role of platelets in the spread of malignant disease. Int. J. Cancer 11:704–718.
Gastpar, H. 1977. Platelet-cancer cell interaction in metastasis formation: A possible therapeutic approach to metastasis prophylaxis. J. Med. 8:103–114.
Giraldi, T., and G. Sava. 1981. Selective antimetastatic drugs. Anticancer Res. 1:163–174.
Gorelick, E., M. Feldman, and S. Segal. 1982. Selection of 3LL tumor sublines resistant to natural effector cells concomitantly selected for increased metastatic potency. Immunol. Immunother. 12:105–109.
Gorelick, E., M. Fogel, M. Feldman, and S. Segal. 1979. Differences in resistance of metastatic tumor cells and cells from local tumor growth to cytotoxicity of natural killer cells. JNCI 63:1397–1404.
Gospodarowicz, D., G. Greenburg, J. M. Foidart, and N. Savion. 1981. The production and localization of laminin in cultured vascular and corneal endothelial cells. J. Cell. Physiol. 107:171–183.
Hagmar, B., and K. Norrby. 1973. Influence of cultivation, trypsinization and aggregation on the transplantability of melanoma B16 cells. Int. J. Cancer 11:663–675.
Hanna, N. 1982. The role of natural killer (NK) cells in the control of tumor metastasis, *in* Tumor Invasion and Metastasis, L. A. Liotta and I. R. Hart, eds. Martinus Nijhoff Publishers, The Hague, pp. 29–41.
Hanna, N., and I. J. Fidler. 1981. Relationship between metastatic potential and resistance to NK cell-mediated cytotoxicity in three murine tumor systems. JNCI 66:1183–1190.
Hart, I. R. 1982. Seed and soil revisited: Mechanism of site specific metastasis. Cancer Met. Rev. 1:5–16.
Hart, I. R., and I. J. Fidler. 1980. Role of organ selectivity in the determination of metastatic patterns of B16 melanoma. Cancer Res. 40:2281–2287.
Hart, I. R., and I. J. Fidler. 1981. The implications of tumor heterogeneity for studies on the biology and therapy of cancer metastasis. Biochim. Biophys. Acta 651:37–50.
Höök, M., Å. Wasteson, and Å. Oldberg. 1975. A heparan sulfate degrading endoglycosidase from rat liver tissue. Biochem. Biophys. Res. Commun. 67:1422–1428.
Howard, B. V., E. J. Macarak, D. Gunson, and N. A. Kefalides. 1976. Characterization of the collagen synthesized by endothelial cells in culture. Proc. Natl. Acad. Sci. USA 73:2361–2364.
Irimura, T., R. Gonzalez, and G. L. Nicolson. 1981. Effects of tunicamycin on B16 metastatic melanoma cell surface glycoproteins and blood-borne arrest and survival properties. Cancer Res. 41:3411–3418.
Irimura, T., M. Nakajima, N. Di Ferrante, and G. L. Nicolson. 1983a. High-speed gel permeation chromatrography of glycosaminoglycans: Its application to the analysis of heparan sulfate of embryonic carcinoma and its degradation products by tumor cell derived heparanase. Analyt. Biochem. 130:461–468.
Irimura, T., M. Nakajima, and G. L. Nicolson. 1983b. Metastatic tumor cell attachment to vascular endothelial cells and destruction of their basal lamina-like matrix. Gann Monogr. Cancer Res. (in press).

Irimura, T., and G. L. Nicolson. 1981a. The role of glycoconjugates in metastatic melanoma blood-borne arrest and cell surface properties. J. Supramol. Struct. Cell. Biochem. 17:325–336.
Irimura, T., and G. L. Nicolson. 1981b. Affinity isolation of cell surface sialoglycoproteins from metastatic B16 melanoma cells and their interaction with endothelial cell basal lamina. J. Cell Biol. 91:118a.
Jones, P. A. 1979. Construction of an artificial blood vessel wall from cultured endothelial and smooth muscle cells. Proc. Natl. Acad. Sci. USA 76:1882–1886.
Joseph, J., T. Miao, L. Alby, J. Grieve, B. Houser, L. Kubai, L. Morrissey, Y. A. Sidky, S. L. Watt, and G. Auerbach. 1983. Immunological probes for the study of endothelial cell diversity, *in* Endothelial Cell Identification and Culture Methods, D. Thilo, ed. Karger, Basel (in press).
Kinjo, M., K. Oka, S. Naito, S. Kohga, K. Tanaka, S. Oboshi, Y. Hayata, and K. Yasumoto. 1979. Thromboplastic and fibrinolytic activity of cultured human cancer cell lines. Br. J. Cancer 39:15–23.
Kinsey, D. L. 1960. An experimental study of preferential metastasis. Cancer 13:674–676.
Klein, U., H. Kresse, and K. von Figura. 1976. Evidence for degradation of heparan sulfate by endoglycosidases: Glucosamine and hexuronic acid are reducing terminals of intercellular heparan sulfate from human skin fibroblast. Biochem. Biophys. Res. Commun. 69:158–166.
Klein, U., and K. von Figura. 1976. Partial purification and characterization of a heparan sulfate specific endoglucuronidase. Biochem. Biophys. Res. Commun. 73:569–576.
Kramer, R. H., R. Gonzalez, and G. L. Nicolson. 1980. Metastatic tumor cells adhere preferentially to the extracellular matrix underlying vascular endothelial cells. Int. J. Cancer 26:639–645.
Kramer, R. H., and G. L. Nicolson. 1979. Interactions of tumor cells with vascular endothelial cell monolayers. A model for metastatic invasion. Proc. Natl. Acad. Sci. USA 76:5704–5708.
Kramer, R. H., and G. L. Nicolson. 1981. Invasion of vascular endothelial cell monolayers and underlying matrix by metastatic human cancer cells, *in* International Cell Biology 1980–1981, S. Schweiger, ed. Springer-Verlag, Heidelberg, pp. 794–799.
Kramer, R. H., K. G. Vogel, and G. L. Nicolson. 1982. Solubilization and degradation of subendothelial matrix glycoproteins and proteoglycans by metastatic tumor cells. J. Biol. Chem. 257:2678–2686.
Liotta, L. A., J. Kleinerman, and G. L. Saidel. 1976. The significance of hematogenous tumor cell clumps in the metastatic process. Cancer Res. 36:889–894.
Liotta, L. A., V. P. Thorgeirsson, and S. Garbisa. 1982. Role of collagenases in tumor cell invasion. Cancer Metastasis Rev. 1:277–288.
Liotta, L. A., S. Tryggvason, S. Garbisa, I. Hart, C. M. Foltz, and S. Shafie. 1980. Metastatic propensity correlates with tumor cell degradation of basement membrane collagen. Nature 284:67–68.
Ludatsher, R. M., S. A. Luse, and V. Suntzeff. 1967. An electron microscopic study of pulmonary tumor emboli from transplanted Morris hepatoma 5123. Cancer Res. 1939–1952.
Miner, K. M., T. Kawaguchi, G. W. Uba, and G. L. Nicolson. 1982. Clonal drift of cell surface, melanogenic and experimental metastatic properties of in vivo-selected, brain meninges-colonizing murine B16 melanoma. Cancer Res. 42:4631–4638.
Murray, J. C., L. A. Liotta, S. I. Rennard, and G. R. Martin. 1980. Adhesion characteristics of murine metastatic and non-metastatic tumor cells in vitro. Cancer Res. 40:347–351.
Nakajima, M., T. Irimura, D. T. Di Ferrante, N. Di Ferrante, and G. L. Nicolson. 1983. Heparan sulfate degradation correlates with tumor invasive and metastatic properties of B16 melanoma sublines. Science 220:611–613.
Nakamura, K., T. Kawaguchi, S. Asahina, T. Sakurai, Y. Ebina, S. Yokoya, and M. Morita. 1977. Electron microscopic studies on extravasation of tumor cells and early foci of hematogenous metastases. Gann Monogr. Cancer Res. 20:57–71.
Neri, A., D. Welch, T. Kawaguchi, and G. L. Nicolson. 1982. Development and biologic properties of malignant cell sublines and clones of a spontaneously metastasizing rat mammary adenocarcinoma. JNCI 68:507–517.
Nicolson, G. L. 1978. Cell and tissue interactions leading to malignant tumor spread (metastasis). Am. Zool. 18:77–86.
Nicolson, G. L. 1982a. Cancer metastasis: Organ colonization and the cell surface properties of malignant cells. Biochim. Biophys. Acta 695:113–176.
Nicolson, G. L. 1982b. Cell surface properties of metastatic tumor cells, *in* Tumor Invasion and Metastasis, L. Liotta and I. R. Hart, eds. Martinus Nijhoff Publishers, The Hague, pp. 57–59.

Nicolson, G. L. 1982c. Metastatic tumor cell attachment and invasion assay utilizing vascular endothelial cell monolayers. J. Histochem. Cytochem. 30:214–220.

Nicolson, G. L., T. Irimura, R. Gonzalez, and E. Ruoslahti. 1981. The role of fibronectin in adhesion of metastatic melanoma cells to endothelial cells and their basal lamina. Exp. Cell Res. 135:461–465.

Nicolson, G. L., T. Irimura, M. Nakajima, T. V. Updyke, and G. Poste. 1983. The cellular interactions of metastatic tumor cells with special reference to endothelial cells and their basal lamina-like matrix, *in* Hemostatic Mechanisms and Metastasis, K. V. Honn and B. F. Sloane, eds. Martinus Nijhoff Publishers, The Hague (in press).

Nicolson, G. L., and G. Poste. 1982. Tumor cell diversity and host responses in cancer metastasis. I. Properties of metastatic cells. Curr. Prob. Cancer 7(6):1–83.

Nicolson, G. L., and G. Poste. 1983a. Tumor cell diversity and host responses in cancer metastasis. II. Host immune responses and therapy of metastases. Curr. Prob. Cancer 7(7):1–43.

Nicolson, G. L., and G. Poste. 1983b. Tumor implantation and invasion at metastatic sites. Int. Rev. Exp. Pathol. 25:77–181.

Nicolson, G. L., and J. L. Winkelhake. 1975. Organ specificity of blood-borne tumour metastasis determined by cell adhesion? Nature 255:230–232.

Ögren, S., and U. Lindahl. 1975. Cleavage of macromolecular heparin by an enzyme from mouse mastocytoma. J. Biol. Chem. 250:2690–2697.

Oosta, G. M., L. V. Favreau, D. L. Beeler, and R. D. Rosenberg. 1982. Purification and properties of human platelet heparitinase. J. Biol. Chem. 257:11249–11255.

Pearlstein, E., P. L. Salk, G. Yogeeswaran, and S. Karpatkin. 1980. Correlation between spontaneous metastatic potential, platelet-aggregating activity of cell surface extracts, and cell surface sialylation in 10 metastatic-variant derivatives of rat renal sarcoma cell line. Proc. Natl. Acad. Sci. USA 77:4336–4339.

Phondke, G. P., K. R. Madyastha, P. R. Madyastha, and R. F. Barth. 1981. Relationship between concanavalin A-induced agglutinability of murine leukemia cells and their propensity to form heterotypic aggregates with syngeneic lymphoid cells. JNCI 66:643–647.

Poole, A. R., K. J. Tiltman, A. D. Recklies, and T. A. M. Stoker. 1978. Differences in secretion of the proteinase cathepsin B at the edge of human breast carcinomas and fibroadenomas. Nature 273:545–547.

Poste, G. 1982a. Experimental systems for analysis of the malignant phenotype. Cancer Met. Rev. 1:141–199.

Poste, G. 1982b. Methods and models for studying tumor invasion, *in* Tumor Invasion and Metastasis, I. R. Hart and L. Liotta, eds. Marcel Dekker, New York, pp. 148–177.

Poste, G., J. Doll, I. R. Hart, and I. J. Fidler. 1980. In vitro selection of murine B16 melanoma variants with enhanced tissue invasive properties. Cancer Res. 40:1630–1644.

Poste, G., and I. J. Fidler. 1980. The pathogenesis of cancer metastasis. Nature 283:139–146.

Poste, G., and G. L. Nicolson. 1980. Arrest and metastasis of blood-borne tumor cells are modified by fusion of plasma membrane vesicles from highly metastatic cells. Proc. Natl. Acad. Sci. USA 77:399–403.

Raz, A., and R. Lotan. 1981. Lectin-like activities associated with human and murine neoplastic cells. Cancer Res. 41:3642–3647.

Roos, E., and K. P. Dingemans. 1979. Mechanisms of metastasis. Biochim. Biophys. Acta 560:135–166.

Salsbury, A. J. 1975. The significance of the circulating cancer cell. Cancer Treat. Rev. 2:55–72.

Sato, H., and M. Suzuki. 1976. Deformability and viability of tumor cells by transcapillary passage, with reference to organ affinity of metastasis in cancer, *in* Fundamental Aspects of Metastasis, L. Weiss, ed. North Holland Publishing Co., Amsterdam, pp. 311–317.

Schirrmacher, V., R. Cheinsong-Popov, and H. Arnheiter. 1980. Hepatocyte-tumor cell interaction in vitro. I. Conditions for rosette formation and inhibition by anti-H-2 antibody. J. Exp. Med. 151:984–989.

Schlepper-Schafer, J., E. Friedrich, and H. Kolb. 1981. Galactosyl specific receptor on liver cells: Binding site for tumor cells. Eur. J. Cell Biol. 25:95–102.

Sindelar, W. F., T. S. Tralka, and A. S. Ketcham. 1975. Electron microscopic observations on formation of pulmonary metastases. J. Surg. Res. 18:137–161.

Sloane, B. F., J. R. Dunn, and K. V. Honn. 1981. Lysosomal cathepsin B: Correlation with metastatic potential. Science 212:1151–1153.

Sloane, B. F., K. V. Honn, J. G. Sadler, W. A. Turner, J. J. Kimpson, and J. D. Taylor. 1982. Cathepsin B activity in B16 melanoma cells: A possible marker for metastatic potential. Cancer Res. 42:980–986.

Sugarbaker, E. V. 1979. Cancer metastasis: A product of tumor-host interactions. Curr. Prob. Cancer 3(7):3–59.

Sugarbaker, E. V. 1981. Patterns of metastasis in human malignancies. Cancer Biol. Rev. 2:235–278.

Sugarbaker, E. V., A. M. Cohen, and A. S. Ketcham. 1971. Do metastases metastasize? Ann. Surg. 174:161–166.

Sugarbaker, E. V., N. Weingard, and J. M. Roseman. 1982. Observations on cancer metastasis in man, *in* Tumor Invasion and Metastasis, L. A. Liotta and I. R. Hart, eds. Martinus Nijhoff Publishers, The Hague, The Netherlands, pp. 427–465.

Terranova, V. P., L. A. Liotta, R. G. Russo, and G. R. Martin. 1982. Role of laminin in the attachment and metastasis of murine tumor cells. Cancer Res. 42:2265–2269.

Terranova, V. P., D. H. Rohrbach, and G. R. Martin. 1980. Role of laminin in the attachment of PAM212 (epithelial) cells to basement membrane collagen. Cell 22:719–726.

Vaage, J., and S. Agrawal. 1976. Stimulation or inhibition of immune resistance against metastatic or local growth of a C3H mammary carcinoma. Cancer Res. 36:1831–1836.

Vlodavsky, I., and D. Gospodarowicz. 1981. Respective roles of laminin and fibronectin in adhesion of human carcinoma and sarcoma cells. Nature 289:303–306.

Warren, B. A. 1973. Environment of the blood-borne tumor embolus adherent to vessel wall. J. Med. 4:150–177.

Warren, B. A. 1981. Origin and fate of blood-borne tumor emboli. Cancer Biol. Rev. 2:95–169.

Wasteson, Å., B. Glimelius, D. Bush, B. Westermark, C.-H. Heldin, and B. Norling. 1977. Effect of a platelet endoglycosidase on cell surface associated heparan sulfate of human cultured endothelial and glial cells. Thromb. Res. 11:309–311.

Wood, S., Jr. 1964. Experimental studies of the intravascular dissemination of ascitic V2 carcinoma cells in the rabbit, with special reference to fibrinogen and fibrinolytic agents. Bull. Schweiz. Akad. Med. Wiss. 20:92–121.

Zamora, P. O., K. G. Danielson, and H. L. Hosick. 1980. Invasion of endothelial cell monolayers on collagen gels by cells from mammary tumor spheroids. Cancer Res. 40:4631–4639.

Zeidman, I., and J. M. Buss. 1952. Transpulmonary passage of tumor cell emboli. Cancer Res. 12:731–733.

Cancer Invasion and Metastasis: Biologic and Therapeutic Aspects edited by Garth L. Nicolson and Luka Milas. Raven Press, New York © 1984.

Tumor Cell Attachment and Degradation of Basement Membranes

Lance A. Liotta, Nageswara C. Rao, Victor P. Terranova,* Sanford Barsky, and Unnur Thorgeirsson

*Section of Tumor Invasion and Metastases, Laboratory of Pathology, National Cancer Institute; and *Laboratory of Developmental Biology and Anomalies, National Institute of Dental Research, National Institutes of Health, Bethesda, Maryland 20205*

Metastasizing tumor cells must traverse epithelium- and endothelium-derived basement membranes at multiple stages in the metastatic process (Liotta et al. 1977, 1979, 1980, 1981, Liotta and Hart 1982). The first step of this traversal is tumor cell attachment to the basement membrane. The attachment may be mediated through a cell surface receptor binding to laminin, a glycoprotein unique to basement membranes (Timpl et al. 1979, Terranova et al. 1980, 1982, 1983). We have previously shown that laminin-mediated tumor cell attachment can be used to isolate highly metastatic tumor cells from a mixed population (Terranova et al. 1982). We have also shown that human carcinoma cells bind laminin with a high affinity (K_D in nanomolar range) with 10,000–50,000 receptor sites per cell (Rao et al. 1983, Terranova et al. 1983). We now present the isolation of a tumor cell laminin receptor from detergent extracts of BL6 melanoma cell plasma membranes. A fragment of the laminin molecule that binds to the receptor and blocks tumor cell attachment in vitro was studied for its ability to inhibit metastases in vivo.

ISOLATION OF A TUMOR CELL LAMININ RECEPTOR

Materials and Methods

Laminin Binding

BL6 melanoma cells were supplied by Dr. Ian Hart, Frederick, Maryland (Poste et al. 1980). The growth/metastasis rate and attachment properties of these tumor cells have been described (Terranova et al. 1982). BL6 cells were cultivated in RPMI 1640 media with 10% FCS. Plasma membranes were isolated from cells in log phase of growth as described previously (Pilch and Czech 1980). The plasma membrane homogenate was solubilized in 0.1% Triton × 100, 1.0–2.0 mg protein/ml. After centrifugation at 30,000 g for 45 min, the supernatant was collected and incubated with SM2 Biobeads (Bio-Rad) to remove the Triton. Iodination of the laminin ligand and the plasma membrane extract was performed using lactoperoxidase (Thorell and Johansson 1969). Laminin receptors were measured on living cells in suspension (Rao et al. 1983, Terranova et al. 1983). After trypsinization, the BL6 cells were incubated in complete medium under constant agitation at 37°C for 2 h. The labeled ligand with or without a 250-fold excess of unlabeled ligand was added and the incubation was continued for 2 h at 25°C. The cell-bound and -free ligand was separated by centrifugation. Binding assays on plasma membrane extracts were performed using one member of the ligand or receptor pair bound to solid phase nitrocellulose Millipore SCWP circles (Terranova et al. 1983) or cyanogen bromide–activated Sepharose 4B. In the latter case, 25 μg of laminin or plasma membrane extract protein bound to cyanogen bromide–activated Sepharose 4B (100 μl) was mixed with an equal amount of 25 mM Tris, 5 mM $MgCl_2$ and $CaCl_2$, pH 7.4, and 100 μl of this buffer containing 0.1% bovine serum albumin (BSA). ^{125}I-labeled plasma membrane extract (10^8 cpm/mg) or ^{125}I-labeled laminin (10^9 cpm/mg) was added in a total volume of 100 μl, diluted with the buffer. Competition was performed with various concentrations of unlabeled laminin in solution or unlabeled plasma membrane extracts (2 to 20 μg). The binding assay mixture was incubated at 4°C overnight. The laminin-Sepharose beads were collected by centrifugation at 5,000 rpm for 30 min and the pellet was washed twice with 2.0 ml of the buffer containing 0.1% BSA. The proteins in the first-spin supernatant and the pellet were identified by electrophoresis on 7% acrylamide slab gels followed by autoradiography. Laminin affinity chromatography was performed using purified laminin cross-linked to Sepharose 4B. ^{125}I-labeled plasma membrane extract was incubated 15 h in the laminin-Sepharose affinity column (1 × 15 cm) at 4°C. The unbound radioactivity was washed with 40 ml of 25 mM Tris, 5 mM $CaCl_2$, 5 mM $MgCl_2$, 0.9% NaCl, pH 7.4. The bound activity was eluted with 0.2 M glycine HCl, pH 3.5, immediately neutralized with 1.0 M Tris saline, and lyophilized. The proteins were identified by slab gel electrophoresis and autoradiography. The number of laminin receptor sites and the K_D were calculated by Scatchard analysis.

Metastases Studies

Laminin is a cross-shaped molecule with three short arms and one long arm (Rao et al. 1982b). All arms have globular end regions. Protease fragment alpha contains the three intact short arms. Protease fragments P_1 and C_1 contain the intersection region of the short arms. Protease-derived fragments of the laminin molecule were prepared and purified as described previously (Rao et al. 1982a, 1982b). Two million BL6 melanoma cells were preincubated for 30 min in Hanks' balanced salt solution with Ca and Mg and containing 1.0, 10.0, or 100.0 μg/ml of: (a) whole laminin, (b) laminin fragment alpha, or (c) laminin fragment C_1. The preincubated cells were injected in a volume of 0.05 ml into the tail veins of C57BL6 6-week-old, pathogen-free male mice. The laminin was purified from the same strain of mice. Preincubation with the laminin or laminin fragments did not alter cell viability or clumping. Lung metastases were counted 25 days after tail vein injection.

Results

BL6 melanoma cells exhibited saturable binding for laminin. Scatchard analysis demonstrated approximately 110,000 binding sites per cell with a high affinity: $K_D = 2.2$ nM (Figure 1A). Laminin binding to the tumor cells was abolished by extensive trypsinization. The receptor regenerated after 2–4 h incubation in serum-free or serum-containing media. Collagen, denatured laminin, fibronectin, or serum did not compete for binding. Binding of ^{125}I laminin to isolated cell plasma membranes obtained from solid tumors or cultured cells also showed a high affinity: $K_D = 1.5$ nM (Figure 1B). Excess unbound laminin competed for binding of the solubilized membrane receptor to laminin immobilized to a solid phase. Gel electrophoresis of the solubilized membrane proteins bound to laminin before and after competition demonstrated a single molecular weight class for the receptor. Laminin affinity chromatography was therefore used to isolate the receptor (Figure 2), producing a 900-fold purification relative to the crude membrane extract. The receptor's molecular weight was 67,000 after reduction by polyacrylamide gel electrophoresis. The isolated receptor retained a high binding affinity for laminin: $K_D = 2$ nM. Binding of whole laminin to the receptor was competitively abolished by a fragment (P_1 or C_1) of the laminin molecule that retained the intersection region of the short arms and lacked the globular end regions of the laminin molecule (Rao et al. 1982a, 1982b,

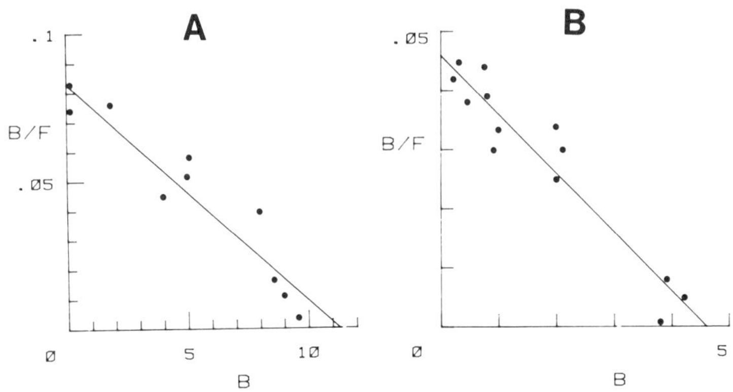

FIG. 1. Scatchard analysis for the specific binding of laminin to suspended BL6 melanoma cells **(A)**, detergent extract of the BL6 plasma membranes **(B)**. For panel A the X-axis units are laminin (ng/ml) and the X intercept is 11.3; $K_D = 2.2$ nM, r = 0.94. For panel B the X-axis units are plasma membrane protein (fmol/mg protein). The X intercept is 4.6, $K_D = 1.5$ nM, r = 0.95.

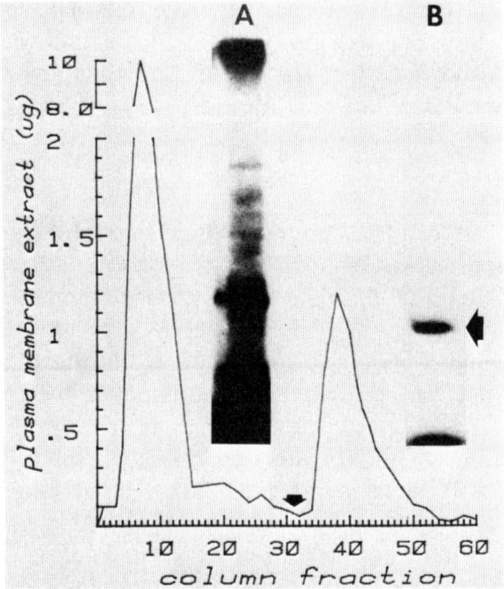

FIG. 2. Isolation of laminin receptor using laminin affinity chromatography. The BL6 plasma membrane extract was applied to the affinity column, and the bound receptor was eluted (*small arrow*) with 0.2 M glycine, pH 3.5. The unbound fraction (95%) is the first peak. Gel electrophoresis followed by autoradiography of the unbound fraction reveals a large series of components **(A).** The bound fraction after elution migrated as a single band (*large arrow*) on polyacrylamide gel electrophoresis **(B)** with a M_r of 67,000 after reduction.

Terranova et al. 1983). Binding of the P_1 or C_1 fragment to the cell inhibits cell attachment to type IV collagen in vitro, whereas the alpha fragment of the laminin molecule, which retained the globular end regions, bound to the receptor and stimulated cell attachment in vitro (Terranova et al. 1983, Rao et al. 1982b). Preincubation of the BL6 cells with the P_1 or C_1 fragment of

TABLE 1. *Inhibition of intravenous metastases by laminin fragments*

BL6 treatment (μg/ml)	Pulmonary metastases (percent change in median compared to control)
Whole laminin	
10	300 Increase
100	340 Increase
Fibronectin	
100	20 Increase
Laminin C_1 fragment	
1	10 Decrease
10	50 Decrease
100	95 Decrease
Laminin alpha fragment	
100	250 Increase

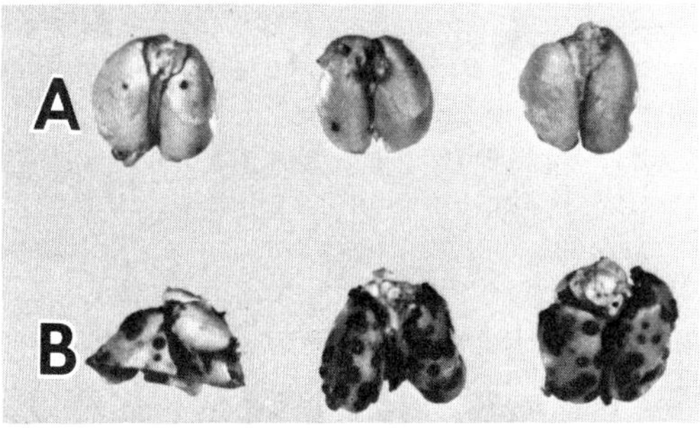

FIG. 3. Representative murine lungs from experiment described in Table 1. **A.** BL6 cells plus laminin C_1 fragment (100 μg/ml), **B.** BL6 cells untreated.

the laminin molecule markedly inhibited i.v. metastasis formation in a dose-dependent manner in seven separate experiments (Table 1, Figure 3) (S. H. Barsky, C. N. Rao, J. B. Williams, and L. A. Liotta, manuscript submitted).

Discussion

Cell receptors for extracellular matrix proteins could play a role in a wide variety of biologic processes, including cell differentiation and neoplasia (Rao et al. 1982b, Terranova et al. 1983, Rao et al. 1983, Hay 1982, Couchman et al. 1983, and Dr. Max Wicha, personal communication). The basement membrane is a ubiquitous extracellular matrix that separates organ parenchymal cells from interstitial stroma. Whenever any cell migrates from one tissue to another, it must traverse the basement membrane. Cell receptors for basement membrane components may be expressed by cells that are anchored to or moving through basement membranes.

We have previously demonstrated the existence of high affinity cell-binding sites specific for laminin on tumor cells (Rao et al. 1982a, 1982b, 1983, Terranova et al. 1983). Using protease fragments of laminin, it was determined that a specific protease-resistant domain of the molecule is necessary for binding to the cell receptor. In this report, we describe the isolation of a tumor cell receptor for laminin. After detergent extraction from plasma membranes and purification using laminin affinity chromatography, the receptor migrates as a single 67,000-M_r band on sodium dodecyl sulfate polyacrylamide gel electrophoresis. (It must be noted that estimations of M_r based on gel electrophoresis alone are sometimes inaccurate.) The isolated receptor retains a high binding affinity. The biochemical characteristics of this isolated receptor and its relative expression in a wide variety of cell types remains to be elucidated.

Hematogenous metastasis formation is obviously a complex and inefficient process. Tumor cells must traverse basement membranes at multiple stages of metastasis. Therefore, biochemical factors that promote or retard interactions of tumor cells with basement membranes may alter the outcome of the metastatic process. A necessary biochemical interaction is tumor cell attachment to the basement membrane. At least for some murine and human tumor cells, laminin may be an important attachment factor in this process. The present study demonstrates that tumor cell interaction with laminin is mediated via a specific plasma membrane receptor. Blocking such receptor-mediated binding by a fragment of the ligand markedly inhibits i.v. metastases formation. The BL6 tumor cells have 110,000 free receptors for laminin. If these receptors are saturated with whole laminin or the laminin alpha fragment, which retains the type IV collagen binding domain (Terranova et al. 1983, Rao et al. 1982b), metastasis is stimulated (Table 1). On the other hand, saturation of the receptor with the cell-binding fragment of laminin inhibits metastasis. Because the laminin was purified from syngeneic mice in these experiments, it is unlikely that aggregation or immunologic factors played a role. Increased clumping or alterations in viability were not noted. Whether the laminin fragments alter metastasis formation in other model systems remains to be determined.

TYPE IV COLLAGENASE IN HUMAN BREAST CANCER

Many invasive tumors elaborate proteolytic enzymes that can degrade basement membrane (BM) components. In some animal models BM degrading activity correlates with metastatic behavior (Liotta et al. 1977, 1980, Liotta and Hart 1982). Type IV collagen is the major structural component of the BM. We have purified a type IV collagenase from a highly metastatic murine PMT sarcoma (Liotta et al. 1981) and raised specific antibodies to both the native and denatured forms of the enzyme in adult white male New Zealand rabbits. These antibodies were found to be specific for type IV collagenase by immunoprecipitation and competition studies.

These antibodies were applied to 25 surgical specimens of human invasive breast carcinoma to determine whether this enzyme is present in situ in human carcinoma and whether its localization would be useful in the detection of tumor invasion.

Materials and Methods

Twenty-five specimens of invasive breast carcinoma (18 infiltrating ductal, 5 infiltrating lobular, 1 colloid, and 1 tubular) were obtained fresh from the operating room and sectioned (5 μm) on a cryostat. They were then stained with a standard immunoperoxidase technique using antibodies to both native and denatured type IV collagenase as the first antibody. The second antibody was goat antirabbit and the third antibody was rabbit peroxidase/antiperoxidase (Cappel Laboratories). Immunoreactivity was detected with 3,3′-diaminobenzidine and hydrogen peroxide (Sigma Laboratories); Hematoxylin was used as counterstain. Specimens of fibroadenoma, fibrocystic disease, and normal breast were used as controls.

Results

Intense cytoplasmic immunoreactivity was demonstrated in all 25 cases of invasive breast carcinoma. Such immunoreactivity was usually frequent only along the invasive borders. Areas of carcinoma in situ and adjacent benign ductal and acinar structures did not demonstrate immunoreactivity. Cases of fibroadenoma, fibrocystic disease, and normal breast were negative. In invasive breast carcinomas, the cytoplasmic immunoreactivity of type IV collagenase was not present in every invasive cell. The percentage of invasive cells that showed staining ranged from 10% to 75% in our 25 cases. Positive cells tended to occur in clusters or groups rather than singly. Cytoplasmic immunoreactivity was demonstrated with antibodies to both denatured and native type IV collagenase; antibody to the denatured enzyme showed significantly higher affinity. These results, summarized in Table 2, have been reported previously (Barsky et al. 1983).

Discussion

Invasive breast carcinoma cells differ from carcinoma in situ and benign epithelium by loss of extracellular BM components (Barsky et al. 1982). One such component is type IV collagen. We now demonstrate that these same invasive carcinoma cells possess specific cytoplasmic immunoreactivity to type IV collagenase. This finding could explain the loss of extracellular type IV collagen in such invasive tumors. We postulate that this type IV collagenase activity is demonstrable in only a percentage of the invasive cells either because the enzyme is heterogeneously distributed among tumor cells or because production of the enzyme is turned on and off at different stages of the invasive process or cell cycle. Demonstration of type IV collagenase immunoreactivity in human breast carcinoma may be useful both in identifying the invasive tumor cells in tissue sections and in gaining insight into the pathophysiology. The relative expression of type IV collagenase antigenicity in other tumor types or disease states remains to be determined. Collagenase expression is not tumor specific. However, proteolysis may be necessary but not sufficient for tumor cell invasion of the extracellular matrix.

TABLE 2. *Type IV collagenase immunoreactivity in breast lesions*

Lesion	No. cases	% Positive cells	Anti-type IV collagenase	
			Denatured	Native
Invasive carcinoma	25	10–75	++++	++
Fibroadenoma	10	0	−−	−
Fibrocystic disease	10	0	−−	−
Normal breast	10	0	−−	−

REFERENCES

Barsky, S. H., G. P. Siegal, F. Jannotta, and L. A. Liotta. 1982. Loss of basement membrane components by invasive tumors but not by their benign counterparts. Lab. Invest. 46:7A.

Barsky, S. H., S. Togo, S. Garbisa, and L. A. Liotta. 1983. Type IV collagenase immunoreactivity in invasive breast carcinoma. Lancet 8319:296–297.

Couchman, J. R., M. Hook, D. A. Rees, and R. Timpl. 1983. Adhesion, growth and matrix production by fibroblasts on laminin substrates. J. Cell Biol. 96:177–183.

Hay, E. D. 1982. Cell Biology of Extracellular Matrix. New York, Plenum Press.

Liotta, L. A., S. Abe, P. Gerhon-Robey, and G. R. Martin. 1979. Preferential digestion of basement membrane collagen by an enzyme derived from a metastatic murine tumor. Proc. Natl. Acad. Sci. USA 76:2268–2272.

Liotta, L. A., and I. R. Hart, eds. 1982. Tumor Invasion and Metastasis. Martinus Nijhoff, The Hague.

Liotta, L. A., J. Kleinerman, P. Catanzaro, and D. Rynbrandt. 1977. Degradation of basement membrane by murine tumor cells. JNCI 58:1427–1431.

Liotta, L. A., K. Tryggvason, S. Garbisa, I. Hart, C. M. Foltz, and S. Shafie. 1980. Metastatic potential correlates with enzymatic degradation of basement membrane collagen. Nature 284:67–69.

Liotta, L. A., K. Tryggvason, S. Garbisa, P. Gehron-Robey, and S. Abe. 1981. Partial purification and characterization of a neutral protease which cleaves type IV collagen. Biochemistry 20:100–104.

Pilch, P. F., and P. M. Czech. 1980. The subunit structure of the high affinity insulin receptor—Evidence for a disulphide linked receptor complex in bat cell and liver plasma membranes. J. Biol. Chem. 255:1722–1731.

Poste, G., J. Doll, I. Hart, and I. J. Fidler. 1980. In vitro selection of murine B16 melanoma variants with enhanced tissue invasive properties. Cancer Res. 40:1636–1644.

Rao, N. A., S. H. Barsky, V. P. Terranova, and L. A. Liotta. 1983. Isolation of a tumor cell laminin receptor. Biochem. Biophys. Res. Commun. 111:804–808.

Rao, C. N., I. M. K. Margulies, R. H. Goldfarb, J. A. Madri, D. T. Woodley, and L. A. Liotta. 1982a. Differential proteolytic susceptibility of laminin alpha and beta subunits. Arch. Biochem. Biophys. 219:65–70.

Rao, C. N., I. M. K. Margulies, T. S. Tralka, V. P. Terranova, J. A. Madri, and L. A. Liotta. 1982b. Isolation of a subunit of laminin and its role in molecular structure and tumor cell attachment. J. Biol. Chem. 257:9740–9744.

Terranova, V. P., L. A. Liotta, R. G. Russo, and G. P. Martin. 1982. Role of laminin in the attachment and metastases of murine tumor cells. Cancer Res. 42:2265–2269.

Terranova, V. P., C. N. Rao, T. Takebic, I. M. K. Margulies, and L. A. Liotta. 1983. Laminin receptor on human breast carcinoma cells. Proc. Natl. Acad. Sci. USA 80:444–448.

Terranova, V. P., D. H. Rohrbach, and G. R. Martin. 1980. Role of laminin in the attachment of PAM 212 (epithelial) cells to basement membrane collagen. Cell 22:719–726.

Thorell, J. I., and B. J. Johansson. 1969. Enzymatic iodination of polypeptides with ^{125}I to high specific activity. Biochim. Biophys. Acta 251:363–369.

Timpl, R., H. Rohde, P. G. Robey, S. T. Rennard, J. M. Foidart, and G. R. Martin. 1979. Laminin—A glycoprotein from basement membranes. J. Biol. Chem. 254:9933–9937.

Cancer Invasion and Metastasis: Biologic and Therapeutic Aspects edited by Garth L. Nicolson and Luka Milas. Raven Press, New York © 1984.

Degradation of Artificial Tissue Substrates

Peter A. Jones,*† Emil Bogenmann,† Yves A. DeClerck,† Walter E. Laug,† Margaret Heisel,† Harry B. Neustein,‡ and Hart Isaacs‡

*Departments of *Biochemistry, †Pediatrics, and ‡Pathology, Childrens Hospital of Los Angeles, Los Angeles, California 90027*

The breakdown of the extracellular matrix is likely to be important during tumor cell invasion. Connective tissue is often destroyed in the vicinity of invasive tumors (Jones and DeClerck 1982), and the proteolytic enzymes associated with tumors may possibly assist in this process (reviewed by Jones and DeClerck 1982).

The extracellular matrix consists of a supramolecular aggregate of connective tissue proteins, including glycoproteins, glycosaminoglycans, collagens, and elastin. These proteins interact with one another through a variety of covalent and noncovalent bonds to form the highly insoluble material recognized as the extracellular matrix. The relative contributions of the constituents vary greatly within an organism, depending on the structural and physiologic functions of the matrix. Several of the components, including glycoproteins, glycosaminoglycans, and collagens, are also part of multiprotein families; consequently, there is no "typical" connective tissue.

Although considerable information is available on the digestion of isolated connective tissue proteins by tumor cell proteases, little is known about the mechanisms by which tumor cells digest highly complex mixtures of these proteins. This is an important consideration because the individual components may interact in ways that alter their susceptibilities to the various classes of degradative enzymes. We have therefore used connective tissue cells grown in culture to synthesize various extracellular matrices in which the components are organized into supramolecular structures, and we have used these in vitro-elaborated matrices as substrates for cells with invasive potentials.

ISOLATION AND CHARACTERIZATION OF EXTRACELLULAR MATRICES

Techniques for isolating labeled extracellular matrices produced by cultured smooth muscle cells (Jones et al. 1979), human fibroblasts (DeClerck and Jones 1980), and bovine endothelial cells (Laug et al. 1983) have been developed. Cultured cells are grown in the presence of [^{3}H]proline (or other label of interest), with daily additions of ascorbic acid. Ascorbic acid is essential for the deposition of insoluble collagen into the extracellular matrix (DeClerck and Jones 1980). Producer cell layers are lysed by the addition of 25 mM of NH_4OH 14 days after seeding to dissolve the cells, but the matrix proteins are left anchored to the bottom of culture dishes. Ammonium hydroxide is used instead of detergents because its volatility and solubility ensure that no residual lysing agent can interfere subsequently with the added tumor cells.

The extracellular matrix elaborated by rat smooth muscle cells is shown in Figure 1. It contains easily identifiable fibers of collagen, microfibrillar and amorphous components of elastin, and granular material that probably corresponds to glycoproteins. Other areas of electron lucency are also present and may represent matrix material not stained by the procedure used to produce

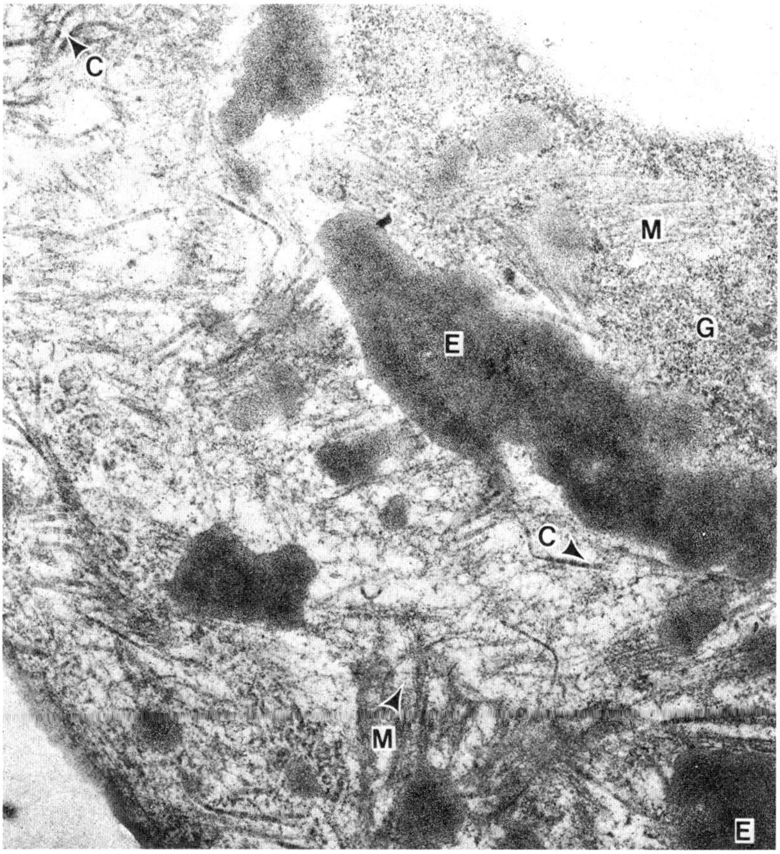

FIG. 1. Electron micrograph of rat smooth muscle cell matrix after NH_4OH lysis of cells. Section has been stained with phosphotungstic acid to highlight matrix components. **C,** banded collagen fibrils; **E,** amorphous elastin; **M,** microfibrillar component (digestible by trypsin); **G,** granular glycoproteins (digestible by trypsin). Reduced from × 35,000. (Courtesy of Dr. Dorothy Bainton, University of California, San Francisco.)

the electron micrograph. Notice also that the matrix contains virtually no residual cellular debris.

The composition of the insoluble matrix can be determined by biosynthetic labeling with either radioactive fucose or proline, followed by sequential enzymatic digestion. Fucose was chosen for its ability to label glycoprotein components preferentially, whereas proline labels all components of the extracellular matrix. The sequence of enzyme digestion is always trypsin, followed by elastase, and finally by collagenase, because cross-linked elastin is not hydrolized by trypsin, and elastase digests proteins other than elastin. Collagenase digestion is always the final treatment used because commercial collagenase preparations are impure and can contain proteolytic activity, which could distort matrix analysis.

The analysis of a typical smooth muscle matrix is shown in Figure 2. Trypsin rapidly solubilized approximately 50% of the radioactivity from a matrix labeled with [^{3}H]proline, whereas approximately 90% of the total matrix radioactivity was solubilized by the same enzyme from a matrix labeled with [^{3}H]fucose. This result shows that trypsin preferentially hydrolyzes fucose-labeled glycoprotein components of the matrix. However, it is also likely that this enzyme removes non-cross-linked precursor molecules of elastin and collagen, which are known to be trypsin sensitive.

Elastase treatment released a further 32% of the proline label, but only 5% of the fucose label. This finding suggests that the trypsin-insensitive material, which was rapidly solubilized by elastase, represented cross-linked elastin and would correspond to the amorphous material seen in Figure 1. The residual 20% of proline radioactivity present after trypsin and elastase treatment was

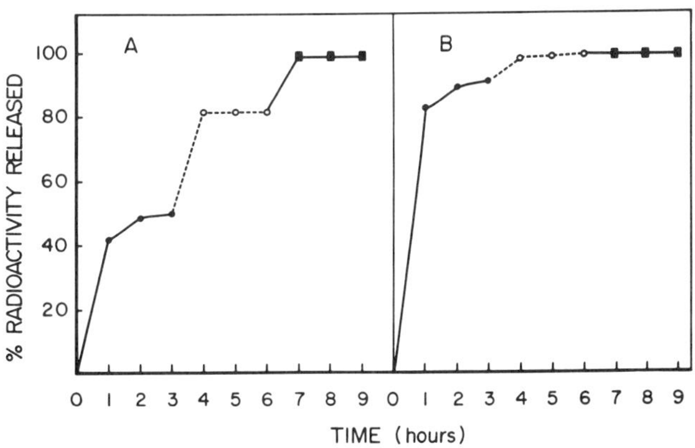

FIG. 2. Sequential release of radioactivity from the rat smooth muscle matrix by trypsin (●——●), pancreatic elastase (O----O), and bacterial collagenase (■——■). Dishes containing matrices labeled with [^{3}H]proline **(A)** or [^{3}H]fucose **(B)** were incubated in phosphate-buffered saline containing 1 mM of $CaCl_2$ and the indicated enzymes (10 μg/ml). Samples were withdrawn at the indicated times for radioactivity determinations.

rapidly solubilized by bacterial collagenase. It contained virtually no incorporated fucose and represents the banded collagen molecules seen in Figure 1 and contains hydroxyproline (DeClerck and Jones 1980). Amino acid analyses of the material solubilized by sequential trypsin, elastase, and collagenase treatments are in good agreement with published values for matrix glycoproteins, elastin, and collagen, respectively (Werb et al. 1980a).

The technique of sequential enzyme analysis therefore allows for correlations between morphologic and biochemical observations on the matrix composition. It also allows one to assess quantitatively which components have been digested from complex mixtures of connective tissue proteins by comparing the matrix composition before and after incubation with cells under a variety of conditions. The matrix composition may be varied by treating it with enzymes before it is presented to degradative cells, so that the influence of each matrix component on the digestion of the others may be determined. A similar type of analysis can be applied to the matrix elaborated by human fibroblasts and bovine endothelial cells, although elastin is not found to be a significant component of these extracellular matrices.

DESTRUCTION OF THE EXTRACELLULAR MATRIX BY HUMAN TUMOR CELL LINES

The rat smooth muscle cell extracellular matrix is susceptible to degradation by several human tumor cell lines (Jones and DeClerck 1980). The human sarcoma cell line HT1080, which was used for most of these experiments, demonstrated elastolytic and collagenolytic activity, in addition to a plasmin-induced hydrolysis of matrix glycoprotein(s). The localization of the tumor cell proteases and the part played by plasminogen activator in matrix degradation were investigated in the experiment shown in Figure 3. Complete or glycoprotein-depleted matrices (prepared by trypsin treatments of complete matrices) were prepared on 25-mm plastic discs, and the HT1080 cells were cultured in different sera, either in direct contact with the matrices or with the discs floating (matrix side down) in 35-mm dishes containing HT1080 cells.

Removal of plasminogen from acid-treated fetal bovine serum decreased the rate of hydrolysis of the complete matrix by HT1080 cells grown in direct contact with the proteins (Figure 3A). The rate of digestion was, however, stimulated when human plasminogen was restored to the plasminogen-depleted serum, although some plasminogen-independent hydrolysis also occurred. Plasminogen was absolutely required for digestion if the matrix was not in direct contact with the tumor cells (Figure 3B). The floating matrix was not digested when the cells were cultured in plasminogen-depleted serum, although digestion did occur with acid-treated serum and with plasminogen-reconstituted serum. Since glycoprotein components of the matrix are plasmin-sensitive (Werb et al. 1980a), the results suggest that the plasmin generated by the HT1080 cell plasminogen activator may have removed these components from the matrix.

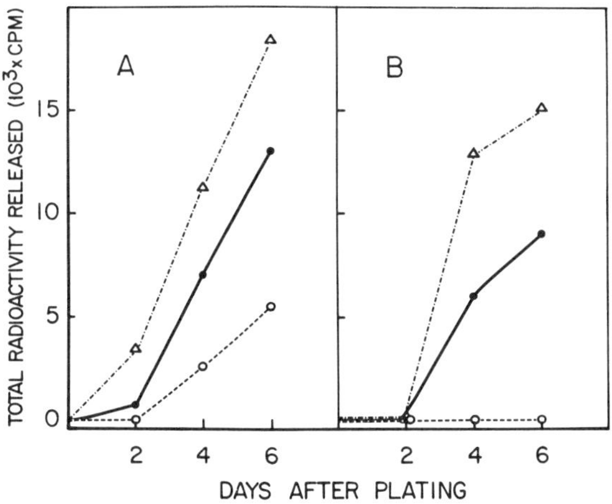

FIG. 3. Effect of plasminogen on the digestion of complete extracellular matrices in contact with or separated from HT1080 cells. Cells were grown in contact with the matrix **(A)** or with the matrix floating above the cells **(B)** in medium containing 10% acid-treated fetal calf serum (●), plasminogen-depleted acid-treated serum (○), or plasminogen-reconstituted acid-treated serum (△). The medium was changed every two days, and the release of radioactivity from the matrix was then determined at the indicated times. Results given are the mean values for duplicate samples; similar results were obtained in a separate experiment. (Reprinted from Jones and DeClerck 1980, with permission from *Cancer Research.*)

The localization of the HT1080 elastolytic and collagenolytic activity was investigated in experiments similar to those shown in Figure 3, by using glycoprotein-depleted matrices as the substrate for the tumor cells (not shown). In contrast to the situation with the complete matrix, plasminogen had no stimulatory effect on the degradation of elastin and collagen when the tumor cells were in direct contact with the matrix. Also, no elastin and collagen degradation occurred when matrix was floating above the tumor cells and was not in direct contact with the HT1080 cells. These enzyme activities were, therefore, probably localized to the tumor cell surface or were rapidly inactivated after secretion into the culture medium.

More recently, we investigated the degradation by HT1080 cells of the subendothelial matrix elaborated by bovine endothelial cells (Laug et al. 1983). The tumor cell plasminogen activator was again found to play a role in glycoprotein hydrolysis from the subendothelium after active plasmin was generated. Some plasminogen-independent hydrolysis of glycoproteins was also evident, and the sarcoma cells were also able to degrade the cross-linked collagen in the endothelial matrix.

The results of these experiments therefore demonstrated that several different tumor cells' proteases may participate in the degradation of discrete matrix components and that synergistic activities among these enzymes may facilitate matrix degradation during tumor invasion in vivo.

DESTRUCTION OF LIVING CULTURES OF RAT SMOOTH MUSCLE CELLS BY HUMAN SARCOMA CELLS

Further studies were conducted using living cultures of rat smooth muscle cells that had not been pretreated with ammonium hydroxide to remove the producer cells. These experiments showed that HT1080 cells were capable of a rapid and efficient degradation of smooth muscle cells and their associated extracellular matrix. Thus, the degradation of a radioactive "tissue" under a variety of experimental conditions could be studied (Jones et al. 1981).

Bovine aortic endothelial cells were able to inhibit markedly the degradative activity of tumor cells (Figure 4). Thus, radioactively labeled rat smooth muscle cells covered with a layer of endothelial cells were almost completely refractory to tumor cell–induced hydrolysis. Detailed morphologic studies indicated that this did not result from the HT1080 cells' failure to penetrate the endothelium, but rather from a curtailment of their degradative activity in the subendothelial area of the artificial vessel wall cultures. Endothelial cells were even able to inhibit the tumor cell destructive activity if they were added simultaneously or up to 7 days after the invasive cells were added.

More recently, we showed that endothelial cells secrete a factor into the culture medium that is capable of inhibiting HT1080 cells' ability to degrade

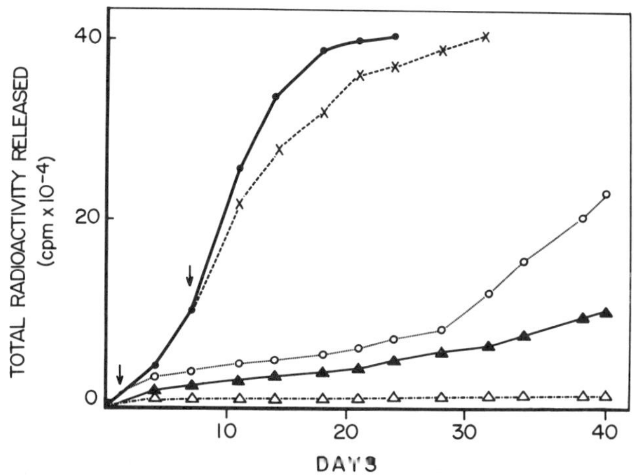

FIG. 4. Degradation of rat smooth muscle cultures by HT1080 cells in the presence or absence of bovine endothelial cells. HT1080 cells (2×10^5 cells/ 35-mm dish) were added to smooth muscle layers prelabeled with [^{3}H]proline one day after (△), simultaneously with (▲), one day before (○), seven days before (×), or in the absence of (●) 10^6 bovine endothelial cells. The total radioactivity of the supernatant medium was determined every three to four days at medium change, and values for control cultures incubated without tumor cells have been subtracted from the values given. Results are expressed as cumulative releases of radioactivity. *Arrows* indicate when endothelial cells were added. (Reprinted from Jones et al. 1981, with permission of *Cancer Research.*)

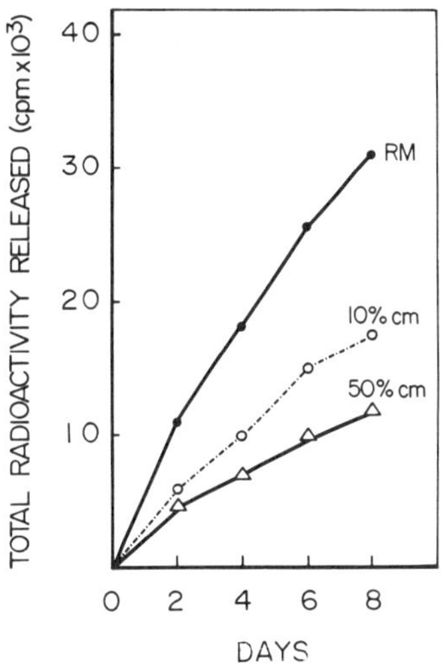

FIG. 5. Inhibition of HT1080 cells' degradation of extracellular matrix proteins by endothelial cell-conditioned medium. HT1080 cells were plated on [^{3}H]-proline–labeled extracellular matrices previously produced by smooth muscle cells. The rates of matrix degradation in fresh regular medium (●) and in fresh medium diluted 9:1 (○) or 1:1 (△) with medium previously conditioned by bovine endothelial cells were then determined.

extracellular matrix (Heisel et al. 1983). Thus, the fibrosarcoma cells' ability to degrade extracellular matrix was inhibited substantially if the cells were cultured in medium that had been mixed with endothelial cell–conditioned medium (Figure 5). Further experiments to characterize this factor have suggested that it is a heat-stable, nondialyzable factor that inhibits plasminogen activator production by the HT1080 cells.

INVASIVENESS OF PRIMARY PEDIATRIC NEOPLASMS

We have recently developed a new system for growing and maintaining primary explants of human pediatric neoplasms (Bogenmann et al. 1983). Primary

TABLE 1. *Correlation of in vivo and in vitro behavior of tumor explants*

Tumor number	Tumor	Invasion in vivo*	Mitotic figures in vitro	Invasion in vitro†	Destruction of smooth muscle cell in vitro†	% Degradation of matrix‡
$HTLA_4$	Osteogenic sarcoma	+	+	+	−	7
$HTLA_3$	Medulloblastoma	+	+	+	+	14
$HTLA_{44}$	Yolk-sac carcinoma	+	+	+	−	1
$HTLA_{19}$	Renal tumor (Wilms')	+	+	+	+	9
$HTLA_7$	Ewing's sarcoma	+	−	+	+	4
$HTLA_{39}$	Neuroblastoma	+	−	+	+	5

* Analyzed by light microscopy on histologic sections of the patient's primary tumor.

† Determined by light and electron microscopy of tumor cells cultured on smooth muscle cells (SMC).

‡ Percentage of radioactivity released from a radiolabeled SMC matrix after nine days in culture.

explanted neoplasms are cultured on either radioactively labeled smooth muscle cell matrix or nylon meshes previously covered with rat smooth muscle cells. The system allows in vitro invasion and the abilities of the explanted tumors to degrade extracellular maxtrix proteins to be assessed simultaneously (Table 1). More than 80% of the most common solid neoplasms in childhood routinely survived or grew in long-term cultures when they were cultured on these substrates. Both substrates were effective in promoting survival or growth or both, and the tumor cells maintained their characteristic cellular and subcellular morphology when compared with that of the in vivo lesions. Several neoplasms were also capable of degrading connective tissue protein, as indicated by the hydrolysis of radioactively labeled smooth muscle cell matrices. However, simple correlations between the extent of matrix degradation and invasive abilities could not be drawn. Further work will therefore be required to determine whether or not matrix degradation is a requirement for invasive activity.

CONCLUSIONS

These experiments suggest mechanisms by which tumor cells degrade extracellular matrix and show that normal cells, such as endothelial cells, can modulate the aggressive behavior of tumor cells. Understanding these phenomena may enable us to limit the invasive process in patients with malignant disease.

ACKNOWLEDGMENTS

This research was supported by grants CA-25397 and HL23500 and fellowship F32CA06995 from the National Institutes of Health and the Ariel Kaare Rosholt Weathers-Lowin Foundation. The excellent assistance of Mary Peer and Felicidad Gonzales is also acknowledged.

REFERENCES

Bogenmann, E., C. Mark, H. Isaacs, H. B. Neustein, Y. A. DeClerck, W. E. Laug, and P. A. Jones. 1983. Invasive properties of primary pediatric neoplasms *in vitro*. Cancer Res. 43:1176–1186.

DeClerck, Y. A., and P. A. Jones. 1980. The effect of ascorbic acid on the nature and production of collagen and elastin by rat smooth muscle cells. Biochem. J. 186:217–225.

Heisel, M., W. E. Laug, and P. A. Jones. 1983. Bovine endothelial cells inhibit the degradation by HT1080 sarcoma cells of extracellular matrix proteins. JNCI (in press).

Jones, P. A. 1979. Construction of an artificial blood vessel wall from cultured endothelial and smooth muscle cells. Proc. Natl. Acad. Sci. USA 76:1882–1886.

Jones, P. A., and Y. DeClerck. 1980. Destruction of extracellular matrices containing glycoproteins, elastin and collagen by metastatic human tumor cells. Cancer Res. 40:3222–3227.

Jones, P. A., and Y. A. DeClerck. 1982. Extracellular matrix destruction by invasive tumor cells. Cancer Metastasis Rev. 1:289–317.

Jones, P. A., H. B. Neustein, F. Gonzales, and E. Bogenmann. 1981. Invasion of an artificial blood vessel wall by human fibrosarcoma cells. Cancer Res. 41:4613–4620.

Jones, P. A., T. Scott-Burden, and W. Gevers. 1979. Glycoprotein, elastin and collagen secretion by rat smooth muscle cells. Proc. Natl. Acad. Sci. USA 76:353–357.

Laug, W. E., Y. A. DeClerck, and P. A. Jones. 1983. Degradation of the subendothelial matrix by tumor cells. Cancer Res. 43:1827–1834.

Werb, Z., M. J. Banda, and P. A. Jones. 1980a. Degradation of connective tissue matrices by macrophages. I. Proteolysis of elastin, glycoproteins, and collagen by proteinase isolated from macrophages. J. Exp. Med. 152:1340–1357.

Werb, Z., D. F. Bainton, and P. A. Jones. 1980b. Degradation of connective tissue matrices by macrophages. III. Morphological and biochemical studies on extracellular, pericellular, and intracellular events in matrix proteolysis by macrophages in culture. J. Exp. Med. 152:1537–1553.

Cancer Invasion and Metastasis: Biologic and Therapeutic Aspects edited by Garth L. Nicolson and Luka Milas. Raven Press, New York © 1984.

Proteases, Angiogenesis, and Invasion

Daniel B. Rifkin, David Moscatelli, Janet Gross, and Eric Jaffe*

*Department of Cell Biology, New York University School of Medicine, New York, New York 10016 and *Department of Medicine, Cornell University School of Medicine, New York, New York 10021*

A number of invasive processes occur within higher organisms. Some are normal, such as neovascularization, trophoblast implantation, and leukocyte infiltration, and some are not normal, such as tumor invasion. One of the more intensively studied of these normal processes is neovascularization, which is the controlled formation of new capillaries by endothelial cells as they grow into a specific region or tissue. The initial stages of neovascularization, which have been studied through microscopic techniques, appear to occur in the following sequence (Ausprunk et al. 1975, Ausprunk and Folkman 1977). The first observable morphologic event in parent capillaries is the dissolution of the basement membrane underlying the endothelial cells closest to the inducer of angiogenesis. These endothelial cells then migrate into the new tissue space, while adjacent endothelial cells move into the space vacated by the invading endothelial cells. Only those cells at the base of the new capillary divide; the invasive cells do not appear to divide.

Although this sequence of morphologic events during angiogenesis has been described, the biochemical mechanisms controlling this process are not understood. Based on the morphologic analyses, neovascularization can be divided into at least three components, each of which may require a specific set of biochemical processes. One of these is a mitogenic component, necessary to account for the proliferation of the endothelial cells. A second component stimulates a chemotactic response, since the endothelial cells demonstrate directional migration during angiogenesis, and a third component facilitates the invasive aspect of endothelial cell migration. The penetration of capillaries through basement membranes or connective tissue elements or both requires that cells display invasive behavior. Each of these three responses may be attributable to a distinct stimulatory molecule, or a particular molecule may elicit more than one response.

An understanding of angiogenesis at the molecular and biochemical levels has not yet been possible, primarily because of two problems. The first is that the bioassays used, neovascularization of the cornea (Gimbrone et al. 1974) or angiogenesis on the chick embryo chorioallantoic membrane (Armstrong et al. 1982), have been cumbersome and nonquantitative. The second is that little progress has been made in identifying the molecule or molecules responsible for angiogenesis. Recently, several groups have begun to purify potential angiogenic molecules using in vitro assays based on specific features of the angiogenic response. Using the stimulation of endothelial cell proliferation as an assay, two groups (Fenselau et al. 1981, Weiss et al. 1979) have purified or partially purified molecules from tumors that are not only mitogenic in vitro but also angiogenic in vivo. Again, the interpretation of these results is not clear, since the invading endothelial cells at the tip of the capillary do not divide (Ausprunk and Folkman 1977). Only those cells at the base of the sprout divide. Therefore, the cells closest to an inducer, which are theoretically exposed to the highest amount of angiogenic factor, are unaffected by the material. Possibly the cell division that occurs is passive and results from the cells at the base of the sprout dividing to fill in the space created as the invasive cells move toward the source of angiogenesis factor. Thus, the endothelial cells may be stimulated to divide in a passive manner much like the cell division seen after a confluent growth-arrested monolayer of fibroblasts is wounded (Burk 1973). The in vivo angiogenic response of the molecules purified by Weiss et al. (1979) and Fenselau et al. (1981) may result from an inflammatory molecule in their preparations and not from a true angiogenic factor that acts as a mitogen.

The potential exists for a molecule or molecules responsible for the chemotactic component of angiogenesis to be isolated using a chemotaxis or chemokinesis assay, as was described by Zetter (1980). Although this is theoretically possible and has been used to identify potential sources of angiogenic factors (Chodak et al. 1981), no one has, as yet, used this assay to purify an angiogenic factor.

For reasons that will be described, we have decided to attempt to use protease production by endothelial cells to assay for a molecule responsible for the invasive aspect of angiogenesis. The advantage of this approach is that the assays are simple, quick, and *quantitative.* The proteases whose production we have monitored are collagenase and plasminogen activator. The rationale for these choices will be described, with respect to a model we have proposed for the invasive aspect of neovascularization (Rohrlich and Rifkin 1979, Mullins and Rohrlich 1983).

We postulate that when endothelial cells are stimulated by angiogenic factors the cells produce latent collagenase and plasminogen activator (Rohrlich and Rifkin 1979). The plasminogen activator produced would then convert plasminogen to plasmin, an enzyme that is known to be an effective activator of latent collagenase (Werb et al. 1977) and is present in many tissue fluids and spaces (Green 1977, Eigel et al. 1979). A model for the interaction of plasminogen activator, plasminogen, latent collagenase, and plasmin is illustrated in Figure 1.

The central feature of this model is that two proteases are generated: plasmin, which has a broad specificity, and collagenase, which has a limited specificity. We postulate that it is the concerted action of collagenase and plasmin that degrades basement membrane glycoproteins and collagen.

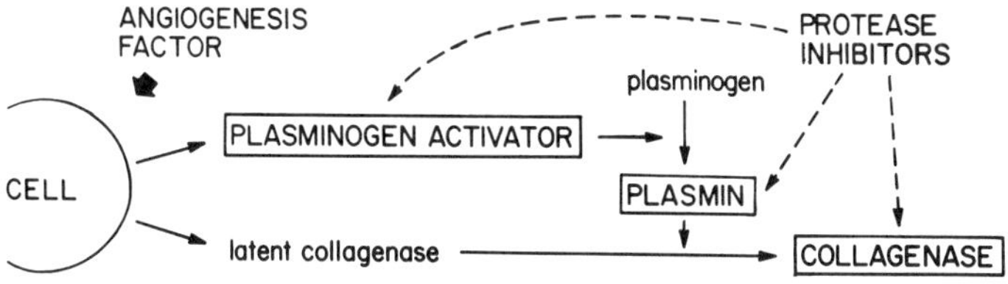

FIG. 1. Model for the mechanism of action of angiogenic stimulators and inhibitors.

The model is based on and supported by the following facts. First, the production of collagenase or plasminogen activator or both is associated with a large number of normal and aberrant processes that involve cellular invasion or degradation (Ossowski et. al. 1979, Rohrlich and Rifkin 1979, Strickland et al. 1976, Vassalli et al 1976, Vassalli and Reich 1977, Mullins and Rohrlich 1983). Second, the avascular nature of certain tissues, such as cartilage, may result from their high levels of specific protease inhibitors (Folkman 1974). Intact cartilage fragments as well as high-salt extracts of cartilage are able to inhibit both angiogenesis (Langer et al. 1976, Langer et al. 1980, Sorgente et al. 1975) and endothelial cell proliferation (Eisenstein et al. 1973). Cartilage extracted with high salt is susceptible to neovascularization (Brem and Folkman 1975). The extract contains high levels of plasmin, collagenase, and thiol protease inhibitors (Kuettner et al. 1974, Rifkin and Crowe 1977, Roughley et al. 1978). Crude preparations of these inhibitors extracted from human or bovine cartilage are also claimed to inhibit several other invasive processes, including tumor cell invasion (Kuettner et al. 1978) and tumor-mediated bone degradation (Horton et al. 1978). Thus, the evidence indirectly indicates an involvement of proteases and their inhibitors in the control of neovascularization. Third, an invasive endothelial cell would have to produce collagenase to degrade the collagen in basement membranes and tissues such as the cornea, since collagen is resistant to most other proteases (Harris and Cartwright 1977). Finally, neovascularization always occurs from venules (Ausprunk and Folkman 1977), structures that are known to leak plasma components. Therefore, the leakage of a specific plasma component, for example, plasminogen, may be required for the invasive process.

The hypothesis that endothelial cells produce latent collagenase and plasminogen activator when exposed to angiogenic factors yields several predictions that can be tested in vitro using cultured endothelial cells as a model: (1) Capillary endothelial cells should be able to produce both latent collagenase and plasminogen activator; (2) capillary endothelial cells should respond to known angiogenic factors by secreting latent collagenase and plasminogen activator; (3) the production of latent collagenase and plasminogen activator should be specific to endothelial cells from the microvasculature and not to endothelial cells found in large vessels, since neovascularization takes place only from the microvasculature; and (4) angiogenic factors can be identified, characterized, and purified using the production of latent collagenase and plasminogen activator as an assay.

METHODS

The bovine adrenal cortex capillary endothelial cells we use were isolated and grown according to procedures developed by Folkman et al. (1979). The human hepatoma cell (HHC) line we shall use to isolate the protease-inducing factor is grown under normal culture conditions (Eagle's medium and calf serum).

To measure collagenase, we have developed an assay (Moscatelli et al. 1980) based on a modification of a procedure we developed to measure elastase (Rifkin and Crowe 1977). Radioactively labeled substrate (^{125}I-labeled native collagen) is coupled to an insoluble matrix (Sepharose beads). The reaction mixture (^{125}I-collagen-Sepharose, collagenase, and buffer) is mechanically agitated at room temperature for a specified time (usually no more than 5 hours). At the end of the incubation, the assay mixture is centrifuged, and the radioactivity of an aliquot of the supernatant is measured. Collagenase activity can be expressed as a percentage of the total radioactivity released into the supernatant. The assay is able to detect as little as 1 ng of collagenase.

Plasminogen activator is assayed by techniques we developed (Unkeless et al. 1973, Ossowski et al. 1973). This assay permits the detection of enzyme in living cells, cell homogenates, or serum-free conditioned medium. The assay consists of coating the surfaces of small Petri dishes with iodinated fibrinogen, activating the thrombin of the fibrin to generate an insoluble film of ^{125}I-fibrin, and subsequent monitoring of the release of soluble ^{125}I-fibrin degradation products from the substance to be tested. The plasminogen activator-induced solubilization of ^{125}I-fibrin is strictly dependent on the addition of purified plasminogen, since plasminogen activator alone has no detectable activity on fibrin. The conversion of plasminogen to plasmin and the subsequent release of ^{125}I-fibrin degradation products have been shown to be dependent on the amount of plasminogen activator present.

To measure bovine capillary endothelial (BCE) cell movement, we shall use an assay similar to the one described by Zetter (1980). In this assay (Albrecht-Beuhler 1977), cells are plated onto coverslips coated with colloidal gold. As the cells move, they phagositize gold particles. After the coverslips have been fixed, the area through which the cells have moved can be visualized under dark-field illumination as a dark area contrasted against the silver-gray background of the remaining colloidal gold. The areas are measured automatically by an image analyzer (Artek Systems).

RESULTS

Cultured Endothelial Cells' Ability to Produce Latent Collagenase and Plasminogen Activator

Using cloned BCE cells, prepared according to the method of Folkman et al. (1979) and shown to be positive by immunofluorescence for factor

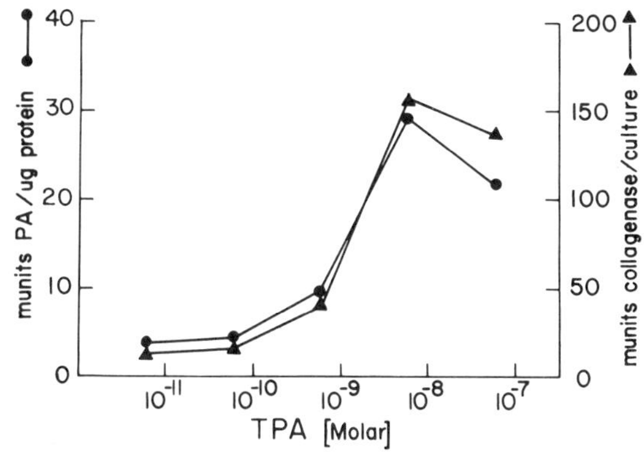

FIG. 2. TPA-induced plasminogen activator collagenase production by BCE cells. BCE cells (passage 8) were grown to confluence in complete tumor-conditioned medium and prepared for experimental use, as described in the Methods section. The cultures were incubated for 23 hours in Dulbecco's modified Eagle's medium (DMEM) with 5% calf serum (depleted of plasminogen) and various concentrations of TPA. The culture fluids from duplicate cultures were collected, activated with trypsin, and assayed for collagenase. The cells from the same cultures were extracted with Triton X-100 and the extracts were assayed for plasminogen activator. (Reprinted from Gross et al. 1982, with permission of the Rockefeller University Press).

VIII-von Willebrand's antigen, we have found (Gross et al. 1982) that the tumor promoter 12-0-tetradecanoyl phorbol-13-acetate (TPA) induces both latent collagenase and plasminogen activator in BCE cells (Figure 2). The maximal response was observed at 2×10^{-7} M of TPA, a dose similar to that found to be effective for TPA induction of latent collagenase in human umbilical cord cells (Moscatelli et al. 1980) and plasminogen activator in rabbit and bovine aortic endothelial (BAE) cells (Loskutoff and Edgington 1977). However, this is the first reported instance of the coordinate induction by TPA of both latent collagenase and plasminogen activator in endothelial cells. The induction of both enzymes is time-dependent (Figure 3) and occurs only with active tumor promoters (Table 1). The inactive analogues of TPA, 4-0-methyl TPA and 4(α) TPA, are ineffective as inducers, whereas the active promoter, phorbol 12,13-didecanoate (PDD) is able to increase latent collagenase and plasminogen activator production.* As in other systems, the latent collagenase can be activated by plasmin, trypsin, or certain mercurials. The collagenase thus generated is a classic vertebrate collagenase, yielding only the TC_A and TC_B pieces when incubated with native collagen (Figure 4). The enzyme effectively degrades types I, II, and III collagens but is unable to degrade types IV and V. The assays

* It should be noted that we use the term "latent collagenase" to denote the inactive form of collagenase produced by cultured cells. Other investigators refer to the collagenase precursor as "procollagenase" (Harris and Cartwright 1977). In fact, the production of collagenase in either a zymogen or a "procollagenase" form would not seriously affect our proposal. Plasmin would then serve to activate the zymogen to the active form.

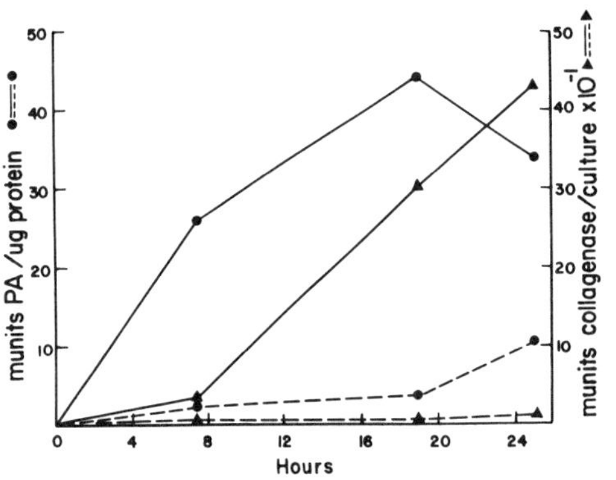

FIG. 3. Time course of TPA stimulation of plasminogen activator and collagenase production by BCE cells. BCE cells (passage 8) were grown to confluence in complete tumor-conditioned medium and prepared for experimental use, as described in the Methods section. Duplicate 35-mm cultures were incubated with or without 2×10^{-7} M TPA in DMEM containing 5% calf serum depleted of plasminogen. At 7.5 hours, 19 hours, and 25 hours after the addition of TPA, culture fluids were collected, activated with trypsin, and assayed for collagenase. The cells from the same cultures were extracted in Triton X-100, and the extracts were assayed for plasminogen activator. *Broken lines* represent untreated cultures; *continuous lines* represent TPA-treated cultures. (Reprinted from Gross et al. 1982, with permission of the Rockefeller University Press).

for type IV collagenase were performed in collaboration with Lance Liotta of the National Institutes of Health (NIH) (Liotta et al. 1979). The failure to detect any type IV collagenase activity was disappointing, given the presence of this protein in basement membranes. However, type IV collagenase has been detected in BAE cells stimulated by an angiogenic factor from bovine retinae. We have found this factor to be effective in stimulating protease production in BCE (vide infra), and, therefore, it may well be that our failure to detect the type IV collagenase was technical in nature.

The plasminogen activator produced is predominantly of the urokinase type, based on molecular weight, lack of binding to concanavalin A (Con A)-Sepha-

TABLE 1. *Effect of TPA analogues on bovine capillary endothelial cell plasminogen activator and collagenase production**

Addition	Plasminogen activator activity (mUnits/μg protein)	Collagenase activity (mUnits/culture)
Control (untreated)	6.6	10.5
TPA†	21.7	136.0
PDD	24.1	131.0
4-0-methyl TPA	6.7	16.5
4-α-PDD	5.8	15.8

* Confluent BCE cell cultures on 35-mm dishes were exposed for 23 hours to TPA or its analogues at a concentration of approximately 2×10^{-7}M. The culture fluids from duplicate cultures were collected, activated with trypsin, and assayed for collagenase activity. The cell layers from the same cultures were extracted with detergent and the extracts were assayed for PA. The data represent the average of duplicate measurements.

† Abbreviations used: TPA, 12-0-tetradecanoyl phorbol-13-acetate; PDD, phorbol 12,13-didecanoate.

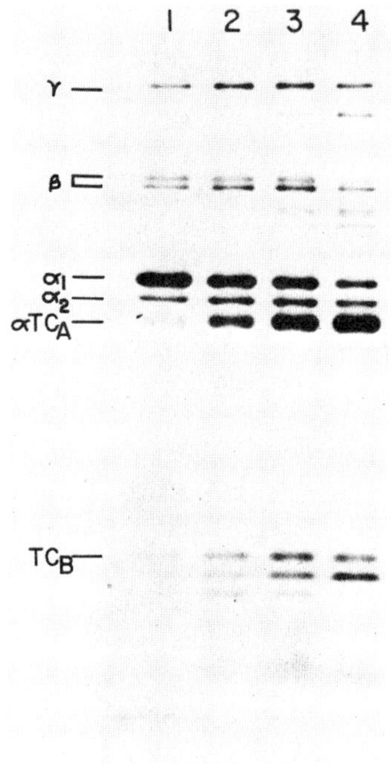

FIG. 4. Digestion of collagen by BCE cell collagenase. BCE cells were incubated with 10^{-7} M TPA for 24 hours. The medium was removed from the cultures and activated with trypsin, and the trypsin was inhibited with a 10-fold excess of aprotinin (Trasylol®). Aliquots of the medium containing 12 mUnits of collagenase activity were mixed with 3×10^{-2} μCi^{125}I-guinea pig skin collagen (0.35 μCi/μg) and incubated at 25°C for various periods of time. The samples were then reduced and boiled, loaded on a sodium dodecyl sulfate (SDS)-5%–16% polyacrylamide gradient gel, and electrophoresed. Kodak X-0 mat film was exposed to the dried gel for 72 hours at −70°C. Lane 1, control; lanes 2–4, samples incubated at 25°C for 2.5, 5, and 12 hours, respectively. (Reprinted from Gross et al. 1982, with permission of the Rockefeller University Press).

rose, and inhibition by antibodies specific for urokinase-type plasminogen activator but not by antibodies specific for tissue activator-type plasminogen activator. Some tissue-type plasminogen activator is produced, but the amount is variable and small relative to the amount of urokinase-type plasminogen activator.

We have performed several studies with specific inhibitors of macromolecule synthesis in an attempt to establish the requirements for the TPA-mediated induction of latent collagenase and plasminogen activator. DNA synthesis is not required, since treatment of the BCE cells with cytosine arabinoside under conditions that inhibit DNA synthesis by more than 95% does not affect enzyme induction upon exposure to TPA. Experiments with inhibitors of protein synthesis and DNA-dependent RNA synthesis have been difficult to perform because the cells are extremely sensitive to the drugs. Upon exposure to cycloheximide, puromycin, or anisomysin at concentrations as low as 0.05 μg/ml, the cells were detached from the surface of the dish within 2 hours. This effect was also observed with actinomycin and daunomycin at low drug concentrations. Thus, we were unable to find concentrations at which these drugs were effective as inhibitors and were not cytotoxic. We were able to examine the effects of mitomycin C on enzyme induction. At mitomycin concentrations of 10 μg/ml, plasminogen activator induction was inhibited whereas induction of latent collagenase was not. This concentration of mitomycin inhibited RNA synthesis by over 90%, a finding that may indicate a fundamental difference in the mechanism of induction for the two proteases or may mean that one comes from a more stable species of message than does the other.

Response of BCE Cells to Angiogenic Factors

Since TPA is not a natural angiogenic factor, we examined the effects of three different preparations of crude angiogenic factors, each of which is known to induce neovascularization in vivo. These included an extract of bovine retinae (Glaser et al. 1980a, D'Amore et al. 1981) sent to us by Patricia D'Amore, culture medium conditioned by mouse adipocytes (F442A cells) sent to us by John Castellot (Castellot et al. 1980), and a cell lysate from a human hepatoma cell culture given to us by Judah Folkman. Each of these preparations induced both latent collagenase and plasminogen activator in BCE cells (Table 2). In each instance, the effect was strictly dose- and time-dependent. A control experiment using medium conditioned by undifferentiated F442A cells showed no induction of latent collagenase or plasminogen activator. However, a control experiment testing a lysate of normal rat hepatocytes indicated that this material was stimulatory in our assay systems. Although this result was somewhat surprising, it is consistent with the observation of Glaser et al. (1980b), who described a potent chemoattractant for vascular endothelial cells in extracts of bovine liver. Further studies on the presence of protease-inducing activities in other cell types are currently in progress.

Specificity of Protease Production by BCE and BAE Cells

When the responses of BCE and BAE cells to TPA were compared (Table 3), we observed that only the BCE cells produced both latent collagenase and plasminogen activator. BAE cells synthesized more plasminogen activator in

TABLE 2. *Effect of angiogenic stimulators on plasminogen activator and collagenase production by bovine capillary endothelial cells**

	(Fold stimulation over control)	
Addition	Plasminogen activator	Collagenase
Hepatoma lysate (0.86 mg)	9.9	55.3
Retinal extract (200 μg)	3.9	8.3
Adipocyte medium (150 μl/ml)	3.3	6.0
TPA† (2×10^{-7} M)	4.8	17.5

* Bovine capillary endothelial cells were grown to confluence in complete tumor-conditioned medium with 10% donor calf serum and treated as previously described (Gross et al. 1982). Cultures were maintained for 24 hours in Dulbecco's modified Eagle medium containing 5% calf serum (depleted of plasminogen) with or without the additions described above. The culture fluids (1.5 ml/plate) and cell layers were assayed for collagenase and PA respectively as in the legend to Table 1.

† Abbreviations used: TPA, 12-0-tetradecanoyl phorbol-13-acetate.

TABLE 3. *BCE and BAE response to angiogenic preparations**

	(Fold stimulation over control)			
	Plasminogen activator		Collagenase	
Addition	BCE† cells	BAE cells	BCE cells	BAE cells
Hepatoma lysate (0.86 mg)	9.9	4.3	55.3	2.4
Retinal extract (200 μg)	3.9	1.0	6.3	0
Adipocyte medium (150 μg/ml)	3.3	0.8	6.0	0
TPA (2×10^{-7} M)	4.8	2.3	17.5	0.9

* Bovine capillary endothelial cells were grown to confluence in complete tumor-conditioned medium with 10% donor calf serum. Bovine aortic endothelial cells were maintained until confluence in Dulbecco's modified Eagle's medium with 10% donor calf serum. The cells were then treated as described in the footnote to Table 2.

† Abbreviations used: BCE, bovine capillary endothelial; BAE, bovine aortic endothelial; TPA, 12-0-tetradecanoyl phorbol-13-acetate.

the presence of TPA, but latent collagenase production was not significantly increased. This difference in the responses of BCE and BAE cells was also observed when the effects of the other angiogenic preparations on BAE cells were examined (Table 3). It should be noted that both BCE cells and BAE cells were prepared from the same animals and treated identically throughout the experiment. The lack of response from the BAE cells is not the result of overproduction of a collagenase inhibitor, since mixing experiments (Figure 5) revealed no increase in collagenase inhibition in TPA-treated cultures. However, we cannot rule out the coordinate production of equivalent amounts of collagenase and collagenase inhibitor.

We have also examined the effect of retinal extract, adipocyte-conditioned

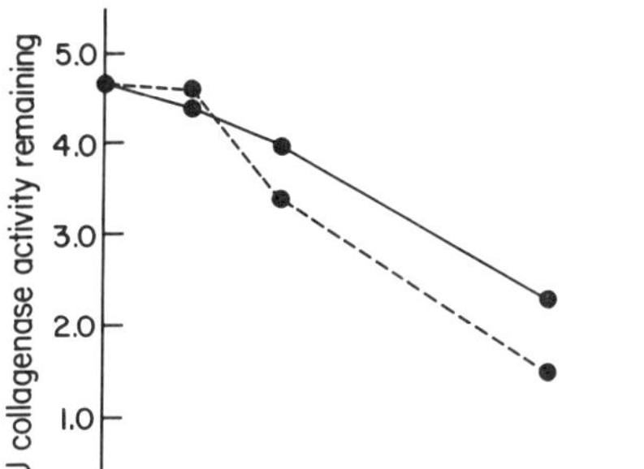

FIG. 5. Inhibition of BCE collagenase by BAE post-culture medium. BAE cells were grown to confluence and prepared for experimental use as described in the methods section. Four plates of BAE cells were incubated for 24 hours in DMEM without serum. The medium on two of the plates also contained 10^{-7} M TPA. The culture fluids were collected, dialyzed, concentrated 10-fold, and assayed for collagenase inhibitory activity. The concentrated post-culture medium was mixed with 4.6 mUnits of trypsin-activated BCE collagenase in 0.4 ml of 0.1 M N'-2-hydroxyethylpiperazine-N'-ethanesulfonic acid buffer HEPES (pH 7.6), 5mM $CaCl_2$, and 0.5 mg/ml bovine serum albumin (BSA) and incubated at room temperature for 30 minutes. The collagenase activity remaining in the sample was determined. The *continuous line* represents the residual collagenase activity in samples containing concentrated post-culture medium from untreated BAE cells. The *broken line* represents the residual collagenase activity in samples containing concentrated post-culture medium from TPA-treated BAE cells. (Reprinted from Gross et al. 1982, with permission of the Rockefeller University Press).

medium, and hepatoma lysate on human umbilical vein endothelial cells. Only the hepatoma lysate was able to increase collagenase production, and none of these preparations stimulated plasminogen activator levels. These findings are consistent with what we had reported previously on the effect of TPA on human endothelial cells (Moscatelli et al. 1980).

Protease Production as an Assay for Angiogenic Factors

Production of latent collagenase and plasminogen activator by BCE cells provides a relatively simple yet quantitative assay for potential angiogenic factors. We have checked a number of known growth factors and hormones to determine whether or not they can elicit the protease response observed earlier with the angiogenic preparations. Insulin, platelet-derived growth factor, epidermal growth factor, endothelial cell growth stimulator, and fibroblast growth factor had no effect on these cells with respect to protease stimulation. Sarcoma growth factor (SGF) (DeLarco and Todaro 1978) has been reported to be angiogenic (Judah Folkman, personal communication), and crude SGF does stimulate enzyme production by BCE cells. However, when crude SGF was fractionated by P-6 chromatography and the individual fractions were assayed [sent to us by Joseph DeLarco and George Todaro (NIH)], the protease-inducing activity eluted at a position that was clearly distinct from that of the SGF. The elution position indicated a molecular weight for the inducing factor that was considerably higher than that of the SGF activity, a finding consistent with our own estimate of the molecular weight of the factor obtained from HHC (see below).

Azizkhan et al. (1980) have reported that heparin may promote angiogenesis. In collaboration with Robert Rosenberg (Harvard Medical School), we have explored this possibility and found that, although the heparin that binds to antithrombin-III will induce plasminogen activator in BCE cells, it does not

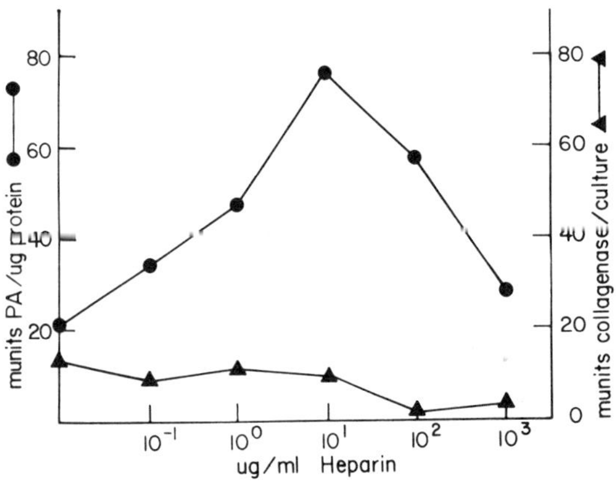

FIG. 6. Stimulation of BCE protease production by heparin. BCE cells were exposed to heparin for 24 hours. The next day the levels of plasminogen activator and collagenase were measured.

induce latent collagenase (Figure 6). Heparin that does not bind to antithrombin-III is ineffective as an inducer of both plasminogen activator and latent collagenase in BCE cells. Other glycosaminoglycans have been tested by this assay, and only dermatan sulfate, which may be contaminated with heparin, was able to induce plasminogen activator in BCE cells. All other glycosaminoglycans were ineffective. This result, which shows the stimulation of plasminogen activator but not collagenase by heparin, is consistent with the proposal of Judah Folkman (personal communication) that heparin is not angiogenic by itself but is a potentiator of angiogenesis. We have also found that protamine, a potent antagonist of heparin, does not affect collagenase or plasminogen activator production at doses that are nontoxic to the cells. The relation of this result to Taylor and Folkman's finding (Taylor and Folkman 1982) that protamine inhibits tumor growth by preventing neovascularization must be evaluated further.

We have also used the protease induction assay to initiate a characterization of the active principle in the HHC extract. This activity is nondialyzable, is stable at 50°C for 30 minutes but is inactivated at 60°C after 30 minutes, and is stable between pH 6 and 9. At pH 5 and below, a rapid loss of activity occurs. The HHC extract has been chromatographed on a Sephadex G-150 after centrifugation at 10,000 × g for 30 minutes (Figure 7). Several peaks of plasminogen activator-inducing activity were found, but only one region was able to induce both plasminogen activator and latent collagenase. This peak had a high molecular weight and eluted slightly behind the void volume of the column. This result, which suggests a high molecular weight for the HHC factor, is consistent with the results obtained with the crude SGF preparations. However, if the HHC extract is chromatographed on the G-150 in the presence of 1M of guanidine, the active fractions elute at a lower molecular weight position of approximately 40,000 daltons.

The protease-inducing factor appears to be in a soluble form in the cell sonicate,

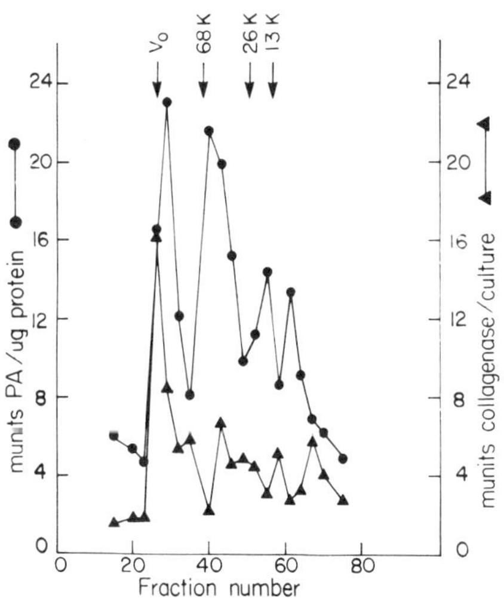

FIG. 7. Sephadex chromatography of human hepatoma lysate. The active fraction of a lysate from a human hepatoma after chromatography on Sephadex G-150 was assayed for plasminogen activator and latent collagenase.

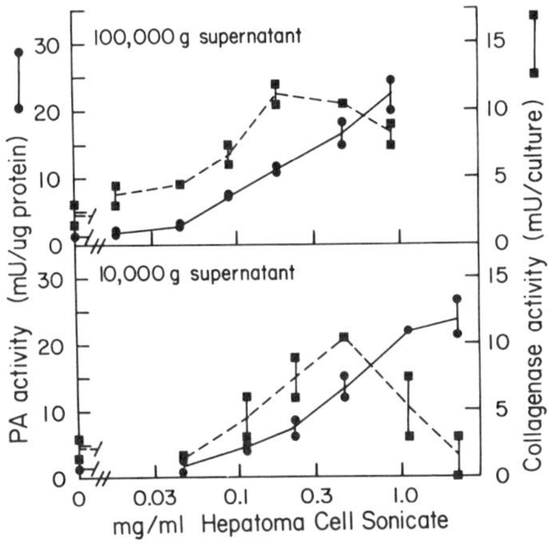

FIG. 8. Stimulation of BCE cell plasminogen activator and collagenase production by HHC sonicate supernatants. Confluent cultures of SK-HEP-1 cells were harvested in phosphate-buffered saline and sonicated. One half of the cell sonicate was centrifuged at 10,000 × g for 30 minutes, and one half was centrifuged at 100,000 × g for 60 minutes. Various concentrations of each of the supernatants were added to fresh medium containing 5% calf serum depleted of plasminogen. These media were put on confluent cultures of BCE cells on 35-mm dishes. After a 24-hour incubation at 37°C, the culture medium was collected and assayed for latent collagenase, and the cell layer was harvested and assayed for plasminogen activator. **A,** plasminogen activator and collagenase activity in BCE cultures treated with 100,000 × g supernatant. **B,** plasminogen activator and collagenase activity in BCE cultures treated with a 10,000 × g supernatant.

since centrifugation of the sonicate at 100,000 × g for one hour fails to deplete the supernatant of its inducing activity (Figure 8). In fact, the specific activity is increased after centrifugation, and the inhibition of collagenase induction that occurs after large amounts of the 10,000 × g supernatant are added is diminished after centrifugation at 100,000 × g, perhaps because an inhibitor is removed. Thus, after sonication, the inducing factor does not appear to be associated with any membrane fragment or organelle.

DISCUSSION

These studies indicate that: (1) bovine capillary endothelial cells have the potential to produce latent collagenase and plasminogen activator in vitro; (2) in the bovine system, this appears to be a unique property of capillary endothelial cells; (3) all bona fide angiogenic preparations tested to date contain molecules that can induce the production of these proteases; and (4) the ability to induce latent collagenase and plasminogen activator production may be used as an assay for isolating those factors. Although the correlation between protease induction and angiogenesis is strong, we have presented no proof that the in vitro assay of protease production is equivalent to the in vivo assay.

The ability to test quantitatively for specific biochemical changes that occur after cells are exposed to defined stimuli should permit potential in vivo angiogenic factors and inhibitors of angiogenesis to be isolated.

ACKNOWLEDGMENT

This investigation was supported by grants CA 23753, CA 09161, and CA 06515, awarded by the National Cancer Institute; HL 18828, awarded by the

National Heart, Lung and Blood Institute; and CD-77, awarded by the American Cancer Society and a grant from the Kroc Foundation.

REFERENCES

Albrecht-Beuhler, G. 1977. The phagokinetic tracks of 3T3 cells. Cell 11:395–404.

Armstrong, P. B., J. P. Quigley, and E. Sidebottom. 1982. Transepithelial invasion and intramesenchymal infiltration of the chick embryo chorioallantois by tumor cell lines. Cancer Res. 42:1826–1837.

Ausprunk, D., and J. Folkman. 1977. Migration and proliferation of endothelial cells in preformed and newly formed blood vessels during tumor angiogenesis. Microvascular Res. 14:53–65.

Ausprunk, D. H., D. R. Knighton, and J. Folkman. 1975. Vascularization of normal and neoplastic tissues grafted to the chick chorioallantois. J. Pathol. 79:597–618.

Azizkhan, R. G., J. C. Azizkhan, B. R. Zetter, and J. Folkman. 1980. Mast cell heparin stimulates migration of capillary endothelial cells in vitro. J. Exp. Med. 152:931–944.

Brem, H., and J. Folkman. 1975. Inhibition of tumor angiogenesis mediated by cartilage. J. Exp. Med. 141:427–439.

Burk, R. R. 1973. A factor from a transformed cell line that affects migration. Proc. Natl. Acad. Sci. USA 70:369–374.

Castellot, J. J., M. J. Karnovsky, and B. M. Spiegelman. 1980. Patent stimulation of vascular endothelial cell growth by differentiated 3T3 adipocytes. Proc. Natl. Acad. Sci. USA 77:6007–6011.

Chodak, G. W., C. J. Scheiner, and B. R. Zetter. 1981. Urine from patients with transitional-cell carcinoma stimulates migration of capillary endothelial cells. N. Engl. J. Med. 305:869–874.

D'Amore, P. A., B. M. Glaser, S. K. Brunson, and A. H. Fenselau. 1981. Angiogenic activity from bovine retina: Partial purification and characterization. Proc. Natl. Acad. Sci. USA 78:3068–3072.

DeLarco, J. E., and G. J. Todaro. 1978. Growth factors from murine sarcoma virus-transformed cells. Proc. Natl. Acad. Sci. USA 75:4001–4006.

Eigel, W. N., C. J. Hofmann, B. A. K. Chobber, J. M. Tomich, T. W. Keenan, and E. T. Mertz. 1979. Plasmin-mediated proteolysis of casein in bovine milk. Proc. Natl. Acad. Sci. USA 76:2244–2248.

Eisenstein, R., K. E. Kuettner, C. Neopolitan, L. W. Soble, and N. Sorgente. 1973. Am. J. Pathol. 73:765–774.

Fenselau, A., S. Watt, and R. J. Mello. 1981. Tumor angiogenic factor. Purification from the Walker 256 rat tumor. J. Biol. Chem. 256:9605–9611.

Folkman, J. 1974. Tumor angiogenesis, *in* Advances in Cancer Research, G. Klein and S. Weinhouse, eds., vol. 19. Academic Press, New York, pp. 331–354.

Folkman, J., C. Haudenschild, and B. Zetter. 1979. Long-term culture of capillary endothelial cells. Proc. Natl. Acad. Sci. USA 76:5217–5221.

Gimbrone, M. A., R. S. Cotran, S. B. Leapman, and J. Folkman. 1974. Tumor growth and neovascularization: An experimental model using the rabbit cornea. J. Natl. Cancer Inst. 52:413–427.

Glaser, B. M., P. A. D'Amore, R. G. Michaels, A. Patz, and A. J. Fenselau. 1980a. Demonstration of vasoproliferative activity from mammalian retina. J. Cell Biol. 84:298–304.

Glaser, B. M., P. A. D'Amore, H. Seppa, S. Seppa, and E. Schiffman, 1980b. Adult tissues contain chemoattractants for vascular endothelial cells. Nature 288:483–484.

Green, H. 1977. Terminal differentiation of cultured human epidermal cells. Cell 11:405–416.

Gross, J. L., D. Moscatelli, E. A. Jaffe, and D. B. Rifkin. 1982. Plasminogen activator and collagenase production by cultured capillary endothelial cells. J. Cell Biol. 95:924–931.

Harris, E. D., Jr., and E. C. Cartwright. 1977. Collagenase, *in* Proteinases in Mammalian Cells and Tissues, A. J. Barrett, ed. North Holland Publishing Company, Amsterdam, pp. 249–284.

Horton, J. E., F. H. Wezeman, and K. E. Kuettner. 1978. Inhibition of bone resorption in vitro by a cartilage-derived anti-collagenase factor. Science 199:1342–1344.

Kalebic, T., S. Garbisa, B. Glaser, and L. A. Liotta. 1982. Degradation of type IV and V collagen by migrating endothelial cells. J. Cell Biol. 95:128a.

Kuettner, K. E., R. L. Croxen, R. Eisenstein, and N. Sorgente. 1974. Proteinase inhibitor activity in connective tissues. Experientia 30:595–597.

Kuettner, K. E., J. Hiti, R. Eisenstein, and E. Harper. 1976. Collagenase inhibition by cationic proteins derived from cartilage and aorta. Biochem. Biophys. Res. Commun. 72:40–46.

Kuettner, K. E., B. V. Pauli, and L. Soble. 1978. Morphological studies on the resistance of cartilage to invasion by osteosarcoma cells in vitro and in vivo. Cancer Res. 38:277–287.

Langer, R., H. Brem, K. Falterman, M. Klein, and J. Folkman. 1976. Isolation of a cartilage factor that inhibits tumor neovascularization. Science 193:70–72.

Langer, R., H. Conn, J. Vacanti, C. Haudenschild, and J. Folkman. 1980. Control of tumor growth in animals by infusion of an angiogenesis inhibitor. Proc. Natl. Acad. Sci. USA 77:4331–4335.

Liotta, L. A., S. Abe, P. C. Robey, and G. R. Martin. 1979. Preferential digestion of basement membrane collagen by an enzyme derived from a metastatic murine tumor. Proc. Natl. Acad. Sci. USA 76:2268–2272.

Loskutoff, D. J., and T. J. Edgington. 1977. Synthesis of a fibrinolytic activator and inhibitor by endothelial cells. Proc. Natl. Acad. Sci. USA 74:3903–3907.

Moscatelli, D., E. Jaffe, and D. B. Rifkin. 1980. Tetradecanoyl phorbol acetate stimulates latent collagenase production by cultured human endothelial cells. Cell 20:343–351.

Mullins, D., and S. T. Rohrlich. 1983. Proteases and cellular invasion. Biochim. Biophys. Acta Reviews in Cancer (in press).

Ossowski, L., D. Biegel, and E. Reich. 1979. Mammary plasminogen activator: Correlation with involution, hormonal modulation, and comparison between normal and neoplastic tissues. Cell 16:929–940.

Ossowski, L., J. C. Unkeless, A. Tobia, J. P. Quigley, D. B. Rifkin, and E. Reich. 1973. An enzymatic function associated with transformation of fibroblasts by oncogenic viruses. II. Mammalian fibroblast cultures transformed by DNA and RNA viruses. J. Exp. Med. 137:112–126.

Rifkin, D. B., and R. M. Crowe. 1977. Isolation of a protease inhibitor from tissues resistant to tumor invasion. Hoppe-Seylers Z. Physiol. Chem. 358:1525–1531.

Rohrlich, S. T., and D. B. Rifkin. 1979. Proteases and cell invasion, *in* Annual Reviews in Medicinal Chemistry. F. Clarke, ed., vol. 14. Academic Press, New York, pp. 229–239.

Roughley, P. J., G. Murphy, and A. J. Barrett. 1978. Proteinase inhibitors of bovine nasal cartilage. Biochem. J. 169:721–724.

Sorgente, N., K. E. Kuettner, L. W. Soble, and R. Eisenstein. 1975. The resistance of certain tissues to invasion. II. Evidence for extractable factors in cartilage which inhibit invasion by vascularized mesenchyme. Lab. Invest. 32:217–222.

Strickland, S., E. Reich, and M. Sherman. 1976. Plasminogen activator in early embryogenesis: Enzyme production by trophoblast and parietal endoderm. Cell 9:231–240.

Taylor, S., and J. Folkman. 1982. Protamine is an inhibitor of angiogenesis. Nature 297:307–312.

Unkeless, J. C., A. Tobia, L. Ossowski, J. P. Quigley, D. B. Rifkin, and E. Reich. 1973. An enzymatic function associated with transformation of fibroblasts by oncogenic viruses. I. Chick embryo fibroblast cultures transformed by avian RNA tumor viruses. J. Exp. Med. 137:85–111.

Vassalli, J.-D., J. Hamilton, and E. Reich. 1976. Macrophage plasminogen activator: Modulation of enzyme production by anti-inflammatory steroids, mitotic inhibitors and cyclic nucleotides. Cell 8:271–281.

Vassalli, J.-D., and E. Reich. 1977. Macrophage plasminogen activator: Induction by products of activated lymphoid cells. J. Exp. Med. 145:429–437.

Weiss, J. B., R. A. Brown, S. Kumar, and P. Phillips. 1979. An angiogenic factor isolated from tumors: A potent low-molecular weight compound. Br. J. Cancer 40:493–495.

Werb, Z., C. L. Mainardi, L. A. Vater, and E. D. Harris. 1977. Endogenous activation of latent collagenase by rheumatoid synovial cells. Evidence for a role of plasminogen activator. N. Engl. J. Med. 296:1017–1023.

Zetter, B. R. 1980. Migration of capillary endothelial cells is stimulated by tumor-derived factors. Nature 285:41–43.

Cancer Invasion and Metastasis: Biologic and Therapeutic Aspects edited by Garth L. Nicolson and Luka Milas. Raven Press, New York © 1984.

Angiogenesis: Initiation and Modulation

Judah Folkman

Department of Surgery, Children's Hospital Medical Center, and the Departments of Anatomy and Surgery, Harvard Medical School, Boston, Massachusetts 02115

Angiogenesis, the growth of new capillary blood vessels, occurs in a variety of normal processes such as wound healing (Knighton et al. 1981) and ovulation (Gospodarowicz and Thakral 1978). There is also increasing evidence that angiogenesis is important to the progressive growth of solid tumors (Folkman 1972, 1974, Folkman and Cotran 1976; Maiorana and Gullino 1978). Angiogenesis also dominates a variety of pathological processes such as chronic inflammation (Polverini et al. 1977) and immune reactions (Sidky and Auerbach 1975, Auerbach 1981). It has become possible in recent years to explore the underlying mechanisms because of new techniques developed during the 1970s to study tumor angiogenesis.

NEW METHODS FOR STUDYING ANGIOGENESIS

Angiogenesis is more inaccessible to study than, for example, blood coagulation. Histologic sections of tumors show an intermingling of new capillaries with tumor cells but reveal little about the effect of one cell type upon the other.

A variety of transparent chambers have been implanted into rabbit ears or hamster cheek pouches (Algire 1943, Greenblatt and Shubik 1968) to observe the growth of capillaries toward tumor implants. Descriptive information can be obtained, but it is difficult to quantitate, and it is restricted to the very few tumors that grow in these species. By 1970, we began to realize that further progress in uncovering the mechanisms of tumor angiogenesis, and perhaps angiogenesis in general, would require new techniques whose results could be quantitated, and that would permit the study of angiogenic stimulatory or inhibitory activity of biochemical compounds. Four methods, subsequently developed, are now used by many investigators who study angiogenesis.

The Corneal Micropocket

The corneal micropocket technique permitted the linear measurement of individual growing capillaries. Tumor implants (1 mm^3) are inserted into a pocket made in the cornea of a rabbit at a distance of 1 to 2 mm from the edge of the cornea and the normal vascular bed (Gimbrone et al. 1974). New capillaries grow at right angles from the edge of the cornea, and elongate toward the tumor at approximately 0.2 mm/day. They are measured with a slit-lamp stereoscope. With this method, it is possible to interpose other tissues between the tumor and its vascular bed. For example, the angiogenesis inhibitory property of cartilage was demonstrated in this way (Brem and Folkman 1975). A disadvantage is that tumors other than those of rabbit origin may excite an immune response once they are vascularized. Subsequent immunologic neovascularization may confuse the original experiment. This problem has been overcome at least for mouse tumors by the implantation of tissues into the cornea of inbred mice (Muthukkaruppan and Auerbach 1980). The rat cornea has also been used (Fournier et al. 1981). Another pitfall is nonspecific inflammation: Inflammatory agents usually can be defined by their ability to attract leukocytes (polymorphonuclear neutrophils, lymphocytes, or macrophages). These cells then migrate rapidly into the cornea and may themselves elicit neovascularization. For example, solutions that are hyperosmotic or of abnormally low or high pH are inflammatory. Whenever a new substance is tested for angiogenic activity, it is important to obtain histologic sections to rule out such an inflammatory response.

Sustained-Release Polymer Implants

After the corneal micropocket technique was developed, it became feasible to substitute soluble tumor extracts for tumor implants. However, most of these extracts rapidly diffused away. There was a need for them to be released over a sustained period of time so that a concentration gradient could be established within the cornea. There were two further requirements: (1) The implantable sustained-release vehicle had to be inert and could not itself cause inflammation in the cornea and (2) the implant had to be capable of releasing substances of large molecular weight. After empirical testing of a variety of polymers, we found two that satisfied these conditions: poly-hydroxyethyl-methacrylate and ethylene vinyl acetate copolymer (Langer and Folkman 1976). From such implants it has been possible to release proteins and other macromolecules at approximately zero order kinetics, at micrograms/day and more recently nanograms/day (Murray et al. in press), for periods of weeks to months. Implants can be as small as 1 mm^3 and are well tolerated in the cornea and other tissues.

Chick Embryo-Chorioallantoic Membrane

As biochemists attempted to purify angiogenic fractions from tumor and normal tissues, a need arose for a rapid screening assay for large numbers of test fractions that would be less expensive than rabbits and would avoid the problem of immunologic reactions. A method of dropping the chorioallantoic membrane and opening the egg shell to reveal a large expanse of vascular membrane was previously described by Leighton (1967). We learned that the vessels of the chorioallantoic membrane grow rapidly until day 11, after which endothelial proliferation rapidly decreases (Ausprunk and Folkman 1977). Tumors or tumor fractions implanted on day 9 gave the most reproducible angiogenic response within 48–72 h. This response could be recognized under a 6× stereoscope as new capillary loops converging on the implant (Knighton et al. 1977, Klagsbrun et al. 1976). We found two optimum vehicles for the delivery of small quantities (1 μg to 50 μg) of test material over these relatively brief periods of time. One is to use methylcellulose (4,000 centipoise), 0.3–0.5%, to make disks of about 2 mm diameter. The other is to dry the test substance in 5–10 μl of distilled water on a Thermanox plastic coverslip (Taylor and Folkman 1982). Either is then applied to the chorioallantoic membrane.

Cloned Capillary Endothelial Cells

Recently we have developed a way to isolate cloned capillary endothelial cells and passage them in vitro for long periods of time (Folkman et al. 1979). This finding permitted screening for endothelial cell mitogens. It has also confirmed in vivo observations implying that capillary growth is a multistep program that requires an orderly sequence of events.

CAPILLARY GROWTH: A PROCESS OF MULTIPLE STEPS

By using all of these techniques to study angiogenesis, it is becoming clear that capillary growth takes place by a series of steps that are much the same regardless of the type of angiogenic stimulus. These steps can be summarized as follows: (1) New capillaries originate from small venules. Larger vessels with layers of smooth muscle do not usually give rise to capillary sprouts. (2) Local degradation of the basement membrane on the side of the venule closest to the angiogenic stimulus (Ausprunk and Folkman 1977) is one of the earliest events. Capillary endothelial cells stimulated in vitro by angiogenic substances secrete high concentrations of collagenase and plasminogen activator (Moscatelli et al. 1981). These findings suggest that the local degradation of basement membrane seen in vivo is carried out directly by endothelial cells once they receive an angiogenic stimulus. (3) Through this opening in the basement membrane, endothelial cells begin to migrate toward the angiogenic stimulus (Ausprunk and Folkman 1977). (4) Endothelial cells that follow the leaders align in a bipolar fashion as the first sprout begins to form. (5) Lumen formation begins. In most examples of postembryonic angiogenesis, a lumen appears to be produced by a curvature that develops in the capillary endothelial cell as if the cytoskeleton itself were undergoing curvature. This phenomenon has been observed in vivo in the cornea (Ausprunk and Folkman 1977) and also in vitro (Folkman and Haudenschild 1980). However, during early embryonic angiogenesis, lumen formation may take place by vacuole formation. This has also been observed in vivo (Bär and Wolff 1972) and in vitro (Folkman and Haudenschild 1980).

(6) Endothelial cells in the mid-section of the sprout begin to undergo mitosis. The leading capillary endothelial cells at the very tip of the sprout continue to migrate, but usually do not divide. (7) Loop formation occurs next, as individual sprouts join or anastomose with each other. These loops then elongate and may be the origin of additional sprouts. The loops continue to converge upon the angiogenic target. (8) Flow begins slowly after loops have formed. (9) Pericytes emerge along the length of the capillary sprout. (10) Synthesis of new basement membrane follows.

When cloned capillary endothelial cells were studied in vitro, most of these same events were observed. Entire capillary networks were built up in culture dishes including lumena, branches, and multiple layers (Folkman and Haudenschild 1980). Maciag, using umbilical vein endothelial cells, has shown that these in vitro "tubes" are hollow and will carry fluid (Maciag et al. 1982). Pericytes were not present in vitro. When the observations from in vivo and in vitro studies are taken together, they suggest that the vascular endothelial cell expresses a defined program of events to generate a capillary network. The program seems to be the same regardless of whether the angiogenic signal is from a tumor or from an inflammatory agent or immunologic stimulus.

MODULATION OF THE RATE OF CAPILLARY GROWTH

Although the information for constructing a new capillary network appears to be expressed by the vascular endothelial cell, the *rate* at which this endothelial program unfolds, once stimulated, appears to be modulated by an elaborate system of external controls. Two such controls are now being studied in some detail. One of these is mast cell heparin, which can amplify or increase the rate of capillary growth once neovascularization has been initiated by an angiogenic stimulus such as a tumor. The other is platelet factor 4, which appears capable of inhibiting capillary growth.

Mast Cells Promote Angiogenesis

The density of mast cells in the chick embryo chorioallantoic membrane was 40-fold higher at the site of implantation of a tumor fragment than in normal tissue. This rapid increase in mast cell density near the tumor site occurred within about 24 h after tumor inoculation (Kessler et al. 1976). Furthermore, the accumulation of mast cells near the avascular tumor *preceded* the appearance of new blood vessel sprouts that were converging upon the tumor. In subsequent studies of other types of neovascularization, we found that mast cells often seemed to move in advance of capillary sprouts. However, mast cells could not initiate angiogenesis themselves. Packed mast cells placed on the chorioallantoic membrane did not cause angiogenesis. These findings suggested that mast cells might play an amplifying or a potentiating role in the growth of new capillaries toward a tumor. It is not known whether inflammatory or immune angiogenesis might also be potentiated by mast cells.

Heparin is the Mediator by Which Mast Cells Amplify Capillary Growth

After capillary endothelial cells were successfully carried in long-term culture (Folkman et al. 1979), Zetter (1980) developed an assay to measure their in vitro migration (chemokinesis). This method was based upon the phagokinetic tracks that cells make as they move over colloidal gold (Albrecht-Buehler 1977). Azizkhan et al. (1980) then showed that culture medium conditioned by rat mast cells stimulated *migration* of capillary endothelial cells in vitro in a dose-dependent manner. While tumor-conditioned medium could stimulate both migration and proliferation of capillary endothelial cells, mast cell–conditioned medium could stimulate only migration. Other cell types such as aortic endothelium, smooth muscle cells, and 3T3 cells were not stimulated by the mast cell–conditioned medium nor could their conditioned medium cause capillary endothelial cells to migrate. These results suggested that mast cells may enhance angiogenesis by increasing the rate of directional migration of capillary endothelial cells toward an angiogenic stimulus such as a tumor.

When many mast cell products were tested, only heparin significantly stimulated capillary endothelial cell migration. Heparin could completely substitute for mast cell–conditioned medium. Heparin antagonists such as protamine and heparinase were found to block the stimulatory effect of heparin on capillary endothelial cell migration (Azizkhan et al. 1980). When heparin was applied to the chorioallantoic membrane of the chick embryo at the time of implantation of tumor or tumor extract, angiogenesis was enhanced (Taylor and Folkman 1982). There was intense neovascularization at the site of tumor extracts by 24 h instead of the 3 days shown previously. Also, lower concentrations of tumor angiogenesis activity were detectable. Nonanticoagulant heparin lacking anti-thrombin III activity (supplied by Dr. Robert Rosenberg) also enhanced angiogenesis. Furthermore, neither heparin nor its nonanticoagulant subcomponents could initiate angiogenesis over a wide range of concentrations up to 500 times the enhancing dose.

Platelet Factor 4 Inhibits Angiogenesis

Platelet factor 4 had the opposite effect of mast cells or heparin; that is, it suppressed angiogenesis in the presence of an angiogenic substance. This finding was made by following up the use of protamine as a control in the original in vitro experiments in which heparin stimulated migration of capillary endothelial cells. Protamine in a 2:1 ratio (wt/wt) inhibited the stimulatory effect of heparin.

We then added protamine to the chorioallantoic membrane after heparin and tumor extracts had been placed on the membrane (Taylor and Folkman 1982). As expected, protamine applied at twice the heparin concentration prevented heparin enhancement of tumor angiogenesis. However, a surprising finding was that further increments of protamine eliminated angiogenesis on the membrane even in the absence of exogenous heparin. Therefore, protamine sulfate was tested in a variety of model systems of angiogenesis. Protamine is an arginine-rich basic protein of 4,300 m.w. found only in sperm and used clinically to neutralize heparin after open heart surgery or renal dialysis. Protamine was found to inhibit embryonic angiogenesis in the developing chick embryo (Taylor and Folkman 1982). It was also found to inhibit inflammatory angiogenesis, immunologic angiogenesis, and tumor angiogenesis in the rabbit cornea. When protamine was administered systemically to mice, it suppressed the growth of pulmonary metastases. This growth suppression was demonstrated to be due to antiangiogenesis (Taylor and Folkman 1982).

However, systemically administered, protamine also had toxic side effects unrelated to its antiangiogenic activity. Therefore, other heparin-neutralizing compounds were studied. Platelet factor 4 and major basic protein (from eosinophils) are both known to bind to heparin and neutralize its anticoagulant activity. When these compounds were tested in the chick embryo, both showed angiogenesis inhibitory activity. While major basic protein was very toxic, platelet factor 4 had little, if any, toxicity and was less toxic than protamine at concentrations that maximally inhibited angiogenesis.

Platelet factor 4 is localized in the alpha granules of platelets (Rucinski et al. 1979). The protein has been completely sequenced (Deuel et al. 1981). It is a 70-residue polypeptide with a pI of 7.6 and a calculated molecular weight of 7767. We found that 25 μg of purified platelet factor 4 (obtained courtesy of Dr. Robert Handin of Brigham and Women's Hospital, Boston) produced the same avascular zone in the chick embryo within 48 h as approximately 50 μg of protamine. Platelet factor 4 is obtained from outdated platelets, and because of the short supply it has not been possible to administer it systemically to tumor-bearing mice.

DISCUSSION AND CONCLUSION

It is too early to say just how mast cell heparin and platelet factor 4 might function in vivo (if at all) in the episodes of angiogenesis that take place during normal repair such as wound healing or pathologic states such as tumor growth or chronic inflammation. Nevertheless, our current conceptual framework is to think of angiogenesis as a program of events expressed by vascular endothelial cells and especially capillary endothelial cells upon direct stimulation by a very small family of angiogenic substances. It appears that the rate of this expression may be amplified or suppressed by various natural compounds within the body. Mast cell heparin and platelet factor 4 may possibly be the effector candidates for two such modulating systems.

Future progress in the field of angiogenesis may require that such external control systems be understood in some detail, not only for the identification of angiogenic factors but also for the isolation and demonstration of angiogenesis inhibitors.

ACKNOWLEDGMENT

Parts of the work described in this review were supported by USPHS grant R01-CA14019 from the National Cancer Institute and by a grant provided to Harvard University by Monsanto Co. I thank Rita Marlowe for typing the manuscript.

REFERENCES

Albrecht-Buehler, G. 1977. The phagokinetic tracks of 3T3 cells. Cell 11:395–404.

Algire, G. H. 1943. An adaptation of the transparent-chamber technique to the mouse. JNCI 4:1–11.

Auerbach, R. 1981. Angiogenesis-inducing factors: A review. Lymphokines 4:69–88.

Ausprunk, D. H., and J. Folkman. 1977. Migration and proliferation of endothelial cells in preformed and newly formed blood vessels during tumor angiogenesis. Microvasc. Res. 14:53–65.

Azizkhan, R. G., J. C. Azizkhan, B. R. Zetter, and J. Folkman. 1980. Mast cell heparin stimulates migration of capillary endothelial cells in vitro. J. Exp. Med. 152:931–944.

Bär, Th., and J. R. Wolff. 1972. The formation of capillary basement membranes during internal vascularization of the rat's cerebral cortex. Z. Zellforsch. 133:231–248.

Brem, H., and J. Folkman. 1975. Inhibition of tumor angiogenesis mediated by cartilage. J. Exp. Med. 141:427–439.

Deuel, T. F., R. M. Senior, D. Chang, G. L. Griffin, R. L. Heinrikson, and E. T. Kaiser. 1981. Platelet factor 4 is chemotactic for neutrophils and monocytes. Proc. Natl. Acad. Sci. USA 78:4585–4587.

Folkman, J. 1972. Anti-angiogenesis: New concept for therapy of solid tumors. Ann. Surg. 175:409–416.

Folkman, J. 1974. Tumor angiogenesis factor. Cancer Res. 34:2109–2113.

Folkman, J., and R. S. Cotran. 1976. Relation of vascular proliferation to tumor growth. Int. Rev. Exp. Pathol. 16:207–248.

Folkman, J., and C. Haudenschild. 1980. Angiogenesis in vitro. Nature 288:551–556.

Folkman, J., C. C. Haudenschild, and B. Zetter. 1979. Long-term culture of capillary endothelial cells. Proc. Natl. Acad. Sci. USA 76:5217–5221.

Fournier, G. A., G. A. Lutty, S. Watt, A. Fenselau, and A. Patz. 1981. A corneal micropocket assay for angiogenesis in the rat eye. Invest. Ophthalmol. Vis. Sci. 21:351–354.

Gimbrone, M. A., Jr., R. S. Cotran, and J. Folkman. 1974. Tumor growth and neovascularization: An experimental model using rabbit cornea. JNCI 52:413–427.

Gospodarowicz, D., and K. K. Thakral. 1978. Production of a corpus luteum angiogenic factor responsible for proliferation of capillaries and neovascularization of the corpus luteum. Proc. Natl. Acad. Sci. USA 75:847–851.

Greenblatt, M., and P. Shubik. 1968. Tumor angiogenesis: Transfilter diffusion studies in the hamster by the transparent chamber technique. JNCI 41:111–124.

Kessler, D. A., R. S. Langer, N. A. Pless, and J. Folkman. 1976. Mast cells and tumor angiogenesis. Int. J. Cancer 18:703–709.

Klagsbrun, M., D. Knighton, and J. Folkman. 1976. Tumor angiogenesis activity in cells grown in tissue culture. Cancer Res. 36:110–114.

Knighton, D. R., I. A. Silver, and T. K. Hunt. 1981. Regulation of wound healing angiogenesis—Effect of oxygen gradients in inspired oxygen concentration. Surgery 90:262–270.

Knighton, D. R., D. Ausprunk, D. Tapper, and J. Folkman. 1977. Avascular and vascular phases of tumor growth in the chick embryo. Br. J. Cancer 35:347–356.

Langer, R., and J. Folkman. 1976. Polymers for the sustained release of proteins and other macromolecules. Nature 263:797–800.

Leighton, J. 1967. The Spread of Cancer. Academic Press, New York.

Maciag, T., G. A. Hoover, J. van der Spek, M. B. Stemerman, and R. Weinstein. 1982. Growth and differentiation of human umbilical-vein endothelial cells in culture, *in* Growth of Cells in Hormonally Defined Media, Book A, G. H. Sato, A. B. Pardee, and D. A. Sirbasku, eds. Cold Spring Harbor Laboratory, Cold Spring Harbor, New York, pp. 525–538.

Maiorana, A., and P. M. Gullino. 1978. Acquisition of angiogenic capacity and neoplastic transformation in the rat mammary gland. Cancer Res. 38:4409–4414.

Moscatelli, D., J. L. Gross, and D. B. Rifkin. 1981. Angiogenic factors stimulate plasminogen activator and collagenase production by capillary endothelial cells. (Abstract) J. Cell Biol. 91:201.

Murray, J. B., L. Brown, R. Langer, and M. Klagsbrun. 1983. A micro sustained release system for epidermal growth factor. In Vitro (in press).

Muthukkaruppan, V., and R. Auerbach. 1980. Angiogenesis in the mouse cornea. Science 205:1416–1417.

Polverini, P. J., R. S. Cotran, M. A. Gimbrone, Jr., and E. R. Unanue. 1977. Activated macrophages induce vascular proliferation. Nature 269:804–806.

Rucinski, B., S. Niewiarowski, P. James, and D. A. Walz. 1979. Antiheparin proteins secreted by human platelets, purification, characterization, and radioimmunoassay. Blood 53:47–62.

Sidky, Y., and R. Auerbach. 1975. Lymphocyte-induced angiogenesis: A quantitative and sensitive assay of the graft-vs.-host reaction. J. Exp. Med. 141:1084–1100.

Taylor, S., and J. Folkman. 1982. Protamine is an inhibitor of angiogenesis. Nature 297:307–312.

Zetter, B. R. 1980. Migration of capillary endothelial cells is stimulated by tumour-derived factors. Nature 285:41–43.

Tumor Heterogeneity

Cancer Invasion and Metastasis: Biologic and Therapeutic Aspects edited by Garth L. Nicolson and Luka Milas. Raven Press, New York © 1984.

Mammary Tumor Heterogeneity

Gloria H. Heppner, Scott E. Loveless, Fred R. Miller, Keith H. Mahoney, and Amy M. Fulton

Department of Immunology, Michigan Cancer Foundation, Detroit, Michigan 48201

The observations that individual cancers are made up of subpopulations of tumor cells and that these subpopulations may be of clonal origin have been broadcast so effectively that researchers who study tumor heterogeneity are presented with a new problem. We no longer face audiences of nonbelievers who need to be convinced that tumors are heterogeneous; instead, we are now often confronted with superzealots for whom all facets of tumor growth and behavior are reduced to the level of a grade B western: there are the good guys and the bad guys, and all we need do is find ways to look at their "hats" (i.e., "markers") and then direct our magic bullets to the ones in black. Unfortunately, real life is not as simple as the Saturday matinees of our childhood. In real life, good guys also do bad things, especially when they are in bad company. Their well-intentioned behavior may have untoward effects on their environment and on the noncowboys who live there. Good guys do not always have good children. Furthermore, bad guys can have good sides, too. Real life is a dynamic process characterized by change and social interaction. The purpose of this presentation is to present results from our work on mammary tumor heterogeneity, a phenomenon which shares these characteristics.

A MODEL OF MAMMARY TUMOR HETEROGENEITY

Our model system for studying mammary tumor heterogeneity has been described elsewhere (Dexter et al. 1978, Heppner et al. 1978, Miller et al. 1983). Briefly, it consists of five tumor subpopulation lines and clones of these lines, all of which were derived from the same, spontaneously arising, strain BALB/cfC_3H mouse mammary tumor. As shown schematically in Figure 1, four of the subpopulation lines (no. 66, 67, 168, and 68H) were isolated from early monolayer cultures of the autochthonous tumor. The fifth subpopulation (no. 4.10) was isolated from a single lung metastasis of the parent tumor that had been serially passaged in vivo for 10 generations. All five of the subpopulations are of epithelial origin (Hager et al. 1981b), and all are tumorigenic in normal, syngeneic hosts. There are marked differences among them in morphology, karyotype, expression of mammary tumor virus–associated antigens, growth

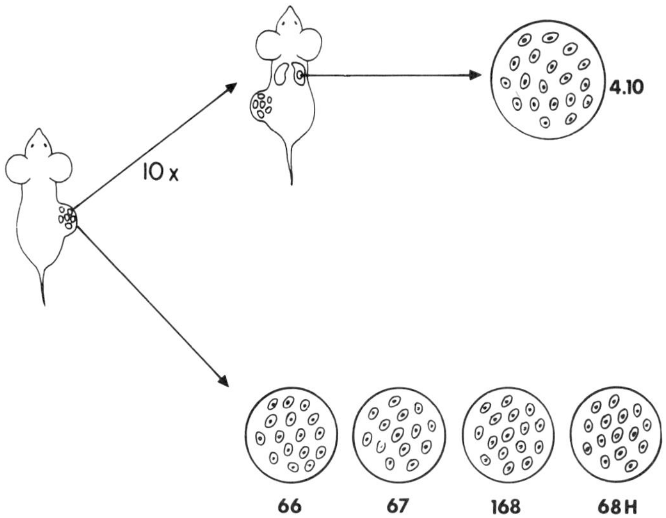

FIG. 1. Mammary tumor subpopulations. (Reproduced from Heppner 1982, with permission of Academic Press.)

properties in vitro and in vivo, sensitivity to chemotherapeutic agents, immunogenicity, and ability to metastasize (Dexter et al. 1978, Heppner et al. 1978, Miller and Heppner 1979, Hager and Heppner 1982, Miller et al. 1983). We use these subpopulations as tools to study the possible origins and consequences of tumor heterogeneity.

INTERACTIONS BETWEEN MAMMARY TUMOR SUBPOPULATIONS

The ability to isolate tumor cell subpopulations that differ in such clinically important characteristics as drug sensitivity and metastatic potential has led to the suggestion that one need only be concerned with the "relevant" subpopulations, that is, the "bad actors," in a tumor, since, for example, the slow-growing or nonmetastatic subpopulations do not pose a threat to the patient's survival. This suggestion assumes that the behavior of tumor subpopulations or clones is the same when studied with isolated populations as when the cells are growing together in a complete tumor. That this is not necessarily so is evident from the work of Hauschka (1953) and the Kleins (1956), as well as from more recent studies by Jansson and Revesz (1976), Keyner et al. (1978), Newcomb et al. (1978), and Poste et al. (1981).

Our laboratory has reported a series of interactions among our mammary tumor subpopulations. The ability of some subpopulations to alter the in vivo take rate or the latency period of other subpopulations has been demonstrated (Miller et al. 1980), as have interactions affecting growth in vitro (Heppner et al. 1980). We have also described subpopulation interactions that redirect the induction of cell-mediated immunity from an otherwise immunogenic tumor to a tumor that, by itself, is nonimmunogenic (Miller and Heppner 1980, Miller et al. 1980). Thus, "slow-growing" subpopulations may keep up with their faster-growing companions, or, alternatively, "fast-growing" subpopulations may be held back by the presence of slower-growing subpopulations. Furthermore, some subpopulations produce factors that inhibit other cells (Heppner et al. 1980). We have also shown, using both in vivo and in vitro protocols, that the degree of sensitivity of a subpopulation to a chemotherapeutic drug can be altered by the presence of another, differentially sensitive subpopulation (Miller et al. 1981).

A further example of subpopulation interactions has recently been described by Fred Miller (1983). Of relevance to the theme of this symposium, Miller's example involves the metastatic phenotype. A diagram of his experiment, which is described below, is shown in Figure 2.

Tumors of subpopulation 168 do not metastasize spontaneously in normal mice from a s.c. implant, although 168 cells will produce colonies in the lung following i.v. injection of high numbers of cells. Tumors of line 410.4, a derivative of subpopulation 410 (Miller et al. 1983), metastasize to the lung at a high rate from s.c. implants and also form lung colonies after i.v. injection. Syngeneic mice were given line 168 cells s.c. When the resulting tumors were 12 mm in mean diameter, the mice were injected i.v. with saline, 1×10^4 168 cells, or 1×10^4 410.4 cells. Five weeks later, the mice were sacrificed and examined for lung metastases. Not surprisingly, lung colonies were only found in the mice that had received the 410.4 cells. Nine of these metastastic nodules were removed and placed in monolayer culture. Although only 410.4 cells were found in most of the nodules, two of the metastases yielded both 410.4 and 168 cells,

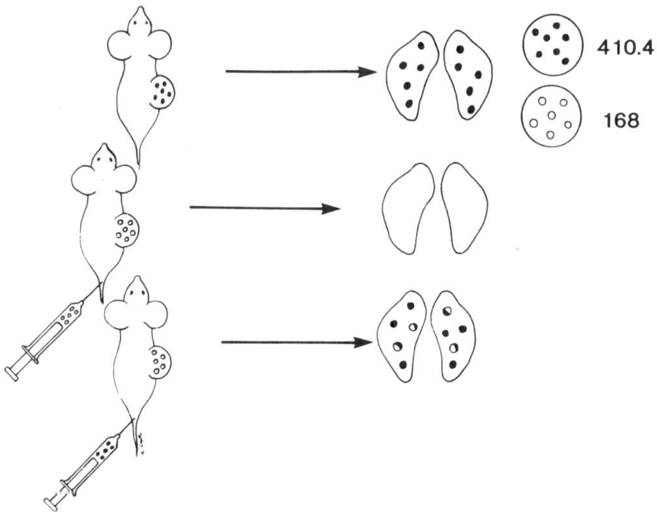

FIG. 2. Metastasis of "nonmetastatic" mammary tumor cells. Line 410.4 cells spontaneously metastasize to lungs, whereas line 168 cells do not. When 410.4 cells are injected i.v. into mice bearing a 168 tumor, lung metastases develop. These metastases contain 410.4 and 168 cells.

as judged by morphological criteria. Both types of cells were capable of further growth in vitro, showing that they were viable. Thus, even though line 168 cells did not metastasize alone, they did do so in the presence of 410.4 cells.

Although the mechanisms by which tumor subpopulations can interact to influence each other's growth and behavior are still being investigated, it is clear that they are many and varied and depend on the particular characteristics of the participating cells. The host may mediate the interaction by, for example, an immune response (Miller et al. 1980) or an effect on drug metabolism (Miller et al. 1981). The tumor cells may carry out the interactions directly through the release of factors capable of being detected in vitro (Heppner et al. 1980). Interactions may or may not require cell contact between the two subpopulations (Heppner 1982). Whatever the mechanisms, the concept of a tumor that is emerging from this work is that of an ecosystem, a cellular society, in which the various subpopulations both influence and are influenced by each other. The behavior of the society transcends the contributions of its individual components.

STABILITY OF MAMMARY TUMOR SUBPOPULATIONS

The fact that one can isolate distinct subpopulations of tumor cells at a particular point in the life of a given neoplasm does not mean that the isolates represent all the subpopulations present at that time, nor that other variants might not be present at other times. The instability of tumor cells is notorious (Nowell 1976). Several investigators have discussed tumor subpopulation instability, particularly in regard to metastasis (Chambers et al. 1981, Neri and Nicolson 1981, Poste et al. 1981). In our experience, the relative stability of a phenotype is yet another characteristic by which tumor subpopulations differ. For example, tumor subpopulation 66 has retained the ability to metastasize at high frequency after several years cultivation in vitro, and subpopulations 67, 168, and 68H have remained poorly metastatic over a similar period of time. Subpopulation 4.10 LM, however, which was originally highly metastatic, lost this ability after only a short time in culture. Unlike the experience with melanoma subpopulations (Poste et al. 1981), clones of the mammary tumor subpopulations are as stable in regards to metastasis as are the subpopulations themselves (Miller et al. 1983).

Heterogeneity in phenotypic stability is also illustrated by subpopulation 68H. Line 68H cells are epithelioid. Unlike our other tumor subpopulations, which remain morphologically stable after passage in vivo and reisolation in vitro, tumor cells that grow in vitro from 68H tumors are heterogeneous in morphology. Cultures of 68H tumors contain both epithelioid and fusiform cells. Jean Hager isolated a series of both epithelioid and fusiform clones from a monolayer culture of a line 68H tumor (Hager et al. 1981a). As diagrammed in Figure 3, the parent 68H line produces tumors in syngeneic mice only after a long latency period. For example, 1×10^6 cells produced palpable tumors after 140 days. All the clones isolated from the 68H tumor were tumorigenic, but their

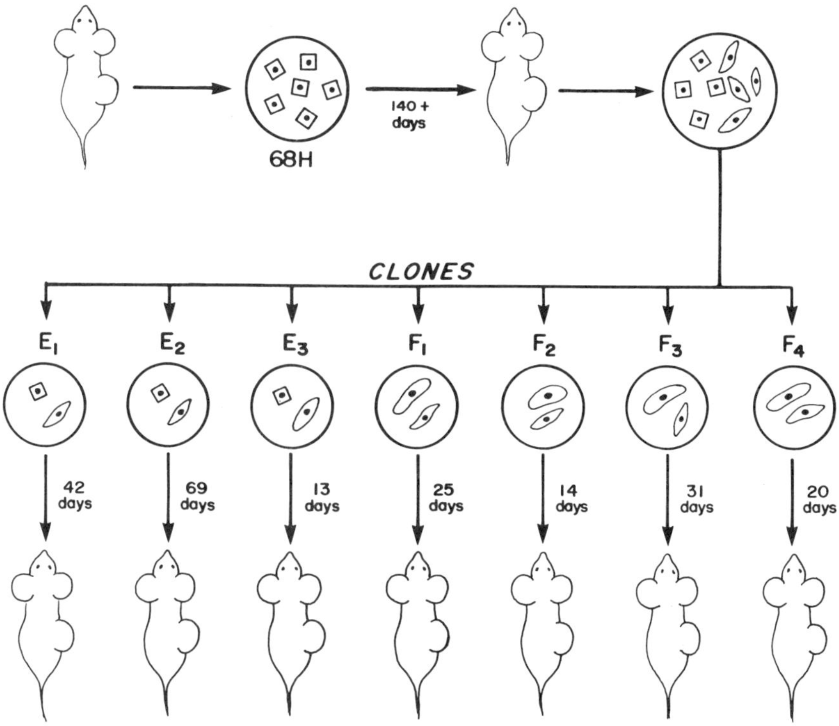

FIG. 3. Variant production by line 68H. See text for details.

latency periods ranged from 13 to 69 days at a 1×10^6 inoculum. Thus, a subpopulation that is itself of low tumorigenicity gave rise to other, more-tumorigenic subpopulations. That these variant subpopulations were of line 68H origin was shown by their sharing of marker chromosomes. The ability to give rise to further variants was differentially distributed among the 68H clones. Epithelioid clones were able to produce fusiform cells in vitro, without the in vivo passage required by parent 68H cells, whereas fusiform clones remained morphologically stable in culture. The high frequency at which 68H tumors generate variants suggests that the mechanism of diversification is akin to differentiation (Rudland et al. 1982), rather than to genetic change. This is not to imply that mutation cannot contribute to variant production (Nowell 1976, Cifone and Fidler 1981; also see below), but to suggest an additional mechanism by which relatively benign subpopulations of tumor cells ("good guys") can have progeny that exhibit considerably more aggressive behavior.

TUMOR HETEROGENEITY AND HOST RESPONSE

Up to now, this discussion has focused on the tumor cell populations of a single mammary cancer. Clearly, however, cancers contain many nonneoplastic cells. Indeed, cancer cells may themselves be in the minority in certain tumors.

Host cells play a major role in the biology of a tumor. We have been interested in how the heterogeneity of tumor cell populations interfaces with one host component, namely infiltrating cells. We found that the heterogeneity of the tumor cell populations is mirrored by heterogeneity in the infiltrating populations.

The first host component we investigated were the T lymphocytes. Previous work in our laboratory (Blazar and Heppner 1978) had established that the predominant lymphocyte population, which could be isolated by isokinetic gradient separation directly from mouse mammary tumors, was either a T (θ antigen positive) or null cell; B cells were seldom found. More recently, Angie Rios has isolated lymphocytes from tumors produced by our mammary subpopulation lines. The data, which have just been published (Rios et al. 1983), show that the different tumor subpopulations are infiltrated in vivo with both qualitatively and quantitatively characteristic T-cell populations. For example, line 168 tumors yield only a fraction of the antilymphocyte serum-positive, Thy 1.2 antigen–positive lymphocytes that can be isolated from 68H and 4.10 tumors. On the other hand, the proportion of Thy 1.2–positive cells from 68H tumors that are also positive for Lyt 1.2 antigen is about three times greater than those positive for Lyt 2.2 antigen, whereas Lyt 2.2 antigen–positive cells greatly outnumber Lyt 1.2–positive cells in tumors of lines 168 and 4.10 and of two 4.10 clones. The T-cell populations of 68H and 168 tumors growing on the same mice show the characteristic distribution for those tumors when they grow alone. Thus, the heterogeneity of a tumor cell population can lead to a heterogeneity in the T-cell component of the host.

A similar picture is beginning to emerge in regard to the macrophage infiltration of the various mammary tumor subpopulations. Tumor-associated macrophages have been isolated from tumor suspensions by trypsin-resistance adherence to plastic. In some experiments, the tumor suspensions were fractionated by centrifugal elutriation prior to the adherence step. We thus obtained data on the total macrophage context of the tumors, as well as on the distribution of these macrophages in regard to size and density. As shown in Table 1, the content of macrophages ranged from 20% to 44% for tumors of lines 168, 68H, 66, 410.4, and 67. As has been reported by others, macrophage content per se did not correlate with any known biological characteristic of the tumors, such as growth rate, immunogenicity, or ability to metastasize. A provocative correlation is apparent, however, in regard to indicators of macrophage maturation: macrophages from the metastatic tumors 66 and 410.4 were found further down the elutriation "gradient" than were macrophages from the nonmetastatic tumors 67 and 168. This difference is indicated in Table 1: at least twice as many macrophages are in fraction 2 as in fraction 3 for tumors 67 and 168, whereas the distribution is more nearly even for 66 and 410.4 tumors. Since size and density is increased in the more-mature macrophages, these data suggest a differential association of macrophage "subpopulations" with mammary tumor cell subpopulations.

TABLE 1. *Tumor-associated macrophages of mammary tumor subpopulations*

Line	Phenotype	Macrophages				
		Content	Distribution 2:3*	LAP concentration† 2:3	PGE distribution‡ 2:3	Cytotoxicity§
66	Metastatic‖	35 ± 4	1.4	0.6 (9.3)	2.5	5/5
410.4	Metastatic	36 ± 9	1.2	n.d.	n.d.	9/9
68H	Nonmetastatic # variant producing	32 ± 7	0.8	1 (6.4)	0.3	5/10
67	Nonmetastatic	44 ± 1	2.4	1 (2.3)	0.1	1/5
168	Nonmetastatic	20 ± 7	2.0	1 (3.7)	0.3	0/2

* Ratio of number of macrophages in elutriation fraction 2 to that in fraction 3. Fractions 2 and 3 contain 75–84% of all tumor-associated macrophages.

† Leucine aminopeptidase-nmole/min/μm^2. Ratio of concentration in elutriation fraction 2 to that in 3 (mean concentration in fractions 2 + 3).

‡ Prostaglandin E. Ratio of concentration in fractions 2:3.

§ Number of experiments in which tumor cell cytotoxicity was detected in vitro/total number of experiments performed.

‖ Metastatic = spontaneous metastases in lungs from s.c. implants in >80% of syngeneic mice.

Nonmetastatic = spontaneous metastases in lungs from s.c. implants in <10% of syngeneic mice.

LAP, leucine amino peptidase; PGE, prostaglandin E.

The above conclusion is strengthened by further data on the characteristics of macrophages isolated from tumors of the different subpopulation lines. Macrophages from line 66 tumors have a higher surface concentration of leucine aminopeptidase (LAP), an ectoenzyme associated with cytotoxic activity (Campbell et al. 1980), than do macrophages from the other tumors, and the LAP activity is especially associated with the fraction 3 macrophages of line 66 tumors, whereas it is evenly distributed between fractions 2 and 3 for the others. In contrast, the distribution of prostaglandin E–producing macrophages is principally into fraction 2 of tumor 66 macrophages and into fraction 3 for the others. In terms of functional activity, macrophages from nonelutriated suspensions of lines 66 and 410.4 tumors are consistently cytotoxic in vitro against mammary tumor target cells, whereas cytotoxicity is rare for macrophages from lines 67 and 168 tumors.

Although macrophages from the metastatic 66 and 410.4 tumors differ in maturational and functional properties from macrophages of nonmetastatic 67 and 168 tumors, Table 1 shows that the correlation with metastatic behavior is not complete. Macrophages from the nonmetastatic line 68H tumors seem to occupy an intermediate position, sharing some properties with 66 and 410.4 tumors and others with 67 and 168 tumors. As described above, line 68H tumors are unique in that they produce variant tumor subpopulations at high frequency. Thus, they are in reality quite heterogeneous themselves, a fact that may be related to the heterogeneity evident in their associated macrophages.

In the aggregate, our data suggest that tumor cell heterogeneity is a determinant in the heterogeneity of at least one normal cell component of tumors, namely infiltrating cells. Again, the concept of a tumor as an ecosystem seems apt. Not only are there multiple interactions among tumor cells but also between tumor cells and other cellular societies in their environment.

HOST RESPONSE AND TUMOR HETEROGENEITY

If tumor cell heterogeneity results in heterogeneity in host cells, it is clear that the opposite can also occur. Host immune responses exert a selective force that influences the composition of cancer cell populations. We have discussed elsewhere how "one-way" immunological cross-reactions between tumor cell subpopulations can, by influencing growth of a nonimmunogenic, immunosensitive tumor subpopulation, maintain the heterogeneity of a tumor in the face of a seeming growth advantage of that subpopulation over its companions (Miller et al. 1980). Recent results of Scott Loveless suggest another way by which the host contributes to tumor heterogeneity.

As described above, macrophages from spontaneously metastatic mammary tumors are routinely cytotoxic in vitro, whereas macrophages from nonmetastatic tumors are cytotoxic only occasionally. In an effort to explain this apparent paradox, we reviewed reports of Weitzman and Stossel (1981, 1982) on the ability of certain human peripheral monocytes to induce mutations in bacteria under conditions of the Ames assay (Ames et al. 1975). These workers have presented evidence that the mutagenic activity is due to products of oxygen metabolism, some of which are known mutagens (Levin et al. 1982). Since products of oxygen metabolism are released by activated macrophages and implicated in their cytotoxic activity (Nathan et al. 1979), we hypothesized that the association of cytotoxic macrophages with metastatic tumors may be a reflection of the affinity of certain tumor cells for macrophage subpopulations that, because of their oxygen metabolism, increase the mutation frequency of those tumor cells through the release of endogenous mutagens. Increasing the mutation frequency would increase the rate of production of tumor cell variants, thus increasing the chance for emergence of metastatic variants. A corollary to this hypothesis is that metastatic tumor subpopulations should be especially likely to be infiltrated with "mutagenic" macrophages. Data supporting this corollary are presented in Table 2 and Figure 4. A flow chart of the methodology is shown in Figure 5.

Whole-tumor suspensions of subpopulations 66, 410.4, 68H, and 168 were tested for mutagenic activity against two *Salmonella typhimurium* tester strains, TA 98 and TA 100. TA 98 detects point and TA 100 detects frame-shift mutations. The assay detects mutants that have reverted from a requirement for exogenous histidine to histidine independence. The tumor cells were mixed with the bacteria and immediately plated in histidine-deficient agar. In order to rule out the possibility that the cells were a source of histidine, rather than of mutagen, revertant colonies from the tumor cell–bacteria plates were isolated and replated in histidine-deficient agar. Their ability to grow indicated that they were truly mutants.

As shown in Table 2, statistically significant mutagenic activity was seen against the TA 98 strain in 9 of 13 experiments with the metastatic tumor suspensions and in 2 of 5 experiments with the nonmetastatic tumors. The degree of activity (revertant index) was greater for the metastatic than for the nonmetastatic tumors. Little or no mutagenic activity was seen with either tumor type against the TA 100 strain.

TABLE 2. *Mutagenicity of mammary tumor suspensions*

	Tester strain			
	TA 98		TA 100	
Tumor phenotype (subpopulations)	Frequency*	Revertant index† (range)	Frequency*	Revertant index† (range)
Metastatic (66, 410.4)	9/13	2.1 ± 0.4 (1.0–5.1)	0/2	1.05 ± 0.5 (1.0–1.1)
Nonmetastatic (68H, 168)	2/5	1.4 ± 0.2 (1.0–2.0)	1/2	1.2 ± 0.05 (1.15–1.25)

* Number of experiments in which number of revertants in test was significantly greater than in background control/total number of experiments performed.

† Number of revertants in test/number of revertants in background control.

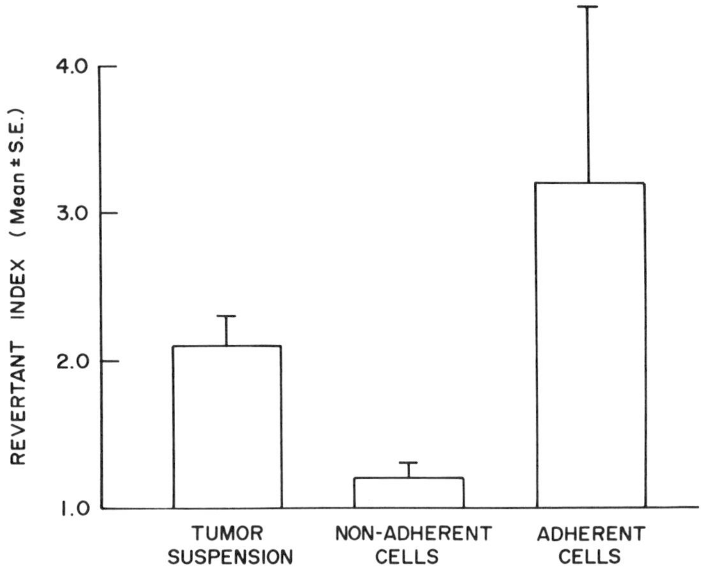

FIG. 4. Association of mutagenic activity with macrophages isolated from mammary tumors of lines 66 and 410.4. Macrophages were isolated from whole tumor suspensions by adherence to plastic.

That the mutagenic activity of the tumor suspensions is due to their macrophages is shown in Figure 4. Macrophages isolated by adherence from metastatic tumors 66 and 410.4 were mutagenic against the TA 98 strain in all experiments. Essentially no activity was seen with the nonadherent cells from the tumor suspensions.

These preliminary data are clearly a long way from proving our principle hypothesis. We do not know whether mammalian cells are susceptible to macrophage-mediated mutation, nor whether the mutagenic activity has any thing to do with oxygen metabolism. We do not know whether macrophages are mutagenic within the environment of the tumor. We also do not know whether our findings with a series of related mammary tumor lines are applicable to any other cancers. Of considerable practical importance, however, is the possibility that macrophages contribute to the heterogeneity of tumor cell populations, not only in regard to metastatic properties but to other differences as well. For example, it may be that immunotherapy directed toward activation of macrophages within tumor masses might, if it is not curative, have the undesirable effect of increasing the frequency of chemotherapy-resistant variants. Design and scheduling of combined chemoimmunotherapy regimens may need to incorporate methods of defusing this problem, such as appropriate administration of free-radical scavengers. It may also be that measurement of the mutagenicity of tumor samples, or of macrophages from them, would be one way of gauging

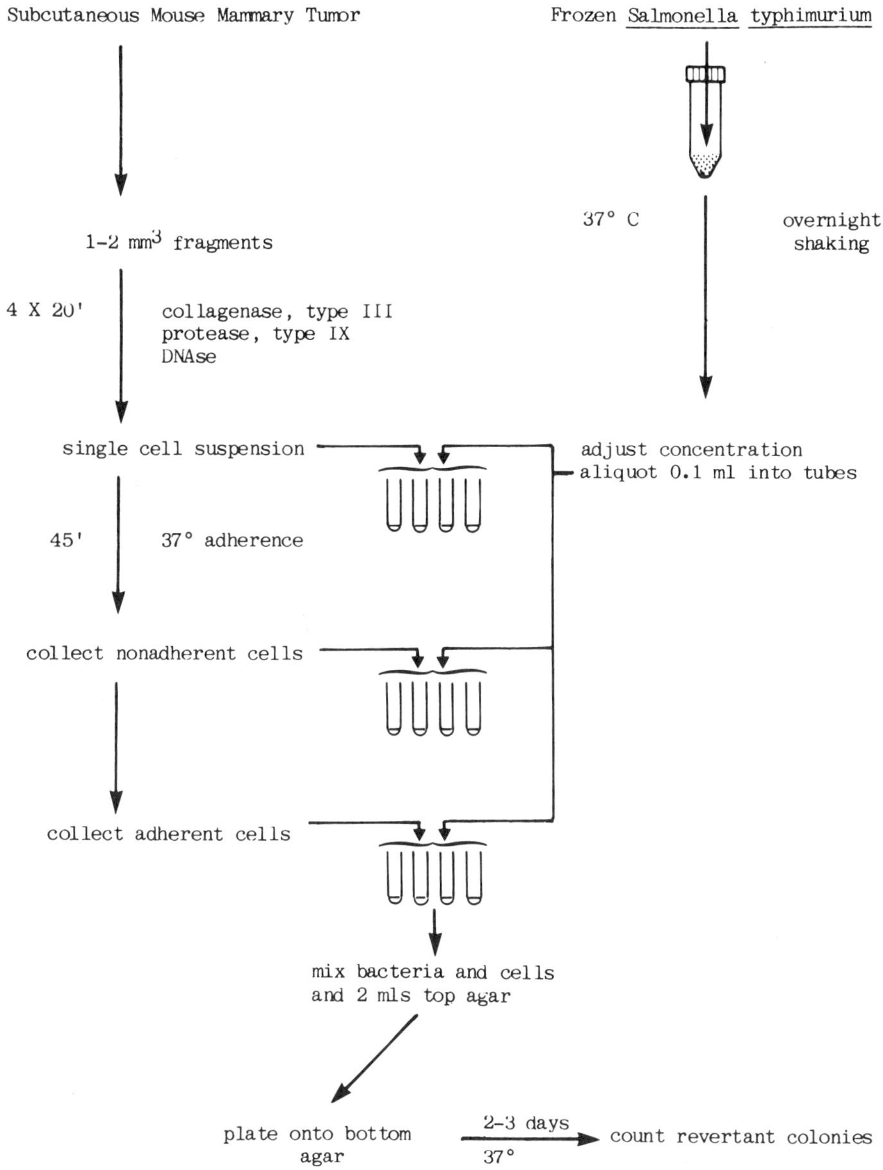

FIG. 5. Procedures used to demonstrate mutagenicity of mammary tumor–associated macrophages.

a tumor's propensity for variability and hence of assessing prognosis. Whatever the ultimate clinical significance of our observations, we believe they illustrate the necessity of viewing cancers not as collections of individual cells, but rather as complex societies with unexpected capacity for interaction, change, and evolution. The fact that tumors are heterogeneous in their cellular components does not mean that these components are independent. To understand the origins and consequences of tumor heterogeneity, we need to trace the cellular networks within individual cancers and to appreciate the complexity of their supracellular organization.

ACKNOWLEDGMENTS

This investigation was supported by grants CA-27437 and CA-27419, awarded by the National Cancer Institute, Department of Health and Human Services, by a grant from Concern Foundation, by the E. Walter Albachten bequest to the Michigan Cancer Foundation, and by the United Foundation of greater Detroit.

REFERENCES

Ames, B. N., J. McCann, and E. Yamasaki. 1975. Methods for detecting carcinogens and mutagens with the *Salmonella*/mammalian-microsome mutagenicity test. Mutat. Res. 31:347–364.

Blazar, B. A., and G. H. Heppner. 1978. In situ lymphoid cells of mouse mammary tumors. II. The characterization of lymphoid cells separated from mouse mammary tumors. J. Immunol. 120:1881–1886.

Campbell, M. W., M. M. Sholley, and G. A. Miller. 1980. Macrophage heterogeneity in tumor resistance: Cytostatic and cytotoxic activity of *Corynebacterium parvum*-activated and protease peptone-elicited rat macrophages against Moloney sarcoma tumor cells. Cell Immunol. 50:153–168.

Chambers, A. F., R. P. Hill, and V. Ling. 1981. Tumor heterogeneity and stability of the metastatic phenotype of mouse KHT sarcoma cells. Cancer Res. 41:1368–1372.

Cifone, M. A., and I. J. Fidler. 1981. Increasing metastatic potential is associated with increasing genetic instability of clones isolated from murine neoplasms. Proc. Natl. Acad. Sci. USA 78:6249–6252.

Dexter, D. L., H. M. Kowalski, B. A. Blazar, Z. Fligiel, R. Vogel, and G. H. Heppner. 1978. Heterogeneity of tumor cells from a single mouse mammary tumor. Cancer Res. 38:3174–3181.

Hager, J., S. Fligiel, W. Stanley, A. M. Richardson, and G. H. Heppner. 1981a. Characterization of a variant producing tumor cell line from a heterogeneous strain BALB/cfC$_3$H mouse mammary tumor. Cancer Res. 41:1293–1300.

Hager, J. C., and G. H. Heppner. 1982. Heterogeneity of expression and induction of mouse mammary tumor virus antigens in mouse mammary tumors. Cancer Res. 42:4325–4329.

Hager, J. C., J. Russo, R. L. Ceriani, J. A. Peterson, S. Fligiel, G. Jolly, and G. H. Heppner. 1981b. Epithelial characteristics of five subpopulations of a heterogeneous strain BALB/cfC$_3$H mouse mammary tumor. Cancer Res. 41:1720–1730.

Hauschka, T. S. 1953. Methods of conditioning the graft in tumor transplantation. JNCI 14:723–736.

Heppner, G. H. 1982. Tumor subpopulation interactions, *in* Tumor Cell Heterogeneity Origins and Implications, A. H. Owens, Jr., D. S. Coffey, and S. B. Baylin, eds. Academic Press, New York, pp. 225–236.

Heppner, G. H., D. L. Dexter, T. DeNucci, F. R. Miller, and P. Calabresi. 1978. Heterogeneity in drug sensitivity among tumor cell subpopulations of a single mammary tumor. Cancer Res. 38:3758–3763.

Heppner, G., B. Miller, D. N. Cooper, and F. R. Miller. 1980. Growth interactions between mammary tumor cells, *in* Cell Biology of Breast Cancer, C. M. McGrath, M. J. Brennan, and M. A. Rich, eds. Academic Press, New York, pp. 161–172.

Jansson, B., and L. Revesz. 1976. A deductive approach to the analysis of the growth of ascites tumor cell populations, *in* Methods in Cancer Research, H. Busch, ed., vol. XIII. Academic Press, New York, pp. 227–290.

Keyner, D., J. Christman, G. Acs, S. Silagi, E. W. Newcomb, and S. C. Silverstein. 1978. Co-cultivation of tumorigenic mouse melanoma cells with cells of a non-tumorigenic subclone inhibits plasminogen activator expression by the melanoma cells. J. Cell Physiol. 95:159–167.

Klein, G., and E. Klein. 1956. Conversion of solid neoplasms into ascites tumors. Ann. NY Acad. Sci. 63:640–661.

Levin, D. E., M. Hollstein, M. F. Christman, E. A. Schwiers, and B. N. Ames. 1982. A new *Salmonella* tester strain (TA 102) with A-T base pairs at the site of mutation detects oxidative mutagens. Proc. Natl. Acad. Sci. USA 79:7445–7449.

Miller, B. E., F. R. Miller, and G. H. Heppner. 1981. Interactions between tumor subpopulations affecting their sensitivity to the antineoplastic agents cyclophosphamide and methotrexate. Cancer Res. 41:4378–4381.

Miller, B. E., F. R. Miller, J. Leith, and G. H. Heppner. 1980. Growth interaction in vivo between tumor subpopulations derived from a single mouse mammary tumor. Cancer Res. 40:3977–3981.

Miller, F. R. 1983. Tumor subpopulation interactions in metastasis. Invasion and Metastasis. (in press).

Miller, F. R., and G. H. Heppner. 1979. Immunologic heterogeneity of tumor cell subpopulations from a single mouse mammary tumor. JNCI 63:1457–1464.

Miller, F. R., and G. H. Heppner. 1980. Intratumor immunologic interactions. (Abstract) Proceedings of the American Association for Cancer Research 21:201.

Miller, F. R., B. E. Miller, and G. H. Heppner. 1983. Characterization of metastatic heterogeneity among subpopulations of a single mouse mammary tumor: Heterogeneity in phenotypic stability. Invasion and Metastasis 3:22–31.

Nathan, C. F., S. C. Silverstein, L. H. Brukner, and Z. A. Cohn. 1979. Extracellular cytolysis by activated macrophages and granulocytes. II. Hydrogen peroxide as a mediator of cytotoxicity. J. Exp. Med. 149:100–113.

Neri, A., and G. L. Nicolson. 1981. Phenotypic drift of metastatic and cell-surface properties of mammary adenocarcinoma cell clones during growth in vitro. Int. J. Cancer 28:731–738.

Newcomb, E. W., S. C. Silverstein, and S. Silagi. 1978. Malignant mouse melanoma cells do not form tumors when mixed with cells of a non-malignant subclone: Relationship between plasminogen activator expression by the tumor cells and the host's immune response. J. Cell Physiol. 95:169–177.

Nowell, P. C. 1976. The clonal evolution of tumor cell populations. Science 194:23–28.

Poste, G., J. Doll, and I. J. Fidler. 1981. Interactions among clonal subpopulations affect stability of the metastatic phenotype in polyclonal populations of B16 melanoma cells. Proc. Natl. Acad. Sci. USA 78:6226–6230.

Rios, A. M., F. R. Miller, and G. H. Heppner. 1983. Characterization of tumor-associated lymphocytes in a series of mouse mammary tumor lines with differing biological properties. Cancer Immunol. Immunother. 15:87–91.

Rudland, P. S., B. A. Gusterson, C. M. Hughes, E. J. Ormerod, and M. J. Warburton. 1982. Two forms of tumors in nude mice generated by a neoplastic rat mammary stem cell line. Cancer Res. 42:5196–5208.

Weitzman, S. A., and T. P. Stossel. 1981. Mutation caused by human phagocytes. Science 212:546–547.

Weitzman, S. A., and T. P. Stossel. 1982. Effects of oxygen radical scavengers and antioxidants on phagocyte-induced mutagenesis. J. Immunol. 128:2770–2772.

Cancer Invasion and Metastasis: Biologic and Therapeutic Aspects edited by Garth L. Nicolson and Luka Milas. Raven Press, New York © 1984.

Interactions Between Tumor Cell Subpopulations in Malignant Tumors

George Poste,* Russell Greig, James Tzeng,* Thomas Koestler, and Steven Corwin

*Smith Kline and French Laboratories, Philadelphia, Pennsylvania 19101, and *Department of Pathology and Laboratory Medicine, University of Pennsylvania, Philadelphia 19104*

Research on the pathogenesis of cancer metastasis has experienced a significant renaissance over the last 5 years as a result of important new insights into the cell biology of cancer. The demonstration in 1977 by Fidler and Kripke that a malignant mouse tumor (B16 melanoma) contained clonal subpopulations of tumor cells with widely differing metastatic abilities, including subpopulations of tumor cells that were tumorigenic but nonmetastatic, was a landmark that has had profound consequences for experimental studies on the pathogenesis of metastatic disease. The finding that tumor cell subpopulations coexisting in the same tumor exhibit heterogeneous metastatic capabilities has now been confirmed in many laboratories using a wide range of experimental animal tumors of different histologic origins (reviews, Poste and Fidler 1980, Nicolson and Poste 1982, 1983, Poste 1982). These studies indicate that only certain subpopulations of tumor cells are endowed with the properties needed to complete the complex sequence of steps in the metastatic process in which tumor cells leave the primary tumor and disseminate to distant organs where they proliferate to form metastatic lesions.

This concept portrays metastasis as being a nonrandom and highly selective process in which only specific subpopulations of tumor cells are capable of forming metastases. This does not imply, however, that metastases will always be caused by subpopulations with the greatest metastatic potential. Analysis of the cellular composition of multiple metastases from the same host has shown that cells with low, medium, and high metastatic capabilities can be recovered from individual metastases (for references, see Poste 1982, Poste et al. 1982a).

The use of the term "nonrandom" to describe the metastatic process is prompted by the need to make a clear distinction from the long-held view in which metastasis was believed to be a random process in which all the cells in a malignant tumor were considered to be endowed with metastatic potential and that any cell "at random" could thus form a metastasis. Referring to metastasis as a nonrandom process does not mean that random (chance) events will not affect the ability of metastatic subpopulations of tumor cells to successfully generate metastases. Subpopulations of tumor cells endowed with metastatic properties will be at constant risk throughout the metastatic process of perishing because of random events. For example, it is easy to envisage a situation in which a metastatic cell in transit in the circulation could be killed as a result of a random collision with a blood cell or the vessel wall; yet the same cell at a different time and place might survive to complete the metastatic process and generate a metastatic tumor.

In addition, the competence of a tumor cell endowed with metastatic properties to complete a specific step in the metastatic process could be subject to reversible impairment imposed by its microenvironment (see Poste and Greig 1982). Conversely, changes in the nature or the intensity of the selection pressures acting at one or more steps in the metastatic process could modify metastatic competence in the absence of any change in cellular properties (see Poste 1982).

Despite the large body of experimental evidence demonstrating metastatic heterogeneity among tumor cell subpopulations isolated from common parent cell populations, the existence of metastatic subpopulations and their role in metastasis has been questioned by Mantovani et al. (1981), by Eccles and Alexander (Eccles et al. 1980, Eccles 1982), and by Weiss (1983). These investigators cite two sets of observations in support of their views.

First, on finding that cells recovered from individual metastases produced by several rodent tumor cell lines produced a broad spectrum of metastatic behavior when reinjected into animals, Mantovani et al. (1981) and Eccles et al. (1980) concluded that metastases did not arise from specific "metastatic" subpopulations. This interpretation is based on their incorrect assumption that cells recovered from metastases should produce more metastases than the original parent cell population. This assumption stems from a fundamental misinterpretation of the concept of metastatic heterogeneity. The basic tenet, at least as proposed by Fidler and Kripke (1977), Nicolson (1983, see pages 1–4, this volume), Poste (1982), and many others (see Hart 1982, Kerbel et al. 1982, Tarin 1982, loc cit) is that malignant neoplasms contain metastatic and nonmetastatic subpopulations of cells and that only the former give rise to metastases. This hypothesis merely proposes that to produce a metastasis tumor cells must be endowed with properties that befit them to complete all of the potentially destructive steps in the metastatic process and that tumor cells that lack these properties will be unable to form metastases. The hypothesis does *not* state that metastases will always arise from subpopulations with the *greatest* metastatic potential.

In showing that tumor cells recovered from different individual metastases in the same host can have low, intermediate, and high metastatic abilities, Mantovani, Eccles, Alexander, and their colleagues have merely confirmed what has been demonstrated by others (see Poste et al. 1980, 1982a). In setting out to test the false premise that cells isolated from metastases should produce *more* metastases than the parent population from which they arose, these investigators have sought to examine a question that only they, and no one else, proposed. On failing to confirm their own erroneous hypothesis (an outcome that was predictable on the evidence available even at the time), these investigators proceeded to attribute their own hypothesis to others, thereby generating one of the more remarkable exercises in self-fulfilling circular logic to be published for some time.

The second line of evidence cited by opponents of the view that metastases are caused by specific subpopulations of tumor cells relates to reports of failure to isolate tumor cells with enhanced metastatic potential from certain malignant tumor cell lines (see Weiss 1983). Such statements have little meaning unless the cellular composition of the cell line being studied is defined. For example, if the majority of subpopulations in a cell line already exhibit high metastatic capabilities, the probability of developing a selection pressure to detect the rare subpopulations with even greater metastatic potential will be low. In contrast, in heterogeneous polyclonal tumor cell lines in which subpopulations with high metastatic abilities are rare, or are at least in the minority, relatively weak selection pressures can increase the fraction of such highly metastatic cells within the overall population (Fidler 1973, Brunson et al. 1978, Kripke et al. 1978, Hart 1979, Poste et al. 1981, 1982a).

This concept is illustrated by recent data from my own laboratory (Poste et al. 1982a). Clonal analysis of a series of uncloned B16 melanoma cell lines revealed that in lines of a low metastatic capacity (B16-F1; B16-F1-CAM10) only 30% of the clones tested produced more metastases than the parent cell line. However, in three (B16-F10; B16-F1-BV8; B16-F1-BL6) cell lines that had been selected for high metastatic properties from the B16-F1 line, 60–70% of the clones tested produced more metastases than the original B16-F1 line (Poste et al. 1982a). In an analogous set of experiments, Talmadge and Fidler (1982) showed that cells recovered from lung metastases arising from s.c. implants of the weakly metastatic B16-F1 cell line produced 25 to 35 times more metastases than the uncloned parent Fl cell line. In contrast, the proportion of metastatic clones isolated from metastases produced by s.c. implants of the highly metastatic B16-F10 and B16-F1-BL6 cell lines did not differ significantly from the parent cell lines. These data demonstrate that when a weakly metastatic cell line is used as starting material (e.g. B16-F1), the process of metastasis selects for subpopulations that have well-developed metastatic abilities even though they represent only a minor fraction of the total parent cell population. However, the highly metastatic B16-F10 and B16-F1-BL6 cell lines already contain a large fraction of highly metastatic cells, and it is therefore difficult, if not impossible, to select for cells that exhibit greater metastatic abilities. Consequently, in starting with cell lines that are already highly metastatic it is not surprising that cells with even greater metastatic proficiency cannot be easily detected.

The issue of whether nonmetastatic cells and subpopulations of tumor cells with differing metastatic abilities coexist within tumors no longer merits serious debate. The more challenging exercise now is to begin to understand how this extensive cellular heterogeneity is generated and controlled. We are also ignorant about when metastatic variants first make their appearance in a tumor. Are they present from the very early life of a tumor? Are variant subpopulations with metastatic potential present in certain tumors from the very outset of neoplastic conversion? Once metastatic subpopulations are present, do they have adaptive advantage over nonmetastatic subpopulations so that their contribution to the overall population will increase with progressive growth of the tumor? Answers to these questions are lacking, and they represent obvious topics for future research.

As discussed in detail elsewhere (Nicolson and Poste 1982, 1983, Poste 1982, Poste and Greig 1982) cellular diversity could arise in tumors by two, nonexclusive mechanisms. For tumors of multicellular origin, diversity would be present from the outset. However, even in these tumors, and certainly for tumors of unicellular origin (believed to be the mode of origin of most human tumors), the available evidence suggests that additional diversity is generated by the emergence of new clones with altered phenotypes during progressive tumor growth.

Nowell (1976), elaborating on the concept advanced earlier by Foulds (1953), has proposed that generation of clonal cell variants is an inevitable and fundamental feature of progressive tumor growth. He proposes that tumor progression occurs via a series of multiple yet independent changes in many different cellular properties, resulting in rapid generation of clonal subpopulations with widely differing phenotypes. This diversity is amplified by the fact that tumor progression toward autonomy from host control may proceed simultaneously along many pathways and need not follow a set "program" of inevitable phenotypic progression.

At any time during progression, the number of subpopulations present in a tumor, and the extent of their phenotypic diversity, will reflect the selection pressures encountered during the lifetime of the tumor. Selection pressures can be natural (e.g., assault by host defense mechanisms, limiting nutritional conditions) or applied (e.g., therapy). Even though the kinetics for the generation of cell variants may vary in tumors of differing histologic origin, as well as in tumors of common histologic origin in different patients, the probability is high that by the time of initial clinical presentation most tumors will exhibit extensive cellular heterogeneity for a wide range of phenotypes.

Nowell's concept of tumor progression also proposes that as successive clonal subpopulations emerge, they will display increasing genetic instability. This, coupled with the selection pressures imposed by host defense and therapy, will favor relentless emergence of new subpopulations with enhanced metastatic capacities.

This chapter describes studies that suggest that the generation of cellular diversity via the emergence of clonal subpopulations of tumor cells with altered (variant) phenotypes is influenced by interactions occurring between constituent cellular subpopulations within the overall cell population. These findings suggest that a tumor is more than simply the sum of its parts and that we must expand our conceptual and technical horizons to accommodate these phenomena. We must begin, as Gloria Heppner has urged (1983, see pages 209–221, this volume) to view tumors as complex "ecosystems" in which the population dynamics of the constituent cellular subpopulations are determined by a complex interplay of endogenous (tumor) and exogenous factors (host, therapy).

THE ROLE OF TUMOR CELL INTERACTIONS IN REGULATING THE FORMATION OF TUMOR CELL VARIANTS: IN VITRO STUDIES

Identification of significant variation in the metastatic properties of cells isolated from the same tumor has important implications for experimental attempts to define which cellular properties correlate with metastatic ability. Hitherto, this question has been investigated by analyzing cultured tumor cell lines or biopsies of tumor tissue derived from lesions in vivo. This method is valid only if the tumor cell population being studied is uniform and the cells are homogeneous for the metastatic phenotype. If, however, extensive cellular heterogeneity exists, and cell subpopulations endowed with metastatic properties represent only a minor fraction of the total population, random analysis of the entire population may prove futile since nonmetastatic subpopulations may create a "background noise" that obscures features unique to metastatic subpopulations.

Whereas the experimental strategy adopted for identifying tumor cell properties that correlate with tumorigenicity involves comparison of nonneoplastic and neoplastic cells, analysis of the metastatic phenotype requires more sophisticated, and technically more demanding, comparison of the following tumor cell subpopulations isolated from the same parent cell population: tumorigenic, noninvasive versus tumorigenic, invasive, nonmetastatic versus tumorigenic, invasive, metastatic. Inclusion of nonneoplastic cells in the comparison may be helpful but is probably not essential for the identification of cellular and subcellular phenotypic traits that correlate with metastatic capacity.

The experimental analysis outlined above requires that cell subpopulations with differing metastatic abilities be isolated. The exact number of phenotypically distinct subpopulations that can exist has yet to be defined for even a single tumor. The number is undoubtedly high. Also, it is probably dynamic, fluctuating in the face of even small changes in growth conditions that may not even be detectable using our present crude assay systems. Subpopulations that express metastatic capacity and subpopulations that are tumorigenic but noninvasive merely represent the two extremes of a broad spectrum of subpopulations in heterogeneous tumors. Tumor cell subpopulations that are invasive but nonmetastatic have already been demonstrated (Poste et al. 1980). The possibility must therefore be considered that additional subpopulations exist that can complete many, but not all, steps in the metastatic process. Coexisting with such subpopulations will be an unknown number of metastatic subpopulations of increasing aggressiveness that produce increasing levels of metastatic disease. At the other extreme, the tumorigenic but noninvasive phenotype may also represent a graded spectrum of phenotypic progression towards the eventual acquisition of invasive potential. Finally, subpopulations defined on the basis of their abilities to complete specific steps in the metastatic process can, in turn, be subdivided further on the basis of their heterogeneity for other phenotypes, including resistance to susceptibility to killing by host defense mechanisms and various therapeutic modalities (reviews, Nicolson and Poste 1982, 1983, Poste 1982).

Cloning provides the most direct and efficient procedure for procuring tumor cell subpopulations with defined metastatic properties from polyclonal tumor cell lines. However, the value of tumor cell clones in analyzing any aspect of tumor cell behavior requires that the phenotypic characters of interest remain stable during serial passage of the clones, whether in vivo or in vitro. Although many cellular properties are highly stable in cloned cells in the absence of specific selection pressures, the metastatic properties of B16 melanoma clones are highly unstable during serial passage. Subclones with different invasive and metastatic properties are generated rapidly on serial passage in vitro and in vivo (Fidler and Nicolson 1981, Poste et al. 1981). In contrast, the metastatic properties of the uncloned parent cell lines remain stable when exposed to the same culture conditions. "Destabilization" of the metastatic phenotype in individual clones does not occur, however, when replicate populations of the same clones are cocultivated. The stability of the metastatic phenotype in individual clones during this experiment was verified by using clones bearing stable, drug-resistant markers and by showing that subclones resistant to particular drugs had metastatic phenotypes identical to those of the original clones with the same drug-resistance phenotype (Poste et al. 1981).

The "stabilizing" effect of clonal interactions on the metastatic phenotype is not produced by mixing clones from tumors of different histologic origin. Single clones of B16 melanoma cocultivated with clones from the Lewis lung carcinoma or UV2237 fibrosarcoma show marked phenotypic instability and rapidly generate subclones with widely different metastatic properties (Poste et al. 1981). Similarly, nonneoplastic cells from syngeneic C57/BL6 mice cannot "quench" the metastatic instability of B16 melanoma clones grown in isolation (Poste 1982).

However, clones isolated from tumors of similar histologic origin arising in different hosts can interact to stabilize their metastatic properties, though the differences in responsiveness of individual clones in these heterologous interactions are greater than those between clones isolated from the same tumor. For example, single clones from the B16 melanoma that exhibit unstable metastatic phenotypes when cultivated as single clones exhibit stable metastatic phenotypes when cocultivated with a series of clones from the mouse K-1735 melanoma (and vice versa), even though these tumors arose in different mouse strains (B16 in C57/BL6N mice and K-1735 in C3H/HeN mice). However, clones have been identified that are unresponsive to regulation by clones from the heterologous tumor. Yet these clones do show stable metastatic phenotypes when cocultivated with clones from their homologous tumor (G. Poste, unpublished observations).

The role of clonal interactions in regulating the stability of the metastatic phenotype is not unique to melanomas. Similar instability of the metastatic phenotype has been identified in clones of the mouse UV2237 fibrosarcoma (Cifone and Fidler 1981), mouse RAW 117 lymphosarcoma, rats 13762 mammary adenocarcinoma (Nicolson 1982, and 1983, see pages 1–4, this volume) and the rat 1AR6 hepatocarcinoma (Talmadge et al. 1981). All of these cell lines share the characteristic, however, of having been maintained in vitro or passaged in vivo for lengthy periods since being isolated from the original tumor-bearing host. To examine whether instability and drift of the metastatic phenotype in tumor cell clones is a peculiarity of the "antique" status of these cell lines, we tested the stability of the metastatic phenotype in clones isolated from a series of newly induced fibrosarcomas induced by irradiating mouse skin with UV light or by painting the skin with methylcholanthrene (MCA). Tumors were excised at intervals after their detection, and a series of clones isolated and assayed for their metastatic abilities. As shown in Table 1, many clones isolated from "early" tumors (excised within 2–3 months after detection) exhibited stable metastatic properties when grown as single clones. In contrast, a significantly greater fraction of clones isolated from "advanced" tumors excised after 6–9 months exhibited unstable metastatic phenotypes when cultivated as single clones.

These data indicate that the instability of the metastatic phenotype in single clones of B16 melanoma and other long-established tumor cell lines is not due to the "antiquity" of these lines. Comparison of the behavior of clones isolated from "early" and "advanced" fibrosarcomas (Table 1) suggests that tumor progression involves initial formation of clonal subpopulations with stable metastatic properties, followed by emergence of clonal subpopulations with unstable metastatic phenotypes. In the majority of clones tested to date, the metastatic properties of individual clones are "stabilized" by cocultivation with other clones. However, a few clones isolated from advanced UV- and MCA-induced fibrosarcomas have been identified that exhibit unstable metastatic properties and are not stabilized by cocultivation with other clones (G. Poste, unpublished observations). This suggests that the sequence of clonal evolution during tumor progression may be as follows:

Phase 1: initial generation and expansion of clones with diverse but stable* metastatic phenotypes;

Phase 2: evolution of clones with unstable* metastatic phenotypes but that are stabilized by interactions with other clones;

* Throughout this article unless stated otherwise the terms stable and unstable metastatic phenotypes refer to the properties of clones grown as single clones in vitro in isolation from other clones.

TABLE 1. *Incidence of unstable metastatic phenotypes in tumor cell clones isolated from tumors of different ages and from tumor cell lines*

Sample	Number of passages*		Number of unstable clones/total clones tested†
	In vitro	In vivo	
B16 melanoma	>40	—	104/114
K1735 melanoma	>40	—	32/36
UV2237 fibrosarcoma	>40	—	21/39
UV2237-HPM fibrosarcoma‡	>40	8	16/18
UV6487-3/12 fibrosarcoma§	3	—	2/14
UV6487-HPC fibrosarcoma‖	>20	—	11/20
UV6487-HPM fibrosarcoma #	5	8	18/19
UV5175-6/12 fibrosarcoma§	4	—	16/23
UV5175-HPC fibrosarcoma‖	>20	—	18/20
MC 118-3/12 fibrosarcoma§	3	—	3/14
MC 118-HPC fibrosarcoma‖	>20	—	10/17
MC 224-5/12 fibrosarcoma§	4	—	15/18
MC 224-HPC fibrosarcoma‖	>20	—	10/16

* The indicated cell populations were serially passaged in vitro or in vivo for the number of transfers shown. The subcultivation interval for the melanoma and fibrosarcoma lines was 5 and 7 days, respectively. For serial passage in vivo, single-cell suspensions (1×10^6 cells) were injected s.c. into the flank of syngeneic mice and nodules excised on reaching a size of 2 cm or greater.

† Clones were classified as exhibiting an unstable metastatic phenotype if they yielded subclones with significantly different metastatic properties within ten serial subcultivations after cloning. Clones were isolated at the end of the indicated period of serial passaging in vitro or in vivo.

‡ HPM, high passage (in the) mouse.

§ 3/12, 5/12, and 6/12 refer to the number of months between initial macroscopic detection of the indicated tumor and its subsequent excision for preparation of cell cultures.

‖ HPC represents the same tumor cell population shown on the line above after passage in vitro for a minimum of 20 subcultivations.

HPM represents the tumor cell population isolated from the indicated tumor after serial passage in syngeneic mice for a minimum of eight transfers [HPM = high passage (in the) mouse].

Phase 3: emergence of clones with unstable metastatic phenotypes that are unresponsive to the stabilizing effects of other clones.

The last category of clones have thus apparently achieved autonomy not only from the homeostatic controls of the host but also from the regulatory interactions operating within the tumor at earlier stages in its evolution.

Further evidence to support the role of clonal interactions in regulating the stability of the metastatic phenotype has come from studies in which B16 melanoma clonal subpopulations bearing specific drug-resistance markers were cocultivated with a series of wild-type B16 melanoma clones and treated with different drugs to restrict subpopulation diversity by killing wild-type clones and clones carrying the inappropriate resistance marker. Following drug-induced elimination of the majority of clones, the surviving one or two clones generated variants with altered metastatic properties at a significantly faster rate than were generated in the original culture containing six clones (Poste et al. 1981). With time, formation of new cell variants re-creates substantial subpopulation diversity, and the rate of variant formation returns to a low level and remains at this low level until another selection pressure is imposed to restrict subpopulation diversity; the cycle then begins again (Poste et al. 1981).

The mechanisms by which clonal subpopulations interact to regulate each others' behavior are not known. As discussed in this book by Gloria Heppner (1983, see pages 209–221), a complex combination of soluble factors released by the cells, cell-to-cell contact, and host cell factors appears to be involved, with different subpopulations exhibiting differing responses to regulation by each mechanism.

The precise extent of subpopulation diversity needed to "stabilize" the metastatic phenotype is not known. In vitro experiments using B16 clones indicate that the exact number varies from clone to clone (G. Poste, unpublished observations). In addition, it may well vary in different tumors and also at different stages in progression of the same tumor.

THE ROLE OF TUMOR CELL INTERACTIONS IN REGULATING THE FORMATION OF TUMOR CELL VARIANTS: IN VIVO STUDIES

Recent studies using tumor cells bearing identifiable biochemical (Poste et al. 1982b) and karyotypic markers (Talmadge and Fidler 1982) have established that the majority of experimental lung metastases are of clonal origin. The use of the term clonal in this context refers to metastases in which a common parent cell marker can be identified in *all* cells recovered from the lesion. Current limitations in technique do not permit resolution of whether such lesions are truly of single-cell origin or arose from a group of tumor cells with the same phenotype. Irrespective of which explanation applies, metastases of homotypic origin, at least in their initial stages, represent a homogeneous cell population and are thus comparable to a cell clone in vitro. After their dissemination, arrest, and localization in a distant organ, tumor cells in an early homotypic metastasis may not be exposed to the same range of interactions with other clonal subpopulations that they would have experienced in the primary lesion. Experiments were therefore undertaken to determine whether progressive growth of individual metastases in vivo was accompanied by evolution of intralesional clonal heterogeneity analogous to the metastatic drift observed in single clones in vitro.

Clonal analysis of individual lung metastases produced by i.v. injection of a series of B16 melanoma clones bearing identifiable drug-resistance (D^r) markers revealed that this was indeed the case (Poste et al. 1982b). As shown in Figure 1, the majority of "early" B16 melanoma metastases are characterized by intralesional clonal homogeneity; i.e., all of the clones isolated from the same metastasis have indistinguishable metastatic profiles and carry the same D^r marker. In

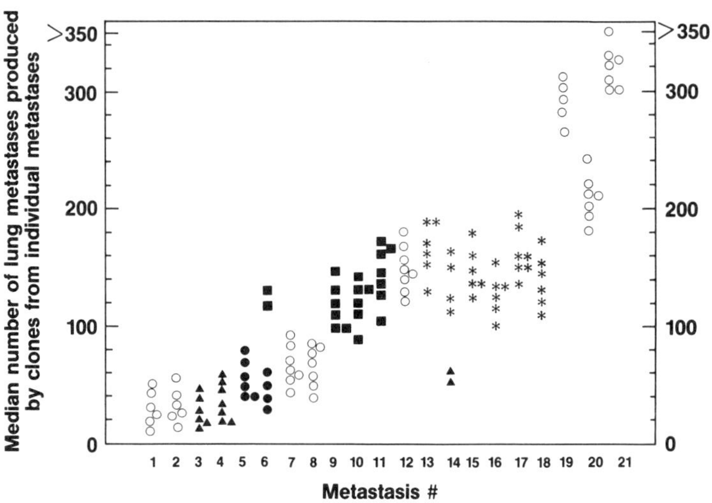

FIG. 1. Drug-resistance phenotypes and metastatic properties of clones isolated from individual B16 melanoma lung metastases 16 days after i.v. injection of tumor cells.

C57BL/6 mice were injected i.v. with a mixture of uncloned *wt* B16-F10 clones resistant to Adriamycin (ADR), diaminopurine (DAP), trifluorothymidine (TFT), or vincristine (VCR). Individual metastases were excised 16 days later. Clones were isolated from the recovered cells and assayed for their metastatic properties and for resistance to 50 ng/ml ADR (*), 47 μM DAP (●), 2 μg/ml TFT (▲), and 20 ng/ml VCR (■). Wild-type cells (○) were identified by their susceptibility to killing by all of these drugs. Wherever possible, a minimum of six clones were isolated from each metastasis. The metastatic properties of individual clones were assayed by i.v. injection of 5×10^4 cells and counting the number of lung metastases after 21 days. The results represent median values from measurements on five mice per clone. The following groups of metastases were produced by injection of different tumor cell preparations: metastases #1, 3, 13, 18, 19; 4, 5, 7, 8, 12, 16; 2, 10, 17; 6, 11, 20; 9, 14, 15, 21. The following metastases were excised from different mice: #1, 3; 13, 18, 19; 4, 7, 8; 5, 12; 16; 2, 10, 17; 6, 11, 20; 9, 21; 14, 15. (Reproduced from Poste et al. 1982b with permission.)

contrast, clonal analysis of "advanced" metastases produced by the *same* preparation of clones used to generate "early" lesions revealed that within as little as 45 days significant intralesional clonal heterogeneity had developed (Figure 2). Different clones isolated from the same metastasis had significantly different metastatic properties, even though they each carried the same D^r marker, which indicated that they had a common parentage.

Our laboratory has also begun to examine the effect of the primary tumor on the generation of tumor cell variants within individual metastases. The metastatic burden arising from s.c. implants of B16 melanoma is enhanced by surgical removal of the implant after initial metastatic dissemination has occurred (Poste et al. 1982a). We have found that the rate of generation of clonal heterogeneity within individual metastases is faster when the implant is removed than when it is allowed to remain (G. Poste and J. Tzeng, unpublished observations).

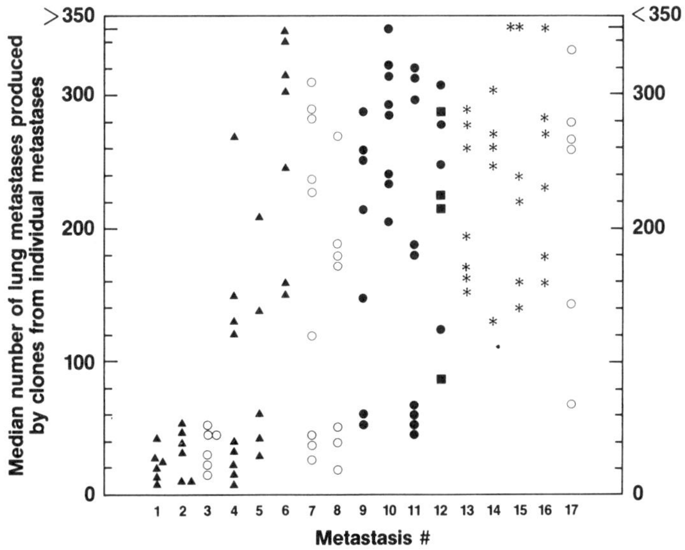

FIG. 2. Drug-resistance phenotypes and metastatic properties of clones isolated from individual B16 melanoma lung metastases 45 days after i.v. injection of a polyclonal suspension of wild-type B16-F10 cells and D^r variants of B16-F10.

The experimental protocol is identical to that described in the legend of Figure 1, as is the legend. The following metastases were produced by injection of different batches of the mixed tumor cell suspension: metastases #1, 7, 13, 16; 2, 4, 6, 10; 3, 9, 11, 12, 15; and 5, 8, 14. These preparations correspond to four of the five batches of tumor cells used in the experiments shown in Figure 1. The following metastases were excised from different animals: #1, 7; 13, 16; 2, 4, 6; 10; 3, 9, 11; 12, 15; 5, 8; and 14. (Reproduced from Poste et al. 1982b with permission.)

CLONAL DIVERSIFICATION AND THE BIOLOGICAL "FITNESS" OF TUMORS

The genesis of cellular diversity within tumors via the generation and expansion of phenotypically different tumor cell clones during tumor progression provides a powerful mechanism for increasing the ability of a tumor to survive a diverse array of destructive selection pressures. The unrelenting emergence of new clonal subpopulations with diverse phenotypes in response to the varied selection pressures increases the probability that one or more subpopulations will possess the phenotypes needed to survive selection pressures mounted by the host and by the oncologist during cancer therapy.

It is now clear, however, that an understanding of malignant tumors will require more than simple cataloging of the number and nature of the cellular subpopulations present at any particular stage in tumor progression. Tumors can no longer be viewed as passive assemblies of different clonal subpopulations. The finding that interactions between the constituent subpopulations of heterogeneous tumors can influence the rate at which new variant subpopulations are generated introduces additional complexity to the experimental study of tumors. At the same time, however, awareness of such interactions provides important clues as to how cellular diversity might be generated and controlled at different stages in tumor progression.

If, as proposed here, the extent of subpopulation diversity within the overall population is important in regulating the rate of formation of new variant subpopulations, a number of situations can be identified in which this mechanism might operate to ensure that significant cellular diversity is maintained in both the primary tumor and in individual metastases.

GENERATION OF CELLULAR DIVERSITY IN PRIMARY TUMORS

During initial formation of the primary tumor, whether it be of monoclonal or polyclonal origin, the level of subpopulation diversity will be low. This low diversity may act as a driving force for rapid formation of new variants and thereby increase cellular diversity. Following initial rapid generation of variants during the earliest stages of tumor progression, a "plateau" phase will be reached in which the rate of new variants will slow, but not necessarily cease (Figures 3 and 4) (see Poste et al. 1981, Poste 1982, Poste and Greig 1982). The exact level of subpopulation diversity needed to achieve the plateau phase is not known. It may well vary in tumors arising in different tissues and at different stages in tumor progression, particularly if clones begin to emerge that are increasingly

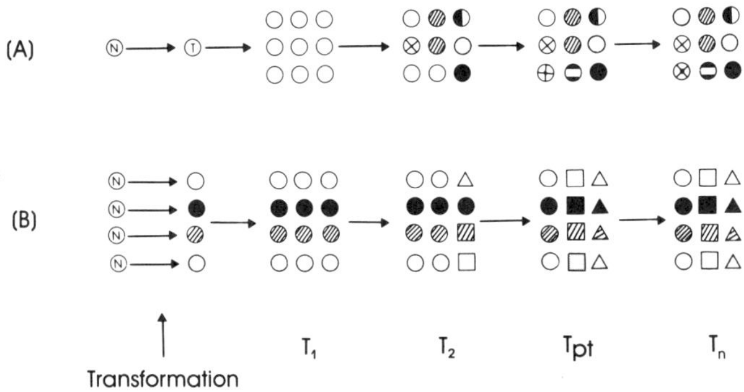

FIG. 3. Possible events in the generation of cellular diversity and metastatic heterogeneity during tumor progression.

Following initial transformation of single **(A)** or multiple **(B)** normal cells (*N*), tumor cells are formed and undergo initial proliferation (T_1). For tumors of multicellular origin **(B),** cellular diversity is present from the outset. With time, progressive growth results in the generation of cell variants with different metastatic phenotypes, as indicated by the different symbols (T_2). The kinetics of the formation of metastatic variants will probably vary between tumors of different histologic origin and between tumors of similar histologic origin in different hosts in which tumors will be exposed to a different array of selection pressures imposed by host defense mechanisms and therapy. (Modified from Fidler and Poste 1982.)

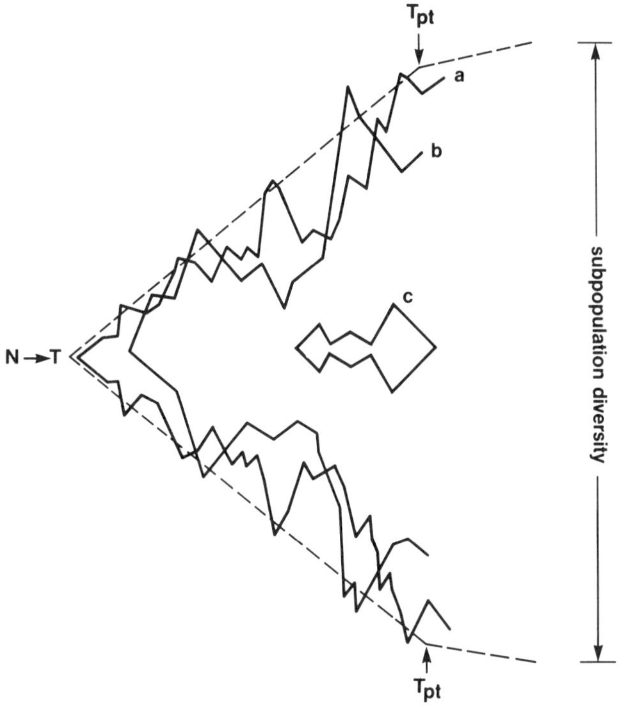

FIG. 4. Fluctuations in the size of different clonal subpopulations of tumor cells during progressive tumor growth. The dynamics of the total tumor cell population is illustrated by the dotted lines. Following conversion of a normal cell (*N*) to a tumor cell (*T*), new clones with variant phenotypes are rapidly generated, producing extensive subpopulation diversity. The formation of new variants slows, however, once a high degree of cellular heterogeneity has been created (T_{pt}). The behavior of the total tumor cell population, portrayed by the dotted lines, represents the collective dynamics of the individual clones. The dynamics of individual clones will fluctuate in response to selection pressures, and this process is illustrated by three clones (*a-c*). Clones a and b arise early in the life of the tumor, and despite fluctuations in the size of each clone (i.e., number of cells) at different times during tumor growth, they continue to expand. Subpopulation c arises later and, despite several clonal expansions and retractions, fails to survive. (Modified from Poste and Greig 1982.)

unresponsive to regulation by interactions with other clones. We refer to the time at which sufficient subpopulation heterogeneity is created within a polyclonal population to limit the rate of formation of new metastatic variants as T_{pt} (pt = plateau) (Figures 3 and 4). In previous publications from this laboratory (Fidler and Poste 1982, Poste 1982, Poste and Greig 1982), the term T_{eq} (eq = equilibrium) had been used. The term "equilibrium" is misleading, however, since it implies that an equilibrium state is reached in which the rate of formation of new cell variants is matched by the demise of a similar number of subpopulations. No experimental evidence is available to suggest that this is occurring. Rather, on achieving a given level of subpopulation heterogeneity, it appears that the rate of formation of new variants establishes a plateau (T_{pt}) relative to the rate in the preceding phase.

The rapid evolution of new variants in newly formed tumors is an example of passive contribution of restricted subpopulation diversity to cellular heterogeneity. In contrast, "active" restriction of subpopulation diversity would apply in the following three situations: initial formation of metastases; domination of a tumor by a single subpopulation or a limited number of subpopulations; and destruction of multiple subpopulations by any potent selection pressure (e.g. host defense reactions, therapy). These are discussed in more detail below.

GENERATION OF CELLULAR HETEROGENEITY IN INDIVIDUAL METASTASES

As discussed earlier, metastatic subpopulations in heterogeneous primary tumors will interact with other clones. However, tumor cells that leave the primary tumor and colonize distant sites to form homotypic metastases will be exposed to a new microenvironment in which the clonal interactions operating in the primary tumor will be lost or at least reduced. The initial cellular homogeneity of homotypic metastases may thus create a permissive condition for rapid formation of new clonal variants. The finding that the rate of clonal diversification of homotypic B16 melanoma lung metastases is slower in mice bearing s.c. tumor implants than in mice whose implant is amputated suggests, however, that some form of long-range regulatory interactions may occur between cells in the primary lesion and cells in distant metastases.

AUTOREGULATION: REGENERATION OF CELLULAR HETEROGENEITY IN RESPONSE TO TUMOR-GENERATED CHANGES IN SUBPOPULATION DYNAMICS

Enhanced formation of tumor cell variants under conditions of restricted subpopulation diversity may allow tumors to regenerate cellular diversity in response to changes in cellular composition resulting from the tumor's own growth dynamics. Specifically, rapid clonal diversification offers tumors protection against domination by a single clone or a few subpopulations. It is likely that new clones generated during tumor progression will have significant adaptive advantages over existing clones and will become the dominant, or even the exclusive, subpopulation within the tumor. Clonal domination could occur via a number of nonexclusive mechanisms; e.g., faster growth rate, more efficient competition for nutrients under rate-limiting conditions, and escape from detection by host-defense mechanisms. Irrespective of mechanism, domination of a tumor by a few subpopulations limits cellular diversity and in so doing stimulates diversification of the dominant clones.

REGENERATION OF CELLULAR HETEROGENEITY FOLLOWING EXPOSURE TO POTENT SELECTION PRESSURE(S)

The last situation in which rapid formation of clonal variants may contribute to tumor survival is under conditions in which subpopulation diversity is restricted by destruction of "unfit" subpopulations by potent selection pressures (Figure 5). A wide range of factors could produce such effects: nonspecific, deleterious growth conditions caused by poor vascularization or tissue necrosis; immunologically nonspecific and specific host defense reactions; and external assaults mounted by the clinical oncologist. The efficiency (potency) of a given selection pressure in eliminating subpopulations of tumor cells will vary depending on the properties of the subpopulations and will also differ in different hosts and at different stages in tumor progression.

The most challenging, and certainly the most disturbing, question arising from this proposal concerns the potential effect of therapy (single/multiagent; single/multimodality) on the dynamics of tumor cell subpopulations. If a particular therapy* were to kill most, but not all, cellular subpopulations in a heterogeneous, polyclonal tumor (as is typically the case), the surviving subpopulations might be rendered phenotypically unstable because of loss of the regulatory interactions between constituent subpopulations.

By restricting subpopulation diversity, therapy may perturb the plateau phase and stimulate rapid formation of new tumor cell variants from the surviving

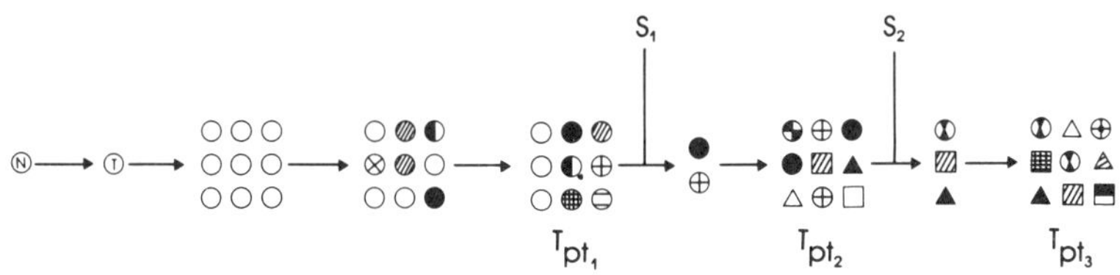

FIG. 5. The possible effect of potent selection pressures in causing cycles of clonal restriction and diversification in tumors.

Following conversion of a normal cell (*N*) to a tumor cell (*T*), additional tumor cell variants arise (depicted by the different symbols) to create a heterogeneous, polyclonal lesion, which eventually reaches a plateau phase (T_{pt_1}), at which time the rate of formation of new variants is reduced (see text). Exposure of a heterogeneous, polyclonal tumor cell population of this kind to a selection pressure (S_1) that eliminates the majority of clones causes rapid formation of a new panel of clonal variants from the surviving clones. With time, sufficient subpopulation diversity is again achieved to establish a new plateau phase population (T_{pt_2}). Exposure of this population to a new (different) selection pressure (S_2) then elicits another cycle of clonal loss and phenotypic diversification of the surviving clones.

* The terms therapy and treatment used here do not refer to any specific anti-cancer agent or modality. The terms apply to multi-agent/multi-modalities as well as single agent/modality treatment protocols.

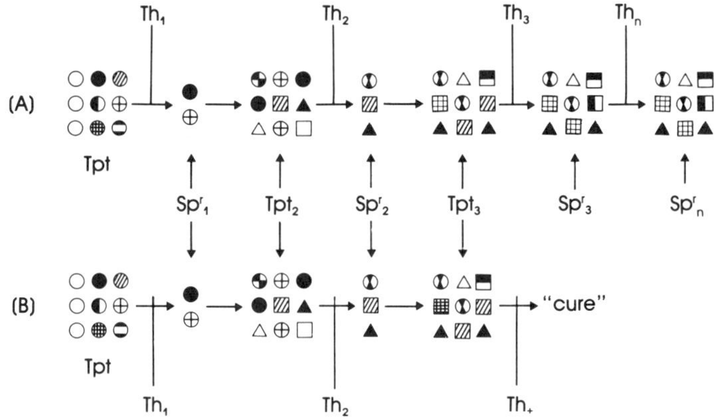

FIG. 6. The possible effects of therapy (*Th*) on subpopulation diversity and stability of the metastatic phenotype in neoplastic lesions. Therapy does not refer to any specific modality or agent or combination of modalities or agents, but only describes a therapeutic intervention that kills some tumor cell subpopulations.

By the time of clinical detection and onset of therapy, the lesion contains multiple tumor cell subpopulations (illustrated by the different symbols). The subpopulations in the lesion have reached the "plateau" phase in which interactions between the various subpopulations limit the rate at which new metastatic variants are generated. Therapy (Th_1) kills susceptible subpopulations, but others survive (SP_1^r). Restriction of subpopulation diversity may render the surviving subpopulations phenotypically unstable and thus stimulate the generation of a new panel of tumor cell variants with widely differing metastatic properties. With increasing diversification, a new plateau state will again be imposed (T_{pt_1}). On subsequent exposure to different treatment regimens (Th_2, Th_3), the cycle of subpopulation restriction and diversification will be repeated until either subpopulations resistant to all therapeutic efforts (SP_n^r) kill the patient **(A)** or a therapeutic modality (Th_+) kills all subpopulations within the lesion **(B)**. (Modified from Poste and Greig 1982.)

subpopulations (Figure 6). Generation of variants would then continue until a sufficient level of subpopulation diversity was achieved to again impose a new plateau. Exposure of the tumor to subsequent treatment regimens would then repeat the cycle (Figure 6) unless a therapeutic regimen eliminated the surviving subpopulations before they had time to generate new variants (Th+ in Figure 6).

If the scheme in Figure 6 is correct, new experimental strategies must be explored with the objective of overcoming the problem of phenotypic instability in tumor cell subpopulations that survive treatment. One approach would be to reduce the time interval between successive treatments with different agents (Figure 7). We have coined the acronym FAST (Fast Accelerated Staging of Therapy) to describe this strategy.

The aim of using a series of different treatment protocols in rapid succession would be to kill not only those subpopulations that survive the previous treatment before they can generate large numbers of new variants, but also new variant subpopulations as soon as they emerge (Figure 7). This contrasts with the practice in many clinical situations in which subsequent treatment regimens using differ-

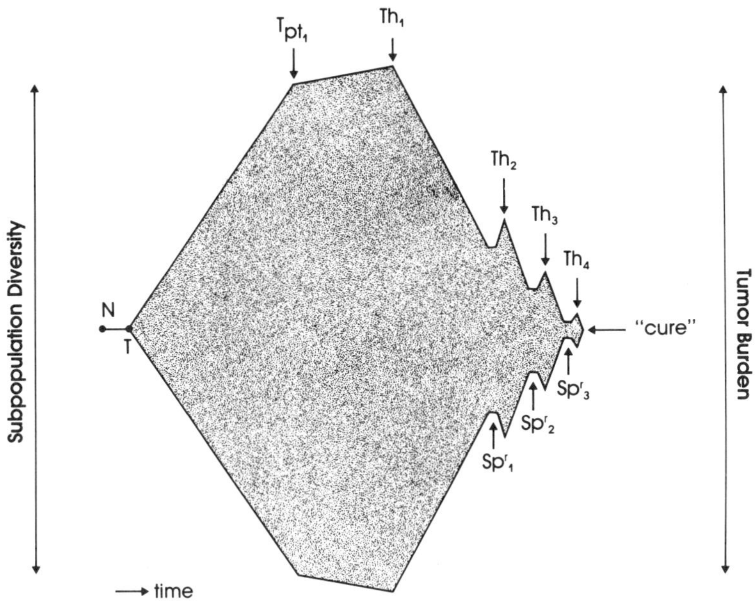

FIG. 7. Schematic illustration of proposed FAST cancer treatment protocol (FAST = Fast Accelerated Staging of Therapy).

Following initial transformation of a normal cell (*N*) to establish an initial focus of tumor cells (*T*), new variants are generated, creating a heterogeneous lesion of diverse subpopulations that eventually establish a "plateau" state (T_{pt}). Therapy (Th_1), reduces the subpopulation diversity and cell mass. The restriction of diversity may stimulate surviving resistant subpopulations (SP^r_1) to rapidly generate new metastatic variants. However, the second treatment regimen (Th_2) is given very shortly after the first treatment protocol even though a residual tumor burden may not be evident clinically. By repeating the process and reducing the interval between successive treatment regimens (Th_1–Th_3), it is intended that each treatment would kill susceptible subpopulations that survive the preceding treatments (SP^r_{1-3}) before they generate a large number of new variants, some of which might prove resistant to all available therapies. It may thus be possible to either eradicate tumor cells entirely or reduce the residual tumor burden sufficiently to allow host defense mechanisms, perhaps augmented by biological response modifier therapy, to kill any remaining tumor cells.

ent agents are often not employed if the first treatment protocol appears successful in eliminating clinically detectable tumor burden; new treatment regimens are implemented only when evidence of a recurrent tumor is detected (Figure 8). By then, phenotypic diversification of the surviving subpopulations may well have taken place, producing new subpopulations with widely differing therapeutic sensitivities (Figure 6).

The heterogeneous response of malignant tumor cell subpopulations to cytotoxic drugs and other therapeutic modalities makes it unlikely that a single treatment regimen will kill all the cells in a tumor, even if several agents are used simultaneously. This problem has been all too familiar to clinicians for a long time. Treatments are available that kill the majority of tumor cells within a tumor. The tumor burden remaining after such treatment is often sufficiently

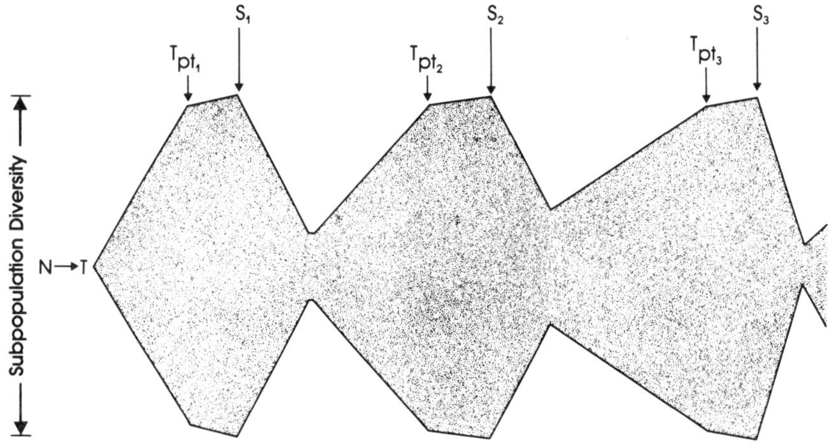

FIG. 8. Schematic illustration of the possible effects of extended staging of successive treatment regimens on subpopulation diversity in neoplastic lesions.

Following initial transformation of a normal cell (*N*) to establish an initial focus of tumor cells (*T*), extensive clonal diversity is generated creating a heterogeneous lesion of diverse subpopulations that interact and reach a "plateau" state (T_{pt}). Treatment (S_1) destroys some subpopulations. This restriction in subpopulation diversity will stimulate the surviving subpopulation (SP_1^r) to generate new variants, culminating in a new "plateau" state (T_{pt2}). By this time, recurrent tumor growth is detectable clinically and a second, different treatment regimen (S_2) is initiated, and another cycle ensues. This process will continue until either the patient dies of a tumor refractory to multiple successive treatments or a therapy eradicates the entire remaining tumor burden.

The term therapy does not refer to any specific anti-cancer agent or modality. The illustrated sequence of events is applicable to treatment regimens using any agent or modality either alone or in combination which fail to kill all of the tumor subpopulations present in the lesion. (Modified from Poste and Greig 1982.)

small that it cannot be detected clinically. In animal tumors, this situation represents the end point of most assays of drug activity. Similarly, in many clinical situations, following completion of a treatment protocol that eliminates clinically detectable tumor burden, further treatment regimens are not implemented routinely. New regimens are implemented (Th_2 in Figure 6) only when a patient presents some time later with clinical evidence of recurrent disease. However, the data discussed in this article suggest that the subpopulations present in the recurrent lesions will not only be resistant to the agents used in the first treatment protocol but will also have a high probability of being resistant to other agents.

Analysis of the validity of this concept requires new experimental systems to investigate two major questions. The first is whether therapy, by restricting subpopulation diversity within a heterogeneous neoplastic lesion (primary tumor or metastases), increases the phenotypic instability of surviving subpopulations and enhances the rate at which new variant tumor cells appear. The second question concerns whether the phenotypic diversification of the residual tumor burden surviving a first treatment protocol (single or multiple modalities) can be blocked by treatment with a series of different treatment regimens administered in rapid succession (Figure 7).

Research on these questions is only just beginning, and considerably more knowledge is needed before accelerated staging of successive treatment cycles could be considered in the clinic. Similarly, in raising the possibility that therapy may stimulate phenotypic diversification and facilitate emergence of increasingly aggressive tumor cell variants, we do not propose that current therapies be withheld or abandoned.

The more immediate issue is to establish whether the problems discussed here are of limited or general significance in the behavior of malignant tumors. This will require further experiments to determine the effects of different therapeutic modalities and their staging on the phenotypic stability and metastatic behavior of tumor cell subpopulations in neoplasms containing different numbers of identifiable subpopulations. The technical difficulties of such experiments are substantial. Most rodent tumors are unsuitable for evaluating the FAST protocol shown in Figure 7, and so alternative test systems are needed. The treatment of canine and feline neoplasms in veterinary clinics may provide such opportunities. The feasibility of this option is now under investigation.

CONCLUSIONS

The extensive phenotypic heterogeneity of tumor cell subpopulations coexisting in the same tumor has emerged as a major focal point for investigations in several areas of cancer research. The problem of tumor cell heterogeneity is also recognized as a major limitation on the success of treatment for solid tumors and their metastases.

The extensive cellular heterogeneity observed in malignant neoplasms is generated by the relentless emergence of new clonal subpopulations of tumor cells expressing phenotypes that render them increasingly unresponsive to host control. Clonal diversification and expansion provides a powerful mechanism for enhancing the biological "fitness" of tumors. The genesis of extensive cellular variation increases the likelihood that at least some tumor cell subpopulations will prove "fit" to survive in the face of the diverse destructive selection pressures a tumor will encounter during its lifetime, whether these be mounted by the host or the clinical oncologist. It is these surviving subpopulations and their variant progeny that are responsible for the problem of recurrent disease in the clinic.

A full understanding of tumor cell heterogeneity will require more than simple cataloging of the number of tumor cell subpopulations in a particular tumor at any given stage in its evolution. Evidence is beginning to emerge that suggests that tumors are more than a passive assembly of constituent cellular subpopulations. We must now begin to view tumors as complex entities in which the number of cellular subpopulations and their properties are changing constantly, not just in relation to selection pressures but also as a consequence of interactions among the subpopulations themselves.

This chapter has provided evidence that interactions between clonal subpopulations exert a significant effect on the rate at which new subpopulations with altered metastatic properties are created. Of particular interest is the finding that events restricting subpopulation diversity in heterogeneous, polyclonal tumor cell populations enhance the rate at which the surviving subpopulations generate new variants. This property affords tumors with an important mechanism for regenerating and sustaining significant cellular heterogeneity in response to both external selection pressures and shifts in subpopulation composition arising from changes in the tumor's own growth dynamics.

REFERENCES

Brunson, K. W., G. Beattie, and G. L. Nicolson. 1978. Selection and altered tumor cell properties of brain-colonising metastatic melanoma. Nature 272:543–545.

Cifone, M., and I. J. Fidler. 1981. Increasing metastatic potential is associated with increasing genetic instability of clones isolated from murine neoplasms. Proc. Natl. Acad. Sci. USA 78:6949–6952.

Eccles, S. A. 1982. Host factors in metastasis, *in* Tumor Progression and Markers, K. Lapis, A. Jeney, and M. R. Price, eds. Kugler, Amsterdam, pp. 183–196.

Eccles, S. A., S. E. Heckford, and P. Alexander. 1980. Effect of cyclosporin A on the growth and spontaneous metastasis of syngeneic animal tumors. Br. J. Cancer 42:252–259.

Fidler, I. J. 1973. Selection of successive tumor lines for metastasis. Nature New Biol. 242:148–149.

Fidler, I. J., and M. L. Kripke. 1977. Metastasis results from pre-existing variant cells within a malignant tumor. Science 197:893–895.

Fidler, I. J., and G. L. Nicolson. 1981. The immunobiology of experimental metastatic melanoma. Cancer Biol. Rev. 2:1–47.

Fidler, I. J., and G. Poste. 1982. The heterogeneity of metastatic properties in malignant tumor cells and regulation of the metastatic phenotype, *in* Tumor Cell Heterogeneity, A. Owens, D. S. Coffey, and S. B. Baylin, eds. Academic Press, New York, pp. 127–145.

Foulds, L. 1953. The histologic analysis of mammary tumors of mice. II. The histology of responsiveness and progression. The origins of tumors. JNCI 17:713–756.

Hart, I. R. 1979. The selection and characterization of an invasive variant of the B16 melanoma. Am. J. Pathol. 97:587–600.

Hart, I. R. 1982. 'Seed and Soil' revised: Mechanisms of site-specific metastasis. Cancer Met. Rev. 1:5–16.

Heppner, G. H., S. E. Loveless, F. R. Miller, K. H. Mahone, and A. M. Fulton. 1983. Mammary tumor heterogeneity, *in* Cancer Invasion and Metastasis: Biologic and Therapeutic Aspects, G. Nicolson and L. Milas, eds. Raven Press, New York, pp. 209–221.

Kerbel, R. S., J. W. Dennis, A. G. Lagarde, and P. Frost. 1982. Tumor progression in metastasis: An experimental approach using lectin resistant tumor variants. Cancer Met. Rev. 1:99–140.

Kripke, M. L., E. Gruys, and I. J. Fidler. 1978. Metastatic heterogeneity of cells from an ultraviolet light-induced murine fibrosarcoma of recent origin. Cancer Res. 38:2962–2967.

Mantovani A., R. Giavazzi, G. Alessandri, F. Spreafico, and S. Garattini. 1981. Characterization of tumor lines derived from spontaneous metastases of a transplanted murine sarcoma. Eur. J. Cancer 17:71–76.

Nicolson., G. L. 1982. Cell surface and cancer metastasis. Hosp. Prac. 18:75–86.

Nicolson, G. L. 1983. An introduction to cancer invasion and metastasis, *in* Cancer Invasion and Metastasis: Biologic and Therapeutic Aspects, G. L. Nicolson and L. Milas, eds. Raven Press, New York, pp. 1–4.

Nicolson, G. L., and G. Poste. 1982. Tumor cell diversity and host responses in cancer metastasis. Part I. Properties of metastatic cells. Curr. Prob. Cancer 7:4–83.

Nicolson, G. L., and G. Poste. 1983. Tumor cell diversity and host responses in cancer metastasis. Part II. Host immune responses and therapy of metastases. Curr. Probl. Cancer 8:4–42.

Nowell, P. C. 1976. The clonal evolution of tumor cell populations. Acquired genetic lability permits stepwise selection of variant sublines and underlies tumor progression. Science 194:23–28.

Poste, G. 1982. Experimental systems for analysis of the malignant phenotype. Cancer Met. Rev. 1:141–200.

Poste, G., J. Doll, A. E. Brown, J. Tzeng, and I. Zeidman. 1982a. A comparison of the metastatic properties of B16 melanoma clones isolated from cultured cell lines, subcutaneous tumors and individual lung tumors. Cancer Res. 42:2770–2778.

Poste, G., J. Doll, and I. J. Fidler. 1981. Interactions between clonal subpopulations affect the stability of the metastatic phenotype in polyclonal populations of B16 melanoma cells. Proc. Natl. Acad. Sci. USA 78:6226–6230.

Poste, G., J. Doll, I. R. Hart, and I. J. Fidler. 1980. In vitro selection of murine B16 melanoma variants with enhanced tissue invasive properties. Cancer Res. 40:1636–1644.

Poste, G., and I. J. Fidler. 1980. The pathogenesis of cancer metastasis. Nature 283:139–146.

Poste, G., and R. Greig. 1982. On the genesis and regulation of cellular heterogeneity in malignant tumors. Invasion and Metastasis 2:137–176.

Poste, G., J. Tzeng, J. Doll, R. Greig, D. Rieman, and I. Zeidman. 1982b. Evolution of tumor cell heterogeneity during progressive growth of individual lung metastases. Proc. Natl. Acad. Sci. USA 79:6574–6578.

Talmadge, J. E., and I. J. Fidler. 1982. Cancer metastasis is selective or random depending on the parent tumour population. Nature 297:593–596.

Talmadge, J. E., J. R. Starkey, and D. R. Stanford. 1981. In vitro characteristics of metastatic variant subclones of restricted genetic origin. J. Supramol. Struct. Cell Biochem. 15:139–151.

Tarin, D. 1982. Investigations of the mechanisms of metastatic spread of naturally occurring neoplasms. Cancer Met. Rev. 1:215–226.

Weiss, L., J. C. Holmes, and P. M. Ward. 1983. Do metastases arise from pre-existing subpopulations of cancer cells? Br. J. Cancer 47:81–89.

Cancer Invasion and Metastasis: Biologic and Therapeutic Aspects edited by Garth L. Nicolson and Luka Milas. Raven Press, New York © 1984.

A New Model for Leukemia-Lymphoma Metastasis: Differential Growth and Rejection of Murine Lymphoid-Leukemia Cell Lines in the Bone Marrow

Borislav Kamenov, Mark W. Kieran, John Barrington Leigh, Arnold H. Greenberg,* and B. Michael Longenecker

*Department of Immunology, University of Alberta, Edmonton, Alberta, Canada, T6G 2H7, and *Manitoba Institute of Cell Biology, University of Manitoba, Winnipeg, Manitoba Canada, R3E 0V9*

The metastatic cascade is known to be a complex series of events that culminate in the formation of secondary and tertiary tumor foci in adjacent tissues and organs distant from the primary tumor. Several good animal model systems utilizing transplantable tumor cell lines as well as clinical observations have recently provided important information on possible mechanisms responsible for various aspects of the metastatic cascade (Fidler 1978, Sugarbaker 1981, Nicolson 1982). Due to the very complex nature of metastasis, it has been difficult to devise model systems that take into account all but a few of the events that probably occur in the metastatic cascade. For example, many models employ cell lines that are injected i.v. to study the organ distribution and number of metastatic lesions (Fidler and Hart 1981). These models have provided valuable information, but fail to take into account several other important aspects of the metastatic cascade such as the circulatory patterns and organ preferences of the tumor lines.

Recently, a great deal of work has been directed to the interesting phenomenon known as organ-specific metastasis (OSM)(Hart 1982, Kieran and Longenecker 1983). The pioneering work of Nowell (1976), Fidler (1978), Nicolson (1982), and many others has enhanced our understanding of the highly heterogeneous and genetically unstable nature of tumor cells evolving within the primary tumor, which serves as the raw material for variant tumor cell populations with differing metastatic potentials. OSM to many organs cannot always be explained by purely mechanical hypotheses. Two additional hypotheses have been formulated: specific tumor cell adherence and "seed and soil." The first hypothesis envisions the existence of a family of specific receptors on tumor cells that interact with specific acceptors or ligands on the target organs (Kieran and Longenecker 1983). The "seed and soil" hypothesis (Paget 1889) postulates the existence of organ-specific growth factors that stimulate the growth of tumor cell variants that have receptors for, and are responsive to, these growth factors (Hart 1982).

At present, little definitive evidence is available to support either of the two latter hypotheses. One obvious difficulty is the apparent lack of relevant model systems that differentiate these two mechanisms. Numerous experiments supporting both hypotheses but proving neither have appeared in the literature. That the two mechanisms are not mutually exclusive is a real possibility and may further complicate our interpretation of available data.

We have recently demonstrated the existence of cell surface molecules on lymphoma cell variants selected for liver metastasis, which may in part be involved in the process of OSM (Shearman and Longenecker 1980, Shearman et al. 1980). We derived a monoclonal antibody that reacted with the liver-selected variant but not with ovary-selected variants. This monoclonal antibody was shown to specifically block liver metastasis in vivo. In addition, the liver-selected variant specificly binds to frozen sections of liver (Kieran and Longenecker 1983, and our unpublished data). These results provide strong evidence for specific tumor cell adherence to explain specific homing to the liver, but they are nevertheless consistent with the existence of receptors on tumor variants for organ-specific growth factors. We have attempted to use the anti–liver metastasis monoclonal antibody to isolate the putative molecule responsible for the observed OSM, but have failed, probably because of the relatively low affinity of the IgM monoclonal antibody.

In the present communication, we describe the development of a new model system for the study of leukemic metastasis in the mouse. The new model attempts to take into account the following aspects of the metastatic cascade: the natural site of leukemogenesis, the bone marrow; the exit site of leukemia cells from the bone marrow; the effect of natural immune mechanisms on leukemic cells in the bone marrow and during metastatic spread in the circulation; the homing of leukemic cells to other organs including the bone marrow; and the growth of metastatic leukemia cells in the bone marrow. We do so by monitoring the growth and spread of lymphatic leukemia (LL) lines injected directly into the bone marrow. We believe that we approach a more realistic starting point for the analysis of leukemogenesis than previously achieved.

MATERIALS AND METHODS

^{131}IUDR Labeling of LL Cells

LL cells were labeled overnight and injected i.v. as described previously (Carlson and Terres 1976). Minimal reutilization of label by normal host cells is an important advantage of this model. All mice were maintained on drinking water supplemented with 0.1% NaI to reduce thyroid uptake of released iodine. Labeling was determined by whole-body counting in a Beckman Gamma 300 counter. For organ distribution, organs were collected in scintilation vials in formaldehyde, and disintegrations counted in a gamma counter.

Complement-Mediated Cytotoxicity Assay

Target cells were incubated at 2×10^7 cells/ml in RPMI, 10% fetal calf serum (FCS), and gentamycin with 200 μCi/ml of $Na_2\,^{51}CrO_4$ for 2 h at 37°C. The labeled cells were washed five times and adjusted to 2×10^6 cells/ml. A mixture of 0.05 ml cells and 0.05 ml test serum at increasing serial dilution was incubated at 37°C for 45 min (three replicate wells per sample). Plates were then centrifuged to remove supernatant, and cells were resuspended in 0.05 ml medium plus 0.05 ml complement (Low-tox, Cederlane Laboratories) per well. After incubation, 0.05 ml medium was added to each well, plates were centrifuged, and 100 μl of supernatant was counted in a gamma counter. Negative controls consisted of cells incubated in medium, and positive controls consisted of cells incubated with 0.5% Triton-X. The percentage of specific ^{51}Cr release was calculated as follows:

$$(\text{experimental release} - \text{control release})/(\text{maximum release} - \text{control release}) \times 100$$

NK Cell ^{51}Cr Release Assay

Target cells were labeled with $Na_2\,^{51}CrO_4$ as described in the previous section. The labeled cells were adjusted to 5×10^5 cells/ml and a mixture of 0.1 ml target cells and 0.1 ml spleen cells were added together (three replicates per sample). The plates were incubated for 12 h and centrifuged, and the specific ^{51}Cr released determined as before. For inhibition of natural killer (NK) cell activity, an anti-NK monoclonal antibody, 49H.8 (unpublished results), was incubated with spleen cells at 4°C for 45 min and lysed with complement at 37°C for 45 min, washed twice, and used in an NK assay.

[^{3}H]Thymidine Incorporation Assay

Standard curve: varying dilutions of leukemia cells were incubated with [^{3}H]thymidine (NEN, 0.625 μCi/well), and after incubation at 37°C for 4 h, cells were harvested on filter discs, placed in scintillation fluid, and counted. The same procedure was used to estimate the number of proliferating leukemia cells in the bone marrow. Groups of irradiated (850 r) mice (five per group) were injected with 10^6 leukemia cells i.v. on day 0. Femoral bone marrow cells were harvested at various time periods after injection in a standard volume of RPMI plus 10% FCS and gentamycin. After washing and counting, 100 μl of the cell suspension was used as previously described (three replicates per sample).

Harvesting Bone Marrow Cells

Bone marrow cells were harvested from femurs. The bone was opened on both ends and perfused with 1 ml of RPMI and 10% FCS.

Intra-Bone Marrow Injections (IBM)

Mice were first anesthetized (Penthrane) and taped in the supine position onto an operating board with legs extended and slightly apart. It was crucial that the leg did not rotate about the hip; i.e., the tibia surface had to be horizontal. The knee was then elevated slightly by insertion of a small cylinder directly underneath it. At the chosen point of insertion (ca. 1 cm distal to the patella), a shortened 26-guage needle of a 25 μl Hamilton syringe was used to make an entrance hole by rotating the needle a few times (as if drilling). The syringe was then aligned along the tibia and inserted at a shallow angle. Injection was done when the tip of the needle was within the bone marrow lumen. The flow had to be easy or no fluid could be moved. The typical volume of injected cells was 5–10 μl. There was no observable leakage or swelling, nor subsequent mortality or mechanical injury, resulting from this procedure. Experimental data (see Results) confirm that at least a useful fraction of the injected cells remained in the bone marrow lumen, while spreading of the cells to other organs also took place. Thus the prerequisite conditions for entry into the hemopoietic system via this route were fulfilled.

Rosettes

Leukemia cells were labeled with fluorescein as previously described (Butcher and Weissman 1980). For rosetting, 100 μl of fluorescein-labeled leukemia cells were mixed with 100 μl of bone marrow or spleen cells (2×10^7 cells per ml) as a negative control. The cells were pelleted, incubated for 2 h at 4°C, and gently resuspended, and rosettes were counted on a hemocytometer.

Cellular Elisa Assay

Gluteraldehyde-fixed spleen cells and lymphoma cells were used in a standard cellular Elisa assay (MacLean et al. 1982) employing peroxidase-labeled goat-anti-mouse IgG.

Dexter Culture and Adherence Assay

Dexter cultures were initiated and maintained as previously described (Dexter 1982, Dexter and Testa 1980); 10^7 leukemia cells were added to flasks containing bone marrow–adherent cell monolayers. After incubation at 37°C for 2 h, the supernatant containing nonadherent cells was removed, the monolayers gently washed, and the percentage of adherent leukemia cells determined by counting the number of adherent leukemia cells. Cultures were reincubated at 37°C for 24 h and adherent cells were recounted.

Mice

Mice syngeneic with the leukemias used in this study were DBA/2J, CBA/CaJ, or C57/B16J and were obtained from Jackson Laboratories or locally from the Medical Science Animal Services, University of Alberta, Edmonton. Mice were 8–10 weeks of age when used for experiments.

Cell Lines

The following leukemia-lymphoma cell lines were used: P388 (Simon et al. 1981); L1210 (Moore et al. 1966); L5178Y (Fisher 1958); L5178Y 1A1 (Young et al. 1981, Young and Hakomori 1981); L5178Y 1A1.616 (Young et al. 1981, Young and Hakomori 1981); RI (Hewitt 1962); EL 4 (Gorer 1950); YAC-1.3 (Chow et al. 1981); SL2.5 (Chow et al. 1981); SL2.9 (Chow et al. 1981); P815.16 (Chow et al. 1981).

RESULTS

Elimination of ^{131}IUDR-Labeled Lymphoma Cells Following I.V. or I.P. Injection

This assay has been shown to be a measure of natural, preexisting immunity, perhaps mediated by natural antibody or NK-like effector mechanisms (Carlson and Terres 1976). Figure 1 shows the relative rates of elimination of three lymphoma cell lines. Two of these cell lines (P388 and L1210) were selected because of their extreme virulence and the third cell line (L5178Y) was selected for comparison because it is a less-virulent line (Table 1). The least-virulent cell line was eliminated much faster than the other two cell lines. It is noteworthy that fully 68% of the injected L5178Y cells were eliminated within 3 h of injection, and by 24 h, only 10% of the injected label remained.

Cells of the fastest-eliminated line, L5178Y, were selected for further elimination studies. Figure 2 demonstrates that i.v. injected cells were eliminated faster than i.p. injected cells. This is an expected result as i.v. injected cells are subjected immediately to the rigors of the circulation, including immediate exposure to "natural" antitumor antibodies. It was also found that cells that had been maintained in vitro were rejected faster than cells that had been passaged in vivo. Again, this is not unexpected as it has been shown previously (Kerbel et al.

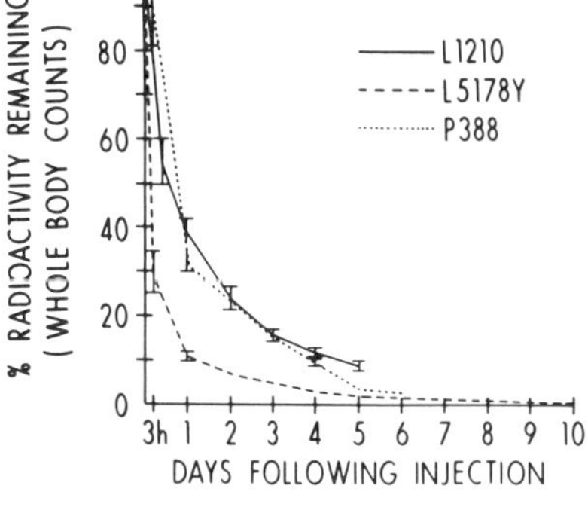

FIG. 1. Elimination of ^{131}IUDR-labeled leukemia cells. The percentage remaining (± 1 S.D., n=5) of each of three labeled leukemia lines, after i.v. injection, as measured by whole body counting, and followed to elimination or death of host (see Methods).

TABLE 1. *Day of death following injection of various LL cell lines by various routes*

Cell line	I.V.	I.P.	IBM
P388	6 ± 0*	8 ± 0	5 ± 0
L1210	5 ± 0	8 ± 0	6 ± 0
L5178Y	12 ± 0	12 ± 0	15 ± 0
RI	14 ± 2	17 ± 1	32 ± 13
EL4	15 ± 1	20 ± 2	30 ± 5

* $\bar{x}$ day of death ± S.D.
IBM, intra-bone marrow.

1982) that lymphoma variants are generated relatively rapidly in vitro and not selected against, as occurs in vivo.

Reactivity of "Natural" Antitumor Antibodies (NAb) with Various Cell Lines

Several additional lymphoma cell lines were selected to determine their susceptibility to killing following incubation with normal serum and complement from syngeneic mouse strains. Figure 3 demonstrates that EL-4 is by far the most

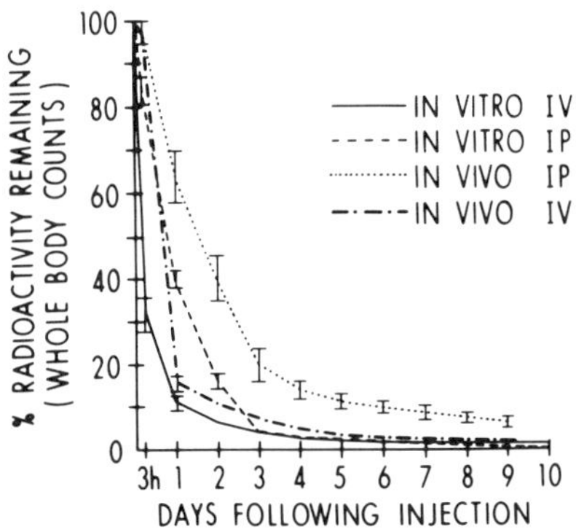

FIG. 2. Elimination of ^{131}IUDR-labeled L5178Y leukemia cells. As for Figure 1, but using single-cell suspensions maintained either in vitro or in vivo and line L5178Y injected either i.v. or i.p.

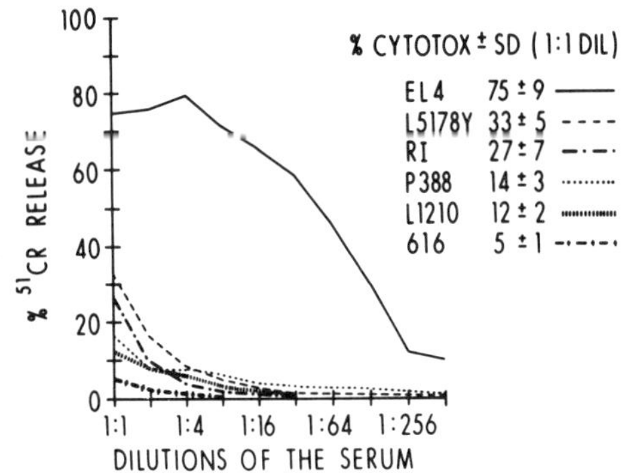

FIG. 3. Cytotoxicity of natural anti-leukemia antibodies. Pooled normal sera from syngeneic mice, assayed by complement-dependent lysis of ^{51}Cr-labeled leukemia lines as a function of dilution (see Methods). Percentage ^{51}Cr release at 1 : 1 dilution is listed for each cell line (± 1.5 S.D., n = 3).

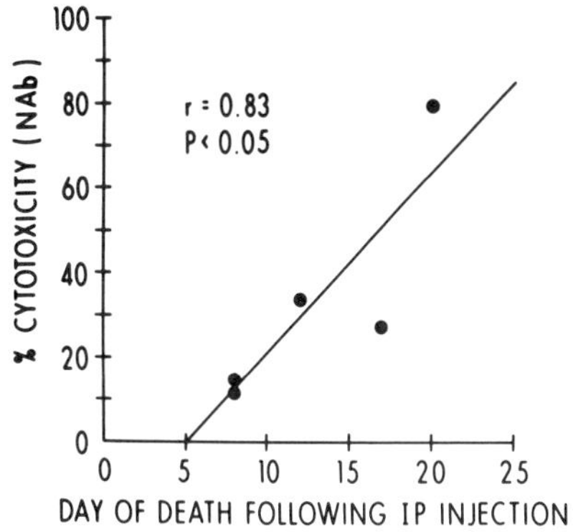

FIG. 4. Inverse correlation of leukemia virulence with susceptibility to natural antibody. Relative virulence of various cell lines measured as time to death after i.v. injection compared with susceptibility to natural antibody as assayed by ^{51}Cr release (see Table 1 and Figure 3).

susceptible to natural antibody–mediated lysis. Interestingly, EL-4 is a relatively nonvirulent cell line (Table 1). The remaining five cell lines varied considerably in their susceptibility to NAb killing. It is noteworthy that L5178Y, which was eliminated faster than P388 and L1210, was also significantly more susceptible to NAb killing than P388 and L1210. There was a significant inverse correlation between NAb killing and virulence (Figure 4).

As serum NAb represent a complex mixture of antibodies of various specificities, we derived a series of monoclonal "natural" antitumor antibodies (MAb) by activating normal spleen B cells with liposaccharide followed by fusion with mouse myeloma cells (Mosmann and Longenecker 1982). Table 2 shows the reactivity of three of our natural MAb with selected lymphoma cell lines. It is noteworthy that the relative susceptibility of the cell lines to NAb was the same as that to the three MAb.

Variant cell lines 1A1 and 616 were derived from L5178Y and were selected for low and high virulence, respectively (Young et al. 1981, Young and Hakomori 1981). Line 1A1 is known to carry glycolipid determinants on the cell surface

TABLE 2. *Natural antitumor monoclonal antibodies: complement-mediated cytotoxicity assay on various murine lymphomas*

	Monoclonal antibody*		
Tumor	106H.26	110H.30	110H.21
EL4	50 ± 3†	75 ± 4	75 ± 4
L5178Y	21 ± 1	50 ± 2	40 ± 2
P388	0.6 ± 0	29 ± 2	31 ± 1
L1210	0.4 ± 0	10 ± 1	10 ± 1
1Λ1	06 ± 3	00 ± 4	100 ± 6
616	2 ± 0	30 ± 2	30 ± 2

* Culture supernatant used at a final dilution of 1:4.
† x̄ % cytotoxicity ± S.D.

that are associated with rapid "natural" immune rejection (Young et al. 1981, Young and Hakomori 1981). Note the marked susceptibility of 1A1 cells to "natural" MAb in comparison to 616 cells (Table 2).

Young and Hakomori (1981) demonstrated that monoclonal antibodies generated to glycolipid determinants on these cells could be successfully used as immunotherapeutic agents against mouse lymphomas. In previous studies, we demonstrated the existence of cryptic carbohydrate antigens on murine lymphoma cells detectable by MAb (Longenecker and Rahman 1983). A MAb called 49H.8 was made following immunization of BALB/c mice with neuraminidase-treated human red blood cells (RBC) (NE-RBC). Interestingly, this MAb shows many of the same characteristics of MAb that detect carbohydrate antigens common to thymocyte precursors and T-lymphoma murine cell lines (Imai et al. 1980). This MAb reacts with neuraminidase-treated murine and human lymphocytes, several murine lymphomas, and certain human T-cell ALL (our unpublished data). Thus, the antigen detected by this MAb is cryptic in normal lymphocytes and fully exposed on certain T-cell leukemias or lymphomas. In addition, cell lines that are most susceptible to "natural" MAb killing are also most reactive with radiolabeled 49H.8 plus complement (Figure 5). Thus, it was of interest to test our "natural" antitumor MAb for reactivity with neuraminidase-treated lymphocytes and lymphoma cells. Lymphocytes and lymphoma cells that showed low reactivity with MAb became significantly more reactive following neuraminidase treatment. Untreated EL-4 cells, which showed extremely high binding, did not show increased binding following neuraminidase treatment (see Table 3).

Susceptibility of LL Cell Lines to NK-Mediated Lysis

Table 4 shows that most of the cell lines used in these studies showed low to moderate susceptibility to NK-mediated lysis in comparison to the "standard" NK target, YAC. Furthermore, susceptibility to NK-mediated lysis showed no correlation with susceptibility or survival to the tumors. Line 1A1 cells demonstrated increased susceptibility in comparison to YAC cells.

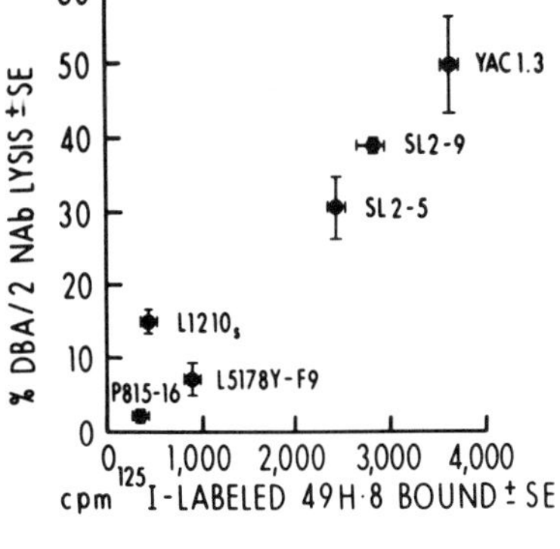

FIG. 5. Positive correlation between susceptibility to natural antibody and surface density of 49H.8 determinant. Susceptibility of the various lines (% ^{51}CR release) compared with target cell surface density, as measured by binding of ^{125}I-labeled monoclonal antibody 49H.8 (Rahman and Longenecker 1982).

TABLE 3. *Crypticity of tumor-associated antigens detected by natural monoclonal antibodies*

Cells	Monoclonal antibody*		
	110H.30	110H.21	110H.26
EL4			
—C†	1.10 ± 0.01‡	0.55 ± 0.01	0.85 ± 0.01
—NE§	0.90 ± 0.01	0.60 ± 0.01	0.80 ± 0.01
L5178Y			
—C	0.20 ± 0.01	0.17 ± 0.00	0.30 ± 0.01
—NE	0.70 ± 0.01	0.62 ± 0.01	0.75 ± 0.01
P388			
—C	0.35 ± 0.01	0.30 ± 0.01	0.25 ± 0.01
—NE	0.60 ± 0.01	0.84 ± 0.02	0.70 ± 0.01
L1210			
—C	0.20 ± 0.01	0.21 ± 0.01	0.25 ± 0.01
—NE	0.80 ± 0.01	0.85 ± 0.01	0.75 ± 0.01
Normal spleen			
—C	0.15 ± 0.00	0.10 ± 0.00	0.10 ± 0.00
—NE	0.53 ± 0.02	0.52 ± 0.01	0.28 ± 0.00

* Used at a concentration of 1:2 in a cellular Elisa assay.
† Control, untreated cells.
‡ Optical density ± S.D.
§ Cells pretreated with neuraminidase prior to sticking to Elisa plate.

TABLE 4. *Susceptibility to NK cells of various murine lymphoma cell lines**

Cell line	Cytotoxicity	Spleen cells treated with anti-NK MAb
YAC	42 ± 3†	6 ± 2
EL-4	11 ± 2	11 ± 2
RI	1 ± 2	0 ± 0
P388	14 ± 1	10 ± 2
L5178Y	11 ± 2	4 ± 1
L1210	12 ± 1	7 ± 1
1A1	60 ± 4	25 ± 1
616	16 ± 2	6 ± 1

* Effector-target ratio = 50%.
† Percent ^{51}Cr release ± S.D.

Organ Distribution of ^{131}IUDR-Labeled LL Cells Following I.V. Injection

The three cell lines used in the elimination study (Figures 1 and 2) were also used for organ distribution studies. Surprisingly, the cell line (L5178Y) that was eliminated most rapidly showed practically no accumulation of label in the liver, whereas the two cell lines that showed a slower elimination demonstrated 40–50% accumulation in the liver (Table 5). Also surprising was that very few cells appeared to accumulate in the lungs, the usual site of nonspecific trapping following i.v. injection (Hart 1982). Most interesting, however, was

TABLE 5. *Organ distribution of ^{131}IUDR labeled lymphoma cells 3 hours following i.v. injection*

	Organ									
Cell line	Brain	Liver	Spleen	Kidney	Lung	Bones	Blood	Intestine	Muscle	Skin
L5178Y	0.08 ± 0.05*	8.2 ± 1.4	5.3 ± 0.5	1.7 ± 0.5	8.8 ± 0.8	17.1 ± 2.1	3.9 ± 0.7	19.8 ± 3.8	9.7 ± 2.4	21.0 ± 4.1
P388	0.03 ± 0.05	47.9 ± 15.1	3.5 ± 0.6	0.6 ± 0.2	24.5 ± 1.7	8.9 ± 1.2	0.3 ± 0.2	5.1 ± 0.8	0.9 ± 0.7	3.3 ± 1.0
L1210	0.05 ± 0.03	50.1 ± 6.7	3.4 ± 0.6	1.6 ± 0.2	8.6 ± 1.6	8.8 ± 0.4	0.6 ± 0.4	9.4 ± 2.2	8.3 ± 2.4	8.9 ± 4.5

* Percent of total label injected ± S.D.

the relatively large number of cells that had apparently migrated to the bone marrow (9–17%).

Homing of Lymphoma Cells to the Bone Marrow

In contrast to their differing susceptibilities to natural immunity in the circulation, no significant differences were noted among LL lines tested for degree of homing to bone marrow following i.v. injection. Generally between 1% and 4% of labeled (either radioactively or fluorescently) cells were found in the femur 3 to 24 h postinjection (see Figures 9–13).

In order to study the growth and rejection of various LL lines in the bone marrow, a variety of approaches were used. The first involved the reculturing of LL lines from various organs as a function of time following i.v. injection. Interestingly, the LL lines showed marked differences in capacity for regrowth in tissue culture from the bone marrow, but generally not from other organs (data not shown). Highly virulent lines (P388 and L1210) could be regrown rapidly from bone marrow in culture after only 3 and 5 days after bone marrow culturing, respectively, whereas the lines with lower virulence took from 10–15 days and one (L5178Y) could never be reestablished in vitro from bone marrow (Table 6).

Many fluorescently labeled P388 cells, which homed to bone marrow following i.v. injection, were contained in rosettes with unlabeled bone marrow cells. This phenomenon could be reproduced in vitro by incubating fluorescent P388 cells with normal bone marrow cells (Figure 6). This phenomenon was further studied using Dexter cultures of normal murine bone marrow. It was found that P388 and L1210 cells adhered firmly to adherent bone marrow cells (Figure 7) (those bone marrow cells that adhere to plastic surfaces), which have been described as the "microenvironment" for growth of hematopoietic progenitor cells. It was also noted that following this attachment, P388 and L1210 cells grew rapidly and eventually detached from the bone marrow–adherent cells, rapidly overgrowing the culture. Collectively, these data suggest that P388 and L1210 cells interact in a novel way with adherent bone marrow cells, and this interaction may be responsible for their rapid stimulation of cell growth.

TABLE 6. *Day after i.v. injection LL line in culture from bone marrow first reestablished*

LL line	Day	LL line	Day
P388	3	EL4	15*
L1210	5	L5178Y	—†
RI	9		

* Once in 5 attempts.
† Not once in 5 attempts.

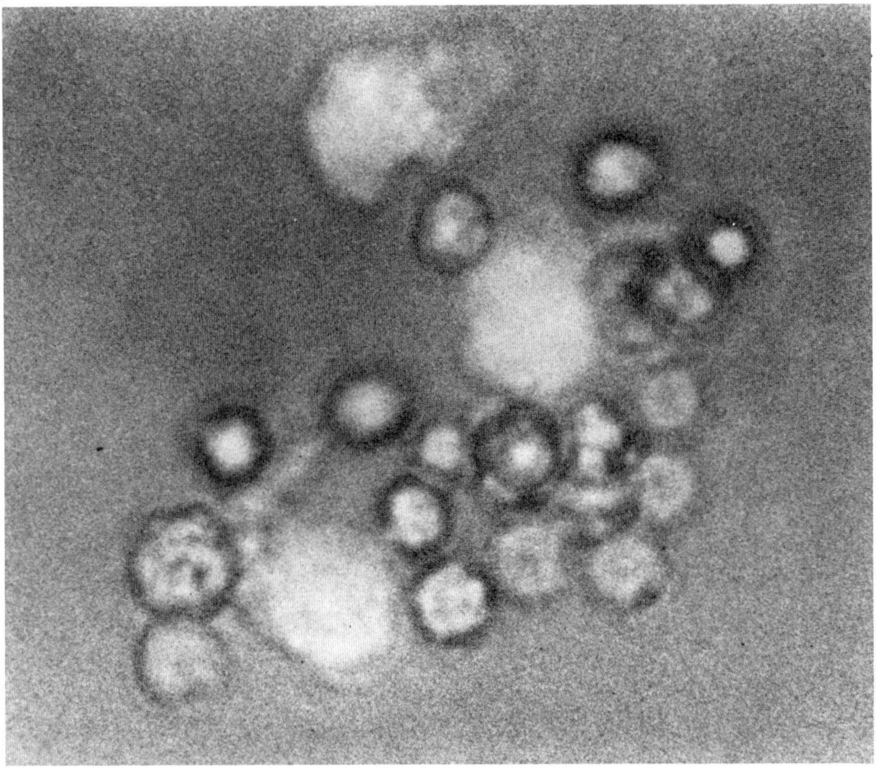

FIG. 6. Affinity of P388 leukemia cells for normal bone marrow cells. Formation of rosettes between fluorescein-labeled P388 and bone marrow cells. See Methods for technique and normal spleen controls.

In Vitro Growth of Various Lymphoma Cell Lines Following Their Recovery from Bone Marrow of I.V. Injected and Irradiated Mice

Tritiated thymidine incorporation into DNA was used as an index of the growth of the lymphoma cells recovered from the bone marrow. Figure 8 demonstrates that the amount of [^{3}H]thymidine incorporated is directly related to the number of EL-4 cells plated per well. This type of direct linear relationship was noted for all five cell lines tested. We have also obtained similar dose-response kinetics from lines newly reisolated from the bone marrow (data not shown), so it is reasonable to assume that this technique provides at least a rough approximation of the number and growth potential of lymphoma cells reisolated from the bone marrow.

Five lymphoma cell lines were injected into five groups of lethally (850 r) irradiated mice. One group of irradiated mice served as a control for background incorporation of [^{3}H]thymidine into normal bone marrow cells. Background incorporation levels dropped to very minimal values within 24 h of irradiation.

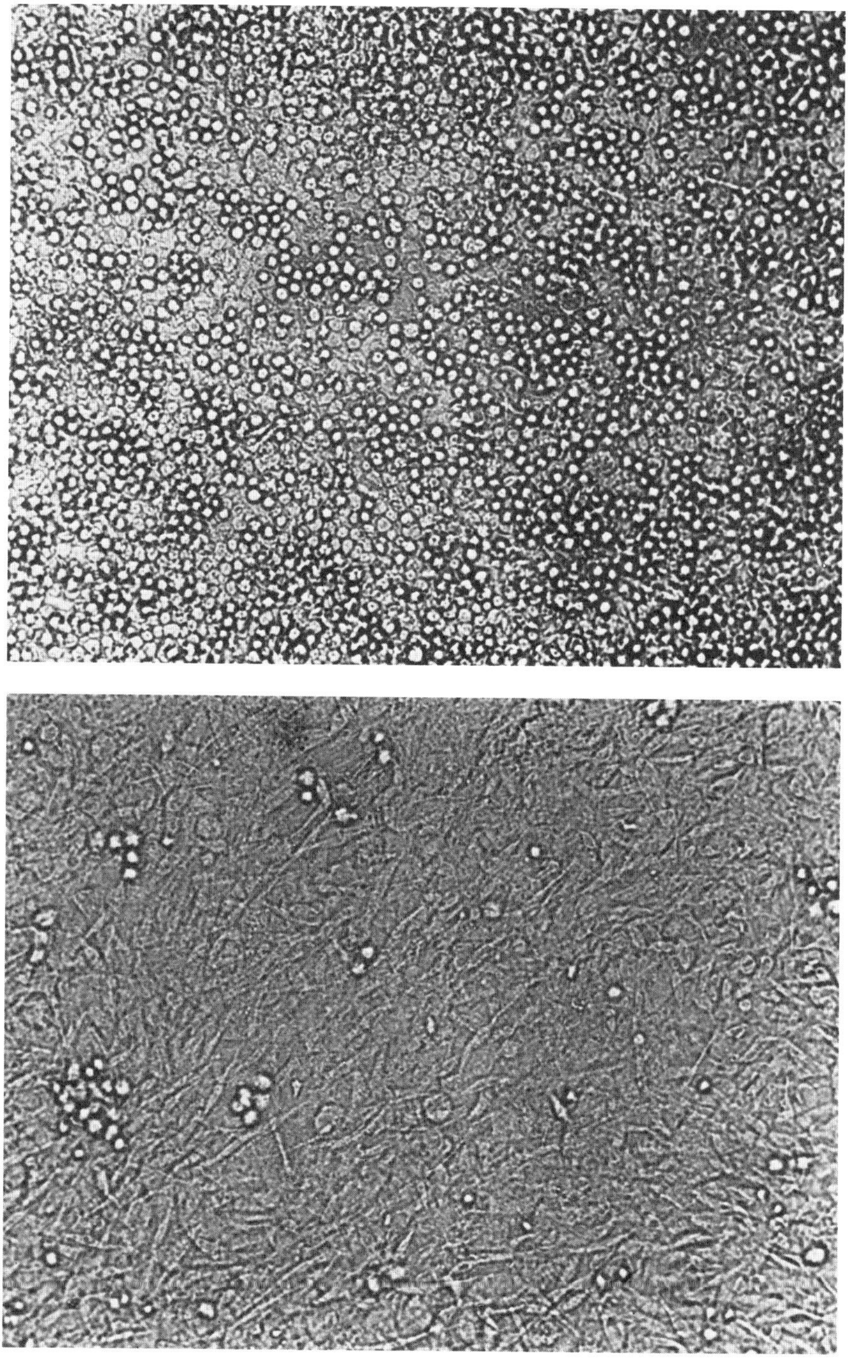

FIG. 7. Top, Adherence of P388 leukemia cells to a bone marrow monolayer in contrast to: **Bottom,** L5178Y as negative control as described in methods.

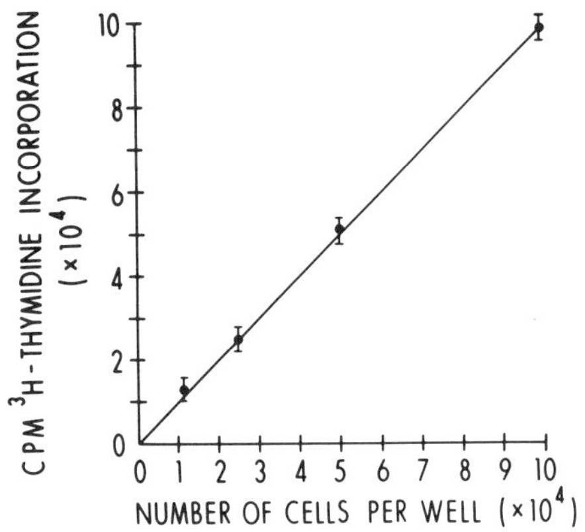

FIG. 8. Linearity of [^{3}H]thymidine incorporation into EL4 versus number of cells/well (see Methods, S.D. < 1%, n=3).

Background incorporation levels were subtracted in order to obtain levels of incorporation into the injected, bone marrow–homed lymphoma cells as a function of time after injection.

Three distinct patterns of incorporation were noted. In the first pattern, which was noted for EL-4 and L5178Y cells, the maximum number of cells was found within 3 h of injection, and this was followed by the rapid elimination of these cells to undetectable levels by day 3 or 4 (Figures 9 and 10). For the second pattern, which was seen only for RI cells, the number of cells fluctuated between 0.1 and 2×10^4 throughout the observation period (Figure 11). The last pattern, noted for L1210 and P388 cells, was the most dramatic. Following an initial decline in cell numbers or their proliferative potential (more noticeable for L1210), there was a dramatic increase in the proliferation of these cells between days 3 and 4 (Figures 12 and 13). For P388 cells, the [^{3}H]thymidine incorporation increased approximately 30-fold over a 24-h period. This tremendous increase in proliferative potential was reflected by the vast numbers of P388 cells noted in the cultures at that time.

Direct Intra–Bone Marrow (IBM) Injection of LL Cells

In order to determine whether the relative growth potential of the LL lines in the bone marrow might be related to virulence, a new technique for direct bone marrow injection of LL cells was devised. To our knowledge, this is the first time this has been accomplished, and we consider it to be an important aspect of the development of a relevant model for leukemogenesis. Interestingly, the differences in virulence among the lines were amplified following IBM injection. The less-virulent lines became even less virulent and the most-virulent lines with tremendous capacity for growth in the bone marrow retained a very high degree of virulence (Table 1).

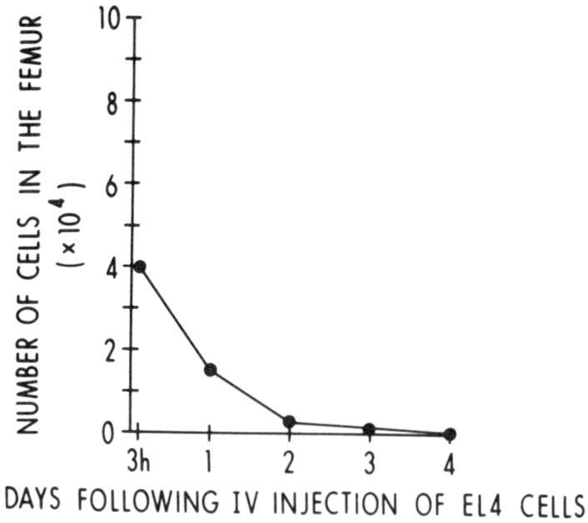

FIG. 9

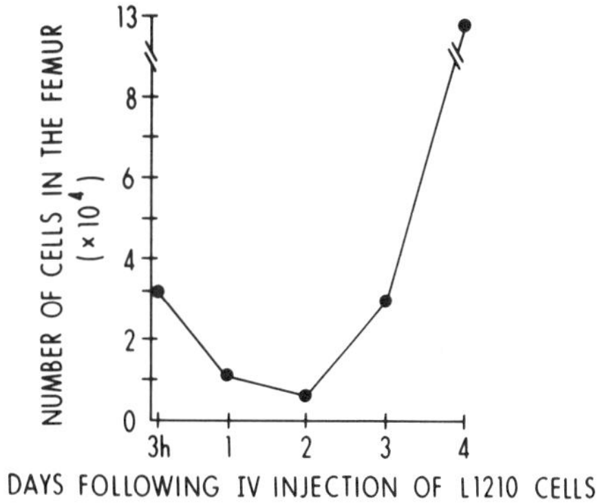

FIG. 12

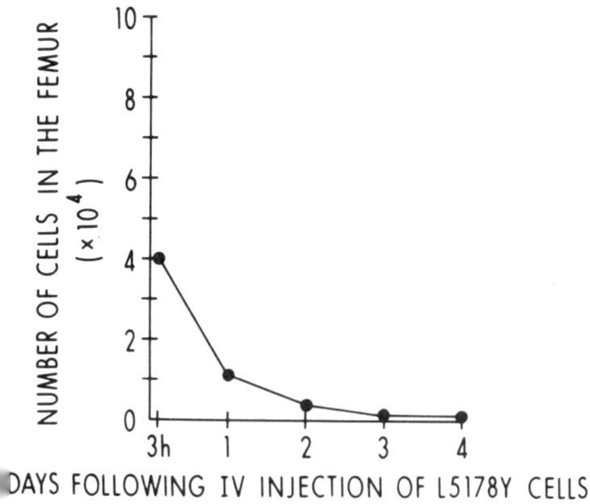

FIG. 10

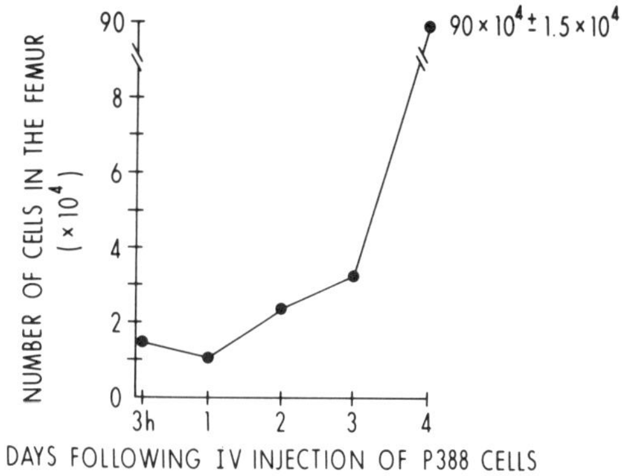

FIG. 13

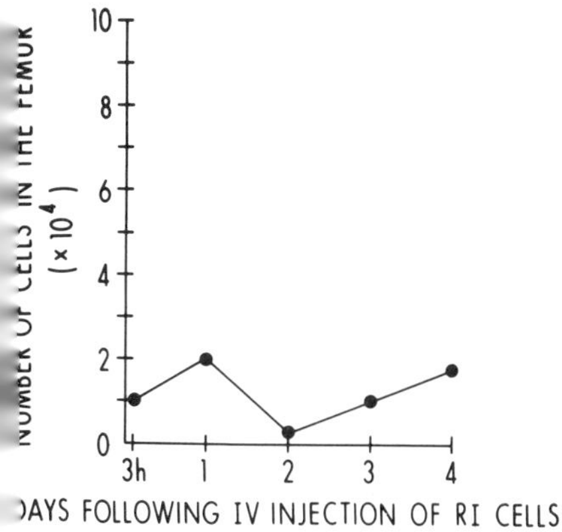

FIG. 11

FIGS. 9–13. Recovery of leukemia lines from bone marrow following i.v. injection. Number of leukemia cells detected in the bone marrow, as assayed by [^{3}H]thymidine incorporation, followed for 5 days after i.v. injection of 10^6 leukemia cells into lethally irradiated syngeneic recipients (see Methods, S.D. $< 1\%$, $n = 5$).

DISCUSSION

We are attempting to develop a valid model system in the mouse for the study of leukemogenesis and metastatic spread of lymphoid leukemia cells. Previous models of murine leukemogenesis have failed to take into account modern principles of metastasis and the natural origin of leukemic cells in the bone marrow as well as their predilection for metastasis and growth in the bone marrow. The presently employed model is far from perfect, but we are attempting to take into account the following aspects of leukemogenesis: (1) its origin in the bone marrow, (2) naturally occurring immunological mechanisms that affect hematogenous metastatic spread, (3) metastatic spread to other organs including other bones in the body, and (4) factors affecting the growth and elimination of leukemic cells in the bone marrow.

Origin of Leukemia in Bone Marrow

Most theories of leukemogenesis assume that this process occurs in the bone marrow and involves transformation of hemopoietic progenitor cells that "freeze" the leukemic cell at a certain stage of differentiation. A clonal proliferation of such leukemic cells results in the destruction of the bone marrow and the generation of leukemic variants with enhanced metastatic potential. We have attempted to inject ^{131}IUDR-labeled leukemic cells into the bone marrow and follow the survival of the animals as well as the spread of the leukemic cells to other organs of the body. Surprisingly, the time of death following IBM injection was relatively rapid, the most virulent cell lines showing the same mortality as that obtained following i.v. injection. This suggests a rapid spread of the leukemic cells from this organ to other parts of the body. Interestingly, the less-virulent lines show decreased virulence following IBM injection, perhaps suggesting the existence of rejection or growth-inhibition mechanisms in the bone marrow. Radiolabeled cells have been localized in several organs following IBM injection (our unpublished data).

Immunological Mechanisms Affecting Metastatic Spread of Leukemic Cells

The present work was limited to an investigation of the role of "natural" defense mechanisms such as natural antibody and NK cells. We measured short-term elimination of i.v. injected ^{131}IUDR-labeled tumor cells, which has been shown to be due to "natural" antitumor immunity. Two highly virulent cell lines, P388 and L1210, were eliminated less rapidly than L5178Y cells, which were eliminated remarkably rapidly. Of these cells, 68% were eliminated within 3 h of i.v. injection and only 10% of the cells remained after 24 h. It is likely that such rapid elimination is mediated by preexisting "natural" antibody. Thus, we investigated the relative susceptibility of these and other lymphoma cell lines to lysis mediated by normal serum plus complement. L5178Y cells were more susceptible to serum NAb lysis than P388 and L1210, but EL-4 cells were by far the most susceptible. We found a direct correlation between a cell line's susceptibility to NAb killing and the time of death following i.p. injection. This observation is consistent with previous work on the role of natural antibody in natural resistance (Chow et al. 1981, Wolosin and Greenberg 1979), including correlative evidence between the NAb phenotype and tumorigenicity (Greenberg and Pohajdak 1982). Interestingly, EL-4 is one of the least-virulent cell lines used in these studies, but could not be used in the elimination studies because of difficulty in labeling it with ^{131}IUDR. These cells were also very susceptible to lysis with "natural" monoclonal antibody plus complement. Line 1A1 cells, a variant line derived from L5178Y cells (Young and Hakomori 1981) selected for low virulence, were almost 100% killed with both serum and the monoclonal MAb, whereas a highly virulent variant (616) of the same cell line was quite resistant to killing. The 1A1 cells were also the most susceptible to NK killing, and no correlation between susceptibility to NK killing and virulence was found.

Antigens recognized by "natural" MAb on tumor cells are often carbohydrate in nature (Imai et al. 1980). The 1A1 and 616 variants of the L5178Y parental line used in this study show differences in cell surface expression of asialo-GM2 glycolipid as well as in resistance to elimination (Young et al. 1979, 1981). We have found that a monoclonal antibody (49H.8), which was made following immunization with neuraminidase-treated human RBC, reacts with carbohydrate antigens that are cryptic in normal lymphocytes and fully exposed on neuraminidase-treated human RBC and on certain lymphomas of both murine and human origin (Longenecker and Rahman 1983). Cell lines that are most susceptible to NAb killing are also the most susceptible to 49H.8 plus complement killing.

Finally, in the present study we have described three additional monoclonal antibodies that appear to detect cryptic carbohydrate antigens on normal lymphocytes. They are revealed following neuraminidase treatment and are expressed at high levels on 1A1 and EL-4 cells. Studies are currently in progress to determine whether "natural" antitumor monoclonal antibodies can serve as effective immunotherapeutic agents against murine lymphoma cell lines. In addition, "natural" antitumor monoclonal antibodies may be valuable reagents for the isolation and chemical characterization of cell surface (carbohydrate), tumor-associated antigens and aid in the determination of the role of these antigens, if any, as targets for immune elimination and spread of metastatic cells.

Homing of Leukemic Cells Back to Bone Marrow

Approximately 50% of P388 and L1210 cells accumulated in the liver by 3 hours postinjection, while little or no accumulation of L5178Y cells was found in the liver. This strongly suggests that the rapid elimination of L5178Y cells does not involve phagocytosis by the reticuloendothelial system.

Most interesting was the unexpectedly high level of homing of lymphoma cells to the bone marrow. This is of potential clinical interest as well, as the bones are the most commonly involved sites of heavy metastatic spread in ALL patients. We are presently attempting to select lymphoma variants for high and low capacity for bone marrow homing to attempt to unravel molecular mechanisms of preferential bone marrow homing.

Growth of Lymphoma Cells in the Bone Marrow Microenvironment

When the various cell lines were compared for ability to home to bone marrow, no detectable differences were found. Despite this, marked differences were found in the growth and rejection of the various cell lines in the bone marrow. Three patterns of "growth" were noted. Approximately 4% of the injected EL-4 and L5178Y cells were detected in the femur 3 h after injection and were rapidly and totally eliminated by day 3 or 4. The mechanisms responsible for this rapid rejection are presently under investigation. In contrast, RI cells showed fluctuations perhaps indicative of rejection followed by selective regrowth. We plan to follow the growth kinetics of this cell line beyond the 4-day period of this study to determine the eventual winner of the apparent "conflict." The last pattern of growth, exhibited by L1210 and P388 cells, was the most striking. Following an initial decrease in cell numbers, a period of extremely rapid growth occurred between days 3 and 4 after injection. This rapid growth of cells in the bone marrow did not reflect a nonspecific capacity for rapid growth by these two cell lines, as their doubling times and [^{3}H]thymidine incorporation levels did not differ from those of the other cells used in this study. Nor does it appear to reflect a differential growth potential of these cells in vivo in general, as lymphoma cells from various lines reisolated from other organs of the mouse appear to grow at about the same rate (our unpublished observations).

The differential growth in the bone marrow of P388 and L1210 cells was investigated further. It was noted that P388 cells have an apparently high affinity for binding to a cell population in the bone marrow. Fluorescent P388 cells, which were reisolated from the bone marrow after i.v. injection, had formed rosettes with bone marrow cells. Furthermore, P388 and L1210 cells adhered firmly to adherent bone marrow cells in Dexter cultures. This was followed by the rapid growth of the P388 and L1210 cells, their detachment from the adherent bone marrow cells, and rapid overgrowth of the culture. None of the other cell lines exhibited this behavior when cocultured in Dexter culture. Adherent bone marrow cells in Dexter cultures are known to provide growth factors for hematopoietic progenitor cells and are thought to represent the cells of the bone marrow "microenvironment" (Dexter 1982). Further work will be required to determine whether such growth factors stimulate the growth of P388 and L1210 cells, and such studies could provide the first definitive evidence supporting the "seed and soil" hypothesis.

ACKNOWLEDGMENTS

Supported by the NCI and MRC of Canada. We thank B. Widtman and M. J. Meeker for valuable technical assistance. M. Kieran is a research student of the Alberta Heritage Savings Trust Fund for Medical Research. J. Barrington Leigh is a Scholar of the MRC, Canada. B. M. Longenecker and A. H. Greenberg are Research Associates of the NCI of Canada.

REFERENCES

Butcher, E. C., and I. L. Weissman. 1980. Direct fluorescent labeling of cells with fluorescein or rhodamine isothiocyanate. I. Technical aspects. J. Immunol. Methods 37:97–108.

Carlson, G., and G. Terres. 1976. Antibody-induced killing in vivo of L1210/MTX-R cells quantitated in passively immunized mice with ^{131}I-iododeoxyuridine-labeled cells and whole-body measurement of retained radioactivity. J. Immunol. 117:822.

Chow, D. A., L. B. Wolosin, and A. H. Greenberg. 1981. Murine natural antitumor antibodies. II. The contribution of natural antibodies to tumor surveillance. Int. J. Cancer. 27:459–469.

Dawe, C. J., and M. Potter. 1957. Morphologic and biologic progression of a lymphoid neoplasm of the mouse in vivo and in vitro. Am. J. Pathol. 33:603.

Dexter, T. M. 1982. Stromal cell associated haemopoiesis. J. Cell. Physiol. (suppl. 1):87–94.

Dexter, T. M., and N. G. Testa. 1980. In vitro methods in haemopoiesis and lymphopoiesis. J. Immunol. Methods 38:177–190.

Fidler, I. J. 1978. Tumor heterogeneity and the biology of cancer invasion and metastasis. Cancer Res. 38:2651–2660.

Fidler, I. J., and I. R. Hart. 1981. The origin of metastatic heterogeneity in tumors. Eur. J. Cancer 17:487–494.

Fisher, G. A. 1958. Studies of the culture of leukemic cells in vitro. Ann. N.Y. Acad. Sci. 76:673–680.

Gorer, P. H. 1950. Studies in antibody response of mice to tumour inoculation. Br. J. Cancer 4:372–379.

Greenberg, A. H., and B. Pohajdak. 1982. The relationship between NK and natural antibody target structures, *in* NK Cells and Other Natural Effector Cells, R. B. Herberman, ed. Academic Press, New York, pp. 719–726.

Hart, I. R. 1982. "Seed and soil" revisited: Mechanisms of site-specific metastasis. Cancer Met. Rev. 1:5–16.

Hewitt, H. B., and C. W. Wilson. 1959. A survival curve for mammalian leukemia cells radioiodinated in vivo. Br. J. Cancer 13:69–75.

Imai, Y., T. Nakano, J. Sawada, and T. Osawa, 1980. Specificity of natural thymocytotoxic autoantibody developed in New Zealand black mice. J. Immunol. 124:1556–1560.

Kerbel, R. S., J. W. Dennis, A. E. Lagarde, and P. Frost. 1982. Tumor progression in metastasis: An experimental approach using lectin-resistant tumor variants. Cancer Metastasis Rev. 1:99–140.

Kieran, M. W., and B. M. Longenecker. 1983. Organ specific metastasis with special reference to avian systems. Metastasis Rev. 12:165–182.

Longenecker, B. M., and A. F. R. Rahman. 1983. Cell surface antigens in TA3-Ha mammary carcinoma model. Hybridoma 2:123.

MacLean, G. D., J. Seehafer, A. R. E. Shaw, M. W. Kieran, and B. M. Longenecker. 1982. Antigenic heterogeneity of human colorectal cancer cell lines analyzed by a panel of monoclonal antibodies. 1. Heterogeneous expression of La-like and HLA-like antigenic determinants. JNCI 69:357.

Moore, G. E., A. A. Sandberg, and K. Ulrich. 1966. Suspension cell culture and in vivo and in vitro chromosome constitution of mouse leukemia L1210. JNCI 36:405–421.

Mosmann, T. R., and B. M. Longenecker. 1982. The high background immune reactivity of mice to polymorphic determinants on xenogeneic erythrocytes: Theoretical and practical implications. J. Immunol. 128:100–104.

Nicolson, G. L. 1982. Cancer metastasis: Organ colonization and the cell surface properties of malignant cells. Biochim. Biophys. Acta 695:113–176.

Nowell, P. C. 1976. The clonal evolution of tumor cell populations. Science 194:23–28.

Paget, S. 1889. The distribution of secondary growths in cancer of the breast. Lancet 1:571–573.

Rahman, A. F. R., and B. M. Longenecker. 1982. A monoclonal antibody specific for the Thomsen-Freidenreich cryptic T antigen. J. Immunol. 129:2021–2024.

Shearman, P. J., W. M. Gallatin, and B. M. Longenecker. 1980. Detection of cell-surface antigen correlated metastasis. Nature 286:267–269.

Shearman, P. J., and B. M. Longenecker. 1980. Selection for virulence and organ-specific metastasis of herpesvirus-transformed lymphoma cells. Int. J. Cancer 25:363–369.

Simon, T. M., D. H. Kunishima, G. J. Vibert, and A. Lorber. 1981. Screening trial with the coordinated gold compound Auranotin using mouse lymphocytic leukemia P388. Cancer Res. 41:94–97.

Sugarbaker, E. V. 1980. Patterns of metastasis in human malignancies, *in* Cancer Biology Reviews 2, J. J. Marchalonis, M. G. Hanna, I. J. Fidler, eds. Marcel Dekker, New York, pp. 235–278.

Wolosin, L. B., and A. H. Greenberg. 1979. Murine natural anti-tumor antibodies. I. Rapid in vivo binding of natural antibody by tumor cells in syngeneic mice. Int. J. Cancer 23:519–529.

Young, W. W., J. M. Durdik, D. Urdal, S. Hakomori, and C. Henney. 1981. Glycolipid expression in lymphoma cell variants. Chemical quality, immunologic reactivity, and correlations with susceptibility to NK cells. J. Immunol. 126:1–6.

Young, W. W., and S. Hakomori. 1981. Therapy of mouse lymphoma with monoclonal antibodies to glycolipid: Selection of low antigenic variants in vivo. Science 211:487–489.

Young, W. W., E. M. S. MacDonald, R. C. Nowinski, and S. I. Hakomori. 1979. Production of monoclonal antibodies specific for two distinct steric portions of the glycolipid ganglio-n-triosyl ceramide (asialo GM2). J. Exp. Med. 150:1008–1019.

Cancer Invasion and Metastasis: Biologic and Therapeutic Aspects edited by Garth L. Nicolson and Luka Milas. Raven Press, New York © 1984.

Heterogeneity in Human Colon Cancer

Daniel L. Dexter*

Department of Medicine, Roger Williams General Hospital and Brown University, Providence, Rhode Island 02912

Large bowel cancer is a major health problem in the United States, where colorectal carcinomas are second only to lung cancer in incidence (excluding skin tumors) and in cause of death among all types of neoplasms (1982 American Cancer Society Booklet 1981, Sugarbaker et al. 1982). Despite the availability of excellent surgical procedures, a large number of antineoplastic drugs, ionizing radiation, and well-trained clinicians, our attempts to treat patients with colon cancer have been ineffectual for the most part (Kroener et al. 1982, Sugarbaker et al. 1982). Our inability to treat these patients successfully suggests that the biology itself of colorectal and other solid tumors is frustrating our therapists.

A key element responsible for this frustration is the phenomenon of intratumor heterogeneity. Numerous studies in the last 5 to 10 years have presented overwhelming evidence that most, if not all, animal and human solid tumors are each heterogeneous tissues (Hart and Fidler 1981, Heppner et al. 1981, Dexter and Calabresi 1982a). Experimental and medical oncologists now appreciate that intraneoplastic diversity is one of the most important aspects of cancer biology. Indeed, tumor heterogeneity provides an explanation of the origins and development of metastatic potential in primary tumors. It is the process of metastasis that is responsible for the demise of the great majority of patients who succumb to colorectal cancer and the other carcinomas responsible for most of the cancer-related deaths in this country and abroad. Progress in our treatment of solid tumors, including large bowel cancer, will depend on how successfully clinicians develop efficacious protocols for patients with disseminated disease. That success will be predicated on our ability to understand tumor heterogeneity, which is the root problem in metastasis.

HETEROGENEITY WITHIN TUMORS

Several laboratories have reported intratumor heterogeneity for a variety of human solid tumors. Vindeløv et al. (1980) demonstrated karyotypic heterogeneity in metastases from each of 6 of 29 patients with small cell carcinoma of

* *Present address:* Du Pont Company, Glenolden Laboratories, Glenolden, Pennsylvania 19036

the lung. Abeloff et al. (1979) have also described heterogeneity in small cell lung cancer. Shapiro et al. (1981) have shown that eight individual human gliomas were karyotypically and morphologically heterogeneous. Two groups (Brennan et al. 1979, Allegra et al. 1980) have reported that single human breast cancers are heterogeneous for expression of estrogen receptor. Heterogeneity has also been demonstrated for ovarian carcinoma (Siracky 1979), testicular cancer (Bronson et al. 1980), and melanoma (Tsuruo and Fidler 1981) in humans.

Human and murine tumors have been shown to be heterogeneous for a variety of phenotypes, including marker production (Gray and Pierce 1964, Abeloff et al. 1979), antigen profile (Prehn 1970, Sugarbaker and Cohen 1972, Pimm and Baldwin 1977, Miller and Heppner 1979), and karyotype (Mitelman et al. 1972, Dexter et al. 1978, Shapiro et al. 1981). One conclusion from these studies is that tumor heterogeneity must be defined in relationship to the phenotypic characteristic being studied. When multiple properties have been examined in heterogeneous melanoma and colon and mammary tumor systems, intraneoplastic diversity has been demonstrated for many of the characteristics studied (Dexter et al. 1978, 1981, Heppner et al. 1978, Hart and Fidler 1981). This kaleidoscopic pattern of multiple variations among subpopulations of individual tumors is undoubtedly a major factor in the success of cancer and in our failure to treat the patient effectively (Hart and Fidler 1981, Dexter and Calabresi 1982a).

Variability for aggressive behavior within a tumor, that is, the ability of certain subsets of cells to invade or metastasize or both, is now considered to be crucial to the successful evolution of the tumor and, ultimately, to the death of the patient. This type of diversity, sometimes referred to as functional heterogeneity, was first reported by Fidler and Kripke (1977) and has subsequently been demonstrated in several laboratories (Fidler and Kripke 1977, Nicolson et al. 1977, 1978, Kripke et al. 1978, Liotta et al. 1980, Poste et al. 1980). Such heterogeneity is of obvious importance for the cancer patient, as metastasis is frequently the cause of death.

However, the implications of functional heterogeneity for successful treatment are based on another major premise as well. Cells within a primary tumor can differ markedly in their sensitivities to various treatments (Barranco et al. 1972, 1973, Hakansson and Trope 1974, Siracky 1979, Dexter et al. 1981, Yung et al. 1982). Moreover, differential drug sensitivities between a primary tumor and its metastases have been found (Slack and Bross 1975, Trope 1975, Fugmann et al. 1977, Heppner et al. 1978, Lotan and Nicolson 1979, Biorkland et al. 1980). Finally, heterogeneity for response to chemotherapeutic drugs among metastases from the same primary tumor has also been reported (Siracky 1979, Tsuruo and Fidler 1981). The finding that certain cells within a tumor have an increased propensity for colonizing distant sites has had a profound impact on our thinking. The demonstration that these aggressive cells may also respond differently to drugs when compared with (nonmetastatic) cells in the primary neoplasm or cells in other metastases has ominous implications for our ability to eradicate these cells. The propensity of certain clones to disseminate, together with their differential and unpredictable responsiveness to treatment, defines an enormous problem for the clinician.

INTRANEOPLASTIC DIVERSITY IN HUMAN COLON CANCER

Laboratory Investigations

Some reports have described intraneoplastic diversity in human colon cancers. Petersen et al. (1979) demonstrated that five of six colorectal carcinomas that were operated on consecutively were each karyotypically heterogeneous. Kimball and Brattain (1980) have described the selection of a fluorodesoxyuridine (FUdR) variant from the human colon carcinoma cell line HT29. Brattain et al. (1981) have also isolated three component subpopulations from another heterogeneous colon cancer (HCT 116) using a linear density gradient method. Siracky (1979) reported that cells from different regions of each of two primary human colon carcinomas differed in their response to several antineoplastic agents.

Our laboratory has been investigating heterogeneity in human colon carcinomas for the past several years. The DLD-1 cell line was established from a primary human colon cancer that was histologically heterogeneous at the time of surgical removal. The patient's tumor contained moderately differentiated areas with glandular structures, as well as anaplastic, poorly differentiated regions. The cell line established from this neoplasm contained two morphologically distinct cell types. Early passage DLD-1 cultures consisted of cells that were predominately diploid, but about 5% to 10% of the cells were hyperploid, with chromosome numbers in the range of 60 to 90. Two morphologic types were cloned from soft agar cultures of DLD-1 cells. Clone A cells were hyperploid, resembled morphologically the minority variant in DLD-1 cultures, and produced poorly differentiated, anaplastic carcinomas in nude mice. Clone D cells were diploid, resembled the majority subpopulation in DLD-1 cells, and produced moderately differentiated colon cancers in nude mice. The history and growth characteristics of the DLD-1 system have been described previously (Dexter et al. 1979, 1981, Dexter and Hager 1980).

Clone A and clone D were also antigenically distinct. Clone A cells had significantly more H-gene–determined blood group 0 substance than did clone D. We also determined levels of membrane-associated colonic mucin antigen (CMA), which was originally described by Gold and Miller (1974). Clone A cells had more cell-surface CMA than did clone D cells. Clone D cells expressed more membrane-associated carcinoembryonic antigen (CEA) than did clone A cells after differentiation induction with N,N-dimethylformamide (DMF). The two clones had essentially equivalent amounts of CEA before induction. These results have been reported in detail (Dexter and Hager 1980, Hager et al. 1980) and indicate that the antigenic profiles for these two subpopulations are different.

We have also studied, in the DLD-1 system, two clinically significant phenotypes: treatment (drug, hyperthermia, or irradiation) sensitivity and metastasizing ability. We have tested the sensitivity of DLD-1, clone A, and clone D cells to six chemotherapeutic drugs (Dexter et al. 1981). No difference in response was noted among the three lines to each of three drugs—vincristine, cytosine arabinoside, and methyl chloroethyl cyclohexyl nitrosourea (CCNU). In contrast, differential chemosensitivities were demonstrated among the lines for three other antineoplastic agents. Clone A cells were approximately threefold more sensitive to 5-fluorouracil than were clone D or DLD-1 cells. DLD-1 cells, on the other hand, were about fivefold more sensitive to actinomycin D than were clone A or clone D cells. The most striking difference was seen with mitomycin C. Clone A cells were thirtyfold and fiftyfold more sensitive to mitomycin C than were clone D and DLD-1 cells, respectively. Thus, large differences in responsiveness to anticancer drugs can exist among subpopulations, depending on the agent tested. Furthermore, the direction of the change in sensitivity cannot be predicted.

Our laboratory has also determined the sensitivities of DLD-1, clone A, and clone D cells to the physical treatment methods X-irradiation and hyperthermia. Parent DLD-1 cells were the most sensitive to heat (Leith et al. 1982a) and were the least sensitive to ionizing radiation (Leith et al. 1982b). Thus, as has been reported for drugs, differential responses to heat and X-rays exist among the parent line and subpopulations. The following principle seems to be emerging from work with the DLD-1 system: the ranking of parent and cloned lines in terms of their sensitivities to each of a number of chemical and physical agents will be modality-dependent. Hierarchies of sensitivity exist, and a unique hierarchy can be constructed for each agent employed. The implications for combination chemotherapy and multimodality treatment are obvious.

We have begun to look at metastasis in the DLD-1 system through experiments with the nude mouse. Metastases have occurred more often with clone A xenografts than with clone D tumors. The following experiment was performed recently in our laboratory (E. N. Spremulli et al. 1983a). Xenograft tumors were produced by subcutaneous inoculation of nude mice with a mixture of clone A and clone D cells. The tumors were then continuously propagated in nude mice. The tumors were composed of both A and D cells at each passage generation, as was shown by chromosome analysis. In three instances, hematogenous metastases developed, and in each instance the secondary neoplasm contained only clone A cells. These data indicate that metastases of human tumors can be clonal in origin, and that clone A cells have a greater propensity for metastasis than do clone D cells. Our findings also indicate that metastasis of a heterogeneous human colon cancer can be studied in an experimental setting.

We have also begun studies on a second heterogeneous human colon cancer system (Spremulli et al. 1983b). Biopsies from two distinct metastases were obtained from a woman who had a primary colon carcinoma; the primary tumor was not surgically removed. One metastasis was found in the ovary; the second was growing in the omentum. Transplantable xenograft tumor lines were established from the ovarian (HOT-3) and omental (OM-1) metastases. The OM-1 and HOT-3 cell lines were then established from the initial xenograft tumors that developed from the implanted biopsy material.

We found several similarities between OM-1 and HOT-3 (Table 1). The two metastases from the patient were histologically quite similar to each other and to the primary colon tumor tissue removed by sigmoidoscopy. The HOT-3 and OM-1 xenograft tumors that were either passaged continuously in vivo from the original biopsy materials or were produced by inoculation of cultured HOT-3 and OM-1 cells histologically closely resembled the patient's primary and secondary tumors. OM-1– and HOT-3–cultured cells contained common marker chromosomes (4q– and 6q–); the two cell lines had similar cloning efficiencies in agar; and OM-1 and HOT-3 xenograft tumors contained essentially equivalent amounts of nonspecific cross-reacting antigen (NCA).

Differences between the two metastases were also demonstrated (Table 1). OM-1 cells had a shorter doubling time than did HOT-3 cells. In contrast, HOT-3 cells had a higher saturation density and plating efficiency than did OM-1 cells. Cultured OM-1 cells secreted more CEA into the tissue culture medium than HOT-3 cells did. Colon-specific antigen p (CSAp) was undetectable in OM-1 xenograft tumor tissue; HOT-3 tumor tissue contained 1,200 units of CSAp/g tissue. However, OM-1 xenograft tumors contained considerably more CMA (2,500 μg/g tissue) than did HOT-3 tumors (300 μg/g tissue).

TABLE 1. *Properties of OM-1 and HOT-3 tumor lines*

Properties*	Omental metastasis (OM-1)	Ovarian metastasis (HOT-3)
Similarities		
Histology (xenograft tumors)	Well-differentiated adenocarcinoma	Same as OM-1
Karyotype	4q– and 6q– markers; extra chromosomes in pair 7 of C group; missing chromosomes in pair 18 of E group	Same as OM-1
NCA (nonspecific cross-reacting antigen in xenografts)	20.8 μg/g tumor tissue	21.2 μg/g tumor tissue
Cloning efficiencies (agar)	Low (about 1%)	Low (about 5%)
Differences		
Doubling time (culture)	42 hours	61 hours
Plating efficiency (plastic)	48% (per 1.5×10^5 cells)	65% (per 1.5×10^5 cells)
Saturation density	2.3×10^5 cells/sq cm	4.2×10^5 cells/sq cm
CEA (cultured cells)	518 ng/10^6 cells	92 ng/10^6 cells
CSAp (colon-specific antigen p) in xonografts	Undetectable	1,200 units/g tumor tissue
CMA (colonic mucin antigen) in xenografts	2,500 μg/g tumor tissue	300 μg/g tumor tissue

* Data adapted from Spremulli et al. 1983b.

Therefore, considerable heterogeneity exists between OM-1 and HOT-3 with respect to certain growth characteristics and immunochemical markers associated with human colonic cancer. These phenotypic differences between lines established from two distinct metastatic tumor deposits in one individual could not be predicted from the histopathologies of the primary and secondary neoplasms.

Implications of Laboratory Findings

Data from many laboratories have provided convincing evidence that combination chemotherapy and multiagent therapies should be considered for use against heterogeneous cancers and their metastases (Heppner et al. 1978, Calabresi et al. 1979, Dexter et al. 1981). Our results on responses of clone A, clone D, and parent DLD-1 cells to chemical and physical agents certainly support the conclusion that intraneoplastic diversity justifies the use of multimodality treatment of human colon cancers as well as other solid tumors.

These findings on colon intratumor heterogeneity have important implications for detection and diagnosis of neoplasms using reagents specific for tumor markers. Detection with a single marker will fail unless all the cells in a tumor elaborate the substance (Hart and Fidler 1981, Calabresi and Dexter 1982, Dexter and Calabresi 1982a). A metastasis that does not produce circulating CEA cannot be detected by classic CEA assay methods even if the primary tumor contained many (other) subpopulations that did secrete CEA. Our work with the OM/HOT model has shown that an assay for CMA would detect OM-1 preferentially, as HOT-3 had a greatly reduced level of this mucin. The situation would be more dramatic if CSAp were used. With this marker, HOT-3 would be identified, whereas OM-1 would probably escape detection altogether. The conclusion from such considerations would be that a multiple panel of marker-detectors must be used in order to identify the presence of multiple metastases in a patient. In summary, primary colon and other tumors contain subsets of cells, some of which metastasize. Panels of reagents will be needed to detect these secondary tumors, and multiple agents will be required to eradicate them.

HETEROGENEITY, METASTASIS, AND TREATMENT

The consensus among clinicians is that the bottom line on cancer is metastasis. The great majority of cancer patients who are not cured die of disseminated disease, not of their primary tumor. This is certainly true in the case of colorectal carcinomas, in which most patients who fail therapy succumb to liver or lung metastases (Sugarbaker et al. 1982). Thus, metastasis has become the central clinical issue in cancer and the focus of much recent experimental research directed toward the treatment of neoplastic disease.

The approaches available to experimental and medical oncologists and radiotherapists must be examined in light of what is known about the natural history of solid tumors in patients. Some tumors remain localized in individuals. The salient finding, however, which is widely accepted among clinicians, is that, in most instances, the tumor has already metastasized by the time the cancer patient seeks treatment. At the time of surgery, micrometastases are present in distant organs, and macroscopic secondary tumors are often apparent (Fisher et al. 1975, Golinger et al. 1977, Sugarbaker 1979). Therefore, approaches that would interfere with the process of metastasis could not be applied successfully to most patients at the time their primary tumor is diagnosed (Sugarbaker 1979). Interesting information will be generated from studies with animal tumor models, which focus on arresting or inhibiting invasion of the primary tumor, or aggregation of emigrating cancer cells with platelets in the circulation, among others. Patients might accrue some benefit from interference with cells released from primary tumors through surgical manipulation (Foss et al. 1966, Sugarbaker and Ketcham 1977) or from inhibition of the dissemination of the metastases themselves (Bross et al. 1975). However, for most individuals, this kind of information will have little relevance to their treatment. Metastases already present at diagnosis will have to be successfully eradicated if the patient is to survive; at that point, it is too late to interfere with the dissemination process, which has already occurred.

Compelling documentation now confirms that a critical problem in the treatment of micro- and macrometastases is the heterogeneity of these secondary tumors in a single patient. Distinct metastases in the same patient can respond differently to chemotherapuetic drugs (Siracky 1979). The existence of estrogen-positive as well as estrogen-negative secondary tumors within the same individual with breast cancer indicates that hormonal therapy will not be effective against all metastatic foci in that individual (Brennan et al. 1979, Allegra et al. 1980). Our work with colon carcinoma shows that OM and HOT colon cancer cells and xenograft tumors differ in a number of properties. Kinetic differences alone would lead one to predict that these two lines would respond dissimilarly to cycle-active agents. Clone A cells have quite different responses to a number of drugs compared to clone D cells, and clone A cells also have a greater tendency to metastasize in nude mice. Therapy against the majority of cells in the DLD-1 tumor almost by definition should be effective against clone D. Whether such therapy would also succeed in eradicating clone A cells is an open question. Yet, experimental evidence suggests that clone A cells should be the target for therapy, not clone D cells.

An important implication of the finding, reported by many laboratories, that metastases from a tumor differ in their drug sensitivities compared with that of the primary tumor is that information gained from studies of primary neoplasms may not be useful in the treatment of disseminated cancer. This is particularly important in evaluating the usefulness of the stem cell, or clonogenic, assay (Salmon et al. 1978) as a routine test for determining chemotherapeutic regimens for individual patients. Knowledge of tumor heterogeneity would lead one to think that the clonogenic assay performed on cells from a primary tumor might not accurately predict the sensitivity of cells in metastases from the same patient, and this is precisely the result obtained by Schlag and Schreml (1982). These investigators compared the sensitivities of cells from a series of primary cancers and their corresponding metastases, as assessed by the clonogenic assay. They found a discordance in results from cells of a primary tumor and a metastasis from each of several patients. One conclusion from this study is that the stem cell test should be performed with metastases, not primary tumors, since the patients are dying of metastases. However, this would be impractical or impossible in many instances because the secondary tumors would not be detectable or accessible. Furthermore, the finding that distinct metastases in a host can differ among themselves in sensitivity to drugs indicates that *all* the metastases in a patient would have to be examined in the clonogenic assay. This would clearly be impossible for the great majority of patients. Certainly, the general and routine use of the stem cell assay must be carefully considered in light of what has been revealed by investigations of heterogeneity for drug sensitivity among cells from a primary tumor and its metastases (Tsuruo and Fidler 1981, Calabresi and Dexter 1982).

FUTURE APPROACHES

Tumor heterogeneity presents monumental problems to the clinician. The differences among subpopulations within a primary tumor, between a primary and its metastases, among metastases in a given patient, and even among clones within one secondary tumor seem to constitute an almost insurmountable obstacle preventing the detection, diagnosis, and treatment of disseminated disease. Nevertheless, an understanding of these complex solid tumors and the design of efficacious protocols for their treatment are possible provided the right approaches can be found.

A careful review of the phenomenon and implications of intraneoplastic diversity leads one to the following hypothesis. The answer to attacking this array of phenotypes that coexist within single neoplasms and among their metastases is perhaps not to focus on the differences, that is, on the heterogeneity. Rather, efforts should be made to look for similarities among subpopulations. It is the common denominator that, if it can be identified, will provide us with the rational approach to detection and treatment. We should emphasize finding commonalities, rather than continue to document differences, among subpopulations. Of particular importance will be the identification of properties shared by all metastases in a patient, which then could be exploited clinically. Sugarbaker (1979) and Hart and Fidler (1981) are among those who have emphasized that it will be necessary to treat all the metastases in an individual in order to achieve a cure. The identification of a common denominator among a patient's metastases may well be a prerequisite for designing an efficacious treatment protocol for his disseminated disease.

This approach can be extended further and can be stated as follows: To detect and treat disseminated disease, some common feature shared by the metastases must be identified. This feature need not be found in most of the cells in the primary tumor. If the commonality is a marker, occult disease can be detected for all metastases in an individual. If the shared property is a characteristic associated with the growth or function of cells in metastases, a treatment could be designed to interdict this function or proliferation. Perhaps no one common denominator exists. However, several features or properties could be identified that would each be shared by most of the metastatic tumors in an individual. Then, a combination treatment could be planned so that all the secondary tumors would be affected by at least one of the components of the multimodality therapy. The same reasoning could be applied to markers. If any one of several substances is present on most cells in metastases, and at least one of these markers is expressed by any given cell in the secondary tumors growing in a patient, detection is possible. A cocktail containing a battery of reagents able to detect these several markers is needed. Thus, even if commonalities in an absolute sense do not exist, the collection of several properties shared by a majority of cells in all metastases in a patient can be used to design detection or treatment protocols. The demonstration that a set of features or characteristics shared among metastases in an individual are also shared among metastases in a series of patients with one tumor type would be even more important. A further goal would be the identification of commonalities among secondary tumors in patients suffering from any one of a number of types of cancers. The ultimate aim of this approach is to identify common denominators among secondary neoplasms in patients in order to design detection and treatment protocols that will be generally useful for individuals with all types of cancer.

Is there any reason to believe that such an aim is achievable? Do commonalities exist? Is it going to be possible to describe and exploit a common denominator shared among metastases? There is, in fact, some evidence that such an approach might be feasible. Investigators have demonstrated that activated macrophages specifically discriminate and attack tumor cells, including those in secondary neoplasms, as opposed to normal cells (Fidler 1974, 1980, Hibbs 1974, Liotta et al. 1977, Fidler et al. 1978). Hart and Fidler (1981) concluded that a common feature of all tumor cells, including cells in metastases, is that they are each sensitive to activated macrophages. Obviously, this discovery could be a basis for therapy that might be effective against disseminated or inoperable neoplastic disease in all patients.

Our laboratory has reported extensively on the induction of differentiation in human colon cancer cells using polar solvents as maturational agents (Dexter and Hager 1980, Hager et al. 1980, Dexter et al. 1979, 1982a, 1982c, Leith et al. 1982c). We have hypothesized that the use of differentiation-inducing chemicals such as DMF and N-methylformamide (NMF) could force a convergence of phenotypes existing in a heterogeneous solid tumor (Calabresi et al. 1979, Calabresi and Dexter 1982, Dexter and Calabresi 1982b). This conversion of distinct subpopulations to one better-differentiated, more benign phenotype could simplify therapy because fewer "bullets" would be required in a "homogenized" tumor. Certainly, one method of eliminating differences among clones and causing any commonalities of a patient's neoplastic cells to appear is to attack and limit the heterogeneity via a maturational therapy. This idea is still quite speculative and will require experimentation to determine whether it has merit. However, the recent introduction of the differentiation-inducing agent NMF into clinical trials makes this hypothesis quite timely. Our laboratory is currently studying the effects of NMF and DMF on the phenotypes of subpopulations from the DLD-1 and OM/HOT systems.

Rabotti (1959) has reported that ploidy differences exist between cells in human primary tumors and cells in metastases. Cells in metastases from each of five breast cancers and a nasopharyngeal carcinoma had higher numbers of chromosomes than did the corresponding primary tumor cells. The opposite relationship has been described with methylcholanthrene-induced murine primary neoplasms and their metastases (Sugarbaker et al. 1979). We have established a number of cell lines from both primary and secondary human tumors. Examination of the modal chromosome number and range of these lines supports the view that cells in metastases have a higher ploidy than do cells in primary human tumors. Table 2 shows the results obtained when ten lines from our laboratory were examined. Cell lines established from the primary colon cancers, HCT-15 and DLD-2, are diploid. The great majority of cells (clone D cells) of the DLD-1 heterogeneous colon tumor line are diploid. Clone A cells isolated from the DLD-1 line are hyperploid; the modal chromosome number for this line is 76. However, clone A tumors have been found to have a higher frequency of metastasis in nude mice than do clone D, HCT-15, or DLD-2 tumors. Moreover, our recent data have shown that when artificially constructed A/D tumors

TABLE 2. *Modal chromosome numbers for human tumor cell lines*

Cell line	Tumor type	Tumor location	Modal chromosome number
HCT-15	Colon carcinoma	Primary colon	45
DLD-2	Colon carcinoma	Primary colon	47
DLD-1	Colon carcinoma	Primary colon	46 and 76
Clone D	Colon carcinoma (DLD-1)	Primary colon	46
Clone A	Colon carcinoma (DLD-1)	Primary colon	76
OM-1	Colon carcinoma	Omental metastasis	61
HOT-3	Colon carcinoma	Ovarian metastasis	64
RWP-1	Pancreatic carcinoma	Liver metastasis	64
RWP-2	Pancreatic carcinoma	Liver metastasis	62
H-Mel-3	Melanoma	Superficial nodule (metastasis)	79

were produced in nude mice, the spontaneous hematogenous metastases that appeared were clonal in origin and consisted of A cells. Since our results indicate that clone A has a greater propensity for dissemination than do the diploid lines, one is tempted to speculate that perhaps clone A cells were responsible for the metastases ultimately observed in the DLD-1 tumor patient.

Results from studies of the lines established from metastases clearly indicate that, for the five secondary tumors studied, cells in metastases have a higher ploidy. The OM/HOT system has been described in this report. RWP-1 and RWP-2 are lines that were established from liver metastases from two patients with primary pancreatic carcinomas (Dexter et al. 1982b). H-Mel-3 was established from a superficial nodule from a patient with malignant melanoma (Spremulli et al. 1982). In all five instances, the modal chrosome number is between 60 and 80. Although secondary human tumors with normal ploidy undoubtedly occur, our results do suggest that one property that several metastases may share is a higher DNA content. Moreover, primary human tumors will perhaps be characterized as generally having a lower (diploid) number of chromosomes. The point to be made is that cells in a series of five metastases in four different sites from several distinct human primary tumor types share a feature. Investigators should be able to design and test protocols that could exploit increased polidy in these secondary cancers. Agents that have DNA as their target can be carefully examined to see whether they are preferentially active against metastases compared with diploid tumors or normal tissues.

Investigations with activated tumoricidal macrophages, differentiation-inducing chemicals, and DNA content of tumor cells, therefore, suggest that a search for a common denominator in the cells of metastases may be fruitful. Careful examination of metastases for shared properties may be a viable approach to solving the riddle posed by tumor heterogeneity. Although the differences among subpopulations for a variety of phenotypes have been extensively documented, it may be that those few similarities that can be identified will provide the clue to effective therapeutic strategies.

CONCLUSION

Heterogeneity within human solid tumors presents a major challenge to experimental and medical oncologists. Several groups have demonstrated intraneoplastic diversity in colorectal cancers. In our laboratory, we have developed two models for studying heterogeneity within neoplasms using human colon carcinoma cell lines and xenografted tumors. Differential sensitivities of clonal lines in the DLD-1 system to a variety of drugs, X-irradiation, or hyperthermia have been reported. Moreover, one of the clones has a higher rate of spontaneous metastasis in nude mice. Therefore, variability in two of the most clinically relevant phenotypes, response to treatment modalities and metastatic potential, has been demonstrated in a heterogeneous human colon cancer model. Investigation of the OM-1 and HOT-3 cell lines and xenograft tumors, obtained from two distinct secondary tumor deposits in the same patient, has revealed both similarities and differences between the two metastases. The differences once again underscore the problems that tumor heterogeneity presents to the clinician. The similarities suggest that a search for common denominators shared among metastases might be a worthwhile approach. Commonalities among disseminated tumors could be exploited in diagnostic and treatment protocols. In summary, cell lines and xenograft tumors derived from human large bowel cancers provide material suitable for the design of therapeutic strategies that may be efficacious against secondary as well as primary colorectal neoplasms. It is hoped that any protocols developed for detection and treatment of these cancers will prove useful against other classes of human solid tumors as well.

ACKNOWLEDGMENTS

I wish to acknowledge the superb assistance provided by Judy Wilson in the preparation of this manuscript. This investigation was supported by grants CA-23225, CA-13943, and CA-20842, awarded by the National Cancer Institute, Department of Health and Human Services.

REFERENCES

Abeloff, M. D., J. C. Eggleston, G. Mendelsohn, D. S. Ettinger, and S. B. Baylin. 1979. Changes in morphologic and biochemical characteristics of small cell carcinoma of the lung. Am. J. Med 66:757–764.

Allegra, J. C., A. Barlock, K. K. Huff, and M. E. Lippman. 1980. Changes in multiple or sequential estrogen receptor determinations in breast cancer. Cancer 45:792–794.

American Cancer Society, 1982 Cancer Facts and Figures Booklet. American Cancer Society, New York.

Barranco, S. C., B. Drewinko, and R. M. Humphrey. 1973. Differential responses by human melanoma cells to 1,3-bis-(2-chloroethyl)-1-nitrosourea and bleomycin. Mutat. Res. 19:277–280.

Barranco, S. C., D. Ho, B. Drewinko, M. M. Romsdahl, and R. M. Humphrey. 1972. Differential responses by human melanoma cells grown in vitro to arabinosylcytosine. Cancer Res. 32:2733–2736.

Biorklund, A., L. Hakansson, B. Stenstarn, C. Trope, and M. Ackerman. 1980. Heterogeneity of non-Hodgkin's lymphomas as regards sensitivity to cytostatic drugs. Eur. J. Cancer 16:647–654.

Brattain, M. G., W. D. Fine, F. M. Khaled, J. Thompson, and D. E. Brattain. 1981. Heterogeneity of malignant cells from a human colonic carcinoma. Cancer Res. 41:1751–1756.

Brennan, M. J., W. L. Donagan, and D. E. Appleby. 1979. The variability of estrogen receptors in metastatic breast cancer. Am J. Surg. 137:260–262.

Bronson, D. L., P. W. Andrews, D. Solter, J. Cervenka, P. H. Lange, and E. E. Fraley. 1980. Cell line derived from a metastasis of a human testicular germ cell tumor. Cancer Res. 40:2500–2506.

Bross, I. D., E. Viadana, and J. Pickren. 1975. Do generalized metastases occur directly from the primary? J. Chron. Dis. 28:149–159.

Calabresi, P. and D. L. Dexter. 1982. Clinical implications of cancer cell heterogeneity, *in* Tumor Cell Heterogeneity: Origins and Implications, Fourth Annual Bristol-Myers Symposium on Cancer Research, A. H. Owens, Jr., D. S. Coffey, and S. B. Baylin, eds. Academic Press, New York, pp. 181–201.

Calabresi, P., D. L. Dexter, and G. H. Heppner. 1979. Clinical and pharmacological implications of cancer cell differentiation and heterogeneity. Biochem. Pharmacol. 28:1933–1941.

Dexter, D. L., J. A. Barbosa, and P. Calabresi. 1979. N,N-Dimethylformamide-induced alteration of cell culture characteristics and loss of tumorigenicity in cultured human colon carcinoma cells. Cancer Res. 39:1020–1025.

Dexter, D. L., and P. Calabresi. 1982a. Intraneoplastic diversity. Biochim. Biophys. Acta. 695:97–112.

Dexter, D. L., and P. Calabresi. 1982b. Cancer cell differentiation, *in* Pancreatic Tumors in Children (Vol. VIII of Cancer Treatment and Research), G. B. Humphrey, G. B. Grundey, L. P. Dehner, R. T. Acton, and T. J. Pysher, eds. Martinus Nijhoff Publishers, Boston, pp. 45–66.

Dexter, D. L., and J. C. Hager. 1980. Maturation-induction of tumor cells using a human colon carcinoma model. Cancer 45:1178–1184.

Dexter, D. L., H. L. Kowalski, B. A. Blazar, Z. Fligiel, R. Vogel, and G. H. Heppner. 1978. Heterogeneity of tumor cells from a single mouse mammary tumor. Cancer Res. 38:3174–3181.

Dexter, D. L., J. T. Leith, G. W. Crabtree, R. E. Parks, Jr., A. S. Glicksman, and P. Calabresi. 1982a. N,N-dimethylformamide-induced modulation of responses of tumor cells to conventional anti-cancer treatment modalities, *in* Maturation Factors and Cancer, M.A.S. Moore, ed. Raven Press, New York, pp. 105–114.

Dexter, D. L., G. M. Matook, P. A. Meitner, H. A. Bogaars, G. A. Jolly, M. D. Turner, and P. Calabresi. 1982b. Establishment and characterization of two human pancreatic cancer cell lines tumorigenic in athymic mice. Cancer Res. 42:2705–2714.

Dexter, D. L., E. N. Spremulli, Z. Fligiel, J. A. Barbosa, R. Vogel, A. VanVoorhees, and P. Calabresi. 1981. Heterogeneity of cancer cells from a single human colon carcinoma. Am. J. Med. 71:949–956.

Dexter, D. L., E. N. Spremulli, G. M. Matook, I. Diamond, and P. Calabresi. 1982c. Inhibition by polar solvents of the growth of human colon cancer xenografts. Cancer Res. 42:5018–5022.

Fidler, I. J. 1974. Inhibition of pulmonary metastasis by intravenous injection of specifically activated macrophages. Cancer Res. 34:1074–1078.

Fidler, I. J., and M. D. Kripke. 1977. Metastasis results from preexisting variant cells within a malignant tumor. Science 197:893–895.

Fidler, I. J., R. O. Robbin, and G. Poste. 1978. In vitro tumoricidal activity of macrophages against virus-transformed lines with temperature-dependent transformed phenotypic characteristics. Cell Immunol. 38:131–146.

Fisher, B., N. Slack, D. Katrych, and N. Wolmark. 1975. Ten-year follow-up results of patients with carcinoma of the breast in a co-operative clinical trial evaluating surgical adjuvant chemotherapy. Surg. Gynecol. Obstet. 140:528–534.

Foss, O. P., I. O. Brennhovd, O. T. Messelt, J. Efskind, and K. Liverud. 1966. Invasion of tumor cells into the bloodstream caused by palpation or biopsy of the tumor. Surgery 59:691–695.

Fugmann, R. A., J. C. Anderson, R. L. Stolfi, and D. S. Martin. 1977. Comparison of adjuvant chemotherapeutic activity against primary and metastatic spontaneous murine tumors. Cancer Res. 37:496–500.

Gold, D. V., and F. Miller. 1974. Characterization of human colonic mucoprotein antigen. Immunochemistry 11:369–375.

Golinger, R. C., R. M. Gregorio, and E. R. Fisher. 1977. Tumors cells in venous blood draining mammary carcinomas. Arch. Surg. 112:707–708.

Gray, J. M., and G. B. Pierce. 1964. Relationship between growth rate and differentiation of melanoma in vivo. JNCI 32:1201–1211.

Hager, J. C., D. V. Gold, J. A. Barbosa, Z. Fligiel, F. Miller, and D. L. Dexter. 1980. N,N-Dimethylformamide-induced modulation of organ- and tumor-associated markers in cultured human colon carcinoma cells. JNCI 64:439–446.

Hakansson, L., and C. Trope. 1974. On the presence within tumors of clones that differ in sensitivities to cytostatic drugs. Acta. Pathol. Microbiol. Scand. (A) 82:35–40.

Hart, I. R., and I. J. Fidler. 1981. The implications of tumor heterogeneity for studies on the biology and therapy of cancer metastasis. Biochim. Biophys. Acta. 651:37–50.

Heppner, G. H., D. L. Dexter, T. DeNucci, F. R. Miller, and P. Calabresi. 1978. Heterogeneity in drug sensitivity among tumor cell subpopulations of a single mammary tumor. Cancer Res. 38:3758–3763.

Heppner, G. H., J. R. Ranken, and W. R. Shapiro. 1981. Tumor heterogeneity, *in* Pediatric Oncology I, G. B. Humphrey, L. P. Dehner, G. B. Grundey, and R. T. Action, eds. Martinus Nijhoff, The Hague, pp. 99–116.

Hibbs, J. B., Jr. 1974. Discrimination between neoplastic and non-neoplastic cells in vitro by activated macrophages. JNCI 53:1487–1492.

Kimball, P. M., and M. G. Brattain. 1980. Isolation of a cellular subpopulation from a human colonic carcinoma cell line. Cancer Res. 40:1574–1579.

Kripke, M. L., E. Gruys, and I. J. Fidler. 1978. Metastatic heterogeneity of cells from an ultraviolet light-induced murine fibrosarcoma of recent origin. Cancer Res. 38:2962–2967.

Kroener, J. F., F. Saleh, and S. B. Howell. 1982. 5-FU and allopurinol: Toxicity modulation and Phase II results in colon cancer. Cancer Treat. Rep. 66:1133–1137.

Leith, J. T., J. K. DeWyngaert, D. L. Dexter, P. Calabresi, and A. S. Glicksman. 1982a. Differential sensitivity of three human colon adenocarcinoma lines to hyperthermic cell killing. JNCI 61:381–383.

Leith, J. T., D. L. Dexter, J. K. DeWyngaert, E. M. Zeman, M. Y. Cha, P. Calabresi, and A. S. Glicksman. 1982b. Differential response to x-irradiation of subpopulations of two heterogeneous human carcinomas in vitro. Cancer Res. 42:2556–2561.

Leith, J. T., L. A. Gaskins, D. L. Dexter, P. Calabresi, and A. S. Glicksman. 1982c. Alteration of the survival response of two human colon carcinoma subpopulations to x-irradiation by N, N-dimethylformamide. Cancer Res. 42:30–34.

Liotta, L. A., C. Gattozzi, J. Kleinerman, and G. Saidel. 1977. Reduction of tumor cell entry into vessels by BCG-activated macrophages. Br. J. Cancer 36:639–641.

Liotta, L. A., K. Tryggvason, S. Garbisa, I. Hart, C. M. Foltz, and S. Shafie. 1980. Metastatic potential correlates with enzymatic degradation of basement collagen. Nature 284:67–68.

Lotan, R., and G. L. Nicolson. 1979. Heterogeneity in growth inhibition by β-transretinoic acid of metastatic B16 melanoma clones and in vivo-selected cell variant lines. Cancer Res. 39:4767–4771.

Miller, F. R., and G. H. Heppner. 1979. Immunologic heterogeneity of tumor cell subpopulations from a single mouse mammary tumor. JNCI 63:1457–1463.

Mitelman, F., J. Mark, G. Levan, and A. Levan. 1972. Tumor etiology and chromosome pattern. Science 176:1340–1341.

Nicolson, G. L., K. W. Brunson, and I. J. Fidler. 1977. Cell interactions in the metastatic process: Some cell surface properties associated with successful blood-borne tumor spread. Soc. Gen. Physiol. Ser. 32:225–241.

Nicolson, G. L., K. W. Brunson, and I. J. Fidler. 1978. Specificity of arrest, survival and growth of selected metastatic variant cell lines. Cancer Res. 38:4105–4111.

Petersen, S. E., P. Bichel, and M. Lorentzen. 1979. Flow-cytometric demonstration of tumor-cell subpopulations with different DNA content in human colorectal carcinoma. Eur. J. Cancer 15:383–386.

Pimm, M. W., and R. W. Baldwin. 1977. Antigenic differences between primary methylcholanthrene-induced rat sarcomas and post-surgical recurrences. Int. J. Cancer 20:37–43.

Poste, G. W., J. Doll, I. R. Hart, and I. J. Fidler. 1980. In vitro selection of murine B16 melanoma variants with enhanced tissue invasive properties. Cancer Res. 40:1636–1644.

Prehn, R. T. 1970. Analysis of antigenic heterogeneity within individual 3-methyl-cholanthrene induced mouse sarcomas. JNCI 45:1039–1045.

Rabotti, G. 1959. Ploidy of primary and metastatic human tumours. Nature 183:1276–1277.

Salmon, S. E., A. W. Hamburger, B. Soehnlen, B. G. M. Durie, D. S. Alberts, and T. E. Moon. 1978. Quantitation of differential sensitivity of human-tumor stem cells to anticancer drugs. N Engl. J. Med. 298:1321–1327.

Schlag, P., and W. Schreml. 1982. Heterogeneity in growth pattern and drug sensitivity of primary tumor and metastases in the human tumor colony-forming assay. Cancer Res. 42:4086–4089.

Shapiro, J. R., W-K. A. Yung, and W. R. Shapiro. 1981. Isolation, karyotype, and clonal growth of heterogeneous subpopulations of human malignant gliomas. Cancer Res. 41:2349–2359.

Siracky, J. 1979. An approach to the problem of heterogeneity of human tumour cell populations. Br. J. Cancer 39:570–577.

Slack, N. H., and I. D. J. Bross. 1975. The influence of site of metastasis on tumor growth and response to chemotherapy. Br. J. Cancer 32:78–86.

Spremulli, E., D. Dexter, K. McCarthy, G. Matook, P. Libbey, and P. Calabresi. 1982. Characterization of two new human melanoma cell lines. (Abstract) Clin. Res. 30:423A.

Spremulli, E. N., D. L. Dexter, P. Young, D. Campbell, and P. Calabresi. 1983a. Clonal origin of spontaneous metastases of a human colon carcinoma xenografted in nude mice. (Abstract) Proc. Am. Assoc. Cancer Res. 24:28.

Spremulli, E. N., C. Scott, D. E. Campbell, N. P. Libbey, D. Shochat, D. V. Gold, and D. L. Dexter. 1983b. Characterization of two metastatic subpopulations originating from a single human colon carcinoma. Cancer Res. 43:3828–3835.

Sugarbaker, E. V. 1979. Cancer metastasis: A product of tumor-host interactions. Curr. Probl. Cancer 3:1–59.

Sugarbaker, E. V., and A. M. Cohen. 1972. Altered antigenicity in spontaneous pulmonary metastases from an antigenic murine sarcoma. Surgery 72:155–161.

Sugarbaker, E. V., and A. S. Ketcham. 1977. Mechanisms and prevention of cancer dissemination: An overview. Semin. Oncol. 4:19–32.

Sugarbaker, P. H., J. S. MacDonald, and L. L. Gunderson. 1982. Colorectal cancer, *in* Cancer: Principles and Practices of Oncology, V. DeVita, Jr., S. Hellman, and S. A. Rosenberg, eds. J. B. Lippincott Co., Philadelphia, pp. 643–723.

Sugarbaker, E. V., J. T. Thornthwaite, and A. S. Ketcham. 1979. Transient changes in tumor-cell characteristics during spontaneous pulmonary metastasis formation. Surg. Forum 30:134–136.

Trope, C. 1975. Different sensitivity to cytostatic drugs of primary tumor and metastasis of the Lewis carcinoma. Neoplasma 22:171–180.

Tsuruo, T., and I. J. Fidler. 1981. Differences in drug sensitivities among tumor cells from parental tumors, selected variants and spontaneous metastases. Cancer Res. 41:3058–3064.

Vindeløv, L. L., H. H. Hansen, S. J. Christensen, M. Spang-Thomsen, F. R. Hirsch, M. Hansen, and N. I. Nissen. 1980. Clonal heterogeneity of small-cell anaplastic carcinoma of the lung demonstrated by flow-cytometric DNA analysis. Cancer Res. 40:4295–4300.

Yung, W-K. A., J. A. Shapiro, and W. R. Shapiro. 1982. Heterogeneous chemosensitivities of subpopulations of human glioma cells in culture. Cancer Res. 42:992–998.

Cancer Invasion and Metastasis: Biologic and Therapeutic Aspects edited by Garth L. Nicolson and Luka Milas. Raven Press, New York © 1984.

The Spectrum of Human Lung Cancer Cells in Culture: A Potential Model for Studying Molecular Determinants of Tumor Progression and Metastasis

Stephen B. Baylin, Rebecca H. Jackson, William Lennarz, Jr., and Joel H. Shaper*

*The Oncology Center, and the Departments of Medicine, and *Pharmacology and Experimental Therapeutics, The Johns Hopkins University Medical Institutions, Baltimore, Maryland 21205*

The complex bronchial mucosa of man gives rise to four major histologic types of lung cancer. These human tumors are potentially useful models for studying the mechanisms that account for tumor cell heterogeneity, tumor progression, resistance to therapy, and the variable metastatic behavior of different tumor cell populations. As yet, relatively few studies have been aimed directly at investigating these facets of lung cancer biology. However, recent investigations of lung cancer cells in culture, matched with the known clinical behavior of these tumors, suggest possibilities for further delineating biochemical properties of the different populations of lung cancer cells that play critical roles in the behavior of these neoplasms. It is the purpose of this brief review to highlight aspects of the biology of human lung cancer that relate to the clinical course of the disease, including the process of metastasis. It is hoped that the data discussed may stimulate a more direct investigation of properties of the different types of lung cancer cells, which might in turn explain their widely divergent metastatic potentials.

THE CLINICAL BEHAVIOR OF THE MAJOR TYPES OF HUMAN LUNG CANCER

Pathologists generally place the different human lung carcinomas into four major histologic classifications (Carter and Eggleston 1980). For the purposes of clinical and biologic behavior, the tumors can be contrasted as non-small cell (squamous, adeno- and large cell undifferentiated carcinomas) versus small (oat) cell lung carcinoma (SCC). SCC is an extremely virulent neoplasm, and relatively small primary lesions are often present when metastases occur, early in the course of disease. This early metastasizing activity dictates that patients with SCC are not candidates for surgical cure at the time of clinical presentation (Cohen and Matthews 1978, Greco and Oldham 1979, 1981). In contrast, the non-SCC lung cancers, although they metastasize, appear to do so later and less aggressively than SCC tumors. Consequently, much larger primary lesions can be seen prior to the appearance of overt metastases. Patients with SCC who present with stage I disease (tumor localized to one lung) have virtually no chance for a 5-year survival and only a 6-month average survival in the untreated state. In contrast, patients who undergo surgery for stage I non-SCC lung tumors have a 50% chance for 5-year survival (Mountain 1977).

Despite its more virulent growth behavior, SCC responds, initially, much more dramatically to chemotherapy and radiation therapy than do the non-SCC lung neoplasms. Hence, 40–80% rates of complete and partial remissions can be achieved in patients with SCC using combination drug treatment (for review, see Greco and Oldham 1981). The non-SCC tumors are generally nonresponsive to these same modes of therapy. Unfortunately, tumor almost always returns in all patients with SCC, and the disease is then resistant to further treatment. Hence, SCC remains essentially a lethal disease, and the average life expectancy with today's treatment regimens is approximately 12 months (Greco and Oldham 1981).

The factors that account for the very different growth patterns of SCC and non-SCC lung tumors have not been delineated. Recently, however, several groups have begun to study the biology and biochemistry of lung cancer cells in culture, and the data emerging may be highly relevant to the growth characteristics of these tumor cells in the human host. It is the purpose of the remainder of this review to highlight data that suggest that the spectrum of human lung carcinomas, studied in culture, may provide a valuable model for understanding further the properties of human cancer cells that exhibit a high metastatic potential and clinically significant tumor progression.

THE BEHAVIOR OF HUMAN LUNG CANCER CELLS IN CULTURE

Growth Characteristics of Small Cell Versus Non-Small Cell Human Lung Cancer

At least three laboratories have now had a number of years of experience in growing human SCC and non-SCC lung tumors in cell culture (Gazdar et al. 1980, Luk *et al.* 1981, Pettengill and Sorensen 1981). A number of well-established culture lines, plus documentation of tumor histology acquired by heterotransplants of the cells in the athymic nude mouse, have been derived. In all instances, the differences between SCC and non-SCC tumor cells have been striking for a number of parameters (summarized in Table 1). First, SCC cells in culture generally contain a high degree of neuroendocrine differentiation properties, including high activity of enzymes such as L-dopa decarboxylase and neuron-specific enolase (Baylin et al. 1980, Gazdar et al. 1980, Marangos

TABLE 1. *Comparisons between the types of human lung cancer in culture*

Properties	SCC	Large cell of SCC lineage	Non-SCC
Growth characteristics	Suspended cell aggregates	Monolayer	Monolayer
Neuroendocrine features (L-dopa decarboxylase, neuron-specific enolase, small polypeptide hormones, neurosecretory granules)	+	−	−
3p Chromosome deletion	+	+	−
Cell surface protein phenotype	SCC specific	SCC specific + several non-SCC proteins	Non-SCC specific
Radiation sensitivity	Sensitive	Resistant relative to SCC	?

Data compiled from: Baylin et al. 1982a, Gazdar et al. 1980, Goodwin and Baylin 1982, Goodwin et al. 1983, Marangos et al. 1982, Minna et al. 1982, Pettengill and Sorenson 1981, Whang-Peng et al. 1982.

et al. 1982), ultrastructural features of neuroendocrine differentiation (Gazdar et al. 1981, Pettengill and Sorenson 1981), and a higher content of several small polypeptide hormones (Gazdar et al. 1981, Pettengill and Sorensen 1981). Second, a specific karyotypic marker chromosome has been defined for SCC cells (Whang-Peng et al. 1982).

Finally, and perhaps most important to the subject of this review, there are significant differences in the growth patterns between SCC and non-SCC lung cancer cells; these differences may be most revealing for considering the metastatic potential of these neoplasms. Lines of non-SCC human lung cancers grow as typical monolayers in culture (Gazdar et al 1980, 1981). In contrast, a high percentage of SCC lines lack anchorage dependency over the first year or two of growth in culture. The lines of SCC tumors grow as suspended aggregates of cells with varying degrees of intercellular adhesiveness and morphologies (Gazdar et al. 1980, 1981, Pettengill and Sorensen 1981). In some lines, such as OH-1 developed in our laboratories (Francis et al. 1983, Luk et al. 1981), the cell-cell surface contact in the early passages is extensive. The floating aggregates of cells in this line spontaneously form tight spheroidal aggregates (Francis et al. 1983, Luk et al. 1981).

Factors That Potentially Mediate the Aggregate Growth Pattern of SCC Cells

Cell Surface Morphology of SCC Cells

We have investigated the degree of cell-cell surface contact within aggregates of OH-1 SCC cells at the level of the electron microscope. Although most of the results are to be published in detail elsewhere, they can be summarized briefly as follows. As visualized by transmission electron microscopy, there is extensive contact between adjacent cells over the total area of the surface membranes (Goodwin and Baylin 1982). The shape of one cell appears to be molded to the shape of its neighboring cell. More recent scanning electron microscopy studies reveal that these membrane interactions are mediated by contact of numerous cytoplasmic processes. These processes, or filopodia, extend irregularly from the surface of a given cell and extensively engage the cytoplasmic processes of neighboring cells.

Cell Surface Protein Phenotype of Human Lung Cancer Cells

Over the past 2 years, our laboratory has worked to establish whether differences in the cell surface protein phenotype might exist between SCC and non-SCC human lung cancer cells in culture. By a combination of cell surface iodination and two-dimensional polyacrylamide gel electrophoresis, we have shown that the cell surface protein pattern for SCC is distinct from that for the non-SCC tumor cells (Baylin et al. 1982a). This work has been reviewed in detail elsewhere (Baylin et al. 1982b), and we will only comment briefly on the differences here. For SCC cells, iodination studies reveal a group of surface proteins with monomer subunit sizes ranging between 30 and 100 kilodaltons (kD). Twelve of these proteins appear to be unique to the SCC cells compared with non-SCC lung cancer cells. The non-SCC tumor cells (including adenocarcinoma, squamous carcinoma, and some types of large cell undifferentiated carcinoma), which show anchorage dependency in culture, are characterized by a predominance of the surface iodination labeling in a series of proteins of greater than 100 kD, absence of the 12 unique SCC proteins, and the presence of another 9 proteins of between 30 and 100 kD that are not seen on the SCC cells.

The functional role of the cell surface proteins we have thus far identified remains to be established. Whether one or more of these proteins may mediate, at the molecular level, intercellular adhesion of SCC cells merits serious consideration and further investigation. We are currently preparing specific antibodies to a number of the SCC and non-SCC cell surface proteins to directly probe these interesting questions.

A Potential Role for Carbohydrate Moieties in Intercellular Adhesion of SCC Cells

We have obtained initial evidence that surface glycoproteins or glycolipids may be important to the growth of the suspended cell aggregates formed by the OH-1 line of SCC. The details of these studies have been given in abstract form (Jackson et al. 1981) and are to be published elsewhere. In brief, treatment of SCC cell aggregates with the antibiotic tunicamycin—a specific inhibitor of N-glycosylation of proteins and, as shown recently, of incorporation of carbohydrate moieties into glycosphingolipids (Guarnaccia et al. 1983)—can alter the morphology and the maintenance of SCC spheroids. When early passage OH-1 cultures are treated at the time of single-cell seeding, a specific block in protein glycosylation precedes inhibition of protein and DNA synthesis by 48–72 h. The apparent loss of N-linked carbohydrate moieties on cell surface proteins and/or on glycolipids leads to disruption of the spheroidal aggregates of OH-1 cells. By 48 h, the aggregates begin to show progressive disorganization, leading to cell death. It is not known whether the block by tunicamycin affects: (a) carbohydrate moieties in proteins or lipids that are specifically responsible for cell-cell adhesion or (b) the rate of turnover of membrane proteins that become more susceptible to proteolysis owing to the absence of carbohydrate moieties (for review, see Olden et al. 1982).

POTENTIAL DIFFERENTIATION RELATIONSHIPS BETWEEN SCC AND NON-SCC LUNG CANCERS THAT MAY DETERMINE THE COURSE OF SCC TUMOR PROGRESSION

Clinical and Biological Background

An important development in the study of human lung cancers over the past decade has been the accumulating evidence that all of the major types, including SCC, may be linked to one another through a common differentiation cell lineage within the bronchial mucosa. We have reviewed these concepts in detail elsewhere (Baylin 1983, Baylin et al. 1982b, Gazdar et al. 1981) and can summarize them briefly as follows.

SCC tumors, because of their expression of neuroendocrine differentiation features, have been thought to arise in a small population of endocrine cells present in the bronchial mucosa of man and other species (Cutz et al. 1975, Terzakis et al. 1972). In turn, some investigators have postulated that these endocrine cells may be of neuroectodermal embryologic origin (Pearse 1969), in contrast to the other cell types in the bronchial mucosa that are endodermally derived. However, it is now apparent that, in the host, neuroendocrine properties are not restricted to SCC among the human lung cancers (Baylin and Gazdar 1981, Berger et al. 1981, McDowell et al. 1981) and that mixtures of SCC and non-SCC histologies can be found within the same patient and even within the same tumor lesion (Abeloff et al. 1979, Berger et al. 1981, Brereton et al. 1978, McDowell et al. 1981).

Most important, there is also evidence that time-dependent transitions in tumor types may occur within patients, and the vector appears to involve the loss of SCC features and appearance of non-SCC features. Thus, some patients with well-confirmed initial diagnoses of SCC may, after initial treatment response and relapse, have only non-SCC tumor histologies at autopsy (Abeloff et al. 1979, Brereton et al. 1978).

Studies of Tumor Progression in Culture

Implications for Treatment Response

The change from SCC to a type of non-SCC lung cancer, specifically large cell undifferentiated carcinoma (see summary in Table 1), has now been documented in cell culture (Gazdar et al. 1981). Over time, a significant number of well-established SCC cultures lose their neuroendocrine differentiation features and change, as evaluated by heterotransplants in the nude mouse, from SCC to large cell undifferentiated tumors (Gazdar et al. 1981). The large cell tumor that evolves in culture is composed of a cell type found in patients (Goodwin et al. 1983). Analyses of the surface protein phenotype of clones of these cells show them to have an apparently totipotent differentiation capability with respect to all of the major types of human lung cancer (Goodwin et al. 1983).

The potential for interchange between the types of human lung carcinomas, along a cell differentiation lineage operative within the cells from which these tumors arise, could have significant consequences for the treatment response of SCC cells. We now know that even a slight progression of SCC towards the non-SCC phenotype in culture, which involves a loss of neuroendocrine features but little change in histologic appearance of the cells, can increase the radiation resistance of such cells (Goodwin and Baylin 1982). These studies were performed in OH-1 cells, which, after 16 months in culture, showed a rapid loss of neuroendocrine differentiation features but retained, in cytology studies and in nude mouse heterotransplants, the SCC histologic phenotype.

Relationships Between the Changing Phenotype of SCC Cells, Cell-Cell Contact, and Cell Surface Morphology

When most lines of SCC cells lose their endocrine phenotype and assume large cell undifferentiated histology in nude mouse heterotransplants, they dramatically alter their growth characteristics in culture. Anchorage dependency usually appears, and the cells grow as monolayers rather than suspended aggregates (Gazdar et al. 1981, Goodwin et al. 1983).

Our electron microscopy studies have documented that even the loss of neuroendocrine phenotype in OH-1 cells, without a change in histology or appearance of anchorage dependency, can coincide with dramatic changes in cell surface morphology. Intercellular contact is much reduced as viewed by transmission electron microscopy (Goodwin and Baylin 1982). At the level of scanning electron microscopy, this change becomes even more apparent. The late passage OH-1 cells are more rounded and exhibit much less contact between neighboring cells. The surfaces of the late passage OH-1 cells, compared with the early passage cells, have become much smoother and the cytoplasmic extensions are much narrower. Also, these cytoplasmic extensions are much more regularly spaced along the surface of the cells, and the degree of contact between processes from one cell to another is significantly reduced.

Implications of Studies of Cultured Human Lung Cancer Cells for In Vivo Behavior

The data we reviewed above suggest many analogies between cultured human lung cancer cells and the behavior of the corresponding tumor types in the human host. Of particular interest is the conversion of SCC toward the non-SCC phenotype, which may be an integral feature of (a) the cellular heterogeneity seen in SCC lesions within individual patients and between patients (Baylin et al. 1982b, Berger et al. 1981) and (b) the overlapping of characteristics between SCC and non-SCC tumors. In turn, given the different characteristics of SCC and non-SCC tumors, including treatment sensitivity and metastasizing potential, the drift of SCC toward the non-SCC phenotype in culture could have profound implications for the in vivo behavior of SCC tumors.

At present, precise extrapolation from the culture data to the metastatic behavior of lung cancer in the human host is not possible. However, the data invite such speculation and, most important, more direct studies. For example, apparent avidity of individual cells for each other in the aggregate growth of most culture lines of SCC may relate to a process that contributes significantly, in vivo, to the highly metastatic nature of this neoplasm. Many investigators of the metastatic process have stressed the importance of such homotypic cell-cell adhesion (for review, see Nicolson and Poste 1982, also Nicolson 1978a, 1978b, Fidler 1973). Single tumor cells, when migrating from the area of primary growth, may have far less chance of establishing residence in other parts of the body than do small, tightly adherent cell aggregates.

Indeed, where specifically studied in nonhuman tumors, increased cell-cell adhesion tendencies are most characteristic of cell populations with high metastatic behavior. Small clumps of tumor cells have more probability than do single cells of arresting in small capillaries or lymph channels and thus setting up a condition favorable for a metastatic lesion to form (for review, see Nicolson and Poste 1982, also, Fidler 1973, Liotta et al. 1976). Also, the clump of cells so trapped establishes an initial microenvironment of tumor cells capable of interacting with one another in a manner favorable for allowing these "foreign cells" to establish a nidus of growth in the microvascular or lymph channel areas in which they are trapped.

It is significant that the aggregate growth of SCC cells in culture is not dissimilar to that seen in the human host. The metastatic lesions of SCC also grow as generally well circumscribed nodules scattered in small metastatic deposits. This pattern is often seen best in the hepatic metastases from these tumors, which are characterized by circular lesions, often with a central necrotic core.

The changes in the cell surface morphology coincident with the loss of the neuroendocrine phenotype of late-passage OH-1 cells could also have consequences for the differences in metastatic behavior between SCC and non-SCC lung cancer cells in the context of our discussions above. While individual cells can separate more easily from late passage than from early passage OH-1 cells—which might favor metastatic potential—the cell clumps that do break off from such aggregates would contain fewer cells and be much less susceptible to trapping in microvascular or microlymphatic channels. Therefore, these changes in the surface properties of the OH-1 cells and of other SCC culture lines that lose SCC properties could provide a valuable model for studying molecular events that may be instrumental in determining the metastasizing capacity of human cancer cells.

The molecular events that may mediate these changes in cell-cell adhesion between early and late passages of SCC culture lines remain to be determined. Studies are under way in our own laboratory to investigate whether changes in the cell surface proteins we have described may accompany the loss of SCC features with time. Specifically, we need to know whether the proteins characteristic of the non-SCC lung tumor types are acquired by SCC cells during the time of their transition to large cell carcinoma. Our studies of a line of large cell undifferentiated tumor cells that apparently arose from cells of SCC lineage indicates that the cell surface protein phenotype can, in single clones of such cells, be characteristic of both SCC and non-SCC tumor cells (Goodwin et al. 1983).

Chemical manipulations of early and late passages of SCC cells may also prove revealing. Use of agents such as retinoids, phorbol esters, etc., may prove valuable for further exploring the precise differentiation relationships between large undifferentiated cells and the major differentiated forms of human lung cancer. Such studies are ongoing in our laboratory.

Also, further studies of the effects of tunicamycin on SCC cells in culture may prove rewarding for exploring the relationships between the growth properties of these cells and their in vivo behavior. Results of such studies could be compared to the known effects of tunicamycin in altering the metastasizing capacity of nonhuman cancer cells (for review, see Nicolson and Poste 1982, also Irimura and Nicolson 1981, Irimura et al. 1981).

The change from SCC non-SCC tumor in culture may, then, provide a useful model for investigating properties that mediate cell-cell adhesion and various aspects of the metastatic process. One important component, however, is necessary for direct implementation of such studies. A model must be developed wherein the direct correlation between the biochemical properties of cultured lung cancer cells and their metastatic behavior can be examined. To date, we are not aware of attempts to construct such models. Perhaps recent maneuvers with nude mice (Hanna 1983, see pages 309–319, this volume), which may make possible the direct study of human tumor metastasis, would prove ideal for this type of work. We think such investigations will be most rewarding for correlating the findings reviewed in this manuscript with the processes of tumor progression and metastasis in human neoplasms.

SUMMARY

We have reviewed the behavior of human lung cancer cells in culture. We have considered the implications of cell biology and biochemistry studies of the cultured cells for the in vivo behavior of lung neoplasms, including the metastatic potential of the different tumor types. Among the human lung cancers, SCC, which grows in culture as suspended aggregates of adherent cells, metastasizes earlier in the life cycle of the tumor and more widely than the major types of non-SCC lung cancers. These latter tumors grow as anchorage-dependent cells in culture. We have pointed out that ultrastructural studies of cultured human lung cancer cells reveal dramatic changes in cell surface membrane morphology coincident with progressive loss of SCC features and intercellular adhesion. We have stressed the potential value of these cultures of human lung cancer cells for studying the molecular determinants of intercellular adhesion and their importance to the process of metastasis. In this context, we have stressed that a different cell surface protein phenotype exists between SCC and non-SCC lung cancer cells in culture and that some of these proteins could be intimately involved in the different growth behavior patterns of these tumor cells. Finally, we have pointed out the need to construct models in which the growth characteristics and biochemical properties of cultured lung cancer cells can be *directly* compared in vivo with their metastatic potential.

ACKNOWLEDGMENTS

We appreciate the secretarial assistance of Ms. Alverta Fields in preparation of the manuscript. Portions of the studies cited were supported by grants CA18404 and CA30471 from the National Cancer Institute, grant ACS-PDT108 from the American Cancer Society, and a gift from the W. W. Smith Foundation.

REFERENCES

Abeloff, M. D., J. C. Eggleston, G. Mendelsohn, D. S. Ettinger, and S. B. Baylin. 1979. Changes in morphologic and biochemical characteristics of small cell carcinoma of the lung—A clinicopathologic study. Am. J. Med. 66:757–764.

Baylin, S. B. 1983. Biochemical markers of small (oat) cell lung carcinoma—Biological and clinical implications, *in* Oncodevelopmental Markers, W. H. Fishman, ed. Academic Press, New York, pp. 259–277.

Baylin, S. B., M. D. Abeloff, G. Goodwin, D. N. Carney, and A. F. Gazdar. 1980. Activities of L-dopa decarboxylase and diamine oxidase (histaminase) in human lung cancers and decarboxylase as a marker for small (oat) cell cancer in cell culture. Cancer Res. 40:1990–1994.

Baylin, S. B., and A. F. Gazdar. 1981. Endocrine biochemistry in the spectrum of human lung cancer: Implications for the cellular origin of small cell carcinoma, *in* Small Cell Lung Cancer, F. A. Greco, R. K. Oldham, and P. A. Bunn, Jr., eds. Grune and Stratton, New York, pp. 123–143

Baylin, S. B., A. F. Gazdar, J. D. Minna, S. D. Bernal, and J. H. Shaper. 1982a. A unique cell surface protein phenotype distinguishes human small-cell from non-small cell lung cancer. Proc. Natl. Acad. Sci. USA 79:4650–4654.

Baylin, S. B., G. Goodwin, and J. H. Shaper. 1982b. Analysis of cell surface proteins as a means to study differentiation in the spectrum of human lung cancers, *in* 18th Symposium Medicum Hoechst—Systemic Role of Regulation Peptides, S. Bloom, J. Polak, and E. Lindenlaub, eds. F. K. Schattauer, Verlag, Stuttgart, pp. 307–328.

Berger, C. L., G. Goodwin, G. Mendelsohn, J. C. Eggleston, M. D. Abeloff, S. Aisner, and S. B. Baylin. 1981. Endocrine-related biochemistry in the spectrum of human lung carcinoma. J. Clin. Endocrinol. Metab. 53:422–429.

Brereton, H. D., M. M. Matthews, J. Costa, H. Kent, and R. E. Johnson. 1978. Mixed anaplastic small-cell and squamous-cell carcinoma of the lung. Ann. Intern. Med. 88:805–806.

Carter, D., and J. C. Eggleston. 1980. Tumors of the lower respiratory tract, *in* Atlas of Tumor Pathology, 2nd Series—Fascicle 17. Armed Forces Institute of Pathology, Washington, D.C., pp. 59–69.

Cohen, M. H., and M. J. Matthews. 1978. Small cell bronchogenic carcinoma: A distinct clinicopathologic entity. Semin. Oncol. 5:234–243.

Cutz, E., W. Chan, and V. Wong. 1975. Ultrastructure and fluorescence histochemistry of endocrine (APUD-type) cells in tracheal mucosa of human and various animal species. Cell Tissue Res. 158:425–437.

Fidler, I. J. 1973. The relationship of embolic homogeneity, number, size and viability to the incidence of experimental metastasis. Eur. J. Cancer 9:223–227.

Francis, J., R. Thompson, S. D. Bernal, G. D. Luk, and S. B. Baylin. 1983. Effects of dibutylryl cyclic adenosine 3′:5′-monophosphate on the growth of cultured human small-cell lung carcinoma and the specific cellular activity of L-dopa decarboxylase. Cancer Res. 43:639–645.

Gazdar, A. F., D. N. Carney, J. G. Guccion, and S. B. Baylin. 1981. Small cell carcinoma of the lung: Cellular origin and relationship to other pulmonary tumors, *in* Small Cell Lung Cancer, F. A. Greco, R. K. Oldham, and P. A. Bunn, Jr., eds. Grune and Stratton, New York, pp. 145–175.

Gazdar, A. F., D. N. Carney, E. K. Russell, H. L. Sims, S. B. Baylin, P. A. Bunn, Jr., J. G. Guccion, and J. D. Minna. 1980. Establishment of continuous clonable cultures of small-cell carcinoma of the lung which have amine precursor uptake and decarboxylation cell properties. Cancer Res. 40:3502–3507.

Goodwin, G., and S. B. Baylin, 1982. Relationships between neuroendocrine differentiation and sensitivity to γ-radiation in culture line O-H-1 of human small cell lung carcinoma. Cancer Res. 42:1361–1367.

Goodwin, G., J. H. Shaper, M. D. Abeloff, G. Mendelsohn, and S. B. Baylin. 1983. Analysis of cell surface proteins delineates a differentiation pathway linking endocrine and nonendocrine human lung cancers. Proc. Natl. Acad. Sci. USA. 80:3807–3811.

Greco, F. A., and R. K. Oldham. 1979. Small cell lung cancer. N. Engl. J. Med. 301:355–358.

Greco, F. A., and R. K. Oldham. 1981. Clinical management of patients with small cell lung cancer, *in* Small Cell Lung Cancer, F. A. Greco, R. K. Oldham, and P. A. Bunn, Jr., eds. Grune and Stratton, New York, pp. 353–379.

Guarnaccia, S. P., J. H. Shaper, and R. L. Schnaar. 1983. Tunicamycin inhibits ganglioside biosynthesis in neuronal cells. Proc. Natl. Acad. Sci. USA 80:1551–1555.

Hanna, N. 1983. Role of natural killer cells in host defense against cancer metastasis, *in* Cancer Invasion and Metastasis: Biologic and Therapeutic Aspects, G. Nicolson and L. Milas, eds. Raven Press, New York, pp. 309–319.

Irimura, T., and G. L. Nicolson. 1981. The role of glycoconjugates in metastatic melanoma blood-borne arrest and cell surface properties. J. Supramol. Struct. Cell. Biochem. 17:325–336.

Irimura, T., R. Gonzalez, and G. L. Nicolson. 1981. Effects of tunicamycin on B16 metastatic melanoma cell surface glycoproteins and blood-borne arrest and survival properties. Cancer Res. 41:3411–3418.

Jackson, R. D., G. Goodwin, J. H. Shaper, and S. B. Baylin. 1981. A loss of neuroendocrine differentiation accompanies a conversion of small cell cancer to its large cell variant in culture. (Abstract) Proceedings of the 63rd Annual Meeting of the Endocrine Society 61:Abs. p. 127.

Liotta, L. A., J. Kleinerman, and G. M. Saidel. 1976. The significance of hematogenous tumor cell clumps in the metastatic process. Cancer Res. 36:889–894.

Luk, G. D., G. Goodwin, L. J. Marton, and S. B. Baylin. 1981. Polyamines are necessary for the survival of human small-cell lung carcinoma in culture. Proc. Natl. Acad. Sci. USA 78:2355–2358.

Marangos, P. J., A. F. Gazdar, and D. N. Carney. 1982. Neuron specific enolase in human small cell carcinoma cultures. Cancer Lett. 15:67–71.

McDowell, E. M., T. S. Wilson, and B. F. Trump. 1981. Atypical endocrine tumors of the lung. Arch. Pathol. Lab. Med. 105:20–28.

Minna, J. D., D. N. Carney, R. Alvarez, P. A. Bunn, F. Cuttitta, D. C. Ihde, M. J. Matthews, H. Oie, S. Rosen, J. Whang-Peng, and A. F. Gazdar. 1982. Heterogeneity and homogeneity of human small cell lung cancer, *in* Tumor Cell Heterogeneity—Origins and Implications, A. H. Owens, Jr., D. S. Coffey, and S. B. Baylin, eds. Academic Press, New York, pp. 29–52.

Mountain, C. F. 1977. Biologic, physiologic and technical determinants in surgical therapy for lung cancer, *in* Lung Cancer—Clinical Diagnosis and Treatment, M. S. Strauss, ed. Grune and Stratton, New York, pp. 185–198.

Nicolson, G. L. 1978a. Cell and tissue interactions leading to malignant tumor spread (metastasis). Am. Zool. 18:77–86.

Nicolson, G. L. 1978b. Experimental tumor metastasis: Characteristics and organ specificity. Bioscience 28:441–447.

Nicolson, G. L., and G. Poste. 1982. Tumor cell diversity and host responses in cancer metastasis. Current Problems in Cancer 7:54, 57–58.

Olden, K., J. B. Parent, and S. L. White. 1982. Carbohydrate moieties of glycoproteins: A reevaluation of their function. Biochim. Biophys. Acta 650:209–232.

Pearse, A. G. E. 1969. The cytochemistry and ultrastructure of polypeptide hormone-producing cells of the APUD series and the embryologic, physiologic, and pathologic implications of the concept. J. Histochem. Cytochem. 17:303–313.

Pettengill, O. S. and G. D. Sorenson. 1981. Tissue culture and in vitro characteristics, *in* Small Cell Lung Cancer, F. A. Greco, R. K. Oldham, and P. A. Bunn, Jr., eds. Grune and Stratton, New York, pp. 51–77.

Terzakis, J., S. Sommers, and B. Andersson. 1972. Neurosecretory appearing cells of human segmental bronchi. Lab. Invest. 26:127–132.

Whang-Peng, J., C. S. Kao-Shan, E. C. Lee, P. A. Bunn, D. N. Carney, A. F. Gazdar, and J. D. Minna. 1982. Specific chromosome defect associated with human small-cell lung cancer: Deletion 3p (14–23). Science 215:181–182.

Host Factors and Metastasis

Cancer Invasion and Metastasis: Biologic and Therapeutic Aspects edited by Garth L. Nicolson and Luka Milas. Raven Press, New York © 1984.

Host-Mediated Mechanisms in the Elimination of Circulating Cancer Cells

Peter Alexander and Suzanne A. Eccles*

*Department of Medical Oncology, University of Southhampton, Southampton General Hospital, Hants S09 4XY England, and *Institute of Cancer Research, Sutton, Surrey, SM2 5PX England*

One of the key features of tumor metastasis is the relative inefficiency of the process. It has been calculated from both the survival of i.v. inoculated cells (Weiss 1980, 1982) and the disparity between cells spontaneously shed from a growing tumor and the number of overt metastatic colonies yielded (Butler and Gullino 1975, Schirrmacher and Waller 1982) that the survival of disseminated cells may be considerably lower than 1%. Although mechanical trauma may be a major cause of death of circulating tumor cells, there are many experimental systems in which host defense mechanisms are implicated in the failure of a tumor to produce overt metastases. Such processes can be inferred from systems in which tumors are "cured" by local therapy, yet the malignant cells that compose the tumor are shown to possess all of the properties required for invasion, dissemination, and metastatic growth.

Several mechanisms can be envisaged by which the host prevents disseminated cancer cells from expressing their metastatic potential: (1) Destruction of circulating cells by specific (T-cell-dependent) cellular or humoral effector mechanisms directed against immunogenic cell membrane constituents (e.g., tumor-specific transplantation antigens, viral antigens); (2) Loss of clonogenic potential and/or establishment of a dormant state because of terminal differentiation occurring within the microenvironment of the host, induced either by hormones or by the local absence of appropriate growth factors; (3) Death of tumor cells in capillary beds before extravasation is achieved (perhaps a result of oxygen toxicity).

In this report, we will summarize data from experimental tumor systems in which host immune mechanisms play a critical role in determining the incidence of metastatic disease and discuss those in which metastasis fails for other reasons. We will then describe preliminary results from experiments aimed at limiting the growth of micrometastases by treatments that promote cellular differentiation. Finally, we will summarize data that suggest that oxygen toxicity plays a part in the rapid death of tumor cells arrested in capillary beds.

IMMUNE FACTORS IN THE PREVENTION OF METASTASIS

We have demonstrated that for chemically induced sarcomas in the rat and in some mouse strains (vide infra), T-cell-dependent immune reactions determine the incidence of overt spontaneous metastases. Comparable results were obtained with mouse lymphomas.

The experimental protocol consisted of transplanting non-enzyme-treated tumor cells intramuscularly in the thigh, or subcutaneously in the flank, and allowing them to grow for 14–28 days to an average diameter of 2 cm in rats or 1 cm in mice, at which point they were surgically removed. The animals were observed for 6–12 months to allow the natural development of disseminated tumor cells. Animals could be immunosuppressed during or after the local tumor growth period to determine the influence of host immunity on tumor cell shedding and dissemination or on subsequent colonization and growth phases. Tumor immunogenicity was assessed from the relative increase in the number of tumor cells required to induce a tumor (TD_{50} values) in animals preimmunized by tumor growth and excision compared with normal animals.

The evidence for immunological control of metastasis in these tumor systems is as follows:

1. There was an inverse correlation between the immunogenicity of rat and mouse sarcomas and their metastatic capacity (Eccles and Alexander 1974, Eccles 1982a, 1982b). Similar relationships have been reported for a series of chemically induced rat mammary carcinomas (Kim 1970), mouse sarcomas (Fidler et al. 1979), mouse lymphomas (Davey et al. 1979), and mouse colorectal carcinomas (Belnap et al. 1979), indicating that this property is not peculiar to rat sarcomas. However, it may best be demonstrated with chemically induced tumors whose potential spectrum of immunogenicity seems to be greater than for other (e.g., virally associated or spontaneous) tumors.

2. Poorly metastatic or nonmetastatic tumors yielded widespread disseminated disease in various categories of immunosuppressed hosts (Eccles and Alexander 1975, Eccles et al. 1979, 1980, Eccles 1980, 1982b). Immunosuppressive procedures we have successfully employed to promote metastases from sarcomas and lymphomas include whole-body x-irradiation and cortisone administration, which nonspecifically damage immunocyte precursors in the marrow; use of thymectomized and congenitally athymic animals, which are deficient in thymocytes; administration of a variety of drugs that show degrees of selectivity against T-lymphocytes (e.g., asparaginase, deoxycoformycine, cyclosporin A), and use of silica, which abrogates macrophage function.

Since some of the procedures employed may affect nonimmunological aspects of the host's physiology, we investigated the possibility that these influence the outcome of metastatic disease. We found, however, that the blood coagulability was unaffected in most cases (P. Hilgard, personal communication) and that all of these tumors were resistant to natural killer (NK) cell cytotoxicity (I. Parr, personal communication). In addition, we were able to reconstitute the animal's ability to inhibit metastasis development with lymphoid cells, and in some cases with serum from immunized or tumor-bearing animals (Eccles 1978, Proctor et al. 1973). Table 1 shows that in the case of HSN rat sarcoma, tumor-bearer serum was more effective than thoracic duct lymphocytes in restoring resistance to lung metastases following immune suppression by prolonged draining of thoracic duct lymph. Others have shown that the enhanced metastasis induced by thymectomy (with or without irradiation) from Lewis lung carcinoma (Carnaud et al. 1974) or epidermoid carcinoma (Suurkula and Boeryd 1975) could be reversed by spleen cells and that of murine fibrosarcomas by thymocytes (Kearney et al. 1975).

Athymic animals fail to produce specific antibodies against growing tumors, and this failure may contribute to the more widespread disseminated disease in these animals than in immunocompetent controls (Eccles et al. 1979). Recent experiments have shown that i.v. administration of tumor-specific monoclonal antibodies produced by the fusion of syngeneic tumor-bearer spleen cells and the Y3 myeloma can prevent overt metastasis in over 50% of animals treated (North and Dean 1983).

The effector mechanisms that control the development of spontaneous tumor metastases in immunocompetent animals is not clear, since different experiments implicate T lymphocytes, mononuclear phagocytes, or humoral antibodies. In

TABLE 1. *Effect of immunosuppression and cellular or humoral reconstitution on spontaneous tumor metastasis**

			Metastases	
Tumor	Immuno-suppression	Reconsti-tution	Incidence (%)	Weight (g)
HSH†	None	None	0	—
	TDL depletion	None	100	3.0–4.6
	TDL depletion	TDL	100	1.8–2.7
	TDL depletion	NS	100	2.4–3.4
	TDL depletion	TBS	0–10	0–0.1
HSBPA‡§	None	None	10–14	NT
	TDL depletion	None	72	NT
	X-irradiation	None	75	NT
	X-irradiation	LNC	15	NT
	X-irradiation	TBS	52	NT
				No. nodules
MC24″	nu/nu athymic	None	100	>200
	nu/nu athymic	MAb	47	0–200

* All tumors are chemically induced fibrosarcomas in Lister hooded/Cbi rats.
† Proctor et al. 1973
‡ Eccles and Alexander 1974.
§ Eccles 1978.
″ North and Dean 1983.
TDL, thoracic duct lymphocytes; LNC, lymph node cells; NS, normal rat serum; TBS, tumor-bearer rat serum; MAb, syngeneic tumor-specific monoclonal antibody M10/76; NT, not tested.

a model experiment (Denham et al. 1980) in which an alloantiserum was used against a rat leukemia growing in immunosuppressed allogeneic hosts, antibody caused the elimination of circulating tumor cells by immunophagocytosis; complement-dependent lysis played no part.

In other systems, it has been shown that antibody can suppress tumor growth if sufficient macrophages are present at the site (Johnson et al. 1979), and recently Herlyn and Koprowski (1982) have implicated Fc receptor–bearing mononuclear cells in the antibody-mediated inhibition of growth of human xenografts in nude mice. Taken together, the data suggest to us that mononuclear phagocytes in the circulating blood and within the tumor mass cooperate with humoral antibodies to destroy immunogenic tumor cells and prevent their successful dissemination and colonization of distant sites. T lymphocytes are required for antibody production, and also release factors that activate macrophages, and they are therefore required for the induction of the antitumor response.

Less work has been done on the role of immunity in the control of carcinoma metastasis. Carnaud et al. (1974) showed that thymectomy and irradiation could increase the number and weight of Lewis lung carcinoma metastases, and the same procedures have been shown to enhance metastasis of a murine mammary adenocarcinoma (Parthenais and Haskill 1979), murine hepatoma (Makidono et al. 1976), and epidermoid carcinoma (Suurkula and Boeryd 1975). Also, Agosin et al. (1952) found that cortisone induced metastases from a "nonmetastatic" murine mammary carcinoma.

We have investigated spontaneous metastasis in a series of murine mammary carcinomas and a series of chemically induced squamous cell carcinomas for its susceptibility to immune-mediated control. These tumors differed from the rat and mouse sarcomas and lymphomas already described in that, although only weakly or moderately immunogenic, they did not generally (in early in vivo transplant generations) yield widespread spontaneous metastases. Also, when three different mammary carcinomas and three squamous cell carcinomas were grown in cyclosporin A–immunosuppressed recipients, no significant increase in metastatic disease was seen (Eccles et al. 1980). We have since extended these observations, and the results to date are shown in Tables 2 and 3. These data by and large confirm our earlier findings that, in general, metastasis of syngeneic carcinomas of recent origin is not significantly enhanced by a number of immunosuppressive maneuvers, especially in the case of mammary carcinomas, where only ST4 shows any suggestion of increased metastasis following host immunosuppression.

In squamous cell carcinomas, however, two tumors responded to host immunosuppression by an increased incidence of spontaneous metastasis. CA6 is a moderately well differentiated tumor that was demonstrably more immunogenic than the other tumors in the CA series. (The TD_{50} increased by 2–3 logs in immunized mice.) DM6 originally was a well-differentiated keratinizing squamous cell carcinoma that likewise showed significant levels of immunogenicity (up to 1½ logs), but at passage 3 did not respond to host immunosuppression. However, at

TABLE 2. *Effects of host immunocompetence on murine mammary carcinoma metastasis*

Tumor	Host	Immunosuppression	Incidence metastasis (%)
MT1	CBA	None	0–10
		Cyclosporin A	0
		Cortisone	0
MT3	CBA	None	10–20
		Cyclosporin A	10
		Cortisone	10
		Nu/nu athymic	0
MT5	CBA	None	0–10
		Cyclosporin A	10
		Cortisone	0
SM1	C57	None	100
		Cyclosporin A	100
		Nu/nu athymic	100
ST4	CBA	None	0–20
		Cyclosporin A	30
		Cortisone	10
		TXI	40
		Nu/nu athymic	40

TXI, neonatal thymectomy plus whole-body X-irradiation; cyclosporin A: 80 (CBA) and 200 (C57) mg/kg s.c.; cortisone: 80 mg/kg i.p./wk × 3.

TABLE 3. *Effects of host immunocompetence on murine squamous cell carcinoma metastasis*

Tumor	Host	Immunosuppression	Incidence metastasis (%)
DM1	C57	None	40
		Cyclosporin A	20
DM2	C57	None	10–20
		Cyclosporin A	10
		Nu/nu athymic	30
DM6, p3	C57	None	0
		Cyclosporin A	20
DM6, p6	C57	None	20
		Cyclosporin A	90
		TXI	70
CA2	C57	None	20
		Cyclosporin A	20
		TXI	10
CA4	C57	None	0
		Cyclosporin A	0
CA6	C57	None	10
		Cyclosporin A	90

DM series; induced by skin painting of mice with dimethylbenzanthracene.

CA series; induced by skin painting of mice with methylcholanthrene and promotion with croton oil.

TXI, neonatal thymectomy + whole-body X-irradiation.

Cyclosporin A: 200 mg/kg s.c.

the sixth transplant generation, the tumor gave metastases in 20% of control animals and 70–90% of immunosuppressed animals. During this period, the tumor had retained a degree of immunogenicity, but showed a much less well differentiated morphology; keratin was absent and the cells less well organized and more anaplastic.

We have previously reported that with serial transplantation in syngeneic recipients, originally well-differentiated carcinomas can become progressively less differentiated and that this progression is associated with an increase in tumorigenicity and metastatic capacity (Eccles at al. 1980, Eccles 1982b). This phenomenon was marked in MTI mammary carcinoma, since by passage 17 the metastatic incidence had risen from 0% to 40%, and by passage 30 the tumor was anaplastic and gave widespread metastases in 100% of mice. On the other hand, after 20 serial passages ST4 retained a relatively well differentiated acinar structure, and the spontaneous metastasis incidence has not significantly increased. SM1 mammary carcinoma presented as a poorly differentiated tumor that on its first passage became totally anaplastic; and metastases developed in 100% of the host animals.

We believe two factors complicate the picture of chemically induced squamous cell carcinomas: the degrees of (1) histological differentiation and (2) immunogenicity of the tumor. It seems that CA6 is an inherently metastatic tumor whose incidence of metastasis is determined largely by the host immune response (as are the sarcomas in C57/B1 mice), whereas DM6 acquires an immune-dependent capacity for metastasis, as its differentiated phenotype tends toward anaplasia.

One other point of interest is that those mouse tumors in which immunological control of metastasis has been demonstrated were all syngeneic with C57/B1 and DBA/2 mice, whereas the mammary carcinomas in which no such phenomenon was observed were syngeneic with CBA mice. We have investigated to a limited extent the biology of chemically induced sarcomas in this latter strain to determine whether a genetic difference in sensitivity of tumor cells to immune destruction exists.

Table 4 lists the properties of three CBA fibrosarcomas. The tumors showed varying degrees of immunogenicity, but universally low incidences of metastasis, unlike comparable C57/B1 sarcomas in which a 1-log increase in immunogenicity (e.g. FS6M1) did not protect against widespread disseminated disease. Neither

TABLE 4. *Properties of chemically induced CBA carcomas*

Tumor	Immunogenicity*	Metastatic capacity (%)	
		Normal mice	Immunosuppressed mice†
FS12	2 Logs	0–10	(A)0 (B)0 (C)N.T.
FS13	1 Log	0–10	(A)10 (B)0 (C)20
FS19	3 Logs	0–20	(A)10 (B)0 (C)60

* Difference in TD_{50} between normal and immunized mice.
† (A) Cycloleucine 150 mg/kg i.p. (B) Cyclosporin A 80 mg/kg s.c. (C) TXI.

cycloleucine nor cyclosporin A immunosuppression significantly increased their metastatic capacity, and thymectomy and irradiation increased it only in the case of FS19.

These data suggest a genetic component is responsible for the differential behavior and responsiveness to immunosuppression of C57 and CBA sarcomas. Whether the differences are due to variations in sensitivity of the immunogenicity assays in the two strains, differential susceptibility to immunosuppressive procedures (CBA mice did not tolerate 200 mg/kg/day cyclosporin A, whereas C57 mice were given this dose), or inherent differences in the metastatic potential of the tumor cells remains to be elucidated.

DIFFERENTIATION AND SPONTANEOUS METASTASIS OF CARCINOMAS

Reference has already been made to the fact that there is no correlation between immunogenicity (as assessed by increases in TD_{50} in immunized animals) and spontaneous metastasis in a series of CBA mammary carcinomas. There is, however, an association between the degree of differentiation of these tumors and metastasis in that the more anaplastic the tumor the greater the incidence of metastasis (see Table 5). Similar correlations have been noted by Belnap et al. (1979), Sordat et al. (1977), and Calabresi et al. (1979). It has been suggested that induced redifferentiation of anaplastic tumor cells might limit their malignancy and control their propensity for metastasis (Calabresi et al. 1979). Retinoic acid and its analogs are known to play a role in cellular differentiation of normal epithelia (Bollag 1983); hence a study has been made of the effects of a retinoid on the growth and metastasis of a variety of tumors. The retinoid chosen was an aromatic analogue of retinoic acid (Ro 10-9359, also called Etrinate), which Bollag (1975) had found to have the highest therapeutic index in relation to antitumor activity and toxicity due to hypervitaminosis A.

No evidence of increased cellular differentiation or inhibition of tumor growth and metastasis was obtained in the nonimmunogenic carcinomas tested by us, but both the growth rate of the "primary" and the incidence of secondary disease were reduced in two demonstrably immunogenic carcinomas, the CBA mammary carcinoma ST3 and the C57/Bl squamous cell carcinoma DM6 at passage 10, but not at passage 20 (see Table 5). In vitro, retinoids did not appear to induce differentiation in our carcinomas, and growth inhibition in vitro did not correlate with in vivo tumor responsiveness (Eccles, Barnett, and Alexander, to be published). The data suggest that in these systems the in vivo effects of retinoids on tumors were mediated indirectly via the host, probably in their role as immunopotentiators (Patek et al. 1979, Glaser and Lotan 1979).

To test this hypothesis further, we studied the effect of retinoids on the growth of a series of mouse sarcomas that possess different degrees of immunogenicity (Eccles 1982b, Eccles, manuscript to be published). The most immunogenic tumors (e.g., FS6) regressed under retinoid treatment, moderately immunogenic tumors (e.g., FS29 and FS19) grew more slowly than in control animals, and

TABLE 5. *Effect of retinoid treatment on the growth and metastasis of murine mammary and squamous cell carcinomas*

Tumor	Immuno-genicity	Treatment	Degree of differentiation	Tumor diameter (mm)	Metastasis incidence (%)
SM1	−	None	−	11.2 ± 1.7	100
		Retinoid	−	10.4 ± 1.8	100
MT3	−	None	++	8.3 ± 1.2	35
	−	Retinoid	++	8.9 ± 0.5	30
MT1	−	None	±	7.9 ± 1.1	70
		Retinoid	±	8.4 ± 1.2	60
ST4	−	None	+++	7.2 ± 0.7	10
		Retinoid	+++	6.8 ± 0.8	10
ST3	±	None	++	10.4 ± 0.7	30
		Retinoid	++	8.0 ± 0.6	20
DM2	±	None	++	9.6 ± 1.0	20
		Retinoid	++	8.5 ± 0.9	30
DM6p10	++	None	++	12.0 ± 0.9	80
		Retinoid	++	6.4 ± 0.6	30
		CyA	++	10.7 ± 1.1	100
		Retinoid + CyA	++	11.2 ± 0.8	100
		X	++	10.4 ± 0.8	100
		Retinoid + X	++	9.2 ± 0.6	60
DM6p20	−	None	±	11.8 ± 1.1	100
		Retinoid	±	10.9 ± 0.8	90
CA1	−	None	±	10.3 ± 0.6	80
		Retinoid	±	11.0 ± 0.8	90

Retinoid treatment: Ro 10–9359 40 mg/kg/day orally throughout tumor growth.
Cyclosporin A: 200 mg/kg/day s.c. throughout tumor growth.
X-irradiation: 500 rad whole-body X-irradiation 1 day before tumor implantation.
Tumors: All tumors were grown s.c. from 5×10^5 cells. Tumor diameter is expressed as the mean (± 1 S.D.) of groups of 10 tumors measured on day 21 except for DM6 p10 and DM6 p20 which were measured on days 17 and 13, respectively.

nonimmunogenic tumors (e.g., FS13 and FS6M1) were unaffected (Table 6) (Eccles 1982). Also, the marked inhibitory effects of retinoids on sarcoma and carcinoma growth and (sometimes) metastasis seen with FS6, FS19, and DM6 were reduced or abolished by immunosuppression of the host (Tables 5 and 6). We conclude that in the systems we have studied so far, there is no evidence that retinoids reduce the growth rate or incidence of metastasis of transplanted tumors by directly promoting differentiation but rather that they can influence the behavior of demonstrably immunogenic tumors via the host. The mechanisms underlying this phenomenon and the host cells involved are currently being investigated.

ROLE OF OXYGEN IN THE DESTRUCTION OF TUMOR CELLS WITHIN CAPILLARY BEDS IN WHICH THEY ARE ARRESTED

The hypothesis we wish to advance is that for many types of tumors the cancer cells shed into the blood are killed as a result of the toxic action of oxygen (associated perhaps with changes in pH) in capillary beds where the

TABLE 6. *Effect of retinoid treatment on the growth and metastasis of murine sarcomas*

Tumor	Immunogenicity*	Treatment†	Tumor diameter (mm)‡	Metastasis incidence (%)
FS6	++++	None	10.6 ± 0.7	10
		Retinoid	0.7 ± 0.4	0
		CyA	9.9 ± 0.9	60
		CyA + retinoid	11.0 ± 0.6	40
FS29	++	None	8.9 ± 0.7	40
		Retinoid	5.4 ± 0.8	15
FS6M1	±	None	11.6 ± 0.9	60
		Retinoid	11.0 ± 1.0	70
FS19	++	None	11.3 ± 1.0	20
		Retinoid	5.1 ± 0.4	0
		TXI	10.4 ± 1.0	60
		TXI + retinoid	11.1 ± 0.8	30
FS13	±	None	12.2 ± 0.8	10
		Retinoid	11.6 ± 1.0	10

* Each + represents a 1-log (10) difference in TD_{50} between immunized and normal hosts (see text).

† For retinoid and cylcosporin A (CyA) treatment, see Table 5 notes. TXI, animals were neonatally thymectomized and given 900 rad whole-body X-irradiation 2 days after priming with 200 mg/kg cytosine arabinoside.

‡ All tumors grown s.c. from 5×10^5 cells. The tumor diameter is expressed as the mean (± 1 S.D.) diameter of groups of 10 tumors measured on day 15–16 except the FS6 groups, which were measured on day 20.

oxygen concentration is in equilibrium (or close to it) with that of the atmosphere (i.e., a partial pressure produced by 18% 0_2). The cancer cells are killed in the capillaries in which they have been arrested before they have succeeded in penetrating the extravascular spaces (Jones et al. 1971, Wallace et al. 1978) where the oxygen concentration is not toxic, i.e., corresponding to an atmosphere containing 3–5% 0_2 (Derrick and Russell 1964). Evidence in support can be adduced from a number of quite different approaches. Firstly, there are the comprehensive human studies that show that the frequency within different organs of metastases derived from cancer cells that have entered the arterial circulation after passing through the lung bears no relation to cardiac blood flow (Weiss et al. 1980). Secondly, hyperbaric oxygen can be shown to inhibit the growth within the lung of cancer cells injected i.v. into mice. Thirdly, cells in vitro taken from tumors growing in vivo grow better at oxygen concentrations below those in equilibrium with an atmosphere of 18% 0_2. Finally, the rate of lysis of radiolabeled tumor cells in different organs varies, and as yet limited data are consistent with the concept that this difference may be related to oxygen tension.

Distribution of Metastases Arising from Cancer Cells That Have Passed Through the Lung

Primary cancers growing above the diaphragm will shed their cells into the vena caval system, and the first capillary beds these cells meet are in the lungs.

Such tumors do yield metastases in organs other than the lung, however, and these must derive from cells that have passed through the lung and thence traveled through the arterial system. Detailed postmortem studies (Willis 1964, Weiss et al. 1980) show that the organ distribution of such metastases is not related to the fraction of cardiac output received by the organs. In general, metastases are rare in some organs that receive a major part of the cardiac output, such as the gut, skin, muscles, and kidney. The organs most frequently involved are the liver, bone, and adrenal gland. In the liver, the microcirculation deriving from the portal vein is hypoxic. The sinusoidal circulation in the bone marrow is very hypoxic, and indeed bone marrow stem cells do not survive at atmospheric oxygen concentrations (Bradley et al. 1971). It is possible that parts of the microcirculation of the kidney are at relatively low oxygen concentrations, as it is sinusoidal. On the other hand, in the organs with high arterial blood flow and low susceptibility to metastasis, circulating tumor cells will be trapped in oxygen-rich capillary beds. It would be interesting to determine whether the anatomical distribution of metastases within the brain is related to oxygen concentration. In this connection, the pituitary, which has a portal circulation, deserves study.

Oxygen and Lung Metastases

The fact that the lung is the most common site for metastases of tumors that discharge cells into the vena cava may not only be due to hemodynamic considerations. Cancer cells shed into the vena cava gain access to the lung via the pulmonary artery and this is, of course, the one arterial supply where the blood is hypoxic. Hence, in the pulmonary microcirculation, cancer cells will only be exposed to high (i.e., approaching atmospheric) concentrations of oxygen if they have been trapped at the tips of the capillaries, where the blood becomes reoxygenated. If they are arrested in small arteries they will be in an oxygen-depleted environment. Accordingly, if high oxygen concentrations kill trapped cancer cells, metastases will arise more commonly from cancer cells that have been held up within the arterioles than from those arrested in the capillaries.

Two experimental observations are consistent with this prediction: (1) Intravenous injection of emboli of tumor cells (which would be trapped before reaching the capillaries) give rise to a higher incidence of lung tumors than do single-cell suspensions of cancer cells. (2) Admixture of small microspheres of synthetic polymers with cancer cells increases by a factor of between 10 and 100 the number of lung colonies produced by a given i.v. inoculation of cancer cells (Steel and Adams 1975). We are currently testing this hypothesis by examining the cloning efficiency within the lung of cancer cells in strains of mice that are congenitally anemic and consequently have lowered oxygen levels in their blood. We are also following an alternative approach to reducing blood oxygen by lowering the body temperatures pharmacologically. Since the susceptibility of mammalian cells to H_2O_2 depends on their glutathione content, it may be that the toxic effect of oxygen is similarly related. Hence, one might anticipate that the ability of cancer cells to form lung colonies would be reduced by pretreatments that affect intracellular glutathione such as the nitroso alkylating agent bis-chloroethyl nitrosourea (BCNU), which at subcytotoxic levels inhibits glutathione reductase (Nathan and Cohn 1981).

Effect on Tumor Growth in Lung of Exposing Mice to 3 Atmospheres of Oxygen

For many years the effectiveness of local radiotherapy in patients breathing oxygen at 2 to 3 atmospheres in order to decrease the hypoxic, and hence radioresistant, fraction of large tumors has been investigated. A possible objection to this treatment (Glassburn et al. 1977, Dische 1973) was that breathing high-pressure oxygen might facilitate metastatic spread. Two groups investigated this problem in experimental animals and reported briefly that there was no such hazard of hyperbaric oxygen in experimental systems and that, indeed, it could inhibit tumor growth in the lung. Kluft and Boereme (1964) reported without giving any details that exposing mice to 3 atmospheres of oxygen (3ATA) greatly reduced the number of lung colonies following i.v. injection of a syngeneic mammary carcinoma. Shewell and Thompson (1980) found a similar effect with Ehrlich carcinoma cells but not with syngeneic carcinoma cells, although they mention that the suspension of the latter contained aggregates of cells. For reasons already given, our hypothesis would predict that high-pressure oxygen would less affect tumor cell aggregates lodged in small pulmonary arteries than single cells, which would be arrested in capillaries, where breathing hyperbaric oxygen has its most-pronounced effect.

Together with Dr. John Miller, we are currently investigating systematically the effects of hyperbaric oxygen on the growth within the lung of i.v. injected tumor cells. In the first experiment with the chemically induced FS6 sarcoma (syngeneic to C57/B1 mice) we found that following injection of 10^5 sarcoma cells, tumor growth was greatly inhibited if the mice were exposed to 3ATA for 1 h. Thus mice breathing air developed $\gg$ 100 lung colonies per mouse; 9 of 10 mice maintained at 3ATA for 20 min developed $>$100 lung colonies; whereas only 1 of 10 mice maintained at 3ATA for 1 h developed $>$100 lung colonies; the other 9 had an average of 41 (15 to 83) colonies. These findings are consistent with the hypothesis that oxygen can be toxic for cancer cells lodged in capillaries.

Oxygen and the Growth of Cancer Cells In Vitro

There have been several reports, notably from the laboratory of Dr. Sanford at the NCI (Richter et al. 1972, but see also Courtenay 1976, Packer and Fuehr 1977), that some cells directly isolated from animals grow better in cultures exposed to atmospheres containing 5% oxygen than to air. The evaluation of the optimum oxygen concentration for in vitro growth is complicated since the actual oxygen concentration to which the cells are exposed in vitro is in general very much lower than that to which the corresponding cultures are exposed because of consumption coupled with slow diffusion. The magnitude of this effect depends on the seeding density and the metabolic rate of the cells. In a detailed study using micro-oxygen electrodes, Werrlein and Glinos (1974) showed that for liver cells exposed in Petri dishes, with a 0.5-cm fluid overlay the oxygen concentration in contact with the cells was equivalent to an atmosphere of 1% 0_2 for 1.6×10^6 cells/cm^2; 5% for 10^6 cells/cm^2; and 8% for 5×10^5 cells/cm^2. To determine the effect of oxygen tension on growth, therefore, cells need to be seeded at low densities so as to minimize depletion of oxygen. Indeed, at high in vitro cell densities, the oxygen concentration may be below that needed for optimum growth even when the culture is exposed to the atmosphere. With Dr. K. Moore we have studied the in vitro growth at different oxygen concentrations of six different murine sarcomas, two carcinomas, and one culture of mouse embryo fibroblasts immediately after isolation from the animal. Our findings are summarized in Table 7.

So far we have only carried out a limited investigation into the effect of oxygen on the cloning efficiency of cells from tumors in soft agar cultures. Our results with a murine lymphoma are detailed in Table 8.

In as yet very preliminary studies we noted that cancer cells rapidly adapt to oxygen and that sometimes after as few as two passages in vitro and usually

TABLE 7. *Toxic effect of oxygen in cultures containing low numbers of cells*

Seeding density (cells/cm^2)	Cultures exposed to atmospheres containing		
	18% O_2	5% O_2	2% O_2
$>3 \times 10^5$	+++	+	none
$\sim 3 \times 10^4$	+	+++	++
$\sim 3 \times 10^3$	Cell death	++	+++

TABLE 8. *An effect of oxygen concentration in the atmosphere on cloning efficiency of murine lymphoma at low seeding densities*

Seeding density (no. cells/ml)	No. clones in agarose cultures exposed to atmospheres containing	
	18% O_2	5% O_2
10^3	0	53
10^4	21	280
10^5	1,000	1,000
	(inspection suggests no difference)	

after five passages, the cells grow equally well at 18% as at 5% oxygen, even at low densities. However, when cells that have "adapted" to oxygen are grown in vivo then the cells derived from the tumor again show sensitivity to oxygen on return to culture.

Although much work remains to be done it would appear that many cancer cells—before they have adapted following growth in culture—proliferate optimally at oxygen concentrations equivalent to atmospheres of 3% to 5% and die at concentrations greater than 10%. An optimum in the 2% to 5% range is similar to that in extracellular fluid, where cells other than those of the vascular endothelium exist and divide. Cells in vitro seem to divide less than maximally at oxygen concentrations of less than 1%; in this connection the observation by Chance et al. (1964) is relevant: that a pO_2 of 1 mm Hg(equivalent to 0.1% O_2) gives the mitochondria adequate oxygen and that more will not affect the rate of oxygen transport.

Rapid Lysis in the Lung of Radiolabeled Cancer Cells That Have Been Injected I.V.

The observation was made by Hofer et al. (1970) and subsequently confirmed and extended in many laboratories (cf. Weiss 1980, Weiss et al. 1982) that following i.v. injection of cancer cells from carcinomas, sarcomas, and melanomas, the vast majority are retained in the lung where they undergo rapid autolysis. Frequently, at 4 h after injection, half of the cells permanently arrested in the lung have not only been killed but have suffered extensive breakdown of their DNA. The speed of lysis within capillaries is greater than that suffered by the cells when exposed to atmospheres rich in oxygen in vitro, and we suggest that two mechanisms act in conjunction in the destruction of the cancer cells within capillaries. Toxicity associated with oxygen tensions close to those in equilibrium with the air leads to modification of the plasma membrane and this results in the cancer cell's being recognized by the endothelial cells and thus phagocytosed and quickly degraded in a manner analogous to the clearing of effete erythrocytes by the reticuloendothelial system.

One test of such a hypothesis would be to compare the survival of radiolabeled cancer cells in microvasculatures with different oxygen concentrations. The ideal organ for such an experiment is the liver, where cells inoculated via the portal vein will be arrested in the relatively hypoxic environment of venous blood, while cancer cells that reach the liver through the arterial supply of the hepatic artery will be trapped in oxygen-rich capillaries. Weiss (1980) performed such an experiment and found that cancer cells that had gained access to the liver after being injected into the left ventricle of the heart survived for a much shorter time than those put into the portal vein. He, however, attributed the difference to mechanical damage sustained by the cancer cells in the heart. Surgical colleagues at Southampton are trying to eliminate this possibility by injecting cancer cells into the aorta at the point of the coeliac axis; in this way cells would enter the hepatic artery without having passed through the heart. This procedure is fraught with technical difficulties, but the first experiments have shown markedly superior survival of cells inoculated into the portal vein and thus provide support for the hypothesis that oxygen toxicity contributes to the destruction of blood-borne cancer cells within the entrapping tissues.

ACKNOWLEDGMENTS

The work reported has been supported by a grant from the Cancer Research Campaign.

REFERENCES

Agosin, M., R. Christen, O. Badinez, G. Gasic, A. Neghme, O. Pizzaro, and A. Jarpa. 1952. Cortisone-induced metastases of adenocarcinoma in mice. Proc. Soc. Exp. Biol. Med. 80:128–131.

Belnap, Le-G. P., P. H. Cleveland, M. E. M. Colmerauer, R. M. Barone, and Y. H. Pilch. 1979. Immunogenicity of chemically-induced murine colon cancers. Cancer Res. 39:1174.

Bollag, W. 1975. Prophylaxis of chemically induced epithelial tumours with an aromatic retinoic acid analog (RO 10–9359). Eur. J. Cancer, 11:721–724.

Bollag, W. 1983. Vitamin A and retinoids: From nutrition to pharmacotherapy in dermatology and oncology. The Lancet i:860–863.

Bradley, T. R., P. A. Telfer, and P. Fry. 1971. The effect of erythrocytes on mouse bone-marrow colony development in vitro. Blood 38:353.

Butler, T. P., and P. M. Gullino. 1975. Quantitation of cell shedding into efferent blood of mammary adenocarcinoma. Cancer Res. 35:512.

Calabresi, P., D. L. Dexter, and G. H. Heppner. 1979. Clinical and pharmacological implications of cancer cell differentiation and heterogeneity. Biochem. Pharmacol. 28:1933.

Carnaud, C., B. Hoch, and N. Trainin. 1974. Influence of immunologic competence of the host on metastases induced by the 3LL Lewis tumor in mice. JNCI 52:395–399.

Chance, B., B. Schoenes, and F. Schindles. 1964. The intra-cellular oxidation-reduction state, *in* Oxygen in the Animal Organism, F. Dickens and E. Neil, eds. Macmillan, New York, pp. 367–388.

Courtenay, V. D. 1976. A soft agar colony assay for Lewis lung tumour and B16 melanoma taken directly from the mouse. Br. J. Cancer 34:39–45.

Davey, G. C., G. A. Currie, and P. Alexander. 1979. Immunity as the predominant factor determining metastasis by murine lymphomas. Br. J. Cancer 40:590.

Denham, S., J. W. L. Hooton, R. K. Barfoot, P. Alexander, R. Mayol, and A. B. Wrathmell. 1980. Mechanism by which antibodies to non-AgB antigens mediate rejection of rat leukaemia cells. Br. J. Cancer 42:408–415.

Derrick, J. R., and D. Russell. 1964. Oxygen tensions in tissues. Arch. Surg. (Chicago) 88:1059–1062.

Dische, S. 1973. The hyperbaric oxygen chamber in the radiotherapy of carcinoma of the bladder. Br. J. Radiol. 46:13.

Eccles, S. A. 1978. Macrophages and cancer, *in* Immunological Aspects of Cancer, J. E. Castro, ed. Medical and Technical Press, Lancaster, U.K., pp. 123–154.

Eccles, S. A. 1980. Tumour metastasis in thymectomised and athymic rats, *in* Proceedings of Medical Research Council Symposium on Immunodeficient Animals in Cancer Research, S. Sparrow, ed. Macmillan Press, London, pp. 167–177.

Eccles, S. A. 1982a. Host immune mechanisms important in the control of tumor metastasis, *in* Tumor Immunity in Prognosis: The Role of Mononuclear Cell Infiltration, J. S. Haskill, ed. Marcel Dekker Inc., New York, pp. 39–74.

Eccles, S. A. 1982b. Host factors in metastasis, *in* Tumor Progression and Markers. Proceedings of VIth Meeting of the EACR, October 1981. Kugler, Amsterdam, pp. 183–196.

Eccles, S. A., and P. Alexander. 1974. Macrophage content of tumours in relation to metastatic spread and host immune reaction. Nature 250:667.
Eccles, S. A., and P. Alexander. 1975. Immunologically-mediated restraint of latent tumour metastases. Nature 257:52.
Eccles, S. A., S. E. Heckford, and P. Alexander. 1980. Effect of Cyclosporin A on the growth and spontaneous metastasis of syngeneic animal tumours. Br. J. Cancer 42:252–259.
Eccles, S. A., J. M. Styles, S. M. Hobbs, and C. J. Dean. 1979. Metastasis in the nude rat associated with lack of immune response. Br. J. Cancer 40:802–805.
Fidler, I. J., D. M. Gersten, and M. L. Kripke. 1979. Influence of immune status on the metastasis of three murine fibrosarcomas of different immunogenicities. Cancer Res. 39:3816–3821.
Glassburn, J. R., L. W. Brady, and H. P. Plenk. 1977. Hyperbaric oxygen in radiation therapy. Cancer 39:751.
Glaser, M., and R. Lotan. 1979. Augmentation of specific tumor immunity against a syngeneic SV40-induced sarcoma in mice by retinoic acid. Cell. Immunol. 45:175–181.
Herlyn, D., and H. Koprowski. 1982. IgG_{2a} monoclonal antibodies inhibit tumor growth through interaction with effector cells. Proc. Natl. Acad. Sci. USA 79:4761.
Hofer, K. G. 1970. Radiation effects on death and migration of tumor cells in mice. Radiat. Res. 43:663–667.
Johnson, R. J., R. F. Siliciano, and H. S. Shin. 1979. Suppression of antibody sensitized tumour cells by macrophages: Insufficient supply or activation of macrophages within large tumours. J. Immunol. 122:379–382.
Jones, D. S., A. C. Wallace, and E. E. Fraser. 1971. Sequence of events in experimental metastases of Walker 256 tumor: Light, immunofluorescent, and electron microscopic observations. JNCI 46:493–504.
Kearney, R., A. Basten, and D. S. Nelson. 1975. Cellular basis for the immune response to methylcholanthrene-induced tumors in mice: Heterogeneity of the effector cells. Int. J. Cancer 15:438–450.
Kim, U. 1970. Metastasizing mammary carcinomas in rats: Induction and study of their immunogenicity. Science 167:72–74.
Kluft, O., and I. Boereme. 1964. Hyperbaric oxygen in experimental cancer in mice, *in* Clinical Application of Hyperbaric Oxygen, Proceedings of the 1st International Congress. Elsevier, Amsterdam, pp. 126–136.
Makidono, R., K. Nomoto, and K. Takeya. 1976. Enhanced development of metastatic foci in thymectomised irradiated and bone-marrow reconstituted mice. Gann 67:645–649.
Nathan, C. F., and Z. A. Cohn. 1981. Antitumor effects of hydrogen peroxide in vivo. J. Exp. Med. 154:1539–1553.
North, S. M., and C. J. Dean. 1983. Monoclonal antibodies to rat sarcomata. II. A syngeneic IgG_{2b} antibody with antitumour activity. Immunology (in press).
Packer, L., and K. Fuehr. 1977. Low oxygen concentration extends the lifespan of cultured human diploid cells. Nature 267:423–425.
Patek, P. Q., J. L. Collins, G. Yogeeswaran, and G. Dennert. 1979. Antitumor potential of retinoic acid: Stimulation of immune-mediated effectors. Int. J. Cancer 24:624–628.
Parthenais, E., and J. S. Haskill. 1979. Immunity to the T.1699 murine mammary tumor. J. Immunol. 123:1334–1338.
Proctor, J. W., C. M. Rudenstam, and P. Alexander. 1973. A factor preventing the development of lung metastases in rats with sarcomas. Nature 242:29.
Richter, A., K. K. Sanford, and V. J. Evans. 1972. Influence of oxygen and culture media on plating efficiency of some mammalian tissue cells. JNCI 49:1705–1712.
Schirrmacher, V., and C. A. Waller. 1982. Quantitative determination of disseminated tumor cells by ^{3}H-thymidine incorporation in vitro and by agar colony formation. Cancer Res. 42:660.
Shewell, J., and S. C. Thompson. 1980. The effect of hyperbaric oxygen treatment on pulmonary metastasis in the C3H mouse. Eur. J. Cancer 16:253–259.
Sordat, B., C. Merenda, and S. Carrel. 1977. Invasive growth and dissemination of human solid tumours and malignant cell lines grafted subcutaneously to newborn nude mice, *in* Proceedings of 2nd International Workshop on Nude Mice, 1977. Gustav Fischer, Verlag, Stuttgart, pp. 313–326.
Steel, G. G., and K. Adams. 1975. Stem cell survival and tumor control in the Lewis lung carcinoma. Cancer Res. 35:1530.

Suurkula, M., and B. Boeryd. 1975. Tumour metastasis in mice with reduced immune reactivity. IV. Restoration of relative resistance to metastasis formation in thymectomised sub-lethally irradiated mice by spleen cells. Path. Eur. 10:299–305.

Wallace, A. C., E.-C. Chew, and D. S. Jones. 1978. Arrest and extravasation of cancer cells in the lung, *in* Pulmonary Metastasis, L. Weiss and H. A. Gilbert, eds. G. K. Hall and Co., Boston, pp. 26–42.

Weiss, L. 1980. Cancer cell traffic from the lungs to the liver: An example of metastatic inefficiency. Int. J. Cancer 25:385–392.

Weiss, L., K. Haydock, J. W. Pickren, and W. W. Lane. 1980. Organ vascularity and metastatic frequency. Am. J. Pathol. 101:101–113.

Weiss, L., E. Mayhew, D. G. Rapp, and J. Holmes. 1982. Metastatic inefficiency in mice bearing B16 melanomas. Br. J. Cancer 45:44.

Werrlein, R. J., and A. D. Glinos. 1974. Oxygen microenvironment D and respiratory oscillations in cultured mammalian cells. Nature 251:317–319.

Willis, R. A. 1964. Pathology of Tumours, 4th Ed. Butterworth, London, pp. 174–176.

Cancer Invasion and Metastasis: Biologic and Therapeutic Aspects edited by Garth L. Nicolson and Luka Milas. Raven Press, New York © 1984.

Role of Natural Killer Cells in Host Defense Against Cancer Metastasis

Nabil Hanna

Smith Kline and French Laboratories, Department of Immunology
Philadelphia, Pennsylvania 19101

The process of cancer metastasis is a highly complex one in which both tumor cell properties and host factors play decisive roles (Fidler et al. 1978). Multiple host effector mechanisms, immune and nonimmune, are involved in host defense against cancer metastasis. Immune responses mediated by T lymphocytes (Fidler and Kripke 1980), macrophages (Fidler 1980), and natural killer (NK) cells (Hanna and Fidler 1980, Talmadge et al. 1980) participate in host resistance against hematogenous and lymphatic spread of malignant neoplasms. Most tumor cells that enter the circulation are destroyed during the first 24 h, and only a few cells survive, extravasate, and develop into metastatic foci in the organ parenchyma (Fidler 1970). The elucidation of the effector mechanisms that control tumor dissemination is fundamental to the understanding of the biology of metastasis and the design of new approaches for the control of cancer metastasis.

The multiplicity of host effector mechanisms involved in resistance against tumor growth and metastasis already suggests that no single mechanism could be singled out as being solely responsible for the antitumor activity in vivo.

In this chapter, I will discuss the evidence that implicates NK cells in host resistance against hematogenous and lymphatic spread of malignant tumors and will address briefly the following issues: What is the relationship between the levels of NK cell activity in the host and the incidence of tumor metastasis? Are NK cells effective in destroying circulating malignant solid tumor cells in vivo and will activation of NK cells prevent metastasis development? Are NK cells involved in the natural resistance of nude mice against hematogenous metastasis and will experimental depletion of NK cells render the nude mouse susceptible to experimental or spontaneous metastasis of xenogeneic human malignant neoplasms? What is the relationship between resistance to NK cell–mediated cytotoxicity in vitro and the expression of metastatic potential of malignant tumor cells in vivo? Are NK cells activated by biologic response modifiers (BRM) effective in killing tumor cells grown in vivo? Are BRM-activated NK cells effective in immunotherapy of established extravascular tumor metastasis and what are the regulatory mechanisms that control the activation/suppression of NK cells?

In addition to the expression of natural ability to kill tumor cells, NK cells exhibit unique cellular characteristics that distinguish them from other immune effector mechanisms and, therefore, may be exploited in attempts to evaluate their in vivo role in prevention and therapy of tumor metastasis. NK cells express specific antigenic markers (Glimcher et al. 1977, Burton 1980, Young et al. 1980) and exhibit high sensitivity to treatment in vivo with cyclophosphamide (Cy) (Mantovani et al. 1978), 17-β-estradiol (Seaman et al. 1978) and anti-asialo-GMl (Kasai et al. 1981). NK cells could be activated by interferon or interferon inducers and bacterial adjuvants (Gidlund et al. 1978, Wolfe et al. 1976). The expression of NK cell–mediated cytotoxicity is age dependent (Keissling et al. 1975) and is influenced by environmental and genetic factors (Clark et al. 1979, Hanna et al. 1982). Thus, we have investigated the survival and metastatic behavior of NK-sensitive or NK-resistant tumor cells in hosts that exhibit low (3-week-old mice, beige mice, and mice treated with Cy, β-estradiol, or anti-asialo-GMl) or high (nude mice or syngeneic mice treated with interferon inducers) NK cell–mediated cytotoxicity.

Enhancement of Tumor Metastasis in Mice That Exhibit Low Levels of NK Cell–Mediated Cytotoxicity

NK cell–mediated killing of lymphoma and solid tumor target cells (UV-induced fibrosarcomas, K-1735 and B16 melanomas) in vitro is markedly inhibited by treatment of mice with Cy, β-estradiol, or anti-asialo-GMl serum. Studies of the metastatic behavior of tumor cells in mice pretreated 4 days earlier with a single dose of Cy (100–200 mg/kg) (Hanna and Fidler 1980) led to the following findings: (1) Treatment with Cy markedly enhanced the survival of radiolabeled tumor cells during the first 24 h after i.v. inoculation and significantly increased the incidence of pulmonary and extrapulmonary tumor metastasis; (2) Cy treatment increased the number of lung tumor colonies of all progressor metastatic tumor cells, but not of benign, nonmetastatic tumors; and (3) lymphoid reconstitution experiments demonstrated that the Cy-induced enhancement of experimental metastasis may be reversed by adoptive transfer of normal spleen cells 24 h before i.v. tumor cell inoculation. Lymphoid cells transfused 24 h after tumor cell injection were ineffective. These observations suggested that the effector cells responsible for abrogating the Cy effect are active during a short period (24 h) after i.v. tumor cell inoculation, a period that coincides with the presence of tumor cells in the circulation and before their extravasation to the organ parenchyma (Fidler 1970). The effector cells active in the reconstitution experiments were identified as being non-B, non-T, nonmacrophage, Cy-sensitive, NKl-antigen positive, and endowed with the ability to kill tumor cells within a short period of time; they exhibit the strain specificity, organ distribution, and ontogenic development profiles described for NK cells. Indeed, selective depletion of NK cells by anti-NKl serum and complement abolished the in vivo reconstitutive antimetastatic activity of normal spleen cells adoptively transferred into Cy-treated mice (Hanna and Burton 1981) (Table 1). Thus, by depleting immune effector cells (e.g., NK cells) involved in host resistance against tumor metastasis, chemotherapeutic drugs such as Cy may enhance metastatic spread and also may interfere with the antimetastatic effect of immune stimulants. Indeed, NK cell activation by poly I.C or *Corynebacterium parvum* inhibited metastasis development in normal but not Cy-treated mice, unless normal lymphocytes were adoptively transferred to the drug-treated recipients before the administration of the immunomodulators (Hanna and Fidler 1980) (Table 2).

The inverse correlation between the levels of NK cell–mediated cytotoxicity and the incidence of experimental or spontaneous metastasis was substantiated in other animal models. For example, selective in vivo depletion of NK cells by pretreatment of the recipient mice with anti-asialo-GMl serum was associated with increased incidence of pulmonary and extrapulmonary metastasis of i.v. injected B16 melanoma and UV-2237 fibrosarcoma tumor cells. Enhanced survival of radiolabeled tumor cells administered i.v. was described recently in animals pretreated with specific anti-NK serum (Pollack and Hallenbeck 1982).

Three-week-old mice exhibit low levels of NK cell–mediated cytotoxicity against lymphoma (YAC-1) and solid tumor (UV-2237 fibrosarcoma and B16 melanoma) target cells in vitro, which, however, could be boosted readily by treatment with bacterial adjuvants and interferon inducers. Consistent with re-

TABLE 1. *Effect of treatment with anti-NK 1.2 antibodies and complement on the ability of normal spleen cells to inhibit tumor metastases in vivo*

Treatment of recipients*	Median no. (range) of lung tumor colonies in:† Expt. I UV-2237	Expt. II UV-2237	Expt. III B16-F10
None	23 (6–52)	3 (0–10)	32 (13–40)
Cy	203 (29–246)	236 (116–250)	93 (46–112)
Cy-reconstituted with 50 × 10⁶ normal spleen cells incubated with:‡			
NMS + complement	11 (3–90)	16 (3–29)	42 (15–63)
Anti-NK-1.2 serum + Complement	213 (21–272)	186 (62–250)	90 (50–107)
Anti-Thy-1.2 + Complement	34 (0–68)	24 (0–43)	ND§

* Recipients ($C3H^-$ in experiments I and II; C57BL/6 in experiment III) were treated with Cy (200 mg/kg) 4 days before i.v. tumor injection. Lymphoid reconstitution was carried out 24 h before tumor challenge.

† Ten mice/group. Mice were killed 21 days after tumor cell injection (50,000 and 25,000 viable cells per mouse for UV-2237 and B16-F10, respectively), and pulmonary metastases were counted with a dissecting microscope.

‡ NMS and anti-NK 1.2 sera were used at 1:100 final dilution followed by complement at 1:8. The anti-NK 1.2 sera used were CE anti-CBA in experiment I and (CE × NZB)F_1 anti-CBA in experiments II and III.

§ Not done.

(Reproduced from Hanna and Burton 1981, with permission of *Journal of Immunology.*)

TABLE 2. *Effect of* C. parvum *treatment and lymphocyte reconstitution on Cy-induced enhancement of B16-F1 pulmonary metastasis in C57BL/6 mice*

Treatment of recipient*	No. lung colonies median (range)	Extrapulmonary metastases†
None, control	74 (37–98)	None
Control, *C. parvum*	15 (3–23)	None
Cy	272 (195–350)	8/10, liver; 3/10, intestines; 2/10, kidney; 1/10, spleen
Cy + *C. parvum*	251 (176–325)	9/9, liver; 1/9, spleen
Cy + 5 × 10^7 spleen cells	243 (183–322)	7/9, liver; 3/9 intestines; 1/9, kidney; 2/9, spleen; 1/9, lymph node
Cy + 5 × 10^7 spleen cells and *C. parvum*	91 (51–132)	4/9, liver; 1/9, intestines

* Mice were treated with Cy (240 mg/kg) 4 days before tumor injection. *C. parvum* (350 μg/mouse) and/or spleen cells were injected 24 h before injection of 1 × 10^5 B16-F1 melanoma cells.

† Number of mice with organ metastasis/number of mice receiving injections.

(Reproduced from Hanna and Fidler 1980, with permission of JNCI).

sults obtained in these models, metastatic tumor cells produced significantly higher numbers of lung tumor colonies in 3-week-old mice than in 8-week-old mice (Hanna and Fidler 1980) (Table 3). Alternatively, activation of NK cells by treatment with poly I.C or *C. parvum* 1–3 days before i.v. tumor cell inoculation inhibited metastasis formation equally well in both 3- and 8-week-old mice. The antimetastatic activity was most marked when NK cell stimulants were administered shortly before, but not after, tumor cell injection. These findings confirm previous results suggesting that the NK cells are most effective against

TABLE 3. *Enhanced expression of tumor metastatic potential in hosts with low NK cell activity*

Tumor cells	Dose	Number of lung tumor colonies (range)*		
		8-wk-old mice	3-wk-old mice	Cy-treated mice
UV-2237 fibrosarcoma†	50,000	2 (0–16)	52 (22–107)	All > 250
K-1735 melanoma	50,000	15 (3–36)	59 (20–98)	>250 (125–250)
B16 melanoma variants:‡				
F10	50,000	118 (45–198)	All > 250	All > 250
	25,000	44 (20–80)	All > 250	184 (106–250)
F1	50,000	4 (1–13)	196 (90–250)	85 (61–145)
	25,000	2 (0–7)	98 (68–136)	40 (26–85)
$F10^{LR}$	50,000	1 (0–7)	144 (61–178)	54 (33–98)
	25,000	1 (0–3)	81 (38–105)	26 (10–51)

* All lung tumor colonies were counted 3 weeks after tumor cell inoculation. Cy treatment (200 mg/kg) was given 4 days before i.v. tumor cell inoculation (10 mice/group).

† Syngeneic to the C3H mouse

‡ Syngeneic to the C57BL/6 mouse

(Reproduced from Hanna 1982a, with permission of Martinus Nijhoff Publishers).

circulating tumor cells, and they exhibit only a limited effect against tumor cells that already have extravasated and lodged in the lung parenchyma.

Because of the transient effect of Cy or anti-asialo-GMl serum on NK cells in vivo, as well as the maturation of NK cells by 4–5 weeks of age, the above-mentioned animal models are not ideal for long-term studies of spontaneous metastasis, which require prolonged suppression of NK cell activity. For this purpose, beige mice (Roder and Duwe 1979) and β-estradiol-treated mice (Seaman et al. 1978) may provide potentially valuable models. Indeed, we (Hanna and Fidler 1981) and others (Talmadge et al. 1980) have observed a higher incidence of spontaneous and experimental pulmonary metastasis in beige mice injected with NK-sensitive B16 melanoma cell lines than in C57Bl/6 controls. Enhancement of metastasis was also observed in mice whose NK cells were chronically and selectively depleted by treatment with 17-β-estradiol (Hanna and Schneider 1983). Six to 8 weeks after initiation of estrogen treatment, a marked decrease in the level of NK cell–mediated cytotoxicity against YAC-1 lymphoma, UV-2237 fibrosarcoma, and B16 melanoma target cells was observed. The survival of radiolabeled tumor cells injected i.v. and the incidence of experimental and spontaneous metastasis of the solid tumors, UV-2237 fibrosarcoma, and K-1735 and B16 melanomas, were markedly enhanced in β-estradiol-treated recipients compared with sham treated or untreated controls (Hanna and Schneider 1983). It is noteworthy that under the experimental conditions used, the induction of specific T-cell-mediated responses and the activation of tumoricidal macrophages by BRM were not compromised by estrogen treatment. As observed following Cy treatment, the β-estradiol-induced enhancement of metastasis could be reversed by adoptive transfer of spleen cells from normal syngeneic donors. Also, the antimetastatic activity of poly I.C and *C. parvum*, which is markedly depressed in β-estradiol-treated mice, is enhanced by lymphoid reconstitution. Thus, the chronic and selective inhibition of NK cell activity following treatment with β-estradiol may help in establishing models for ascertaining the metastatic potential of NK-sensitive malignant neoplasms and for evaluating the role of other effector mechanisms unrelated to NK cells in the control of tumor dissemination.

The data presented so far demonstrate that host natural resistance against hematogenous metastasis is mediated, at least in part, by NK cells and that the expression of metastatic potential of malignant tumor cells in vivo is highly dependent on the levels of NK cell activity in the recipient host. Just as highly immunogenic tumors metastasize readily in immunosuppressed but not in normal immunocompetent hosts, so do NK-sensitive malignant tumor cells metastasize more readily in NK-deficient recipients than in hosts that exhibit high NK cell–mediated cytotoxicity. Therefore, the suggestion was made that animal models deficient in NK cell– and T-cell–mediated responses will allow the expression of metastatic potential of NK-sensitive and highly immunogenic tumors and thus should be utilized for ascertaining the "true" metastatic potential of tumor cells.

NK Cell–Mediated Resistance of Athymic Nude Mice to Tumor Metastasis

The low incidence of metastasis in nude mice, despite the local progressive growth of transplanted allogeneic and xenogeneic malignant neoplasms, suggested that T-cell–independent mechanisms may be involved in the destruction of tumor cells released into the circulation and the inhibition of metastasis development.

The correlation between low NK cell activity in 3-week-old syngeneic mice and in mice treated with Cy, 17-β-estradiol, and anti-asialo-GM1 serum and the high incidence of experimental and spontaneous tumor metastasis prompted the initiation of similar studies in athymic nude mice (Hanna et al. 1982, Hanna 1980, 1983). The results of these studies may be summarized as follows: (1) Three-week-old nude mice exhibited low levels of NK cell–mediated cytotoxicity, whereas nude mice older than 5 weeks of age exhibited a consistently high NK cell activity. (2) Treatment of young nude mice with poly I.C or *C. parvum* boosted NK cell activity to levels observed in adult mice. (3) Treatment of adult nude mice with Cy, anti-asialo-GM1, or β-estradiol markedly reduced NK cell–mediated cytotoxicity against both lymphoma and solid tumor target cells. (4) The i.v. injection of metastatic allogeneic murine melanomas and fibrosarcomas and xenogeneic rat adenocarcinomas into 3-week-old nude mice or mice pretreated with Cy, anti-asialo-GM1, or β-estradiol resulted in the formation of large numbers of lung colonies. In contrast, very few lung tumor nodules were detected in untreated adult nude mice inoculated i.v. with the same metastatic tumor cells. (5) Activation of NK cells 1–3 days before tumor cell inoculation inhibited the formation of experimental pulmonary metastasis in young nude mice. (6) Only metastatic tumor cells produced lung colonies in young nude mice, whereas nonmetastatic benign tumors did not (Hanna 1982c) (Table 4). Moreover, the metastatic patterns of allogeneic and xenogeneic tumors were similar in both syngeneic hosts and young nude mice, with the exclusion of highly immunogenic tumors that exhibited higher metastatic potential in syngeneic immunosuppressed, but not immunocompetent, mice and young nude recipients. (7) B16 melanoma tumor cells isolated from lung tumor nodules of 3-week-old nude mice were highly metastatic when reinoculated into either young nude mice or syngeneic hosts (Pollack and Fidler 1982). The successful selection of highly metastatic allogeneic tumor cell variants from heterogeneous primary tumors injected into nude mice has significant implications for studies of human malignant neoplasms. Recently, using young nude mice, we were able to select from a human amelanotic melanoma cell line (A375) several cell subpopulations that upon i.v. injection into young nude mice produced 20–100 times more lung colonies than the parent cell line.

These findings strongly suggest that pathogen-free young nude mice with low NK cell activity or adult nude mice experimentally depleted of NK cells may provide valuable in vivo models for ascertaining the metastatic potential of human primary tumors and for selecting metastatic subpopulations that preexist within the primary heterogeneous neoplasms.

TABLE 4. *Experimental pulmonary metastasis of murine tumor cells in syngeneic hosts and in 3- and 6-week-old nude mice*

			Recipients		
Strain	Tumor	Cell dose	6-wk-old syngeneic mice	3-wk-old nude mice	6-wk-old nude mice
C3H	UV-2237 parent	10^5	25 (15–78)*	68 (38–115)	0
	Clone 38	10^5	1 (0–6)	2 (0–14)	0
	Clone 46	10^5	5 (0–16)	96 (55–178)	1 (0–3)
	Clone 25	10^5	35 (17–92)	89 (42–141)	0 (0–2)
	UV-2237-M1	10^5	145 (85–278)	238 (110–300)	0 (0–4)
	UV-2237-M2	10^5	178 (110–300)	All > 300	2 (0–6)
	UV-1591	5×10^5	0	0 (0–1)	0
	UV-1316	5×10^5	0	0	0
	K-1735 parent	10^5	55 (17–98)	165 (75–300)	0
	Clone 16	10^5	0 (0–2)	0 (0–7)	0
	Clone 13	10^5	0 (0–2)	27 (3–68)	0
	Clone 2	10^5	108 (81–210)	156 (65–233)	0
C57BL/6	B16-F1	5×10^4	6 (0–18)	28 (3–55)	0
	B16-F10	5×10^4	62 (21–95)	98 (35–300)	2 (0–4)
	B16-F10^{LR}	5×10^4	2 (0–3)	11 (1–28)	0

* Median number of lung tumor colonies (range).
(Reproduced from Hanna 1982c, with permission of Martinus Nijhoff Publishers).

NK Resistance of Tumor Cells: Effect on Metastatic Potential and Sensitivity to Antimetastatic Activity of BRM-Activated NK Cells

During the metastatic process, NK cells, among other host factors, may exert selective pressure on circulating tumor cells. Therefore, we examined whether metastatic tumor cells that survive the natural host defense mechanisms and succeed to extravasate and develop into metastases are resistant to NK cell–mediating cytotoxicity. The results of those studies (Hanna and Fidler 1981) showed no consistent correlation between NK cell resistance and metastatic potential of more than 30 tumor cell lines and cloned cell populations. In another study, we selected under defined in vitro conditions NK-resistant tumor cell variants and evaluated their survival and metastatic behavior in vivo (Hanna and Fidler 1981). The selection was carried out by repeated incubations of the parent UV-2237 fibrosarcoma with syngeneic spleen cells that exhibit high NK cell activity. Following i.v. injection into adult syngeneic mice, the selected NK-resistant tumor cells produced more lung colonies than the parent cell line. Moreover, the NK-resistant cells readily metastasized in adult nude mice shown to exhibit high NK cell activity and increased resistance to tumor metastasis. It is noteworthy that the NK-resistant cells did not differ from the NK-sensitive UV-2237 parent in immunogenicity, antigenicity, and sensitivity to killing by tumor-specific cytotoxic T lymphocytes, antibody-dependent cell cytotoxicity, or activated cytotoxic macrophages. They did, however, differ in their ability to bind unactivated NK cells. Thus, although metastasis may be the progeny of either NK-sensitive or NK-resistant tumor cells, resistance to NK cell–mediated cytotoxicity enhances the in vivo metastatic expression of malignant tumor cells in hosts that exhibit high NK cell activity.

The sensitivity of tumor cells to NK cell–mediated killing is relevant to the applicability of NK cell activation to prevention and therapy of tumor metastasis. Since resistance to NK cell–mediated cytotoxicity may develop either by adaptation during in vivo growth of tumor cells (Becker et al. 1978) or by selection during the metastatic process (Gorelick et al. 1979), the efficacy of BRM-activated NK cells in inhibiting metastasis of such NK-resistant variants was investigated (Hanna 1982a). Using several cell lines and clones of the parent NK-sensitive UV-2237 fibrosarcoma, we have demonstrated that freshly excised tumor cells grown in vivo exhibit higher resistance to killing by unactivated NK cells in vitro and produce significantly more lung colonies in vivo than their cultured counterparts (Hanna 1982a) (Table 5). The NK-resistant tumor cells, however, were killed effectively by BRM-activated NK cells in vitro and their metastases were markedly inhibited by in vivo activation of host NK cells. Thus, the emergence of resistance to NK cell–mediated killing by either adaptation or selection may not interfere with the efficacy and applicability of in vivo NK cell activation to the control of spontaneous tumor metastasis.

Recently, we have investigated the possible role of BRM-activated NK cells in inhibition of spontaneous lymph node tumor metastasis. For this purpose, protocols for selectively activating NK cells in regional lymph nodes draining the site of tumor inoculation were established (Hisano and Hanna 1982b), and a sensitive method for quantitation of tumor burden in lymph nodes was developed (Hisano and Hanna 1982a). In the course of these studies, it became

TABLE 5. *NK cell sensitivity and metastatic behavior of UV-2237 tumor cells*

Tumor cells	% Cytotoxicity by spleen cells from:*		Median no. lung tumor colonies (range)†	
	Normal mice	*C. parvum*-treated mice	Normal mice	*C. parvum*-treated mice
UV-2237 parent				
In vitro	42	75	12 (5–23)	0 (0–1)
In vivo‡	18	61	119 (88–154)	2 (0–5)
UV-2237-M3				
In vitro	05	68	46 (27–83)	1 (0–3)
In vivo‡	13	53	218 (129–250)	2 (0–3)
UV-2237 NK-5				
In vitro	13	57	98 (65–145)	9 (0–18)

* Percent cytotoxicity measured at 1.5×10^6 per well in a 20-h [$^3H^-$]proline assay.

† Lung tumor colonies were counted 3 weeks after the i.v. injection of 10^5 tumor cells (10 mice/group).

‡ The cells passaged in vivo were maintained 1 day in culture before being tested for their NK sensitivity in vitro or metastatic potential in vivo.

(Reproduced from Hanna 1982a, with permission of Martinus Nijhoff Publishers.)

apparent that the kinetics and organ distribution pattern of NK cell activation varied according to the type, dose, and route of administration of the BRM, and that activated NK cells present in the peripheral blood do not migrate freely into unstimulated lymph nodes. However, by applying protocols that selectively activate NK cells in lymph nodes containing tumor cells, we obtained a rapid destruction of early infiltrating tumor cells and a marked reduction in incidence and tumor burden of lymph node metastasis.

Relevant to the therapeutic application of NK cell activation by BRM are the kinetics and duration of activation and the possible generation of negative feedback suppression mechanisms that might interfere with achieving a persistently high level of activated effector cells. For example, a single injection of *C. parvum* induces a transient (1–5 days) enhancement of NK cell–mediated cytotoxicity that is followed by activation of tumoricidal macrophages (Hanna 1982b) (Figure 1). Recently, we have shown that macrophage activation was associated with the generation of suppressor cell activity and the development of a state of hyporesponsiveness to reactivation of NK cells, i.e., an optimal challenge with *C. parvum* or poly I.C failed to activate NK cells in mice pretreated 2–5 weeks earlier with *C. parvum* (Hanna 1982a). Moreover, treatment with BRM was less effective in inhibiting experimental tumor metastasis in

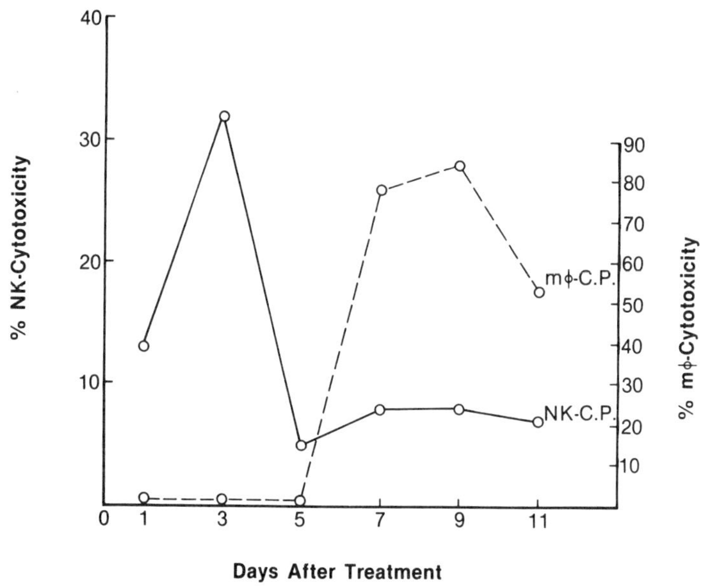

FIG. 1. Kinetics of NK cell and macrophage activation following i.p. injection of 350 μg *C. parvum*. NK cell–mediated cytotoxicity was measured against [^{3}H]proline-labeled B16-F10 melanoma target cells in a 24-h assay. 1 × 10^6 effector spleen cells and 1 × 10^4 tumor cells were added per well. Macrophage tumoricidal activity was assessed against [^{125}I]iododeoxyuridine-labeled B16-F10 melanoma cells in a 72-h assay (1 × 10^5 macrophages/well). (Reproduced from Hanna 1982b, with permission of *Cancer Research*).

mice pretreated with *C. parvum* than in normal controls. Although the mechanism of suppression is not fully understood, the activation of suppressor macrophages by *C. parvum* treatment corresponded with the kinetics of development of hyporesponsiveness. Irrespective of the exact mechanism of suppression, these findings indicate that multiple injections of BRM may not necessarily lead to sustained high levels of activated NK cells. Therefore, the selective activation of NK cells, without subsequent generation of suppressor cells, may prove effective in the control of established extravascular tumor micrometastasis.

REFERENCES

Becker, S., R. Kiessling, N. Lee, and G. Klein. 1978. Modulation of sensitivity to natural killer cell lysis after in vitro explantation of a mouse lymphoma. JNCI 61:1495–1498.

Burton, R. C. 1980. Alloantisera selectively reactive with NK cells: Characterization and use in defining NK cell classes, *in* Natural Cell–Mediated Immunity to Tumors, R. B. Herbermann, ed. Academic Press, New York, pp. 19–36.

Clark, E. A., P. H. Russell, M. Egghart, and M. A. Morton. 1979. Characteristics and genetic control of NK cell-mediated cytotoxicity activated by naturally acquired infection in the mouse. Int. J. Cancer 24:688–699.

Fidler, I. J. 1970. Metastasis: Quantitative analysis of distribution and fate of tumor emboli labeled with ^{125}I-5 iodo-2′deoxyuridine. JNCI 45:733–782.

Fidler, I. J., D. M. Gersten, and I. R. Hart. 1978. The biology of cancer invasion and metastasis. Adv. Cancer Res. 28:149–250.

Fidler, I. J. 1980. Therapy of spontaneous metastases by intravenous injection of liposomes containing lymphokines. Science 208:1469–1471.

Fidler, I. J., and M. L. Kripke. 1980. Tumor cell antigenicity, host immunity and cancer metastasis. Cancer Immunol. Immunother. 7:201–205.

Gidlund, M., A. Orn, H. Wigzell, A. Senik, and I. Gresser. 1978. Enhanced NK cell activity in mice infected with interferon inducers. Nature 273:750–761.

Glimcher, L., F. W. Shen, and H. Cantor. 1977. Identification of a cell-surface antigen selectively expressed on the natural killer cell. J. Exp. Med. 145:1–9.

Gorelick, E., M. Fogel, M. Feldman, and S. Segal. 1979. Differences in resistance of metastatic tumor cells and cells from local tumor growth to cytotoxicity of natural killer cells. JNCI 63:1397–1404.

Hanna, N. 1980. Expression of metastatic potential of tumor cells in young nude mice is correlated with low levels of natural killer cell–mediated cytotoxicity. Int. J. Cancer 26:675–680.

Hanna, N. 1982a. Role of natural killer cells in control of cancer metastasis. Cancer Metastasis Rev. 1:45–64.

Hanna, N. 1982b. Inhibition of experimental tumor metastasis by selective activation of natural killer cells. Cancer Res. 42:1337–1342.

Hanna, N. 1982c. Metastasis of xenogeneic and allogeneic tumors in nude mice, *in* Tumor Invasion and Metastasis, L. Liotta and I. Hart, eds. Martinus Nijhoff Publishers, The Hague, pp. 43–55.

Hanna, N. 1983. Natural killer cell–mediated inhibition of tumor metastasis in vivo. Journal of Survey and Synthesis of Pathology Research 2:68–81.

Hanna, N. and R. C. Burton. 1981. Definitive evidence that natural killer (NK) cells inhibit experimental tumor metastasis in vivo. J. Immunol. 127:1754–1758.

Hanna, N., T. W. Davis, and I. J. Fidler. 1982. Environmental and genetic factors determine the level of NK activity of nude mice and affect their suitability as models for experimental metastasis. Int. J. Cancer 30:371–376.

Hanna, N., and I. J. Fidler. 1980. The role of natural killer cells in the destruction of circulating tumor emboli. JNCI 65:801–809.

Hanna, N., and I. J. Fidler. 1981. Relationship between metastatic potential and resistance to natural killer cell–mediated cytotoxicity in three murine tumor systems. JNCI 66:1183–1190.

Hanna, N., and M. Schneider. 1983. Enhancement of tumor metastasis and suppression of natural killer cell activity by β-estradiol treatment. J. Immunol. 130:974–980.

Hisano, G., and N. Hanna. 1982a. A cytochemical procedure for the in vivo identification of melanoma micrometastases. Journal of Invasion and Metastasis 2:299–312.

Hisano, G., and N. Hanna. 1982b. Murine lymph node natural killer cells: Regulatory mechanisms of activation or suppression. JNCI 69:665–671.

Kasai, M., T. Yoneda, S. Habu, Y. Maruyama, K. Okumura, and T. Tokunaga. 1981. In vivo effect of anti-asialo GMl antibody on natural killer activity. Nature 291:334–335.

Keissling, R., E. Klein, and H. Wigzell. 1975. Natural killer cells in the mouse. a. Cytotoxic cells with specificity for mouse Moloney leukemia cells. Specificity and distribution according to genotype. Eur. J. Immunol. 5:112–117.

Mantovani, A., W. Luini, G. Peri, A. Vecchi, and F. Spreafico. 1978. Effect of chemotherapeutic agents on natural cell-mediated cytotoxicity in mice. JNCI 61:1255–1261.

Pollack, S. B., and L. A. Hallenbeck. 1982. In vivo reduction of NK activity with anti-NK 1 serum: Direct evaluation of NK cells in tumor clearance. Int. J. Cancer 29:203–207.

Pollack, V. A., and I. J. Fidler. 1982. The use of young nude mice to select subpopulations of tumor cells with increased metastatic potential from nonsyngeneic neoplasms. JNCI 69:137–141.

Roder, J., and A. Duwe. 1979. The beige mutation in the mouse selectively impairs natural killer cell function. Nature 278:451–453.

Seaman, W. E., M. A. Blackman, T. D. Gindhart, J. R. Roubinia, J. M. Loeb, and N. Talal. 1978. β-Estradiol reduces natural killer cells in mice. J. Immunol. 121:2193–2198.

Talmadge, J. E., K. M. Meyers, D. J. Prieur, and J. R. Starkey. 1980. Role of NK cells in tumor growth and metastasis in beige mice. Nature 284:622–624.

Wolfe, S. A., D. E. Tracey, and C. S. Henney. 1976. Induction of "natural killer" cells by BCG. Nature 262:584–586.

Young, W. W., S. I. Hakomori, J. M. Durdik, and C. S. Henney. 1980. Identification of ganglio-N-tetraosylceramide as a new cell surface marker for murine natural killer (NK) cells. J. Immunol. 124:199–201.

Cancer Invasion and Metastasis: Biologic and Therapeutic Aspects edited by Garth L. Nicolson and Luka Milas. Raven Press, New York © 1984.

Conditioning of Tissues for Metastasis Formation by Radiation and Cytotoxic Drugs

Luka Milas and Lester J. Peters

Division of Radiotherapy, The University of Texas M. D. Anderson Hospital and Tumor Institute at Houston, Houston, Texas 77030

The metastatic process is analogous in many ways to syngeneic tumor transplantation (which in intact animals is usually very inefficient) in that only a small proportion of the potentially clonogenic cells from solid tumors successfully initiate new growths. Manipulation of the transplant recipient or the tumor cell inoculum can, however, dramatically affect tumor transplantability. For example, to achieve s.c. growth of a syngeneic fibrosarcoma, designated FSa, in normal mice, it is necessary to inject many thousands of cells (Table 1). In contrast, in T-cell-deficient mice, a single FSa cell is sufficient to establish a s.c. tumor when viable tumor cells are injected admixed with heavily irradiated tumor cells. Similar, although quantitatively less striking, results were obtained when tumor cells were injected i.v. in order to generate lung nodules, with or without the manipulations of whole-body irradiation (WBI) and the mixing of viable with heavily irradiated tumor cells.

These experiments illustrate the extent to which factors extrinsic to the tumor cells can affect their ultimate clonogenicity and are therefore of significance in the study of metastasis. In a tumor like FSa, it can be deduced that every or nearly every tumor cell could form a metastatic lesion if, after release from the primary tumor, it escaped or survived all potentially lethal hazards and found an anatomic site fitting its growth needs. Under these circumstances, host systemic and local tissue environment factors play a decisive role in determining whether circulating tumor cells will survive and form metastatic lesions. In this review, we discuss the effect of two iatrogenic factors often used in clinical cancer treatment, namely irradiation and cyclophosphamide, in terms of their ability to condition lung tissue for metastasis formation.

DESCRIPTION OF THE PHENOMENON

Tumor cells injected i.v. into experimental animals previously treated with local thoracic irradiation (LTI) (Withers and Milas 1973, Brown 1973, van den Brenk et al. 1974b, Thompson 1974, Peters et al. 1978, 1980) or cyclophosphamide (CY) (Van Putten et al. 1975, Peters and Mason 1977, Carmel and

TABLE 1. *Enhancement of tumor cell clonogenicity in C_3Hf/Kam murine fibrosarcoma (FSa) system by whole-body irradiation, T-cell deficient state, and admixture of heavily irradiated and viable tumor cells*

Treatment of recipients*	Tumor take	
	s.c.†	i.v.‡
Normal	15,000	2,600
WBI	100	520
Normal + HITC	2,360	270
WBI + HITC	—	40
TIR + HITC	1	—

* Whole-body irradiation with 600 rad gamma rays was delivered 1 day prior to either s.c. or i.v. injection of tumor cells. 5×10^5 heavily irradiated tumor (FSa) cells (HITC) were added to each inoculum. TIR designates thymectomy, whole body irradiation with 900 rad, and reconstitution with syngeneic bone marrow cells.

† The number of tumor cells needed to generate s.c. tumors in 50% of injected mice (TD_{50} values).

‡ The number of tumor cells needed to be injected i.v. to generate one nodule in the lung.

Brown 1977, Milas et al. 1979) generate many times more metastatic nodules in the lungs than if they are injected into untreated animals. Figure 1 illustrates the enhancement of metastasis formation produced in C_3Hf/Kam mice exposed to LTI and in CBA mice treated with CY. In both instances the enhancement of metastasis formation lasted for several days with a peak at 1 day after treatment. However, depending on the tumor-host model, this phenomenon may exhibit some differences in detail. For example, in one system the effect of LTI and CY differed in duration and lasted for weeks (Brown 1973, Carmel and Brown 1977); in another, the difference was in magnitude, with CY increasing lung-colonizing efficiency by up to 1,000 times that in untreated mice (Van Putten et al. 1975). In addition to the acute effect, a second increase in tumor colony growth has been described as late as 9.5 months after LTI (Thompson 1974). As recently demonstrated in our laboratory (Dubravsky et al. 1981), this late enhancement of metastasis was well correlated with the development of radiation-induced fibrosis in the lung.

The magnitude of the metastasis enhancement is dependent on the dose of LTI and CY, so that higher doses produce a larger effect. The dose response is linear over a wide range of doses of both gamma rays and neutrons (Figure 2), and of CY (Figure 3). Figure 3 shows that misonidazole, a selective radiosensitizer of hypoxic cells (Adams 1981), can also promote tumor colony formation in the lung and also augment CY-induced enhancement. The metastasis enhancing effect of misonidazole is described in detail elsewhere (Milas et al. 1983). It should also be mentioned here that many other chemotherapeutic agents can promote tumor colony formation in the lung, but their effect is not as great as that observed for CY (Van Putten et al. 1975).

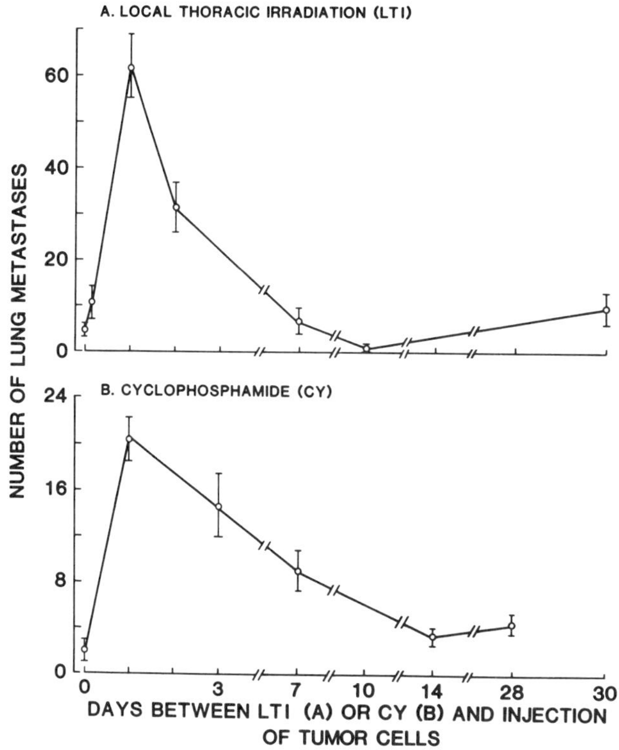

FIG. 1. Effect of time interval between 1,000 rad gamma rays LTI **(A)** or CY treatment **(B)** and tumor cell injection on the number of lung metastases. C_3Hf/Kam mice were injected i.v. with 10^4 fibrosarcoma (FSa) cells at different times after LTI. CY in the dose of 180 mg/kg was given i.p. to CBA mice at different times before i.v. injection of 10^4 syngeneic FSa cells. Number of tumor colonies in the lung of C_3Hf/Kam mice was determined 20 days after and that in the lung of CBA mice 14 days after tumor cell inoculation. (Adapted from Withers and Milas 1973 and Milas et al. 1979.)

MECHANISTIC CONSIDERATIONS

Studies that utilized radioactivity labeled tumor cells (Withers and Milas 1973, Brown 1973, Peters et al. 1978, Brown and Parker 1979) showed that approximately the same percentage of i.v. injected cells initially lodge in the irradiated and the unirradiated lungs. Therefore, both normal and irradiated lungs exhibit similar mechanical trapping of incoming circulating tumor cells; however, the release of tumor cells from the irradiated lungs was not as rapid as that from nonirradiated lungs. About a week following LTI, approximately twice as many cells remained in the irradiated as in the nonirradiated lungs (Withers and Milas 1973). In general, CY treatment affected the retention of tumor cells in the lung in a similar way (Peters and Mason 1977, Grdina et al. 1978). Peters et al. (1978) reported that most of the cells that left the lung

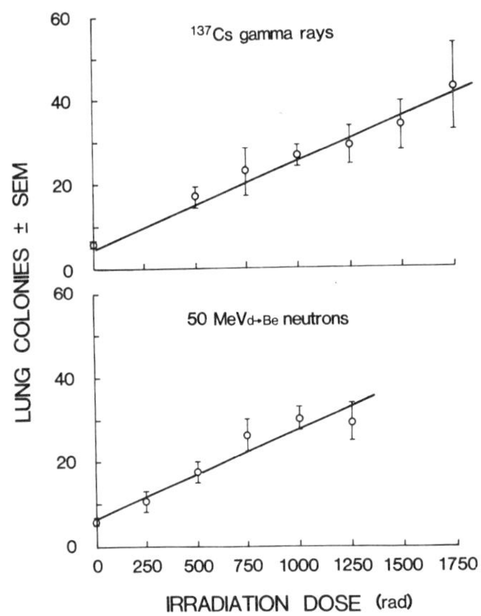

FIG. 2. Dose-response relationships for enhancement of lung colony–forming efficiency by ^{137}Cs gamma rays and by 50-MeV$_{d \to Be}$ neutrons. Single doses of radiation were given to the thorax 1 day before i.v. injection of 2×10^4 fibrosarcoma tumor cells. The number of lung colonies was determined 14 days after i.v. inoculation of tumor cells. (Adapted from Peters et al. 1980.)

were already dead, implying that most of the injected cells die either on their way to the lung or while in the lung. Theoretically, enhancement of lung nodule formation that took place in the lungs of treated mice could result from either systemic or local tissue environment alterations caused by LTI and CY, or from both. We shall briefly review the main conclusions from studies that have considered these mechanistic possibilities.

Systemic Factors

Since ionizing radiation and CY are potent immunosuppressive agents, the possibility that they enhanced metastasis by suppressing immune resistance mechanisms to tumor cells has been considered. Most studies, however, suggest that the phenomenon is nonimmunologic. To begin with, both radiation (Withers and Milas 1973, Brown 1973, Ando et al. 1979) and CY (Van Putten et al. 1975, Peters and Mason 1977, Carmel and Brown 1977, Milas et al. 1979) increase formation of metastases from both immunogenic and nonimmunogenic tumors by a factor that does not correlate with their immunogenicity. Although this lack of correlation excludes suppression by these treatments of the specific antitumor immune reaction mediated by T lymphocytes as a contributing factor in metastasis enhancement of weakly immunogenic tumors, it does not exclude participation of natural killer (NK) cells or macrophages.

NK cells have recently been reported to play an important role in restricting metastatic spread, acting primarily against circulating tumor cells (Hanna and Fidler 1980, Talmage et al. 1980). These cells are sensitive to CY (Hanna and Fidler 1980) (Figure 4), but their sensitivity to ionizing radiation is still a matter

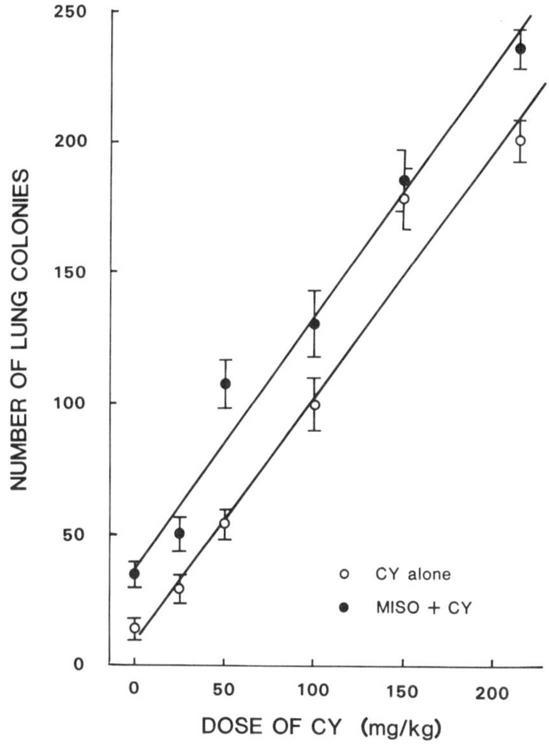

FIG. 3. Effect of different doses of cyclophosphamide (CY) on number of fibrosarcoma (FSa) metastases in C_3Hf/Kam mice. CY was given i.p. one day before i.v. injection of 2×10^4 FSa cells. Misonidazole (MISO) in the dose of 1 mg/g was also given i.p. one day before tumor cells and 30 min before CY. Number of lung metastases was determined 14 days after tumor cell injection.

of controversy (discussed in Milas et al. 1982a). Our recent data (Figure 5) show that WBI, but not LTI, suppresses NK cells, which makes it unlikely that LTI enhancement of lung nodule formation results from interference with NK cell activity. Moreover, CY is still effective in mice immunosuppressed by WBI (Peters and Mason 1977, Milas et al. 1979). Impairment of macrophage function by methylpalmitate (Withers and Milas 1973) or trypan blue (Peters et al. 1978) prior to LTI does not alter the metastasis-enhancing effect of radiation. On the other hand, as described later, preactivation of the macrophage system can impair or abolish the radiation-induced enhancement of metastasis. This suggests an antagonistic but causally unrelated influence of LTI and macrophage activation.

The conclusion that the LTI effect is a nonimmunologic phenomenon is consistent with its localized nature. However, in the case of CY (which enhances tumor transplantation by multiple routes), it appears likely that a component

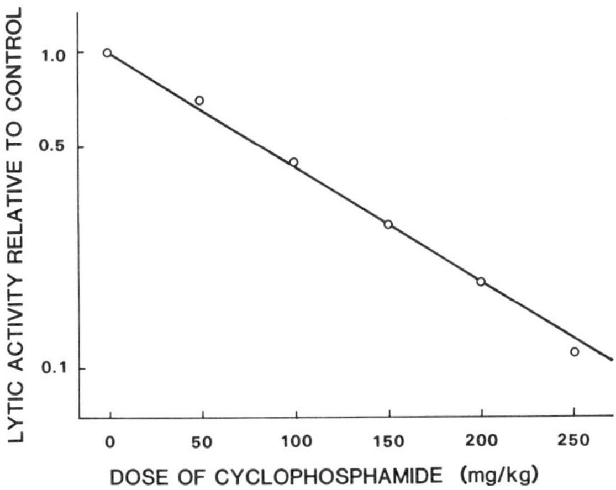

FIG. 4. Dose-dependent cyclophosphamide (CY) reduction in NK cell activity in the spleen of C_3Hf/Kam mice. The activity was measured by the ability of spleen cells from mice treated with CY 1 day earlier to lyse YAC-1 cells cultured in vitro. Spleen-to-target cell ratio was 100:1.

of the effect may be due to depletion of a defensive host-cell population, at least in some circumstances. To demonstrate this, we performed three separate experiments (Figure 6). In the first experiment, CBA mice were treated with CY, and 2 days later, they were given spleen and bone marrow cells i.v. from syngeneic normal or TIR mice (thymectomized, whole-body irradiated, and reconstituted with syngeneic bone marrow). One day after the reconstitution with lymphoid cells, mice were injected i.v. with syngeneic fibrosarcoma cells.

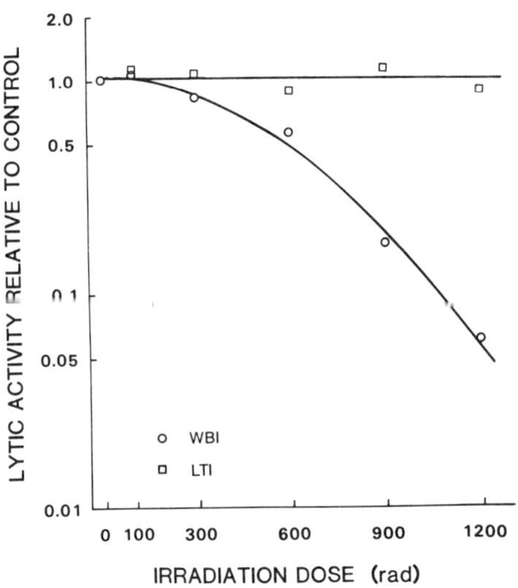

FIG. 5. Effect of local thoracic irradiation (LTI) and whole-body irradiation (WBI) on natural killer cell activity in the spleen of C_3Hf/Kam mice. The activity was measured by the ability of spleen cells from mice treated with radiation 1 day earlier to lyse in vitro cultured YAC-1 cells. Spleen-to-target cell ratio was 100:1.

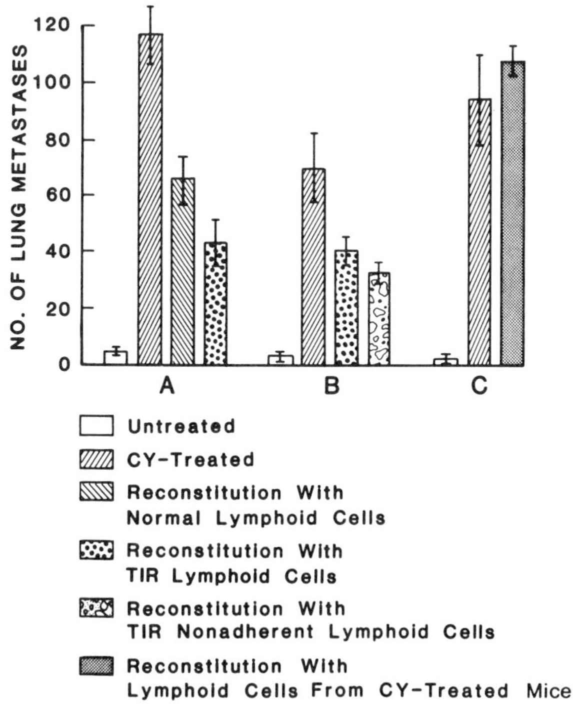

FIG. 6. Effect of reconstitution with syngeneic lymphoid cells on CY-induced enhancement of pulmonary metastases of CBA-FSa in CBA mice. Reconstituting cells were given i.v. 2 days after recipients received 180 mg/kg CY and 1 day before i.v. injection of 10^4 viable tumor cells. TIR, thymectomized, irradiated, reconstituted. (Adapted from Milas et al. 1979.)

Lymphoid cells from normal mice reduced metastasis enhancement by 44%, and cells from TIR mice reduced it by 63% (Figure 6A). In the next experiment, the reconstituting cells were the TIR mouse spleen and bone marrow cells devoid of macrophages. Figure 6B shows that the removal of macrophages from the cell population did not alter the reconstituting capacity of lymphoid cells. If the reconstituting cells were derived from mice treated with CY 3 days earlier, the metastasis-enhancing effect of CY was not affected (Figure 6C). These data indicate that CY-induced enhancement of metastases was caused partially by a systemic effect of CY, which destroyed lymphoid cells responsible for the antimetastatic resistance. In this particular tumor system, these cells were neither T cells nor macrophages, and NK cells are putative candidates.

Local Microenvironment Changes

Based on the data reviewed in the previous section, about 50% of the CY effect and most, if not all, of the effect of LTI should be considered the result of direct damage of lung tissues by these agents or of some other changes in the microenvironment that conditioned this organ for metastasis formation. Ionizing radiation can damage capillary walls and so increase their permeability, which would be expected to lead to transudation of serum into alveolar spaces. However, the histologic and electron microscopic appearance of a mouse lung exposed to 1,000 rad gamma rays LTI 1 day earlier is the same as that of a nonirradiated lung (Peters et al. 1980). In addition, lungs of mice exposed to 1,000 rad LTI showed no change in weight for several days after irradiation, suggesting that no significant transudation into alveolar spaces had occurred. However, in endothelial cell monolayers, retraction from the underlying matrix can be induced by large, single doses of irradiation (see below).

To establish metastases after being arrested in the capillary, tumor cells usually migrate into extracapillary spaces. It is possible that radiation, or CY, or CY metabolites (Peters and Mason 1977) cause subtle changes in the capillary walls, making it easier for tumor cells to pass through. This mechanism is supported by recent in vitro observations by Kramer et al. (1980) concerning interactions of tumor cells with vascular endothelial cell monolayers and the effect of drugs on those interactions. These investigators observed that metastatic tumor cells adhere preferentially to the extracellular matrix underlying vascular endothelial cells, and that EDTA can cause retraction of endothelial cells, thus enabling more tumor cells to adhere to the extracellular matrix. As a consequence of increased capillary permeability, it is likely that more tumor cells would reach extracapillary spaces and "permanently" settle in the lungs of mice exposed to LTI or CY than in the lungs of normal, unexposed mice. Recently, in a preliminary collaborative study with Dr. Nicolson of U. T. M. D. Anderson Hospital, we observed that 1,000 rad gamma rays cause retraction of endothelial cell monolayers in vitro, which led to a higher percentage of seeded tumor cells' attaching to subcellular matrix (G. Nicolson and L. Milas, unpublished observation).

Van den Brenk et al. (1974a, 1974b) proposed that LTI and drugs enhanced tumor cell colony formation by inducing an inflammatory reaction in the lung, which then acted as a stimulating microenvironment for tumor cell proliferation. They supported their view by experimental findings that inhibition of the radiation- or drug-induced enhancement of metastases was achieved by treating rats with antiinflammatory agents a few hours before exposure to radiation or drugs (van den Brenk et al. 1974a). However, Peters et al. (1978), using a mouse tumor system, could not confirm these findings and ascribed their failure to the striking difference in the time interval between LTI and maximum enhancement of colony formation that exists between the rat and mouse. Moreover, in the Peters study, dexamethasone increased the effect of LTI. A more recent attempt to protect against the LTI effect by treating mice with indomethacin, a nonsteroidal antiinflammatory agent, was also unsuccessful. (These results are summarized in Table 2.) Therefore, inflammatory changes produced by radiation or drugs may be one of the mechanisms responsible for the induced metastasis enhancement, but it is not applicable to all animal tumor systems.

TABLE 2. *Effect of steroidal and nonsteroidal antiinflammatory drugs on LTI-induced enhancement of artificial pulmonary metastasis of FSa in C_3Hf/Kam mice*

Experiment	Treatment of recipients	Mean no. lung metastases ± S.E.
1*	None	8.2 ± 1.6
	LTI	30.5 ± 5.1
	LTI + dexamethazone	85.6 ± 9.8
	LTI + phenylbutazone	31.4 ± 3.8
2†	None	29.4 ± 10.2
	Indomethacin	32.0 ± 6.1
	LTI	106.5 ± 7.2
	LTI + indomethacin	109.0 ± 18.5

* Adapted from Peters et al. 1978. Mice were exposed to 1,000 rad gamma rays LTI 1 day before they were given i.v. injections of 10^4 FSa cells. Immediately after irradiation mice were treated i.p. with dexamethazone (10 mg/kg) or phenylbutazone (250 mg/kg).

† LTI (1000 rad) was given 1 day before i.v. injection of 2×10^4 FSa cells. Indomethacin (6 mg/kg) was given i.p. 2 days, 1 day, and 2 hours before LTI. In both experiments the number of lung metastases was determined 14 days after tumor cell injection.

LTI, local thoracic irradiation; FSa, fibrosarcoma.

A further mechanistic possibility is that LTI and CY damaged capillaries and consequently led to local accumulation of platelets and formation of microthrombi, resulting in prolonged retention of tumor cells in the lung. If such a mechanism is operative, then anticoagulants and agents that inhibit platelet aggregation would prevent or reduce metastasis enhancement. However, treatment with anticoagulants such as warfarin provided conflicting data (Brown 1973, Van Putten et al. 1975). A recent discovery that platelet aggregation can be inhibited by prostacyclin (Moncada and Vane 1977) has initiated interest in testing whether stimulation of prostacyclin production can inhibit metastasis formation. Treatment of mice with the prostacyclin-stimulating agent nafazatrom reduced both artificial and spontaneous metastasis formation (Honn 1983). Assuming that the LTI effect might be due to an increase in platelet aggregation, we tested whether nafazatrom given shortly before LTI would reduce metastasis enhancement. Results presented in Table 3 show that, in the schedule used, nafazatrom reduced lung colonization in normal mice, but had no effect on LTI-induced metastasis enhancement.

Two sets of data generated in our laboratory suggest that the mechanism of the LTI effect is independent of radiation cell killing in the lungs. The first evidence is that the metastasis enhancement is equal, if not greater, when radiation is delivered in two equal doses several hours apart rather than as a single dose (Figure 7). If cell killing were responsible for the phenomenon, the split-dose arm would have resulted in a smaller enhancement because of the cell repair that takes place between the two irradiations. The second evidence is the inability of S-2-(3-aminopropylamino)ethylphosphorothioic acid (WR-2721)

TABLE 3. *Effect of prostacyclin-production-stimulator nafazatrom on LTI-induced enhancement of formation of artificial pulmonary metastases of FSa in C_3Hf/Kam mice*

Treatment of recipients	Mean no. lung metastases ± S.E.
None	22.7 ± 1.7
Nafazatrom	9.6 ± 2.4
LTI	62.2 ± 3.6
LTI + nafazatrom	58.7 ± 6.9

Mice were exposed to 1,000 rad gamma rays LTI 1 day before they were given i.v. injections of 4 × 10^4 FSa cells. Nafazatrom (8 mg/kg) was given i.p. 2 days, 1 day, and 1 h before and 4 h and 1 day after LTI. The number of metastases was determined 14 days after tumor cell injection.

LTI, local thoracic irradiation; FSa, fibrosarcoma.

to protect against LTI-induced metastasis enhancement. In fact, the compound had the opposite effect (Table 4). WR-2721 has the ability to greatly protect different normal tissues, including the lung, against early and late radiation damage (Yuhas et al. 1980, Milas et al. 1982b). The radioprotective effect of WR-2721 is considered to be due to its ability to scavange free radicals, making them unavailable to damage DNA.

Thus, although several mechanisms can participate in the pathogenesis of

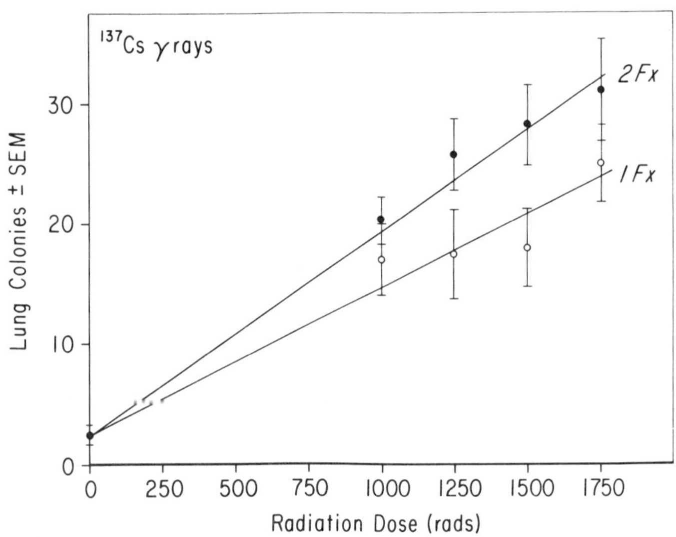

FIG. 7. Effect of dose of gamma rays on number of fibrosarcoma (FSa) metastases in C_3Hf/Kam mice. Radiation was given as a single or split dose (two equal doses separated by 4 h) given 1 day before i.v. injection of 2 × 10^4 FSa cells. Number of tumor nodules was determined 14 days after tumor cell injection. (Adapted from Peters et al. 1980.)

TABLE 4. *Effect of WR-2721 on LTI-induced enhancement of formation of artificial pulmonary metastases of FSa in C_3Hf/Kam mice*

Treatment of recipients*	No. of lung metastases	
	Mean ± S.E.	p†
None	4.3 ± 1.4	(< 0.03)
WR-2721	11.1 ± 2.7	
LTI (1,000 rad)	22.6 ± 3.5	(< 0.001)
WR-2721 + LTI	56.7 ± 6.4	

* LTI and i.p. injection of 400 mg/kg WR-2721 were performed 1 day before i.v. injection of 2×10^4 FSa cells. In combination with radiation, WR-2721 was given 30 min before LTI. Number of FSa nodules in lung was determined 14 days following i.v. injection of tumor cells.

† Mann-Whitney *U* test.

LTI, local thoracic irradiation; FSa, fibrosarcoma.

(Adapted from Milas et al. 1982b.)

LTI- and CY-induced enhancement of metastasis formation, it seems likely that a major mechanism is the damage to capillary walls produced by these agents. It facilitates the crossing of tumor cells into extravascular spaces.

The experiments with labeled tumor cells show that the relative increase in retention of tumor cells in the lungs of treated mice is less than one would expect from the relative increase in the number of lung colonies, which suggests that these treatments make the lung a more suitable environment for proliferation of arrested cells. Peters et al. (1978) and Brown and Parker (1979) suggested that most tumor cells trapped in the lung die in that organ within the first 2 days after tumor cell injection. It is possible, however, that the damaged lung tissue releases factors that increase clonogenicity of tumor cells, a phenomenon similar to the Revesz effect (1956).

CLINICAL RELEVANCE

The clinical relevance of the phenomenon of radiation- and drug-induced enhancement of formation of metastatic foci is uncertain. Radiotherapy for patients with mammary carcinoma was found to be associated with depression of reactivity of patients' lymphocytes to mitogens (Stjernsward et al. 1972). It was even suggested that radiotherapy of mammary carcinoma can enhance the spread of this tumor to the lung (Dao and Kovaric 1962, Stjernsward 1977), and radiation-induced damage of the lungs and radiation-induced immunosuppression were considered underlying mechanisms (Stjernsward 1977). However, recent reviews of the treatment of breast cancer by radiotherapy alone or by surgery followed by radiotherapy at U. T. M. D. Anderson Hospital failed to indicate that radiotherapy increased lung metastases (Peters et al. 1980, Montague and Fletcher 1981). Although radiotherapy can be immunosuppressive and can damage the lung, at the same time it destroys the primary tumor and thus reduces or eliminates the source of circulating tumor cells. Because of the nature of cell killing by radiation, a greater number of tumor cells are eliminated during the first few dose fractions. Thus, when a localized tumor is being treated, the great majority of tumor cells available to seed metastases are killed before significant organ conditioning occurs in a fractionated regimen (Peters et al. 1980).

The difficulty, however, might arise if the treatments exert their deleterious effect on the lung and other tissues in the presence of a growing tumor outside the radiation fields, or if the tumor responds poorly to a therapeutic treatment, especially when tumors are prone to shed tumor cells into circulation. For example, an increased risk for metastasis formation could exist in the case of "prophylactic" irradiation of metastases if the primary tumor were not controlled or undergoing concomitant treatment. The possibility of this danger was shown by Owen and Bostock (1973), who found that irradiation of the lungs of dogs in the presence of growing primary tumors enhanced spontaneous metastasis in the lung. On the other hand, if the elective radiation of the lung was delivered after ablation of the primary tumor, no enhancement of metastasis was observed.

The possibility that chemotherapeutic agents could promote metastatic spread in clinical settings also exists, theoretically more often than for radiotherapy. This enhancement can occur mainly under two circumstances: the antitumor effectiveness of the agents is limited or the tumor cells have developed resistance to chemotherapeutic drugs. It is not a rare observation in clinical chemotherapy practice that the applied agents are ineffective. Also, therapeutic failures of chemotherapy are recently being ascribed more often to the development of tumor cell resistance than to the drugs used. Naturally, under such conditions the undisturbed primary tumor will continue to shed tumor cells into circulation, which will now find remote tissues conditioned for the establishment of secondary growths. However, more studies are necessary to establish the real hazards for enhanced metastasis of both chemotherapy and radiotherapy.

PROTECTION AGAINST METASTASIS ENHANCEMENT

Because of the seriousness of enhanced metastasis formation (regardless of its cause), it is important to find ways to prevent it or reduce its severity. As discussed above, attempts to interfere with putative mechanisms for the LTI and CY effect have mostly been unsuccessful. On the other hand, treatment of animals with agents that stimulate host antimetastatic resistance mechanisms has been successful in counteracting radiation- or drug-induced enhancement of metastasis formation, although, as noted earlier, this protection is not specific.

A few examples illustrate this protection. Anaerobic corynebacteria protected mice against WBI- (Milas et al. 1974) and LTI-induced (Peters et al. 1978) enhancement of metastasis of an immunogenic FSa, but only when given before irradiation. Also, the results presented in Table 5 show that the MVE-2 fraction of pyran copolymer, which is a macrophage activator and stimulator of NK

TABLE 5. *MVE-2-induced protection against LTI- and CY-induced enhancement of NFSa metastases in lungs of C_3Hf/Kam mice*

Experiment*	Treatment of recipients	No. lung metastases Mean ± S.E.	P†
1‡	None	25.3 ± 4.0	
	MVE-2	<1	
	LTI	78.1 ± 9.7	(<0.001)
	MVE-2 + LTI	2.6 ± 0.8	
2	None	6.3 ± 2.2	
	MVE-2	<1	
	CY	95.3 ± 6.0	(<0.001)
	MVE-2 + CY	30.6 ± 2.9	

* *Experiment 1:* Mice were exposed to 1,000 rad gamma rays LTI 1 day before they were given i.v. injections of 2×10^5 NFSa cells. Two days before irradiation, mice were given i.p. 25 mg/kg MVE-2. Number of metastases was determined 12 days after tumor cell injection. *Experiment 2:* Mice were treated i.p. with 25 mg/kg MVE-2, and 6 days later, they were given i.p. 200 mg/kg CY. One day after treatment with CY, mice were given i.v. injections of 5×10^4 NFSa cells. Number of tumor nodules was determined 14 days after tumor cell injection.

† Mann-Whitney *U* test.

‡ (Adapted from Milas et al., 1981.)

LTI, local thoracic irradiation; CY, cyclophosphamide; NFSa, nonimmunogenic fibrosarcoma.

cell activity (Bartocci et al. 1980), can totally abolish the LTI-induced and greatly reduce the CY-induced enhancement of metastasis formation of the weakly immunogenic NFSa. Therefore, a significant protection against metastasis-enhancing effects of radiation and chemotherapy can be achieved by pretreatment with different biological response modifiers that increase the host immune resistance to tumor cells. It is important to emphasize that this effect is not dependent on tumor immunogenicity, which might have importance for human tumors, the majority of which are weakly or not at all immunogenic.

CONCLUSION

Our data show that LTI and CY condition the lungs of experimental animals for the establishment of metastatic foci from circulating tumor cells. The effect is more pronounced as the dose of both radiation and the drug is increased. The effect is also dependent on the time interval between exposure of animals to these treatments and the i.v. inoculation of tumor cells; it peaks 1 day after the treatments, but can last for days and weeks and may show a second wave after many months.

Direct damage to the lung tissue seems to be the major mechanism by which these treatments promote metastasis formation. Although initial trapping is not affected, more tumor cells remain in damaged tissues, which also because of unknown mechanisms stimulate the efficiency of arrested tumor cells to form metastases. CY, however, may act in part by suppressing host antitumor resistance mechanisms mediated by NK cells.

The clinical implications of these findings are uncertain at present. It might be expected that damage to the lung by radiation or drugs would promote spontaneous metastasis if an unsterilized source of circulating tumor cells persists. For example, promotion might occur after prophylactic irradiation in the face of a growing tumor outside the field or when the tumor does not respond to the administered chemotherapeutic agents. When tumors respond to treatments, the source of circulating cells is reduced or eliminated and the probability that the conditioned lung will lead to metastasis enhancement should be reduced or nonexistent.

Several approaches have been tried to prevent or reduce the enhancement of metastasis. Approaches designed to interfere specifically with putative mechanisms of the LTI and CY effect, such as treatments with steroidal and nonsteroidal antiinflammatory drugs, the radioprotector WR-2721, and the prostacyclin-stimulating agent nafazatrom, were ineffective. However, a significant reduction of the metastasis enhancement can be achieved by pretreatment with agents that activate macrophages or stimulate NK cell activity.

Thoracic irradiation and CY treatments are not the only iatrogenic factors that can increase formation of metastases. Many cancer chemotherapy agents and various other drugs, under certain circumstances, share this untoward property. It is important for future research to identify such damaging agents, understand the mechanism of their effect, and develop means of prevention.

ACKNOWLEDGMENTS

This investigation was supported in part by grant number CA-06294 and CA-16672, awarded by the National Cancer Institute.

We wish to thank Drs. H. R. Withers and H. Ito, Mrs. Nancy Hunter, and Ms. Kathy Mason for their collaboration in studies reported herein. We wish to thank Ms. Rozanne Goddard for her assistance in the preparation of this manuscript.

REFERENCES

Adams, G. E. 1981. Hypoxic-mediated drugs for radiation and chemotherapy. Cancer 48:696–707.

Ando, K., N. Hunter, and L. J. Peters. 1979. Immunologically nonspecific enhancement of artificial lung metastases in tumor-bearing mice. Cancer Immunol. Immunother. 6:131–136.

Bartocci, A., V. Papademetriou, and M. A. Chirigos. 1980. Enhanced macrophage and natural killer cell antitumor activity by various molecular weight maleic anhydride divinyl ethers. J. Immunopharmacol. 2:149–158.

Brown, J. M. 1973. The effect of lung irradiation on the incidence of pulmonary metastases in mice. Br. J. Radiol. 46:613–618.

Brown, J. M., and E. T. Parker. 1979. Host treatments affecting artificial pulmonary metastases: Interpretation of loss of radioactively labelled cells from lungs. Br. J. Cancer 40:577–688.

Carmel, J. R., and J. M. Brown. 1977. The effect of cyclophosphamide and other drugs on the incidence of pulmonary metastases in mice. Cancer Res. 37:145–151.

Dao, T. L., and J. Kovaric. 1962. Incidence of pulmonary and skin metastases in women with breast cancer who received postoperative irradiation. Surgery 52:203–212.

Dubravsky, N. B., C. Dubrawsky, S. Jampolis, K. Mason, N. Hunter, and H. R. Withers. 1981. Long-term effects of pulmonary damage in mice on lung weight, compliance, hydroxyproline content and formation of metastases. Br. J. Radiol. 54:1075–1080.

Grdina, D. J., L. Peters, S. Jones, and E. Chan. 1978. Separation of cells from a murine fibrosarcoma on the basis of size. II. Differential effects of cell size and age on lung retention and colony formation in normal and pre-conditioned mice. JNCI 61:215–220.

Hanna, N., and I. J. Fidler. 1980. Role of natural killer cells in the destruction of circulating tumor emboli. JNCI 65:801–809.

Honn, K. V. 1983. Inhibition of tumor cell metastasis by modulation of the vascular prostacyclin/thromboxane A_2 system. Clin. Exp. Metastasis 1:103–114.

Kramer, R. H., R. Gonzales, and G. L. Nicolson. 1980. Metastatic tumor cells adhere preferentially to the extracellular matrix underlying vascular endothelial cells. Int. J. Cancer 26:639–645.

Milas, L., N. Hunter, I. Basic, and H. R. Withers. 1974. Protection by *Corynebacterium granulosum* against radiation induced enhancement of artificial pulmonary metastases of a murine fibrosarcoma. JNCI 52:1875–1880.

Milas, L., B. Malenica, and N. Allegretti. 1979. Enhancement of artificial lung metastases in mice caused by cyclophosphamide. I. Participation of impairment of host antitumor resistance. Cancer Immunol. Immunother. 6:191–196.

Milas, L., E. M. Hersh, and N. Hunter. 1981. Therapy of artificial and spontaneous metastases of murine tumors with maleic anhydride-divinyl ether-2. Cancer Res. 41:2378–2385.

Milas, L., E. M. Hersh, D. A. Stringfellow, and N. Hunter. 1982a. Studies on the antitumor activities of pyrimidinone-interferon inducers. I. Effect against artificial and spontaneous lung metastases of murine tumors. JNCI 68:139–145.

Milas, L., N. Hunter, B. O. Reid, and H. D. Thames, Jr. 1982b. Protective effects of S-2-(3-aminopropylamino)ethylphosphorothioic acid against radiation damage of normal tissues and a fibrosarcoma in mice. Cancer Res. 42:1888–1897.

Milas, L., N. Daly, N. Hunter, R. Meoz, and L. J. Peters. 1983. Enhancement by misonidazole of metastatic tumor nodule formation in the lungs of mice. Clin. Exp. Metastasis 1:61–70.

Moncada, S., and J. R. Vane. 1977. The discovery of prostacyclin—a fresh insight into arachidonic acid metabolism, *in* Biochemical Aspects of Prostaglandin and Thromboxane Research, N. Kharasch and J. Fried, eds. Academic Press, Inc., New York, pp. 155–177.

Montague, E. D., and G. H. Fletcher. 1981. Is irradiation outdated in the primary treatment of nondisseminated breast cancer?, *in* Immunopharmacologic Effects of Radiation Therapy, J. B. Dubois, B. Serrou, and C. Rosenfeld, eds. Raven Press, New York, pp. 389–397.

Owen, L. N., and D. E. Bostock. 1973. Prophylactic X-irradiation of the lung in canine tumours with particular reference to osteosarcoma. Eur. J. Cancer 9:747–752.

Peters, L. J., and K. A. Mason. 1977. Enhancement of artificial lung metastases by cyclophosphamide: Pharmacological and mechanistic considerations, *in* Cancer Invasion and Metastasis: Biologic Mechanisms and Therapy, S. B. Day, W. P. L. Myers, P. Stansly, S. Garattini, and M. G. Lewis, eds. Raven Press, New York, pp. 397–410.

Peters, L. J., K. A. Mason, W. J. McBride, and Y. Z. Patt. 1978. Enhancement of lung colony forming efficiency by local thoracic irradiation: Interpretation of labeled cell studies. Radiology 126:499–505.

Peters, L. J., K. A. Mason, and H. R. Withers. 1980. Effect of lung irradiation on metastases: Radiobiological studies and clinical correlations, *in* Radiation Biology in Cancer Research, R. E. Meyn and H. R. Withers, eds. Raven Press, New York, pp. 515–529.

Revesz, L. 1956. The effect of tumor cells killed by X-rays upon the growth of admixed viable cells. Nature 178:1391–1392.

Stjernsward, J., M. Jondal, F. Vanki, H. Wigzell, and R. Sealy. 1972. Lymphopenia and change in distribution of human B and T lymphocytes in peripheral blood induced by irradiation for mammary carcinoma. Lancet I:1352–1356.

Stjernsward, J. 1977. Radiotherapy, host immunity and cancer spread, *in* Secondary Spread in Breast Cancer, Vol. III, New Aspects of Breast Cancer, B. A. Stoll, ed. Heinemann Medical Books, Ltd., London, pp. 139–167.

Talmage, J. E., K. M. Myers, D. J. Prieur, and J. R. Starkey. 1980. Role of natural killer cells in tumor growth and metastasis: C57Bl/6 normal and beige mice. JNCI 65:929–935.

Thompson, S. C. 1974. Tumor colony growth in the irradiated mouse lung. Br. J. Cancer 30:337–341.

van den Brenk, H. A. S., H. Kelly, and C. Orton. 1974a. Reduction by anti-inflammatory corticosteroids of clonogenic growth of allogenic tumour cells in normal and irradiated tissues of the rat. Br. J. Cancer 29:365–372.

van den Brenk, H. A. S., M. Stone, H. Kelly, C. Orton, and C. Sharpington. 1974b. Promotion of growth of tumour cells in acutely inflamed tissues. Br. J. Cancer 30:246–316.

Van Putten, L. M., L. K. J. Kram, H. H. C. Van Dierendenck, T. Smink, and M. Fuzy. 1975. Enhancement of drugs of metastatic lung nodule formation after intravenous tumor cell injection. Int. J. Cancer 15:588–595.

Withers, H. R., and L. Milas. 1973. Influence of preirradiation of lung on development of artificial pulmonary metastases of fibrosarcoma in mice. Cancer Res. 33:1931–1936.

Yuhas, J. M., J. M. Spellman, and F. Culo. 1980. The role of WR-2721 in radiotherapy and/or chemotherapy. Cancer Clin. Trials 3:211–216.

Cancer Invasion and Metastasis: Biologic and Therapeutic Aspects edited by Garth L. Nicolson and Luka Milas. Raven Press, New York © 1984.

On the Immunogenicity of Tumor Cells and the Pattern of Metastasis

Untae Kim

Department of Pathology, Roswell Park Memorial Institute, New York State Department of Health, Buffalo, New York 14263

All malignant tumors in man have the inherent capacity to invade the underlying soft tissue stroma and metastasize to distant organs via the lymphatic or hematogenous routes. Such tumors do not usually provoke host immune reactions; namely, they are either weakly or not at all immunogenic. This characteristic seems to be produced, at least in part, by the immunological selection pressure on tumor cells over a long period of time. Cancer in man is a relatively late event in life, with enough time for transformed cells to have been subjected repeatedly to various routine selection forces.

In contrast, the common laboratory animal tumors, with the rare exception of spontaneous ones arising among aging retired breeders, are usually induced rapidly with potent oncogenic agents; thus, they lack the capacity to metastasize. During the past 10 years, we have been successful in developing a number of naturally metastasizing rat mammary carcinomas that closely resemble human cancer in that respect. Perhaps it would be useful to examine the origin of these tumors and their metastatic potential in terms of their biological, biochemical, and immunological characteristics.

PATHOGENESIS OF METASTASIZING TUMORS

Table 1 lists nine established rat mammary tumors that metastasize spontaneously via the lymphatic or hematogenous routes. These tumors can be divided into three categories according to their pathogenetic background.

The first group of tumors was induced with 3-methylcholanthrene (MCA) in partially immune "deficient" female rats that were subjected to nonspecific immunostimulation by injecting them i.p. with sheep red blood cells and i.d. with dinitrophenol (DNP)-conjugated bovine gamma globulin during the early phase of carcinogenesis, before tumor development. Then, when the tumors began to develop, the early appearing, putatively more immunogenic tumors were surgically excised to stimulate the production of tumor-specific antibody, yielding spontaneously metastasizing, nonimmunogenic tumors in one third of the animals after a latent period of about 18 months (Kim 1970, 1977). All

TABLE 1. *Biological characteristics of naturally metastasizing mammary carcinomas in W/Fu rats*

Tumor strain	Differen-tiation*	Metastasizing capacity†	Latency‡ (wks)		Metastasizing route and pattern
			Primary	Metast.	
TMT-50	W	±–+	1	7	Hematogenous: lung only
STMT-058	P	+–++	1	4	Hematogenous and lymphatic: lymph node and lung
MT-449	M	++	1.5	5	Hematogenous and lymphatic: lymph node, lung, and liver
DMBA-4	M	++–+++	2	4	Lymphatic and hematogenous: lymph node, lung, liver and bone
MT-450	W	+++	3.5	8	Hematogenous and lymphatic: lymph node and lung
SMT-077	M	++–+++	7	7	Lymphatic: lymph node, bone, lung, and liver
SMT-2B	P	++++	8.5	8.5	Lymphatic: lymph node, bone, lung, liver, spleen, and kidney
TMT-081	P	++++	2.5	3	Hematogenous and lymphatic: lymph node, lung, bone, liver, spleen, and kidney.
SMT-2A	P	++++	2	3	Lymphatic: lymph node, bone, lung, spleen, liver, kidney, and adrenal

* W = well differentiated; M = moderately differentiated; P = poorly differentiated.
† ± = microscopic; + = slight; ++ = moderate; +++ = marked; ++++ = extensive.
‡ Approximate latency when the tumor becomes palpable (3–5 mm).

but three of the tumors—MT-449, MT-450, and DMBA-4—in Table 1 belong to this category.

The second group of tumors, MT-449 and MT-450, were isolated about 5 years apart from the extremely slow growing, well-differentiated, hormone-dependent, nonmetastasizing tumor MT-W9A (Kim and Depowski 1975) after many years of consecutive transplantations in syngeneic rats. No metastasizing tumors have appeared among the rapidly growing, poorly differentiated, hormone-independent, nonmetastasizing tumors that were similarly transplanted during the same period, suggesting that the progression of tumor cells from a well to a poorly differentiated and from a slow- to a fast-growing phase in the evolution of the neoplastic state does not necessarily lead to the development of metastasizing capacity.

The metastasizing tumor DMBA-4 belongs to the third category. It was discovered accidentally in one of 10 rats treated with a large dose of the highly potent chemical carcinogen 7,12-dimethylbenzanthracene (DMBA) to induce rapidly growing, hormone-independent mammary tumors with chromosomal aberrations, under the assumption that the greater the mutagenic power of the carcinogen, the faster the developing tumors would deviate from the usual evolutionary pattern of hormone dependency. DMBA-4 developed in less than 30 days, as most DMBA-induced mammary tumors do, hardly enough time for the host to provide the immunological pressure to select a nonimmunogenic tumor cell clone. Yet it metastasized when transplanted into normal syngeneic rats.

In addition to the three categories described above, there are occasional spontaneous, nonimmunogenic tumors arising in aging animals that seemingly metastasize naturally (Hewitt and Blake 1975, Hewitt et al. 1976). Thus, most metastasizing tumors seem to require, as human cancers do, a prolonged developmental period of immunoselection.

PATTERN OF METASTASIS

As summarized in Table 1, three tumors, SMT-077, SMT-2B, and SMT-2A, metastasize preferentially via the lymphatic route, involving the lymph nodes first and then often disseminating to the bone, bypassing the lung. At later stages, the tumors will involve the lung, liver, and other organs. Five tumors, STMT-058, MT-449, DMBA-4, MT-450, and TMT-081, metastasize by both the hematogenous and lymphatic routes, first to the regional lymph nodes, next to the lung, and then to other organs in the so-called "cascade" pattern. The cells capable of settling in the bone are usually poorly differentiated. TMT-50 is the only tumor that metastasizes exclusively via the hematogenous route; it metastasizes only to the lung by embolizing the small branches of the pulmonary artery, as do most of the established murine tumors that metastasize naturally. Thus, the theory of metastatic cascade may be applicable only to those tumor cells capable of disseminating through the lymphatics.

As illustrated in Figure 1, the nonimmunogenic, antigen-shedding tumor cells enter the afferent lymphatics of the regional lymph node, converge into the caval vein via the efferent lymphatics and thoracic duct, easily traverse the pulmonary capillary network into the left side of the heart, and then spread to various organs, including the bone, by the arterial circulation. The somewhat immunogenic tumor cells with distinct glycocalyx tend to enter into the venous return, perhaps through the blood vessels within the tumor, and directly settle in the lung by embolization, unable to spread beyond it. The mechanism by which the tumor cells are capable of metastasizing to the lymph node and at the same time of developing blood-borne metastases to the lung, whether by entering into the blood stream directly from the blood vessels within or through the intralymphatic veins, is not clear.

Shedding Pattern of Viable Tumor Cells

In order to gain entry into the vascular channel, the metastasizing tumor cells must first detach themselves from the primary mass. However, such a shedding capacity does not seem to be the sole prerogative of metastasizing tumors. As shown in Table 2, some viable tumor cells can be recovered from

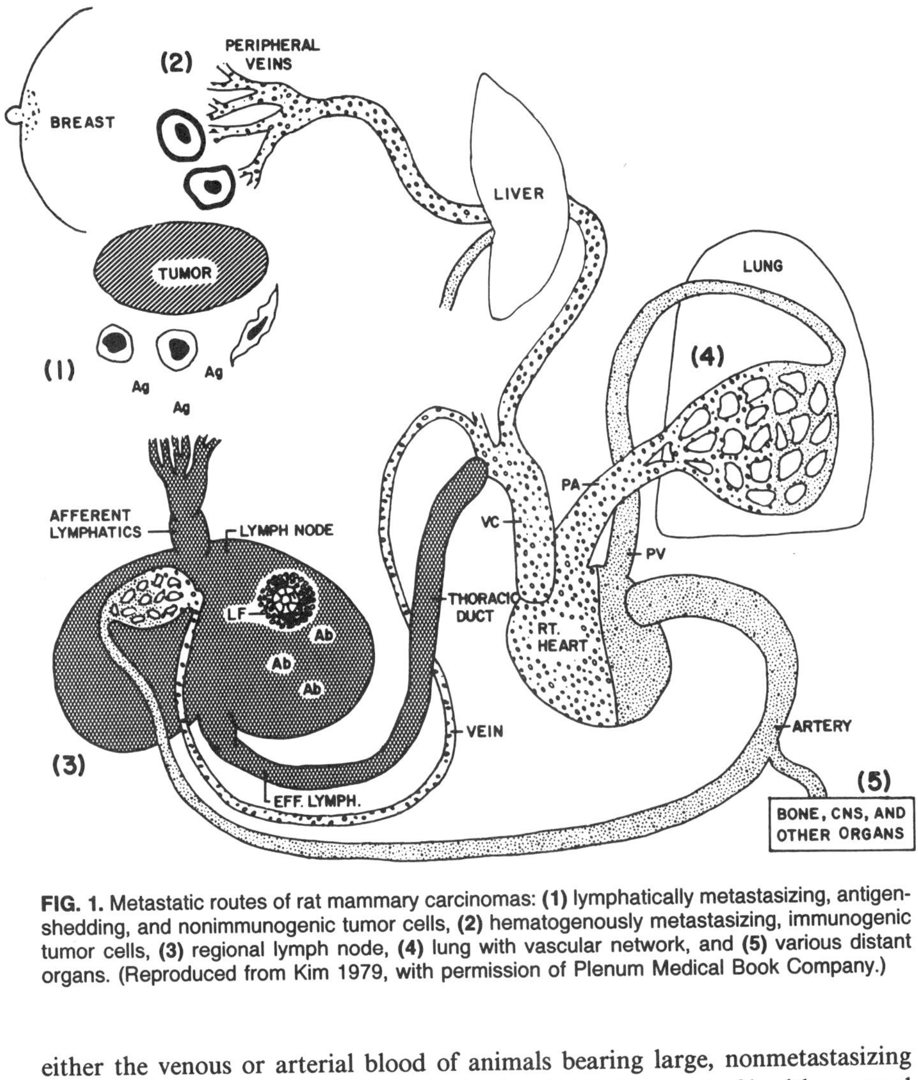

FIG. 1. Metastatic routes of rat mammary carcinomas: **(1)** lymphatically metastasizing, antigen-shedding, and nonimmunogenic tumor cells, **(2)** hematogenously metastasizing, immunogenic tumor cells, **(3)** regional lymph node, **(4)** lung with vascular network, and **(5)** various distant organs. (Reproduced from Kim 1979, with permission of Plenum Medical Book Company.)

either the venous or arterial blood of animals bearing large, nonmetastasizing tumors, but apparently are not able to survive the environment of healthy normal rats or that of their original host, for after a temporary growth they regress completely. On the other hand, all lymphatically and hematogenously metastasizing tumors, with the exception of MT-449 and MT-450, seem to continuously shed a large number of viable tumor cells into the venous return, which pass steadily through the lung into the abdominal aorta. The shedding pattern of MT-449 and MT-450 seems to be somewhat different. The bioassay of both venous and arterial blood from these animals for viable tumor cells did not yield any tumor nodule at the s.c. inoculation site, despite the fact that the rats carried large primary tumors and substantial regional lymph node metastases

TABLE 2. *Bioassay for viable cells in the circulation of mammary tumor hosts*

MT strain	Latency (wks)		MT size (mm) of blood donor*		MT latency (wks) in recipient rats† Venous blood		Arterial blood	
	P	M	P	M	P	M	P	M
Metastasizing								
SMT-2A	2	3	42	35	3	5	4.5	8.5
TMT-081	2.5	3	30	25	6	8	5	7
DMBA-4	2	4	30	20	4	6	4	5
SMT-077	7	7	32	15	25	28	25	25
SMT-2B	8.5	8.5	20	20	8	8	8	8
MT-449	1.5	5	35	10	0	0	0	0
MT-450	3.5	8	43	15	0	0	0	0
TMT-50	1	7	45	(lung)	0	0	0	0
Nonmetastasizing								
MT-100	3	—	35	—	0	—	0	—
MT-W9B	4	—	35	—	0	—	0‡	—
MT-W9D	1	—	36	—	0§	—	0	—

* Heparinized blood was drawn from the inferior caval vein or abdominal aorta.

† Each recipient was inoculated with 1 ml of blood, either venous or arterial, into the right inguinal mammary region and observed for 6 months.

‡ One rat grew an 11-mm tumor in an 8-week period, which then regressed completely.

§ One rat grew a small nodule (2 mm) after 1 week, which disappeared after 3 weeks.

P, primary; M, metastasis (right axillary lymph node); MT, mammary tumor.

when the blood samples were obtained. Whether the failure to produce tumor was due to an insufficient number of viable tumor cells in the blood or to the cells being released at intervals from the primary is not known.

CHARACTERIZATION OF METASTATIC POTENTIAL

Some of the outstanding physicochemical, biological, and biochemical characteristics of the metastasizing and nonmetastasizing tumors are summarized in Table 3. The electrophoretic mobility of these tumor cells was measured in a specially devised glass capillary tube chamber under a light microscope equipped with dark-field illumination. The metastasizing tumor cells manifested more accelerated mobility than the nonmetastasizing ones during a 9-sec period (Park et al. 1982). Increased electrophoretic mobility has been attributed to the greater net negative charge of membrane-bound molecules, and indeed, sialic acid levels have been found to be higher in the metastasizing rat mammary tumor cells (Bernacki and Kim 1977).

The ratio of protein to phospholipid in the plasma membrane is said to be inversely correlated with the membrane fluidity of mammalian cells. It was found to be much lower in some of the rat metastasizing tumors listed in Table 1 (Yatvin et al. 1982). The resulting increased membrane fluidity may represent

TABLE 3. *Characterization of metastatic potential*

Test parameters	Metastasizing	Non-metastasizing
Physicochemical		
Electrophoretic mobility	50% greater	Slower
Plasma membrane fluidity	Twice as high	Lower
Biological		
Growth characteristic:		
In vitro	Noncohesive	Highly cohesive
In vivo	Invasive	Expansive
Surface antigen shedding	Greatly increased	Little or none
Tumor blood flow	Lower, less that ⅓	Higher
Biochemical		
Glycosyltransferases:		
Sialyltransferase	Very high	Lower
Galactosyltransferase	Very high	Lower
Fucosyltransferase	Very high	Lower
Sialic acid	Higher	Lower
Gangliosides	Higher	Lower

the in vivo invasive capacity. When these cells are cultivated in vitro as a suspension culture, they grow as free-floating single cells, while the nonmetastasizing cells grow in large, tight clusters. Such a noncohesive growth pattern in vitro may be due to the constant shedding of cell surface glycoconjugates in the form of tumor-associated antigen, as is the case in vivo (Ghosh et al. 1978, 1979). It may also be partly due to the greater negative electrostatic charge on these cells, causing them to repel each other.

The shed glycoconjugates include glycoproteins as well as glycolipids, and the continuous shedding and renewal of membrane constituents also bring about the elevation of glycosyltransferases in these cells, as well as in their microenvironments (Bernacki and Kim 1977, Chatterjee and Kim 1977, 1978). Contrary to popular belief, the metastasizing tumors contain significantly fewer blood vessels than the nonmetastasizing ones, as measured by infusing radiolabeled latex particles into unanesthetized tumor hosts (Jirtle 1981). It seems, therefore, that solid tumors need only an adequate blood supply to provide nutrients and to remove waste products, but that its quantity is probably not a critical factor in metastasis.

IMMUNOGENICITY

Most of the lymphatically metastasizing tumors are nonimmunogenic, while the ordinary nonmetastasizing ones, particularly those induced by chemical carcinogens, are highly immunogenic, in the sense that only the growth of the latter can be inhibited by prior immunization with radiation-killed tumor cells (Kim 1970). However, the growth and metastasis of some hematogenously metastasizing murine tumors have recently been shown to be inhibited by stimulation of natural killer (NK) cell activity with various biological response modifiers (Hanna and Schneider 1983) and by specific and nonspecific activation of macrophages (Fidler et al. 1981). In order to define the immunogenicity of tumor cells accurately within a standardized system, the "immunological" response of the tumor host to the metastasizing and nonmetastasizing cells were tested.

Immunological Profile of Tumor-Bearing Rats

Weight of Lymphoid Organs in Tumor Hosts

It was earlier demonstrated that nonmetastasizing, chemically induced mammary tumors evoke protective immunity in syngeneic rats, whereas spontaneously metastasizing ones do not (Kim 1970, Kim et al. 1975). In a further study of such divergent effects, the lymph nodes, spleens, and thymuses of tumor-bearing rats were weighed at regular intervals. In the first week after tumor implantation, before the tumors were palpable, the regional lymph nodes of the nonmetastasizing tumor hosts were twice as large as those of normal control rats, while those of the metastasizing ones gained only about 40% over that of the controls. By the fifth week, the splenic weight was increased by 80% in the former, but only 40% in the latter. The thymuses in both groups decreased proportionately with tumor growth. In the enlarged lymph nodes and spleens of the former, there was marked lymphoid follicular hyperplasia, indicating active B-cell response (Yao et al. 1983).

In Vitro Blastogenic Capacity of Spleen Cells and Peripheral Lymphocytes

The spleen cells and peripheral lymphocytes from the nonmetastasizing tumor hosts responded to phytohemagglutinin (PHA) in vitro twice and to concanavalin A (ConA) three times as much as those from the metastasizing tumor–bearing rats. On the other hand, the lymphoid cells from the latter responded slightly better to poke weed mitogen and LPS than those from the former, indicating that the nonmetastasizing tumor cells stimulated T-cell response.

NK Activity and Prostaglandin (PGE_2) Levels

Although the data are few and preliminary, when NK activity in the spleen was measured against YAC-1 cells in vitro by the 4-h chromium-release assay, there was no significant NK activity difference in the two sets of spleens at the early phase of tumor growth. However, in the advanced stages of metastasizing tumor growth, when several lymph nodes were involved, the splenic NK activity was almost twice as high as that of the nonmetastasizing tumor. PGE_2 levels, measured by radioimmunoassay using a commercial radiolabeled PGE_2, were almost twice as high in the metastasizing tumor tissues and host spleens as those in the nonmetastasizing ones. None of the tissue culture tumor cell lines contained any measurable levels, indicating that the PGE_2 in the tumor tissue grown in vivo most likely came from the tissue macrophage. The fact that the metastasizing tumor grows and metastasizes widely in the face of elevated NK activity seems to suggest that NK cells may not be critical in the syngeneic tumor host (Leung and Kim, to be published).

Circulating Immune Complexes (CIC)

CIC in the sera of tumor hosts were measured at various intervals after tumor implantation in 2-month-old W/Fu female rats, using the Raji cell assay technique (Yoo et al. 1983). While none of the sera from rats bearing a nonmetastasizing tumor had CIC levels higher than 30 μg/ml, only a small percentage of the animals bearing the metastasizing tumors had even a slightly higher CIC: there was thus no significant difference between the two groups of tumor-bearing rats. Thus, the role of immune complexes in the pathogenesis of tumor metastasis remains unclear.

Relative Transplantability of Rat Mammary Tumors in Athymic Nude Animals

Since Rygaard (1973) initiated the heterotransplantation of human cancer in athymic nude mice, many investigators have grafted various allogeneic and xenogeneic tumors into these mice with varying degrees of success. However, it was also discovered that many of those solid tumors do not grow when passed directly from the patient to the nude mouse, that is, not without prior cultivation in vitro (Fogh et al. 1977), as though the more malignant the tumor the more difficult its transplantation. The percentage of human tumors that grow in nude mice from primary transplants has been reported as varying from 47% to less than 8% (Fogh et al. 1980). Furthermore, even those human tumors that are successfully grown in nude mice, particularly after cultivation in vitro, seldom metastasize. Sharkey and Fogh (1979) reported that out of 1,045 nude mice implanted by them with 11 different human tumor cell lines, only 14 (1.3%) developed metastasis. Similar results have been obtained even with some hematogenously metastasizing murine tumors.

The failure of virus-infected tumor cells to grow in athymic nude mice was first observed by Stiles et al. (1975). Minato and colleagues (1979) attributed such graft resistance to the increased NK activity in these animals when stimulated by interferon, and they subsequently succeeded in growing the RNA virus–infected hamster BHK21 cells, as well as in inducing metastasis in nude mice by blocking the NK activity with antisera against mouse interferon. Compared with normal mice, nude mice generally have an elevated NK activity (Herberman 1980), which often causes the rejection of syngeneic tumor grafts (Haller et al. 1977). This fact indicates that the natural resistance against tumor outgrowth in vivo may be exerted via the NK cell, outside of conventional T-cell–mediated immunity. Such NK activity can be enhanced by interferon and interferon inducers, such as poly I:C (Gidlund et al. 1978, Djeu et al. 1979a). The removal or inactivation of macrophages prior to poly I:C treatment significantly reduces NK augmentation by the interferon inducer (Djeu et al. 1979b), pointing to a possible helper relationship between the two.

Trichieri et al. (1977) reported that certain human tumor cell lines are capable of stimulating human lymphoid cells to produce interferon in vitro and went on to postulate that the surface antigens of these tumor cells might be responsible for such stimulation, which would seem to explain why human cancer cells are frequently rejected by the nude mouse. Kasai and associates (Kasai et al. 1981, Habu et al. 1981) recently presented evidence for the first time directly linking the level of NK activity and antitumor response in vivo. When nude mice were injected with rabbit antisera raised against an NK marker, asialo-GM1, the number of takes and growth of syngeneic lymphomas, as well as of human tumor xenografts, were greatly increased compared with those in nude hosts receiving only normal rabbit serum (Kasai et al. 1981, Habu et al. 1981).

As frequently observed, the nude mouse not only resists the implantation of malignant tumors, but also prevents their metastasis, even in those few cases when the tumor graft is successful. Despite the large number of viable tumor cells that are continuously being released from the primary, they are somehow blocked in the nude mouse from settling in the secondary organs, even though these cells can be recovered from the blood and organs of the hosts (Simon et al. 1982). NK cells are believed to be responsible for this phenomenon (Hanna and Fidler 1980). Gorelik and colleagues (1979) found that 3LL Lewis lung carcinoma cells growing in a s.c. or i.m. site were more sensitive to NK cytotoxicity than the metastatic 3LL cells in the lung, implying that the metastasizing cells are NK resistant. When NK-sensitive B-16 melanoma cells were implanted into NK-deficient beige mice by Talmadge and associates (1980), the tumor not only grew quickly but also metastasized throughout the lung. Thus, judging from these and other studies, the notion of NK playing a determining role in the control of tumor metastasis seems well founded.

However, the fact that both of these tumors (melanoma and lung tumor) are incapable of metastasizing beyond the lung makes the hypothesis of NK primacy less compelling. If indeed the metastatic 3LL cells are NK-resistant, what prevents them from spreading beyond the lung to other organs, including the spleen? There seem to be other natural cytotoxic cells, besides NK, that control metastasis. Even the work of Habu et al. (1981) supports the latter view, for among the 12 nude mice in which the growth of a xenografted human gastric carcinoma was markedly promoted by the specific suppression of NK activity with rabbit antisera against the asialo-GM1 ganglioside, only one had even a microscopic lymph node metastasis. The detection of normal levels of natural cytotoxic cells against solid tumors in NK-deficient beige mice by Stutman and Cuttito (1981) also supports the supposition that non-NK cytotoxic effector cells participate in the control of tumor metastasis.

Six metastasizing and four nonmetastasizing tumors were used for comparison. The tumors were removed aseptically when they reached 10–15 mm in diameter. Initially, single-cell suspensions were prepared, and about 10^6 viable cells in 0.2 ml of phosphate-buffered saline (PBS) were injected s.c. into the right flank of BALB/c-, C3H-, C57BL-, or Swiss-derived, 6–8-week-old mice of both sexes. Later, the tumors were minced finely and suspended at a 1:1 ratio in tissue culture medium 199 or RPMI-1640 without calf serum, and 0.05 ml was similarly injected into each mouse. Occasionally, mice as old as 3 months were also used. They were kept on a laminar flow rack in a clean room, and a few basic precautions were taken against unnecessary contamination. When necessary, the tumor-implanted mice were kept alive for as long as 6 months, while others were killed when their tumors became very large, usually about 40 mm across.

Thus far, 223 nude mice have been grafted with the metastasizing tumors. Only 58 (26%) accepted the grafts temporarily, whereas of 144 mice implanted with the nonmetastasizing ones, all but three (98%) accepted the grafts, which grew progressively. These results confirm the selective rejection phenomenon encountered with human cancer cells (Fogh et al. 1982). The nude mice temporarily bearing some of the metastasizing tumors showed no regional lymph node involvement or distant metastasis. On the other hand, nearly half of the mice bearing the large, nonmetastasizing tumors, grown for periods of 1 to 4 months, had hematogenous lung metastases in the form of pulmonary emboli of tumor cell clusters and their livers were also mildly involved, containing microscopic foci of tumor cell nests (Kim et al. 1982). These observations seem to indicate that the spontaneously metastasizing, nonimmunogenic, soluble tumor-associated-antigen–shedding tumors may be better defined as "T-independent" tumors that can be better controlled by a T-cell–deficient immunological environment in tumor hosts. Some human carcinomas may indeed belong to this category. The conventional, nonmetastasizing rodent tumors, on the other hand, may be characterized as "T-dependent," for their growth is often successfully controlled by the stimulation of T-cell–mediated immunity.

In order to ascertain that the selective antitumor and antimetastatic response of nude mice is not merely a histoincompatible xenograft rejection event, the metastasizing SMT-2A and TMT-081 tumors and the nonmetastasizing control tumors MT-W9B and MT-100 were allografted into nude rats of the NIH strain. Again, the nude rats rejected the former and accepted the latter. Of course, these phenomena would be best verified in syngeneic W/Fu athymic nude rats (Kim and Shin 1982).

When nude mice and rats that had already rejected the implant of a metastasizing tumor were regrafted with either the same or another metastasizing one, the challenging graft was also rejected. On the other hand, when these mice were challenged with a nonmetastasizing tumor, it was promptly accepted. Such tumor-specific reactions can also be observed by simultaneously transplanting a metastasizing tumor into one flank and a nonmetastasizing one into the other, indicating whether the nude mouse or rat is capable of responding differently to two types of tumor cells at the same time and whether T lymphocytes are involved.

Among the non-NK natural cytotoxic cells, the phagocytic blood monocytes and the tissue-bound macrophages of the reticuloendothelial system, notably those of spleen, lung, and liver, appear to be the most prominent candidates for participating in the control of tumor metastasis. Pim and Baldwin (1975) postulated that the resistance of nude mice against bacillus Calmette-Guérin (BCG)-treated malignant tumor cells from guinea pigs was likely caused by BCG-activated macrophages, and Fidler (1976) found that the i.v. infusion of activated peritoneal macrophages prevented or reduced lung metastasis of blood-borne tumor cells. Riccardi and associates (1981) showed an efficient clearance of radiolabeled tumor cells by the lung, spleen, and liver, and Cohen et al. (1982) demonstrated natural cytotoxicity against YAC-1 and other tumor cells by the isolated hepatic Kupffer cells in vitro. Among the tissue-bound natural cytotoxic cells, the pulmonary alveolar macrophages seem to be the most potent, taking up the first line of defense. Human carcinomas may grow well at the s.c., i.m., or i.p. site, but they are usually promptly rejected when injected i.v. (Stragand et al. 1980). The question remains as to whether the alveolar macrophages are more cytotoxic in the absence of T cells.

On the possible interrelationship between macrophages and NK cells, the findings in the literature are not too clear. Macrophages have been shown to augment NK activity by producing interferon upon exposure to interferon inducers (Djeu et al. 1979a). On the other hand, macrophages often seem to interfere with NK activity (Riccardi et al. 1981), perhaps through prostaglandins released from them (Brunda et al. 1980). The latter view seems to be more compatible with current beliefs about the role of prostaglandins in the development of bone metastasis, in which the osteolytic principle (prostaglandins) is believed to emanate from the tumor-associated macrophages, rather than from the tumor cells themselves. Such a supposition can be tested with one of the bone-metastasizing rat mammary carcinomas listed in Table 1.

It is also possible that the rejection phenomenon is an antibody-mediated process, for nude mice are capable of generating cytotoxic antibodies against allogeneic and xenogeneic skin grafts (Koen et al. 1974, Gerlag et al. 1977, Rygaard 1974), as well as against human tumor grafts (Rygaard 1973). Although the antibody is formed in concentration sufficient to cause rejection after administration of rabbit complement, it is said that rejection does not occur spontaneously in the nude mouse, due to the inefficiency of the mouse's own complement system and to the absence of T cells. This may cause the antibody, even at low levels, to interact with macrophages and carry out the antibody-dependent cell (macrophage)-mediated cytotoxic process against the rat tumors. More qualitative and quantitative analyses of antibody production by the mice that reject the metastasizing rat tumors are necessary.

Abrogation of Selective Antitumor Response in Nude Animals

Suppression of B-Cell Function

Rabbit anti-mouse lymph node serum (ALS) (Microbiological Associates, Bethesda, MD) or rabbit antisera raised against nude mouse spleen cells (ASC) (prepared by Dr. Shin, Albert Einstein College of Medicine, Bronx, NY) were diluted in PBS at a 1:1 ratio, and 0.1 ml was injected i.p. into each nude mouse daily, beginning one day before the tumor transplantation and continuing for 30 days or until the end of the experiment (Simon et al. 1982). The metastasizing tumors grew in both the ALS- and ASC-treated mice, becoming as large as 15–20 mm in some of them in a 30-day period. However, as the tumor implant grew, it gradually became necrotic, with only the periphery of the tumor mass being viable. Some of these mice often developed lymphangitic (perivascular) metastasis to the lung, pericardium, pleura, and, occasionally, the regional lymph node. Such metastasis, however, was not as widespread as that in the intact syngeneic tumor-bearing rats, particularly to the lymph nodes or bones. When the treatment was discontinued, the tumor ceased to grow, turned black, and quickly underwent complete necrosis.

Needless to say, the rabbit sera probably contained various inhibiting factors, including anti-B cell, anti-NK and antimacrophage substances, and more selective suppression is needed to learn the rejection mechanism. In addition, the massive central necrosis developing so rapidly in the tumor suggests a vascular event as the possible cause. Jirtle (1981), who measured the blood flow rate in these metastasizing and nonmetastasizing rat tumors using radiolabeled latex beads, found that the rate in the former was only 25% that of the latter.

Suppression of NK Activity

A small pilot experiment was carried out to test the effect of estrogen on the growth of the metastasizing tumors in athymic nude rats of NIH strain. Diethylstilbestrol (DES) pellets of 1 mg were implanted s.c. in the back of nude rats 1 to 2 days prior to tumor allograft and replaced with new ones every 4 weeks. Of all the nude rats, 15–30%, whether treated or untreated, accepted the tumor grafts initially, but while those in the DES group were quite viable, those in the untreated control group were completely necrotic. No metastasis was detected in either group. The experiment needs to be repeated on a larger scale with a longer period between estrogen treatment and tumor implantation (Kim and Shin 1982).

Antibody Production Against Rat Tumors by Athymic Nude Mice

Surprisingly, as previously described, the sera collected from nude mice that had rejected a metastasizing rat tumor graft contained no detectable tumor-specific antibody against the plasma membrane preparation of such tumor, as tested by the standard Ouchterlony immunodiffusion technique, while the sera of mice bearing a large nonmetastasizing tumor contained a distinct tumor-specific antibody (Kim et al. 1982). Further investigations are needed to determine the significance of these findings.

NK Activity in Nude Mice Implanted with Rat Mammary Tumors

The NK cytotoxicity of spleen cells obtained from nude mice that had rejected or were carrying a rat mammary tumor was tested against YAC-1 mouse lymphoma cells. Whether the spleen cells were from mice that had rejected the tumor immediately after implantation (1–4 weeks after engraftment) or were in the process of rejecting a temporary growth that eventually became completely necrotic (2 months after engraftment), NK activity was not significantly different from that of the control nude mice. The NK activity in mice with nonmetastasizing tumors, whether tested early (tumor not yet palpable), 3 weeks (8 mm), or 5 weeks (16 mm) after implantation, was either slightly decreased or showed no significant change, as compared with that of normal nude mouse spleen cells. The number of nude mice in each group was too small, however, to draw any definitive conclusions.

SELECTIVE SUPPRESSION OF T-CELL FUNCTION IN NORMAL W/Fu RATS WITH CYCLOSPORIN A

When 50-day-old intact W/Fu female rats were thymectomized or given 20 mg of cyclosporin A (Cs-A)/kg body weight three times weekly starting 1 week and 1 day, respectively, prior to the implantation of metastasizing, syngeneic tumors, the growth of these tumors was retarded by 7–10 days and their metastasis by 3 weeks, as compared with those in untreated control rats. Cs-A alone had only an occasional, very slight inhibitory effect, while thymectomy alone had no effect at all. The same combined T-cell-suppression treatment neither inhibited nor stimulated the nonmetastasizing tumors (Kim et al. 1983). Although the degree of tumor inhibition was not remarkable, the fact that selective T-cell suppression alone had some tumor-specific retardation effect is encouraging.

In summary, there has been considerable knowledge gained through the multidisciplinary analysis of this tumor system. It is obvious, however, that more work is needed in order to unravel the complexity of tumor-host interaction in the development of metastasis.

REFERENCES

Bernacki, R., and U. Kim. 1977. Concomitant elevation in sialyltransferase activity and sialic acid content in rats with metastasizing mammary tumors. Science 195:577–580.

Brunda, M. J., R. B. Herberman, and H. T. Holden. 1980. Inhibition of murine natural killer cell activity by prostaglandins. J. Immunol. 124:2682–2687.

Chatterjee, S. K., and U. Kim. 1977. Galactosyltransferase activity in metastasizing rat mammary carcinomas and its possible relationship with tumor cell surface antigen shedding. JNCI 58:273–280.

Chatterjee, S. K., and U. Kim. 1978. Fucosyltransferase activity in metastasizing and nonmetastasizing rat mammary carcinomas. JNCI 61:151–162.

Cohen, S. A., D. Salazar, and J. P. Nolan. 1982. Natural cytotoxicity of isolated rat liver cells. J. Immunol. 129:495–501.

Djeu, J. Y., J. A. Heinbaugh, H. T. Holden, and R. B. Herberman. 1979a. Augmentation of mouse natural killer cell activity by interferon and interferon inducers. J. Immunol. 122:175–181.

Djeu, J. Y., J. A. Heinbaugh, H. T. Holden, and R. B. Herberman. 1979b. Role of macrophages in the augmentation of mouse natural killer cell activity by Poly I:C and interferon. J. Immunol. 122:182–188.

Fidler, I. J., S. Caines, and Z. Dolan. 1976. Survival of hematogenously disseminated allogeneic tumor cells in athymic nude mice. Transplantation 22:208–217.

Fidler, I. J., S. Sone, W. E. Fogler, and Z. L. Barnes. 1981. Eradication of spontaneous metastases and activation of alveolar macrophages by intravenous injection of liposome containing muramyl dipeptide. Proc. Natl. Acad. Sci. USA 78:1680–1684.

Fogh, J., J. M. Fogh, and T. Orfeo. 1977. One hundred twenty-seven cultured human tumor cell lines producing tumors in nude mice. JNCI 59:221–226.

Fogh, J., J. Orfeo, J. Tiso, F. E. Sharkey, J. M. Fogh, and W. P. Daniel. 1980. Twenty-three new human tumor lines established in nude mice. Exp. Cell Biol. 48:229–239.

Fogh, J., J. Tiso, T. Orfeo, J. M. Fogh, W. P. Daniel, and F. E. Sharkey. 1982. Analysis of human tumor growth in nude mice, *in* Proceedings of the 3rd International Workshop on Nude Mice, N. D. Reed, ed. Gustav Fischer, New York, pp. 447–456.

Gerlag, P. G. G., P. J. A. Capel, J. H. M. Barden, and R. A. P. Koen. 1977. Antibody response and skin graft rejection in the nude mouse. Transplant. Proc. 9:1179–1191.

Ghosh, S. K., A. L. Grossberg, U. Kim, and D. Pressman. 1978. Identification and purification of an organ specific, tumor membrane-associated antigen from a spontaneously metastasizing rat mammary carcinoma. Immunochemistry 15:345–352.

Ghosh, S. K., A. L. Grossberg, U. Kim, and D. Pressman. 1979. A tumor associated, organ specific antigen in rat mammary carcinomas, present at high levels in metastatic and at low levels in non-metastatic tumors. JNCI. 62:1229–1233.

Gidlund, M. A., H. Orn, H. Wigzell, A. Senick, and I. Gresser. 1978. Enhanced NK cell activity in mice injected with interferon and interferon inducers. Nature 273:759–761.

Gorelik, E., M. Fogel, M. Feldman, and S. Siegal. 1979. Differences in resistance of metastatic tumor cells and cells from local tumor growth to cytotoxicity of natural killer cells. JNCI 63:1397–1404.

Habu, S., H. Fukui, K. Shimamura, M. Kasai, Y. Nagai, K. Okamura, and N. Tamaoki. 1981. In vivo effect of anti-asialo GMl. Reduction of NK activity and enhancement of transplanted tumor growth in nude mice. J. Immunol. 127:34–38.

Haller, O., M. Hansen, R. Kiessling, and H. Wigzell. 1977. Role of non-conventional natural killer cells in resistance against syngeneic tumor cells in vivo. Nature 270:609–611.

Hanna, N., and I. J. Fidler. 1980. Role of natural killer cells in the destruction of circulating tumor emboli. JNCI 65:801–809.

Hanna, N., and M. Schneider. 1983. Enhancement of tumor metastasis and suppression of natural killer cell activity by β-estradiol treatment. J. Immunol. 130:974–980.

Herberman, R. B. 1980. Natural Cell Mediated Immunity Against Tumors. Academic Press, New York.

Hewitt, H. B., and E. R. Blake. 1975. Quantitative studies of translymphnodal passage of tumour cells naturally disseminated from a non-immunogenic murine squamous carcinoma. Br. J. Cancer 31:25–35.

Hewitt, H. B., E. R. Blake, and A. S. Walder. 1976. A critique of the evidence for active host defence against cancer based on personal studies of 27 murine tumours of spontaneous origin. Br. J. Cancer 33:241–259.

Jirtle, R. L. 1981. Blood flow to lymphatic metastases in conscious rats. Eur. J. Cancer 17:53–60.
Kasai, M., T. Yoneda, S. Habu, Y. Maruyama, K. Okumura, and N. Tamaoki. 1981. In vivo effect of anti-asialo GMl antibody on natural killer activity. Nature 291:334–335.
Kim, U. 1970. Metastasizing mammary carcinomas in rats: Induction and study of their immunogenicity. Science 67:72–74.
Kim, U. 1977. Pathogenesis of spontaneously metastasizing mammary carcinomas in rats. Gann Monogr. 20:73–81.
Kim, U., A. Baumler, C. Carruthers, and K. Bielat. 1975. Immunological escape mechanism in spontaneously metastasizing mammary tumors. Proc. Natl. Acad. Sci. USA 72:1012–1016.
Kim, U., and M. J. Depowski. 1975. Progression from hormone dependence to autonomy in mammary tumors as an in vivo manifestation of sequential clonal selection. Cancer Res. 35:2068–2077.
Kim, U., T. Han, S. Ghosh, V. H. Freedman, S. I. Shin, and D. Pressman. 1982. Immunologic mechanisms of selective graft resistance to certain malignant tumors and prevention of metastases by athymic nude mice, *in* Proceedings of the 3rd International Workshop on Nude Mice, N. D. Reed, ed. Gustav Fischer, New York, pp. 367–377.
Kim, U., and S. I. Shin. 1982. On the T-independent selective anti-tumor immunity in athymic nude rats and mice against spontaneously metastasizing rat mammary carcinomas. Fed. Proc. Abstr. #241.
Kim, U., S. I. Shin, and S. A. Cohen. 1983. Selective suppression of T-cell function in normal rats simulating the T-independent anti-tumor and anti-metastatic reaction of nude mice against metastasizing rat mammary carcinomas, *in* Proceedings of the 4th International Workshop on Immune Deficient Animals in Experimental Research, B. Sordat, ed. S. Karger, AG, Basel, Switzerland (in press).
Koen, R. A. P., P. G. G. Gerlag, J. L. J. Jansen, J. F. H. M. Hagermann, and P. G. A. B. Wijdeveld. 1974. Rejection of skin graft in the nude mouse. Nature 251:69–70.
Minato, N., B. R. Bloom, C. Jones, J. Holland, and L. M. Reid. 1979. Mechanism of rejection of virus persistently infected tumor cells by athymic nude mice. J. Exp. Med. 149:1117–1133.
Park, B. H., R. M. Fike, and U. Kim. 1982. Increased electrophoretic mobility of rat mammary tumor cells: A positive correlation with metastatic potential. IRCS Med. Sci. 10:96–97.
Pim, M. V., and R. W. Baldwin. 1975. BCG immunotherapy of rat tumours in athymic nude mice. Nature 254:77–78.
Riccardi, C., A. Santoni, T. Barlozzari, C. Cesarini, and R. B. Herberman. 1981. Suppression of natural killer (NK) activity by splenic adherent cells of low NK-reactive mice. Int. J. Cancer 28:811–818.
Rygaard, J. 1973. Thymus & Self, Immunology of the Mouse Mutant Nude. Wiley, New York.
Rygaard, J. 1974. Skin grafts in nude mice. Acta Pathol. Microbiol. Scand. 82A:80–112.
Sharkey, F. E., and J. Fogh. 1979. Metastasis of human tumors in athymic nude mice. Int. J. Cancer 24:733–738.
Simon, R. S., A. S. Klein, U. Kim, V. H. Freedman, and S. I. Shin. 1982. Thymus-independent host resistance against the growth and metastasis of allogeneic and xenogeneic tumors in nude mice, *in* Proceedings of the 3rd International Workshop on Nude Mice, N. D. Reed, ed. Gustav Fischer, New York, pp. 379–388.
Stiles, C., W. S. Desmond, G. Sato, and M. H. Saier, Jr. 1975. Failure of human cells transformed by simian virus 40 to form tumors in athymic nude mice. Proc. Natl. Acad. Sci. USA 72:4871–4875.
Stragand, J. J., J. P. Bergerat, R. A. White, J. Hokanson, and B. Drewinko. 1980. Biological and cell kinetic properties of a human colonic adenocarcinoma (LoVo) grown in athymic mice. Cancer Res. 40:2846–2852.
Stutman, O., and M. J. Cuttito. 1981. Normal levels of natural cytotoxic cells against tumours in NK-deficient beige mice. Nature 290:254–256.
Talmadge, J. E., K. M. Meyers, D. J. Prieur, and J. R. Starkey. 1980. Role of NK cells in tumour growth and metastasis in beige mice. Nature 254:622–624.
Trinchieri, G., D. Santoli, and B. B. Knowles. 1977. Tumor cell lines induce interferon in human lymphocytes. Nature 270:611–613.
Yao, L. R., B. H. Park, and U. Kim. 1983. Effects of nonmetastasizing and metastasizing rat mammary tumors on the host immune system. Fed. Proc. 42:516.

Yatvin, M. B., J. Vorpahl, and U. Kim. 1982. Differential response to heat by metastatic and non-metastatic rat mammary tumors, *in* Advances in Medicine and Biology, H. J. Bicher, ed. Academic Press, New York, pp. 177–184.

Yoo, T. J., J. P. Balint, Jr., R. S. Whiteaker, R. A. Floyd, and U. Kim. 1983. Circulating immune complexes in rats with metastasizing or nonmetastasizing mammary tumor. Int. Arch. Allergy Appl. Immunol. 71:224–227.

Cancer Invasion and Metastasis: Biologic and Therapeutic Aspects edited by Garth L. Nicolson and Luka Milas. Raven Press, New York © 1984.

Anticoagulants and Tumor Growth: Pharmacological Considerations

Peter Hilgard

Asta-Werke AG Degussa Pharma Gruppe, D-4800 Bielefeld 14, West Germany

In 1949, Strauss and Saphir demonstrated that dicumarol treatment of rabbits prior to the intravenous injection of a suspension of Brown-Pearce carcinoma cells diminished the incidence of fibrin thrombi associated with intravascular cancer cells in the lungs. Since anticoagulation appeared to permit viable tumor cells to remain free in the circulation for a longer time without becoming entrapped in thrombotic material, the authors speculated that deceleration of blood coagulability might enhance metastasis formation. Three years later, Terranova and Chiossone (1952) showed that anticoagulation of animals with heparin before tumor cell challenge resulted in a significant reduction of subsequent tumor colonies.

The more recent systematic approaches to the evaluation of the effects of anticoagulants on experimental metastasis were based on the observations by Wood (1958) of the intravascular events following the introduction of tumor cells into the circulation. From his in vivo investigations, Wood concluded that the failure of embolic tumor cells to establish metastases may be related to their inability to attach themselves securely to the endothelium and to evoke the formation of a surrounding thrombus. Consequently, the local activation of the coagulation mechanism at the site of tumor cell lodgement was considered to be a prerequisite for metastasis formation from blood-borne cancer cells. Thus, drugs with antithrombotic properties should also generally act as antimetastatic agents.

Initial experimental interest focused on anticoagulants that interfered in one way or another with the formation of fibrin (e.g., heparin, coumarins, snake venoms, fibrinolytic enzymes). Antiplatelet drugs (e.g., aspirin, dipyridamole, prostacyclin) have only recently been investigated more extensively for their effects on tumor dissemination, and new concepts of the specific role of blood platelets are currently emerging.

The approaches to the study of anticoagulants in tumor dissemination have been largely limited to two model systems: (1) The intravenous injection of viable tumor cell suspensions and (2) the transplantation of spontaneously metastasizing solid tumors. Blood coagulability was altered by means of pharmacological interference with the coagulation or fibrinolytic mechanism of the host animal.

The commonly used drugs in these experiments and their targets within the coagulation system are shown in Figure 1. It is beyond the scope of this chapter to review all existing data on each individual compound in relation to its effects on tumor growth and tumor dissemination. Therefore, only a few representative experiments will be discussed, primarily under the aspect of their possible clinical relevance. Since the next chapter will discuss the significance of the platelet-tumor cell interaction for metastasis (Honn 1984, see pages 361–388, this volume), this contribution will be confined to some aspects of the pharmacology of the classic anticoagulants as antimetastatic drugs.

Morphological studies on the fate of intravascular cancer cells following their intravenous injection revealed that thrombus formation around cells adherent to the vascular endothelium is an early event of short duration. Experimentally, fibrin or fibrinlike material and platelets can easily be identified within the first 15 min, but after 6 h the thrombotic material has disappeared even though most tumor cells are still intravascular (Hilgard 1980). From these observations it can be concluded that microthrombosis can be a pathogenic factor only during the very early stage of tumor cell lodgement. Consequently, anticoagulants should exert their "antimetastatic" effects in the lung colony assay primarily during a short period following tumor cell challenge.

Table 1 shows the effects of the pretreatment of C57BL mice with various anticoagulants followed by the intravenous injection of a suspension of viable Lewis lung carcinoma cells. The adequacy of anticoagulation at the time of

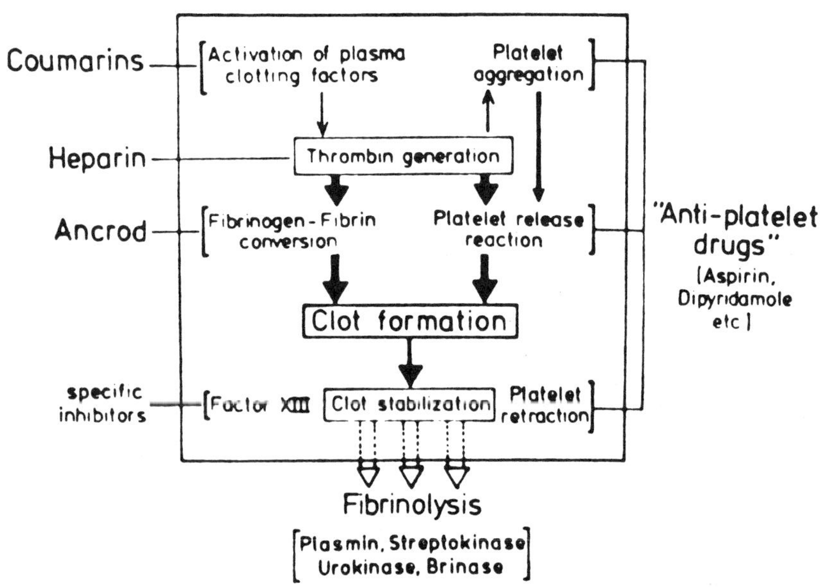

FIG. 1. Pharmacological targets of anticoagulants used to prevent experimental metastases. (Reproduced from Hilgard and Thornes 1976, with permission of the *European Journal of Cancer.*)

TABLE 1. *Effect of pretreatment with hemostatically active drugs on lung colony development after i.v. challenge with Lewis lung carcinoma cells in C57BL mice*

Treatment	No. animals	Lung colonies (percent of control group)	Significance (U test)
Heparin (s.c.)	20	6	P<0.01
Phenprocoumon (oral)	24	3	P<0.01
Ancrod (s.c.)	20	12	P<0.01
Urokinase (i.v.)	18	21	P<0.05
EACA*	12	103	N.S.
Aspirin	25	121	N.S.
Dipyridamole (RA 233)	25	118	N.S.

* epsilon-amino caproic acid.

tumor cell injection was assessed by appropriate laboratory tests. Apart from an antifibrinolytic agent (epsilon-amino caproic acid; EACA) and two platelet aggregation inhibitors (aspirin, RA 233), all drugs reduced the number of lung colonies compared with their corresponding untreated control group. If, however, anticoagulation was initiated 24 h after the tumor cell challenge under otherwise identical experimental conditions, no significant influence on the subsequent development of lung colonies was observed (Table 2). The only exception was the coumarin derivative phenprocoumon, which was as effective as in the previous experiment.

Several conclusions can be drawn from this series of experiments:

1. Anticoagulants preventing fibrin formation are effective in reducing lung colonies after intravenous transplantation of tumor cells, probably through their influence on early tumor cell lodgement.
2. Conventional inhibitors of platelet aggregation failed to reduce lung colonies under the present experimental conditions.
3. Coumarin anticoagulants must exert, in addition to their anticoagulant effects, other pharmacological actions on early "metastatic" tumor growth.

Although these results and conclusions are generally supported by the existing

TABLE 2. *Effect of treatment with hemostatically active drugs 24 h after tumor cell challenge on lung colony development from Lewis lung carcinoma in C57BL mice*

Treatment	No. animals	Lung colonies (percent of control group)	Significance (U test)
Heparin	12	98	N.S.
Phenprocoumon	15	7	P<0.01
Ancrod	12	109	N.S.
Urokinase	10	112	N.S.
Aspirin	14	104	N.S.

literature, conflicting data have also been published: Heparin was shown to decrease lung colonies, but a simultaneous increase of extrapulmonary tumor colonies was frequently observed (Maat 1978). In spontaneously metastasizing tumors, heparin was either ineffective (Maat and Hilgard 1981) or even increased the number of metastases (Hagmar 1970). In accordance with the hypothesis that fibrin formation facilitates the establishment of metastases, fibrinolysis inhibitors were originally found to increase lung colonies in various experiments, whereas fibrinolytic enzymes appeared to reduce "metastases" (Hilgard and Thornes 1976). More recently, however, the opposite effect was described, and fibrin formation around embolic cancer cells was considered to be rather a defense mechanism of the host against tumor metastasis (Tanaka et al. 1982).

These few examples make it already clear that the interrelation between the coagulation mechanism and intravascular tumor cells is more complex than could be anticipated from the original hypothesis. Since most anticoagulants also interact with biological systems other than the coagulation cascade, the interpretation of experimental results is sometimes difficult. The complement system, adhesive glycoproteins of the cell surface, chemotaxis, growth factors, the prostaglandins, and the reticuloendothelial system are just a few examples of other possible pharmacological targets for anticoagulants that could indirectly influence the lodgement and subsequent growth of metastatic tumor cells.

An intriguing fact is the poor reproducibility of the antimetastatic effects of most anticoagulants in spontaneously metastasizing tumor models. Ancrod, a defibrinating viper venom, is highly effective in reducing lung colonies in Lewis lung carcinoma and B16 melanoma. Since daily injections of that compound produced a stable state of anticoagulation in mice, several experiments were carried out to assess its effects on spontaneous metastasis from Lewis lung carcinoma and B16 melanoma (Table 3). In none of the four independent experiments could an antimetastatic effect be documented. Similarly, long-term heparin treatment, although hemostatically active throughout the period of tumor growth, did not prevent the formation of spontaneous metastases from either Lewis lung carcinoma or B16 melanoma. In contrast, long-term treatment with the coumarin derivative phenprocoumon exhibited significant antimetastatic activity in both spontaneously metastasizing tumors (Table 4).

These data suggest a lack of correlation between antithrombotic and antimetastatic activity in spontaneously metastasizing tumors. A review of the current literature on anticoagulants and tumor dissemination confirms the inconsistent effects of heparin, viper venoms, and fibrinolytic enzymes in long-term experiments. In contrast, coumarin anticoagulants are potent antimetastatic agents, and this effect can be reproducibly demonstrated in a great variety of experimental systems (Maat and Hilgard 1981).

Long-term anticoagulation with coumarin derivatives reduced not only metastatic but also primary tumor growth (Hilgard et al. 1977). Hoover and coworkers (1976) succeeded in establishing a dose-response relationship for the antimetastatic effects of sodium warfarin. In therapeutic doses coumarins have

TABLE 3. *Effect of Ancrod on lung colonies and spontaneous metastases from Lewis lung carcinoma and B16 melanoma in C57BL mice*

Tumor	Treatment	No. of animals	Lung: No. colonies	Lung: No. metastases	Significance
Ancrod pretreatment					
Lewis lung	Control	11	41.7 ± 1.5		P < 0.05
	Ancrod	19	9.4 ± 1.1		
B16	Control	14	23.6 ± 1.8		P < 0.05
	Ancrod	16	5.6 ± 0.9		
Continued Ancrod treatment					
Lewis lung					
Exp. 1	Control	14		7.1 ± 1.2	N.S.
	Ancrod	15		6.6 ± 0.1	
Exp. 2	Control	16		2.7 ± 0.5	N.S.
	Ancrod	16		3.2 ± 0.6	
B16					
Exp. 1	Control	16		0.9 ± 0.4	N.S.
	Ancrod	15		0.7 ± 0.2	
Exp. 2	Control	15		4.1 ± 0.8	N.S.
	Ancrod	14		4.4 ± 1.1	

N.S. = not significant.
(Reproduced from Maat and Hilgard 1981, with permission of *Journal of Cancer Research and Clinical Oncology.*)

TABLE 4. *Effect of continued heparin and phenprocoumon treatment on spontaneous metastases in C57BL mice*

Tumor	Treatment	No. animals	No. metastases	Significance
Lewis lung	Control	15	22.7 ± 7.7	N.S.
	Heparin	18	20.8 ± 5.5	
B16	Control	15	12.2 ± 1.3	N.S.
	Heparin	13	10.9 ± 1.4	
Lewis lung	Control	30	7.3 ± 0.5	P < 0.005
	Phenprocoumon	30	1.1 ± 0.2	
B16	Control	15	6.9 ± 0.6	P < 0.005
	Phenprocoumon	17	1.2 ± 0.3	

N.S. = not significant.
(Reproduced from Maat and Hilgard 1981, with permission of the *Journal of Cancer Research and Clinical Oncology.*)

no direct cytotoxic effect: preincubation of Lewis lung carcinoma cells over various periods with phenprocoumon prior to implantation did not alter the kinetics of tumor growth. In addition, coumarin anticoagulation did not influence the mean survival time of L1210 leukemic mice.

The data presented in Table 2 demonstrate that phenprocoumon treatment must affect metastatic tumor growth predominantly after the initial intravascular arrest of the malignant cells, suggesting that its mode of action is not mediated by its antithrombotic action. Further evidence that the reduction of lung colonies caused by oral anticoagulants is independent from their effects on blood coagulability is derived from a series of experiments in which the coumarin-induced coagulation defect was restored by administration of prothrombin complex. The capacity of phenprocoumon to reduce lung colonies was independent from the drug-induced hypocoagulability since it was equally demonstrable in animals with no coagulation defect at the time of tumor cell challenge (Hilgard and Maat 1979).

The finding that warfarin enantiomers act as antimetastatic agents only if they produce a coagulation defect suggested, in light of the above results, that their antimetastatic effect was somehow related to vitamin K antagonism (Poggi et al. 1978). Diet-induced vitamin K deficiency in mice was as effective as coumarin anticoagulation in reducing tumor colonies after i.v. challenge as well as in preventing spontaneous metastasis from transplanted solid tumors (Hilgard 1977). Since the coagulation defect is apparently of minor importance and a direct drug effect could be ruled out, the mode by which coumarin anticoagulants exert their antimetastatic action is likely to involve vitamin K metabolism.

The role of vitamin K in protein synthesis has only recently been elucidated. It has become obvious that this vitamin is not simply the unique coagulation vitamin but that it is also required for a variety of other proteins with hitherto mostly unknown biological functions (Stenflo 1976). Vitamin K is necessary for the postribosomal carboxylation of glutamic acid in these proteins, all of which subsequently exhibit high affinity for calcium and phospholipids. Reduction of these calcium and phospholipid binding sites on the cell membrane through vitamin K antagonists might profoundly influence the function of tumor or certain host target cells.

Evidence that oral anticoagulants (warfarin/phenprocoumon) might indeed alter host factors is derived from the observation of their effects on peritoneal macrophages in mice (Figure 2). Although anticoagulants do not directly stimulate macrophages, they can significantly enhance macrophage activation after stimulation with thioglycolate or *Corynebacterium parvum* (Hilgard 1981).

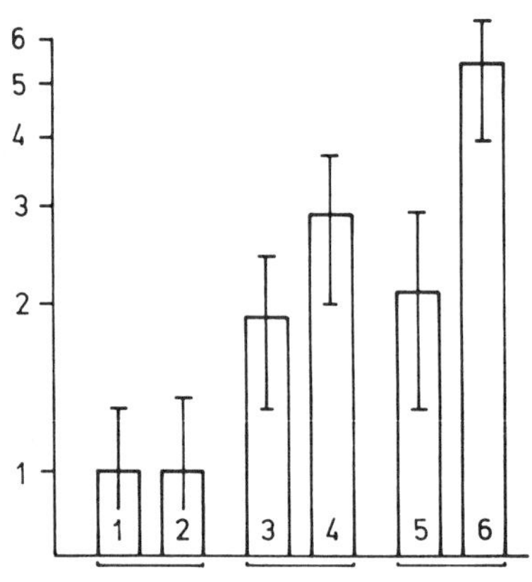

FIG. 2. Phagocytic indices of peritoneal macrophages derived from C57BL mice treated in vivo for 6 days with phenprocoumon and/or a single dose of nonspecific immunostimulants. **1,** control (no treatment); **2,** phenprocoumon; **3,** control plus thioglycolate (i.p.); **4,** phenprocoumon plus thioglycolate (i.p.); **5,** control plus *Corynebacterium parvum* (i.v.); **6,** phenprocoumon plus *C. parvum* (i.v.). (Reproduced from Hilgard 1981, with permission of Raven Press.)

Macrophage poisons such as silica and carrageenan totally abolish the antimetastatic effect of warfarin in Lewis lung carcinoma and B16 melanoma of mice (Maat 1981).

Another experimental finding that could provide a clue to the tumor inhibitory effects of coumarin anticoagulants is the vitamin K dependency of a cancer procoagulant. Lewis lung carcinoma cells contain and secrete under appropriate experimental conditions a cysteine endopeptidase that, by bypassing the classic coagulation pathway, can directly activate coagulation factor X (Hilgard and Whur 1980). Although the biological significance of this enzyme is unknown, its vitamin K–dependent biosynthesis warrants further consideration in the context of the therapeutic efficacy of coumarins.

In summary, the interest in anticoagulants as antimetastatic agents is continuing, but it has become evident that their pharmacological effects may not necessarily be related to their antithrombotic properties. The initial hypothesis that thrombus formation around embolic cancer cells is a consistent part of the pathobiology of metastasis formation clearly requires revision. Morphological evidence of fibrin in association with embolic cancer cells is exclusively derived from experiments with intravenous tumor transplantation, whereas intravascular cancer cells shed from transplanted primary tumors are very rarely associated with fibrin (Maat and Hilgard 1981). Trapping of tumor cell emboli in thrombotic material within lung capillaries after intravenous tumor transplantation is likely to be an unspecific phenomenon, since viable tumor cells as well as killed tumor cells elicit an identical thrombotic response (Hilgard 1973). Furthermore, anticoagulants (heparin) decrease the retention of viable as well as heat-killed osteosarcoma cells in the lungs after intravenous injection in an identical fashion (De Ruiter et al. 1976).

Independent from the validity of the microthrombosis concept, coumarins have emerged as potent antimetastatic drugs. Clinical evidence already exists that suggests a role for oral anticoagulants in the control of human cancer (Hilgard and Thornes 1976, Zacharski et al. 1981).

REFERENCES

De Ruiter, J., T. Smink, and L. M. van Putten. 1976. Studies on the enhancement by cyclophosphamide of artificial lung metastasis after labeled cell inoculation. Cancer Treat. Rep. 60:465–470.

Hagmar, B. 1970. Tumor growth and spontaneous metastasis spread in two syngeneic systems. Influence of heparin, coumarin and ϵ-aminocaproic acid (EACA). Acta Pathol. Microbiol. Scand. 78:131–142.

Hilgard, P. 1973. The role of blood platelets in experimental metastases. Br. J. Cancer 28:429–435.

Hilgard, P. 1977. Experimental vitamin K deficiency and spontaneous metastases. Br. J. Cancer 35:891–892.

Hilgard, P. 1980. Metastatic spread and altered blood coagulability, *in* Metastatic Tumor Growth, E. Grundmann, ed. G. Fischer Verlag, Stuttgart, pp. 107–116.

Hilgard, P. 1981. The use of oral anticoagulants in tumor therapy, *in* Malignancy and the Hemostatic System, M. B. Donati, J. F. Davidson, and S. Garattini, eds. Raven Press, New York, pp. 103–111.

Hilgard, P., and B. Maat. 1979. The mechanism of lung tumour colony reduction caused by coumarin anticoagulation. Eur. J. Cancer 15:183–187.
Hilgard, P., H. Schulte, G. Wetzig, G. Schmitt, and C. G. Schmidt. 1977. Oral anticoagulation in the treatment of a spontaneously metastasising murine tumour. Br. J. Cancer 35:78–85.
Hilgard, P., and R. D. Thornes. 1976. Anticoagulants in the treatment of cancer. Eur. J. Cancer 12:755–762.
Hilgard, P., and P. Whur. 1980. Factor X-activating activity from Lewis lung carcinoma. Br. J. Cancer 41:642–643.
Honn, K. 1984. Role of prostacyclin as a natural deterrent to hematogenous tumor metastasis, *in* Cancer Invasion and Metastasis: Biologic and Therapeutic Aspects, G. L. Nicolson and L. Milas, eds. Raven Press, New York, pp. 361–388.
Hoover, H. C., Jr., D. Jones, and A. S. Ketcham. 1976. The optimal level of anticoagulation for decreasing experimental metastases. Surgery 79:625–630.
Maat, B. 1978. Extrapulmonary colony formation after intravenous injection of tumour cells into heparin-treated animals. Br. J. Cancer 37:369–376.
Maat, B. 1981. Selective macrophage inhibition abolishes warfarin-induced reduction of metastases. Br. J. Cancer 41:313–316.
Maat, B., and P. Hilgard. 1981. Anticoagulants and experimental metastases—evaluation of antimetastatic effects in different model systems. J. Cancer Res. Clin. Oncol. 101:275–283.
Poggi, A., L. Mussoni, L. Kornblihtt, E. Ballabio, G. de Gaetano and M. B. Donati. 1978. Warfarin enantiomers, anticoagulation and experimental tumour metastasis. The Lancet 1:1963.
Stenflo, J. 1976. A new vitamin K-dependent protein. Purification from bovine plasma and preliminary characterization. J. Biol. Chem. 251:355–363.
Strauss, J. F., Jr., and O. Saphir. 1949. The possible significance of altered blood coagulability on the spread of carcinoma cells. PA. Proc. Inst. Med. 17:263.
Tanaka, N., H. Ogawa, M. Kinjo, S. Kohga, and K. Tanaka, 1982. Ultrastructural study of the effects of tranexamic acid and urokinase on metastasis of Lewis lung carcinoma. Br. J. Cancer 46:428.
Terranova, T., and F. Chiossone. 1952. Il fattore coagulazione nell' attachimento delle cellule neoplastiche immesse in circulo. Bull. Soc. Ital. Biol. Sper. 28:1224.
Wood, S., Jr. 1958. Pathogenesis of metastasis formation observed in vivo in the rabbit ear chamber. Arch. Pathol. 66:550.
Zacharski, L. R., W. G. Henderson, F. R. Rickles, W. B. Forman, C. J. Cornell, R. J. Forcier, R. Edwards, E. Headley, S. H. Kim, J. R. O'Donnell, R. O'Dell, K. Tornyos, and H. C. Kwaan. 1981. Effects of warfarin on survival in small cell carcinoma of the lung. Veterans Administration Study No. 75. JAMA 245:831.

Cancer Invasion and Metastasis: Biologic and Therapeutic Aspects edited by Garth L. Nicolson and Luka Milas. Raven Press, New York © 1984.

Role of Prostacyclin as a Natural Deterrent to Hematogenous Tumor Metastasis

Kenneth V. Honn,*,†,‡ David G. Menter,‡ James M. Onoda,* John D. Taylor,*,‡ and Bonnie F. Sloane*,§

*Departments of * Radiation Oncology, † Radiology, ‡ Biological Sciences, and § Pharmacology, Wayne State University, Detroit, Michigan 48202*

A metastatic lesion represents the result of a series of sequential events in which neoplastic cells are released from a primary tumor and disseminate to secondary sites. This process has been termed the "metastatic cascade" (Figure 1). The primary tumor is believed to be initiated by transformation (i.e., chemical, radiation, or viral) of a normal cell, which then proliferates until limited by the blood supply and invasive properties of the tumor. As the tumor grows, the tumor cells release angiogenesis factors, which induce neovascularization. To move to a secondary site, the tumor cells must be able to detach from the primary tumor and invade into the circulatory system (intravasate), where the tumor cells may interact with host platelets and neutrophils during transport. Tumor cells can induce platelet aggregation, and this in turn is thought to facilitate attachment of tumor cells to the endothelium or to areas of exposed basement membrane. Dissolution of the basement membrane by proteolytic enzymes released from the tumor cell then may enable the cells to extravasate at a seondary site, where the processes of proliferation, angiogenesis, invasion, and metastasis (from a metastasis) can reoccur.

Metastasis is an inefficient process, since only 0.001% of cells that detach from the primary tumor are estimated to survive and form a metastasic lesion (Weiss 1980, 1982, 1983). Survival at each step in the metastatic cascade can be altered by pathophysiological properties of the tumor cells (i.e., "pre-existing metastatic phenotype"; Poste and Fidler 1980) or by properties of the host (i.e., tumor cell/platelet interaction; Honn et al. 1983a). Survival of 0.001% of the tumor cells entering the metastatic cascade might also be explained exclusively in terms of random events (Weiss 1983). It is likely that random and nonrandom events act in concert.

The presence of viable circulating tumor cells does not necessarily indicate a poor prognosis (Salsbury 1975). Successful arrest or adhesion of the tumor cells to the vessel wall and the factors (e.g., platelets, endothelial cell surface determinants, tumor cell surface determinants, etc.) that activate or enhance this process may be the most important events in metastasis. Carcinomas were

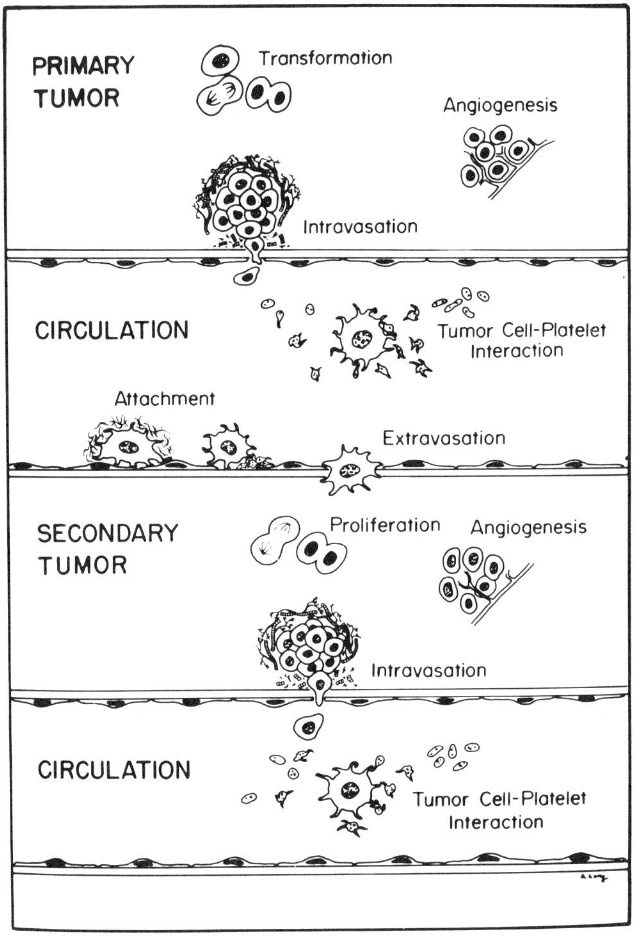

FIG. 1. Overview of the metastatic cascade.

once believed to metastasize via the lymphatics, whereas malignant tumors of mesenchymal origin were believed to spread via the hematogenous route. Hilgard et al. (1972) noted that tumor cells will reach the vascular system when injected initially into the lymphatics. Similar conclusions have been reached by others (del Regato 1977, Fisher and Fisher 1967), and there is now substantial evidence that malignant cells can pass freely between the lymphatics and blood vessels (Weiss 1977, Fidler et al. 1978). It can be concluded that tumor cells disseminate via the hematogenous route at some point in the metastatic cascade.

Once tumor cells have entered the circulatory system, factors such as tumor cell surface properties that may influence tumor cell arrest, attachment to endothelial or de-endothelianized surfaces, and eventual extravasation assume paramount importance (Nicolson 1982). Nicolson and co-workers (Irimura and

Nicolson 1981, Irimura et al. 1981) have described a role for surface sialogalactoproteins in tumor cell binding to endothelial cell monolayers, endothelial extracellular matrix, and immobilized fibronectin. Cells treated with the antibiotic tunicamycin, which inhibits formation of asparagine-linked oligosaccharide chains on glycoproteins (Takacz and Lampen 1975, Takatsuki et al. 1975), demonstrated decreased adhesiveness to the above substrates and decreased lung colony formation in syngeneic mice (Irimura et al. 1981). Others have also found a relationship between sialoglycoproteins and metastatic potential (Raz et al. 1980, Vilarem et al. 1981). Karpatkin and co-workers have demonstrated a correlation between tumor cell sialic acid content, induction of platelet aggregation, and spontaneous metastasis in derivatives of the polyoma virus–induced PW20 Wistar-Furth rat renal sarcoma line (Pearlstein et al. 1980). Recently, Fogel et al. (1983) demonstrated that decreased levels of terminal sialic acid at lectin sites for N-acetylgalactosamine-specific lectins in the ESb lymphoma resulted in decreased metastatic potential.

Malignant cells adhere to vascular endothelium and stimulate endothelial cells to retract, exposing the underlying basal laminalike matrix, whereupon the tumor cells migrate to the subendothelial matrix surface (Kramer et al. 1980, Kramer and Nicolson 1979, 1981, Zamora et al. 1980). Using B16F1 and B16F10 metastatic variants, Nicolson and co-workers demonstrated that tumor cells attached slowly to endothelial cell monolayers, whereas they attached rapidly to the isolated extracellular matrix (Kramer and Nicolson 1979, Kramer et al. 1980), suggesting that damaged or de-endothelianized surfaces may offer preferential attachment sites for circulating tumor cells. The mechanism of tumor cell attachment is a matter of debate. Nicolson et al. (1981) demonstrated that fibronectin may mediate tumor cell attachment to the extracellular matrix. Liotta and co-workers demonstrated that metastatic tumor cells attach preferentially to type IV collagen (Murray et al. 1980) and that this attachment can be enhanced by laminin and blocked by antilaminin antibody, but cannot be enhanced by fibronectin nor blocked by antifibronectin antibody (Terranova et al. 1982). In addition, tumor cells that demonstrated laminin-enhanced attachment to type IV collagen produced more pulmonary tumor colonies in vivo. Lung colony formation was decreased by antilaminin antibody (Terranova et al. 1982). The preferred attachment proteins may vary among tumor types (Vlodavsky and Gospodarowicz 1981). Despite a lack of details on the specific mechanisms, the arrest of circulating tumor cells and the formation of stable adhesions can reasonably be regarded as a critical event in successful metastasis.

PLATELETS, COAGULATION, AND METASTASIS

Patients with malignant neoplasms often demonstrate abnormalities in their blood coagulability (Goodnight 1974, Donati and Poggi 1980, Zacharski et al. 1979, Edwards et al. 1981). These abnormalities include hyperaggregability of platelets (Yahara et al. 1983) with resultant thrombocytopenia (Brain et al.

1970) and a reduction in fibrinogen concomitant with an increase in fibrin-fibrinogen degradation products (Goodnight 1974, Harker and Slichter 1972, Edwards et al. 1981). Tumor cells have been reported to possess both a platelet-activating material (Gasic et al. 1978, Pearlstein et al. 1979, 1980, Karpatkin et al. 1980) and a procoagulant activity responsible for alterations in the fibrin-fibrinogen system (Gordon and Cross 1981, Curatolo et al. 1979, Gordon et al. 1975). These hemostatic alterations have been linked to tumor cell metastasis (for review see Karpatkin and Pearlstein 1981). In addition, many tumor cells have been reported to spontaneously shed membrane vesicles (Black 1980, Liepins and Hillman 1981, Liepins and de Harven 1982), which possess platelet aggregatory (Gasic et al. 1978, K. V. Honn and B. F. Sloane, unpublished observation) and procoagulant activities (Dvorak et al. 1981). Such shed membrane vesicles have been correlated with metastatic potential in the B16F1, B16F10 system (Poste and Nicolson 1980).

Gasic et al. (1968) were the first to provide direct experimental evidence for a role for platelets in tumor cell metastasis. They had noted that pretreatment of mice with neuraminidase resulted in formation of fewer lung colonies following injection of TA3 ascites tumor cells. These results were attributable to induction of thrombocytopenia, and similar antimetastatic effects could be observed when thrombocytopenia was induced with antiplatelet antiserum. Additional evidence was provided by the fact that the antimetastatic effects of neuraminidase could be reversed by platelet infusion.

In a series of follow-up papers, Gasic et al. (1973, 1976, 1978) demonstrated that numerous human and animal tumor cells and plasma membrane vesicles shed from tumor cells were capable of aggregating platelets in vitro with a concomitant stimulation of the release reaction (measured as [^{14}C]serotonin released from prelabeled platelets). Other laboratories have confirmed the in vitro aggregation of platelets by both animal and human tumor cells and the induction of thrombocytopenia following i.v. injection of several tumor lines (Hilgard 1973, Bastida et al. 1981, 1982, Gastpar et al. 1977, Hara et al. 1980, Pearlstein et al. 1980, 1981, Paschen et al. 1979, Skolnik et al. 1980, Tanaka et al. 1982). Recent work from Karpatkin, Pearlstein, and co-workers (Pearlstein et al. 1980) provides more direct evidence that a causal relationship exists. Using ten cell lines derived from the polyoma virus–induced PW20 Wistar-Furth rat renal sarcoma, they found a significant correlation between the ability of the tumor cells to metastasize spontaneously from subcutaneous sites in syngeneic hosts and their platelet aggregating activity in vitro. Recent reviews can be found in Jamieson (1982) and Honn and Sloane (1983a). However, most of the studies to date still only provide circumstantial evidence that host platelets facilitate hematogenous metastasis.

The mechanisms by which platelets might enhance metastasis have not been established. It is generally accepted that tumor cells are damaged during transport from the site of intravasation to the site of extravasation. This circulatory trauma may be due to humoral factors (i.e., macrophages, natural killer cells, antibodies) and physical factors (i.e., shear forces, mechanical trauma due to passage through the microvasculature). Tumor cells shielded within platelet thrombi may be protected from some or all of the above. In addition, platelets may enhance tumor cell adhesion to endothelial or de-endothelianized surfaces via platelet bridges. Recently, Turner et al. (1983) demonstrated that during Walker 256 carcinosarcoma (W256) tumor cell–induced platelet aggregation (TCIPA), fibronectin released from the platelet α-granules becomes associated with the surface of the W256 cells. Prior to TCIPA, the tumor cell surface was devoid of fibronectin. Thus, platelet-derived fibronectin could facilitate tumor cell adhesion (see above).

The contribution of each of the above-suggested mechanisms to platelet enhancement of tumor cell metastasis is not known. However, it is generally accepted that platelets enhance metastasis by facilitating processes that occur during tumor cell arrest and adhesion. Therefore, in an effort to reduce metastasis, cancer therapy aimed at interrupting the metastatic cascade has been attempted with antiplatelet and anticoagulant agents such as heparin (Elias et al. 1973), warfarin (Lione and Bosmann 1978), and dipyridamole (Gastpar 1977). The results to date have been inconsistent, with the exception of those with warfarin (Maat and Hilgard 1981).

PROSTACYCLIN, THROMBOXANES, PLATELETS, AND METASTASIS

Compounds derived from arachidonic acid [prostacyclin (PGI_2) and thromboxane A_2 (TXA_2); Figure 2] have been demonstrated to have a profound but possibly not exclusive (Vargaftig et al. 1981) role in platelet aggregation and normal hemostasis. Hamberg et al. (1975) demonstrated the formation of TXA_2 from the endoperoxide intermediate prostaglandin H_2 (PGH_2) (Figure 2). Subsequently, platelet TXA_2 biosynthesis was found to be stimulated by numerous aggregating agents and was believed to be an absolute requirement for platelet aggregation (Gorman 1979). This view has recently been challenged by the observations that in some cases the endoperoxide PGH_2 can initiate platelet aggregation independent of its conversion to TXA_2 (Heptinstall et al. 1980).

One year following the discovery of TXA_2, Vane and co-workers (Moncada et al. 1976b) discovered PGI_2 as a transformation product of prostaglandin endoperoxides (Figure 2). PGI_2 is produced by vascular tissue of all species so far tested (Moncada and Vane 1980) and is the main product of arachidonic acid metabolism in isolated vascular tissue. It is the most potent endogenous inhibitor of platelet aggregation yet discovered, being 30 to 40 times more potent than prostaglandin E_1 (PGE_1) (Moncada and Vane 1977) and 1,000 times more potent than adenosine (Mullane et al. 1979). In addition, PGI_2 can reverse secondary platelet aggregation in vitro (Moncada et al. 1976a, 1976b) and in the circulatory system of man (Szczeklik et al. 1978). It has been suggested that PGI_2 and TXA_2 play an antagonistic and pivotal role in the control of thrombosis centered upon their bidirectional (PGI_2 increases, TXA_2 decreases)

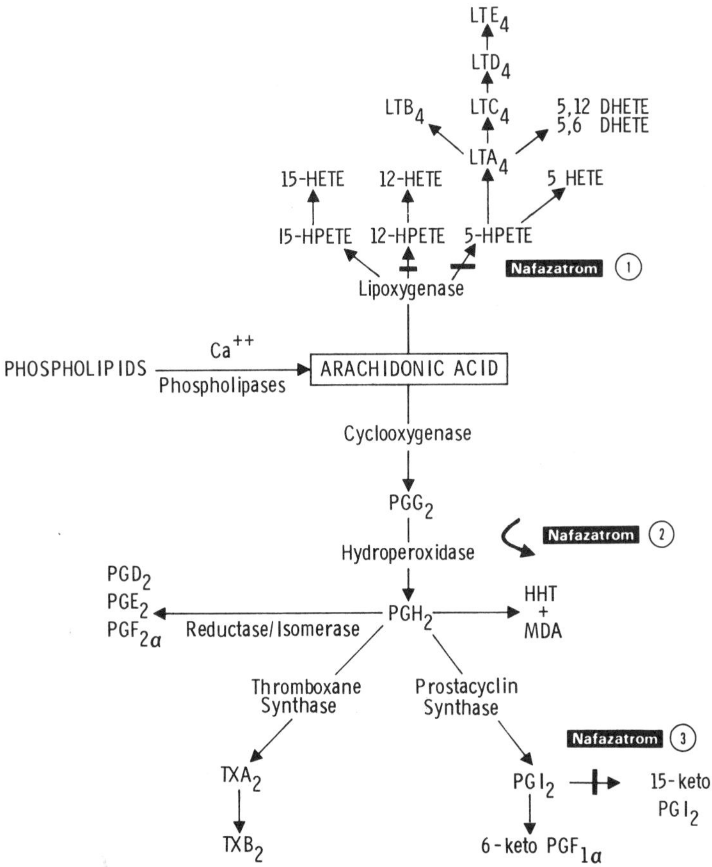

FIG. 2. Arachidonic acid metabolism via the lipoxygenase pathway resulting in hydroperoxy fatty acids and leukotrienes and via the prostaglandin endoperoxide synthetase (cyclooxygenase plus hydroperoxidase) pathway resulting in prostaglandins (including prostacyclin) and thromboxanes. Possible sites of action of nafazatrom include: (1) inhibition of lipoxygenase activity, (2) reducing co-factor for the hydroperoxidase of prostaglandin endoperoxide synthetase, and (3) inhibition of prostacyclin (PGI_2) degradation by 15-hydroxy-prostaglandin dehydrogenase.

effect on platelet cAMP levels. However, proaggregatory agents (i.e., 1-0-alkyl-2-0-acetyl-2sn-glyceryl-3-phosphorylcholine) in addition to TXA_2 should be considered for this pivotal role.

Our working hypothesis has been that the normal intravascular balance between PGI_2 and platelet arachidonic acid metabolites (i.e., TXA_2) can be altered by the presence of a primary tumor or circulating tumor cells and their shed membrane vesicles (Honn et al. 1983a). This hypothesis predicts that arachidonic acid metabolism by the tumor cell, platelet, and vessel wall is a fundamental determinant in the sum total of their interaction and that PGI_2 may be a natural deterrent to metastasis. If this is true, then exogenous PGI_2 should demonstrate some efficacy against metastasis. Given the short physical and biological half-life of PGI_2 (Vane et al. 1982), it would be expected that exogenous PGI_2 may be effective in the tail-vein model (lung colonization) but not in the spontaneous metastasis model. However, the inhibition or stimulation of endogenous PGI_2 production should alter tumor cell metastasis.

Prostacyclin Effects In Vivo and In Vitro

Prostacyclin Effects on TCIPA

In vitro, the addition of elutriated (Sloane et al. 1981) W256 cells to human platelet rich plasma (PRP) resulted in irreversible platelet aggregation after a short lag period of 0.5 to 1 min (Figure 3). This aggregation was inhibited by PGI_2 in a dose-dependent manner; maximal inhibition was observed at a PGI_2 dose of 10 ng/ml (Figure 3). TCIPA may occur via three distinct mechanisms, dependent on tumor type (Pearlstein et al. 1981, Bastida et al. 1982). TCIPA initiated via ADP can be inhibited by apyrase but not by hirudin or DAPA

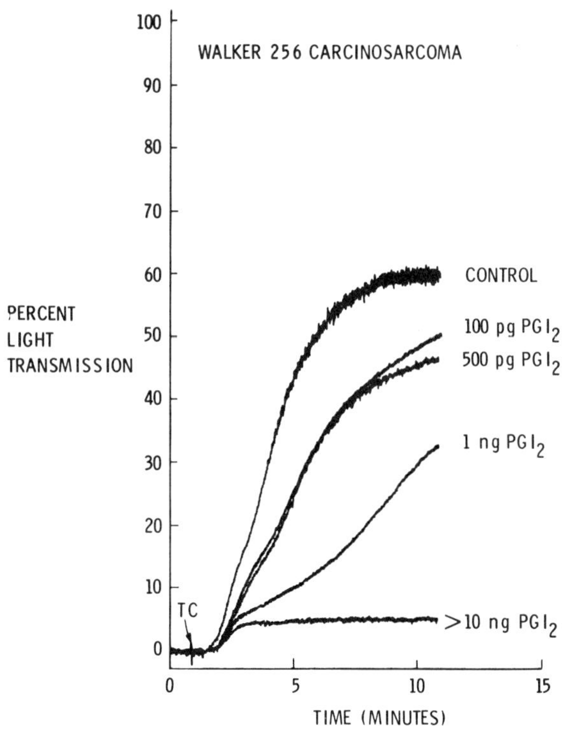

FIG. 3. Effects of PGI_2 on W256-induced aggregation of human platelet-rich plasma. PGI_2 was added 1 min prior to the addition of tumor cells (TC).

[dansylarginine N-(3-ethyl-1, 5-pentanediyl)amide]. However, the reverse is true of tumor cells aggregating platelets via activation of the coagulation pathway (Pearlstein et al. 1981, Bastida et al. 1982).

PGI_2 was therefore tested against a variety of tumor types. Complete inhibition of TCIPA with PGI_2 (10 ng/ml) was observed in the B16 amelanotic melanoma (Honn et al. 1983c), 15091A mammary adenocarcinoma, and Lewis lung carcinoma (Honn and Sloane 1983c). In addition, platelet aggregation in response to spontaneously shed plasma membrane vesicles from 15091A cells (Gasic et al. 1981) was inhibited by 10 ng/ml PGI_2 (K. V. Honn and B. F. Sloane, unpublished observation). PGI_2 was the most potent of the prostaglandins (PG) with respect to inhibition of TCIPA. Two additional PG (PGE_1 and PGD_2) known to inhibit platelet aggregation (Vane et al. 1982) were 100 times less potent than PGI_2 in inhibiting W256-induced platelet aggregation (Honn and Sloane 1983c). The stable metabolite of PGI_2, 6-keto-$PGF_1\alpha$, was effective only at supraphysiological doses (Honn and Sloane 1983c). On the other hand, PGE_2 blocked the inhibitory effects of PGI_2 on TCIPA (D. G. Menter and K. V. Honn, unpublished observation).

Circulating tumor cells may exist as single cells or multicellular clumps. Aggregates of tumor cells have been shown to be more efficient in generating lung colonies than single cells (Watanabe 1954, Fidler 1973, Liotta et al. 1974, 1976). Liotta et al. (1976) demonstrated that the i.v. injection of 10^3 T241 fibrosarcoma cells in clumps of 6 or 7 cells produced ten times as many pulmonary tumors as 10^3 single cells. In these experiments, doubling the size of the homotypic emboli doubled the number of tumors. In in vitro studies in our laboratory, W256 cells spontaneously underwent homotypic adhesion into clumps of 5–10 cells that could be visualized by scanning electron microscopy (D. G. Menter and K. V. Honn, unpublished observation). If W256 cells were placed in a platelet aggregometer, this homotypic aggregation could be measured as an increase in light transmittance (Figure 4). PGI_2 at a dose of 100 ng/ml completely prevented this aggregation (Figure 4). In addition, PGI_2 completely inhibited W256 tumor cell interaction with human neutrophils (R. R. Gorman and K. V. Honn, unpublished observation). The relevance of these observations to PGI_2 effects in vivo are unknown at present. However, it is clear that PGI_2 can prevent various cell-cell interactions involving tumor cells.

Prostacyclin Effects on Tumor Cell–Induced Platelet Release Reaction

During the release reaction, materials stored in platelet granules (dense granules, α granules, and lysosomes) are released into the environment. Not all stimuli provoke release from all three granule compartments (Holmsen and Day 1970). The dense granules contain high concentrations of amines (serotonin), adenine nucleotides, and divalent cations. The α granules contain a variety of proteins, among which are heparin-neutralizing protein (platelet factor 4), β-thromboglobulin, fibrinogen, fibronectin, and platelet-derived growth factors

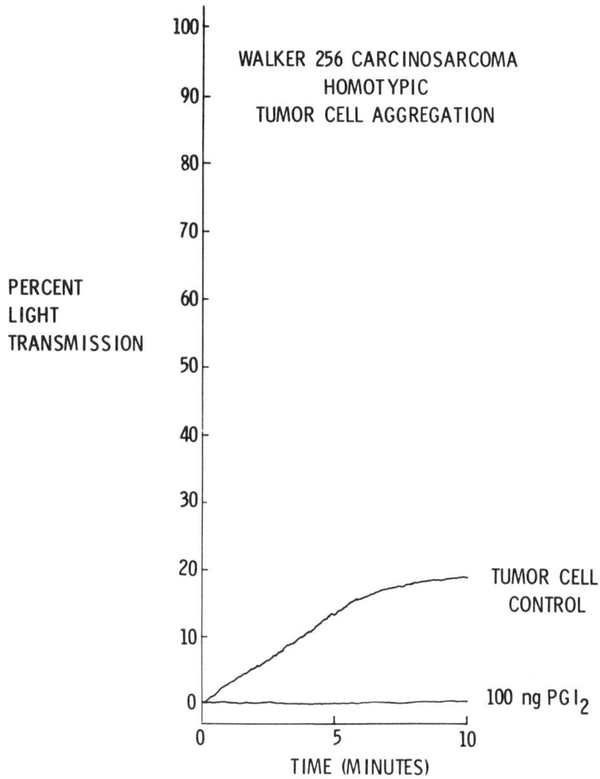

FIG. 4. Effect of PGI_2 on homotypic aggregation of W256 cells. PGI_2 was added at time 0.

(Kaplan 1981). Lysosomes contain acid hydrolases including acid phosphatase, β-N-acetylglucosaminidase, β-glucuronidase, cathepsin D, and collagenase (Gordon 1975, Holmsen and Weiss 1979).

Several of these platelet factors could conceivably aid in tumor metastasis. Dense-granule serotonin is a potent vasoconstrictor and can further stimulate platelet aggregation (Kaplan 1981). Alpha granule–derived β-thromboglobulin inhibits production of PGI_2 by the vascular endothelium (Hope et al. 1979). Platelet-derived fibronectin could coat tumor cells and increase adhesiveness, as discussed above, and could contribute to tumor cell–associated fibrin (Gasic et al. 1976). Platelet-derived growth factors have been demonstrated to be mitogenic for several animal (Lipton et al. 1982) and human tumor cells (Cowan and Graham 1982).

A variety of human and animal tumor cells have been found to evoke the release of platelet-derived dense granules (Gasic et al. 1976). We have demonstrated (Honn et al. 1983c) that PGI_2 inhibits the release of dense granules during TCIPA (measured as release of ^{14}C-labeled-serotonin from prelabeled platelets). In addition, PGI_2 caused a dose-dependent decrease in platelet α granule release (measured as β-thromboglobulin release) induced during W256 TCIPA (Honn et al. 1983c).

The biochemical evidence that tumor cells were inducing release of platelet-derived dense and α granules was confirmed morphologically using transmission electron microscopy (TEM). For the TEM studies of TCIPA, samples of the tumor cells and platelets were fixed at the following times: prior to the first phase of aggregation, during the lag period between the first and second phases of aggregation, and after complete aggregation had occurred. During the initial phase of platelet activation (Figure 5a), the granules became centralized and pseudopods began to form. The platelets formed polar chains leading from the tumor cells. Some initial degranulation had occurred even at this early phase of interaction. At this initial phase of interaction with platelets, the tumor cells had also undergone ultrastructural changes, including sending out pseudopodia (Figure 5a). These pseudopods, in contrast to those of platelets, were thicker and could be distinguished by the presence of ribosomes. The tumor cells also appeared to have shed vesicles containing ribosomes.

By the end of the first phase of TCIPA (Figure 5b), the platelets had released virtually all of their granules (both α and dense) and the pseudopods of adjacent platelets were highly interdigitated. At this stage there appeared to be activation of the tumor cell membrane into blebs with projecting microvilli and increased shedding of vesicles.

Complete aggregation is illustrated in Figures 5c and d. Membranes of the tumor cell and the platelets became closely juxtaposed and the platelet aggregate contracted, thus appearing dense. Fibrin formed upon complete TCIPA (Figure 5d).

In virtually all of the experiments examined thus far, the tumor cell does not appear to be engulfed by platelets. When attachment occurred, it seemed to be between a limited number of platelets and tumor cells. Generally, attachment was followed by activation of surrounding platelets to form aggregates. This scheme does not preclude, of course, that preformed platelet aggregates may also attach to tumor cells. If the attachment of a limited number of platelets to the tumor cells is a selective process, heterogeneous platelet populations may exist. Indeed, there are some recent studies that indicate that functionally heterogeneous platelet populations do exist (Santoro and Cunningham 1981, George et al. 1981, Thompson et al. 1982).

FIG. 5. Interaction of W256 cells and platelets under aggregatory conditions. **a.** Prior to first phase of aggregation, as detected by light transmittance, platelet pseudopods had formed and granules had moved centripetally. Pseudopods also had formed from the tumor cell membrane. (9,590×) **b.** By the end of the first phase of aggregation platelet granules had been released and an aggregate had formed. (10,990×) **c.** At the end of the second phase of aggregation the platelet aggregate had contracted and the membranes of platelets and tumor cells had become closely apposed. (10,290×) **d.** After complete aggregation, fibrin could be seen in association with the tumor cells and platelets (not shown). (13,160×)

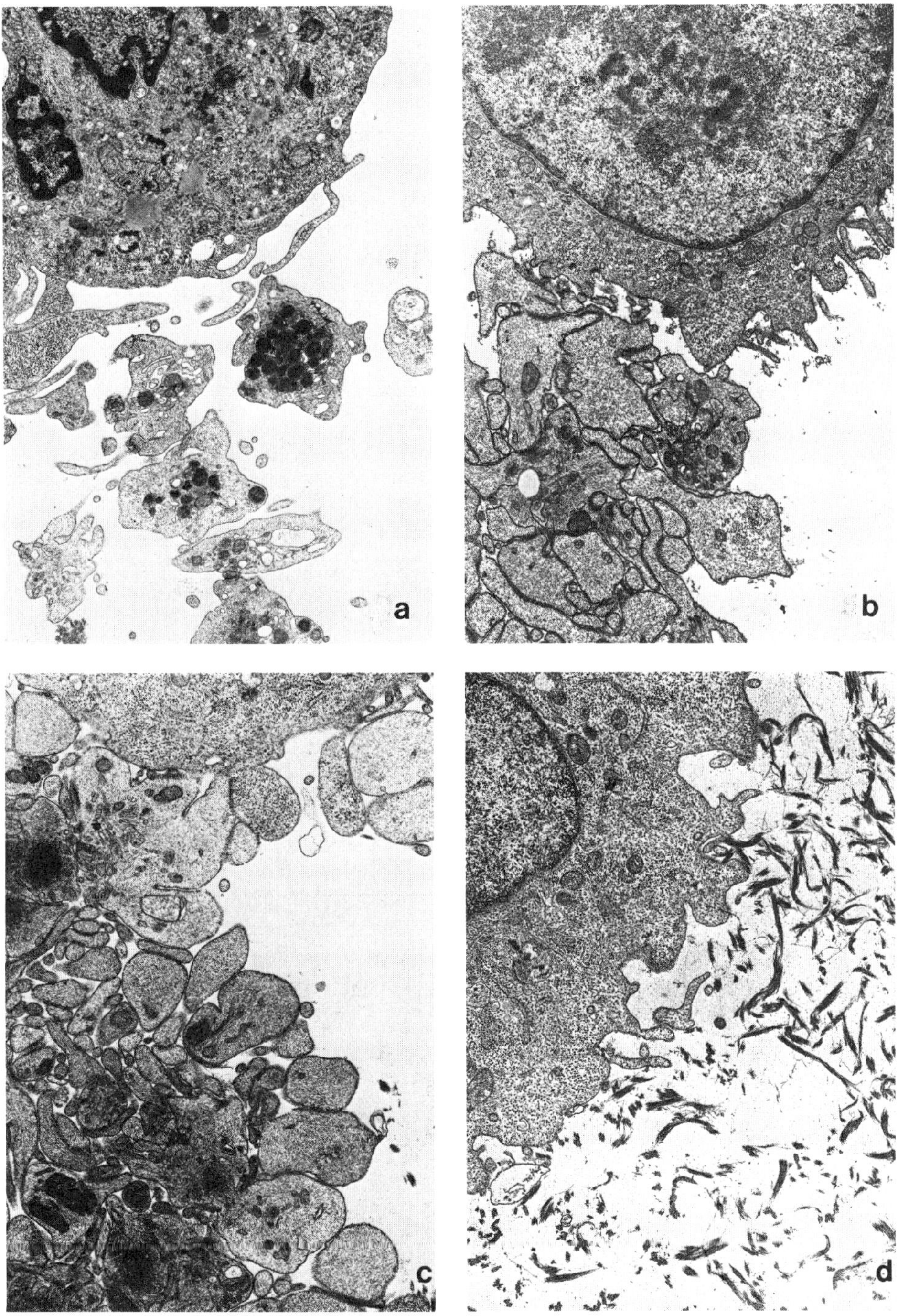
a
b
c
d

In order to more fully examine the possible activation of the tumor cell membrane by platelets, we looked at the interaction between tumor cells and platelets by scanning electron microscopy (SEM) under conditions in which platelet aggregation did not occur (see below). The control tumor cells incubated in the absence of platelets could be characterized by their fine surface microvilli (Figure 6a). After 2 min of coincubation with the tumor cells, platelets that had not undergone shape changes could be seen to be attached to the tumor cells (Figure 6b). At 12 min of coincubation, many more platelets, which had formed pseudopods, were attached to the tumor cells (Figure 6c). In turn, the tumor cell membrane seemed to have lost its fine surface microvilli. These SEM images suggest that there are bidirectional interactions between tumor cells and platelets that may result in modification of the tumor cell membrane and thereby the adhesive properties of the tumor cell.

Prostacyclin Effects on Platelet-Induced Tumor Cell Adhesion In Vitro

Fantone et al. (1982) have recently demonstrated that the adherence of W256 cells to plastic plates or nylon fibers can be stimulated by the tumor promoter phorbol myristate acetate and the chemotactic peptide f-Met-Leu-Phe. PGI_2 directly inhibited this increased adhesion; however, it had no effect on basal (unstimulated) W256 cell adhesion (Fantone et al. 1982). Hara et al. (1980) reported that tumor cells will not aggregate washed platelets. However, the addition of a small amount (2% v/v) of platelet-poor plasma (PPP) restores a full aggregation response, suggesting an absolute requirement for a plasma factor during TCIPA (Hara et al. 1980, D. G. Menter and K. V. Honn, unpublished observation). We have previously demonstrated that platelet–tumor cell adhesion can occur in the absence of overt platelet aggregation and that this interaction results in alterations of the tumor cell surface topology (Figure 6). We therefore explored the possibility that platelets could enhance the adhesion of W256 cells under nonaggregatory (no PPP) and aggregatory (5% PPP v/v) conditions.

The adhesion of W256 cells to plastic plates was increased in the presence of washed rat platelets (Figure 7). This increase varied with platelet preparation but ranged between 100 and 400%. An even larger increase (300–1,400%) was observed if tumor cells were allowed to aggregate (addition of 5% PPP) with platelets (Figure 7). The addition of 30 μg/ml PGI_2 completely abrogated the increased adhesion under both aggregatory and nonaggregatory conditions. The effect was dose dependent both in the presence and absence of PPP; a 40% decrease was observed at 1 μg/ml PGI_2. PGI_2 had no effect on basal (unstimulated) W256 cell attachment (Figure 7).

Rat platelets also enhanced the attachment of W256 cells to cultured rat endothelial cells, a response that can be blocked with PGI_2 (K. V. Honn, unpublished observation). These in vitro results suggest that platelets may increase tumor cell adhesion to endothelium in vivo and PGI_2 may limit the formation of a stable tumor cell–endothelial cell interaction. Support for this concept can

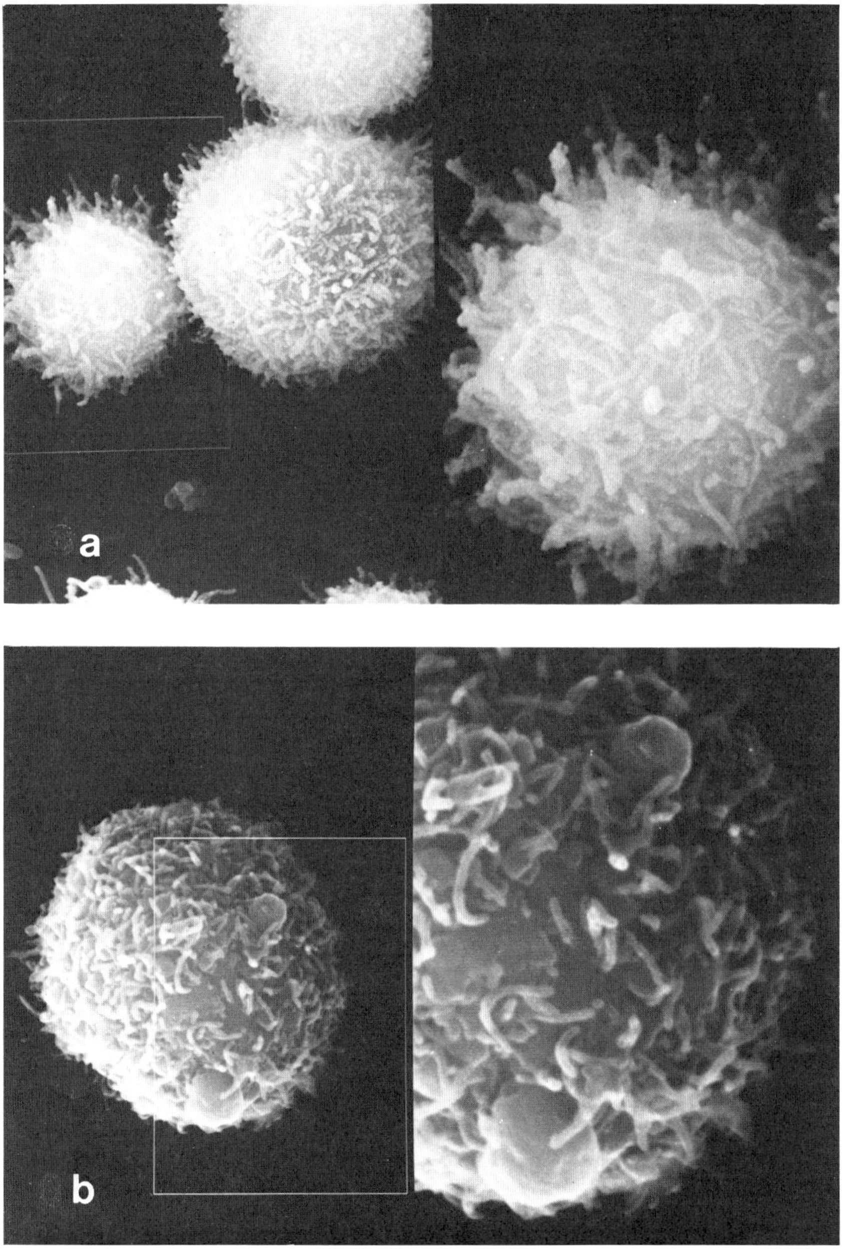

FIG. 6. Interaction of platelets and W256 cells under nonaggregatory conditions. **a.** Normal surface topology of W256 cells with characteristic fine surface microvilli. (*left,* 2,790×; *right,* 6,390×) **b.** Within 2 min of tumor cell–platelet coincubation, platelets have adhered to tumor cells but not undergone pseudopod formation. (*left,* 5,040×; *right,* 13,140×)

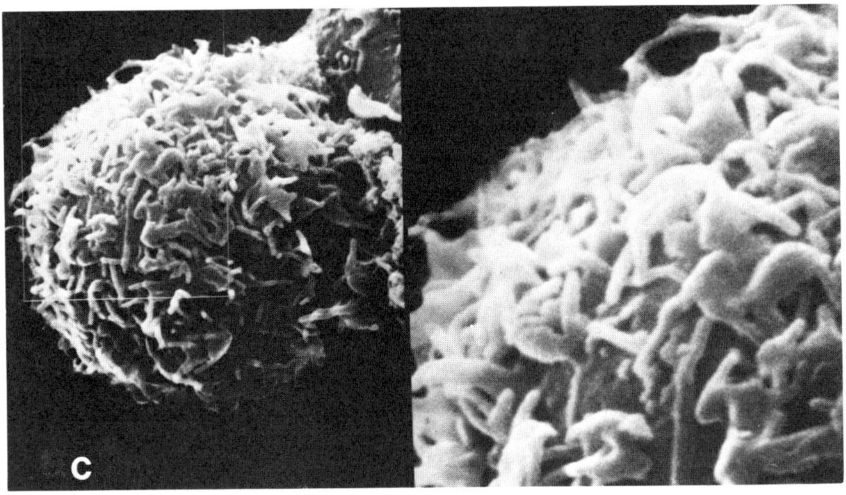

FIG. 6. Cont. c. After 12 min of coincubation, many more platelets have adhered to the tumor cells and have undergone shape changes and formed pseudopods. (*left,* 3,870×; *right,* 8,100×)

be derived from the experiments of Marcum et al. (1980), who utilized rabbit aortic segments in a standard Baumgartner perfusion chamber to study tumor cell (HUT 20)–platelet–endothelial cell and subendothelial interactions. Tumor cells and platelets were perfused in the presence of PGE_1 (30 μg/ml) or PGI_2 (50 ng/ml). Both agents totally inhibited TCIPA and the deposition of both tumor cells and platelets on the vascular surface. Interestingly, perfusion of HUT 20 cells with whole blood deficient in factor VIII/von Willebrand factor (found in normal platelet α granules) resulted in a $>97\%$ inhibition of tumor cell adherence to endothelial and de-endothelianized surfaces, suggesting a role for this platelet protein in tumor cell metastasis.

Prostacyclin Effects on Metastasis In Vivo

We have previously reported that bolus i.v. injection of PGI_2 into mice reduced lung colony formation from tail vein-injected B16a cells by greater than 70%; in combination with a phosphodiesterase inhibitor (theophylline) it reduced such formation by $>93\%$ (Honn et al. 1981b). Prostaglandins E_2 and $F_{2\alpha}$ and the stable hydrolysis product of PGI_2, 6-keto-$PGF_{1\alpha}$, were ineffective (Honn et al. 1981b). PGD_2 is also antimetastatic as reported by Stringfellow and Fitzpatrick (1979); however, we found PGD_2 to be less than ⅓ as effective as PGI_2 (Honn et al. 1981b). These results correlate well with the effects of these various icosanoids on TCIPA (Honn et al. 1983a, 1983c, Honn and Sloane 1983c).

Willmott et al. (1983) recently reported that treatment of animals with the antiplatelet drug RA233 prior to tail-vein injection of S-180 sarcoma cells enhanced extrapulmonary tumor formation. We demonstrated that PGI_2 does not significantly alter tumor cell distribution patterns using [^{125}I]deoxyuridine-

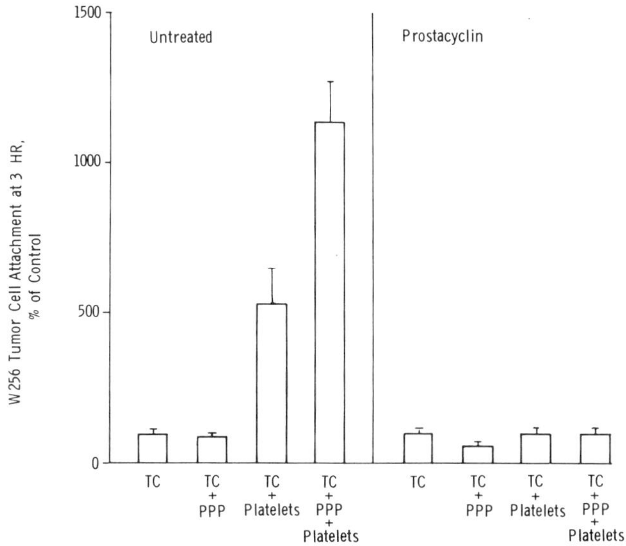

FIG. 7. *Left:* Effect of rat platelets on adhesion of W256 cells to plastic culture dishes under aggregatory (TC + PPP + platelets) and nonaggregatory (TC + platelets) conditions. PPP alone had no effect on basal adhesion. *Right:* Prostacyclin inhibition of platelet-enhanced W256 cell adhesion to plastic. Prostacyclin had no effect on basal adhesion. TC, tumor cell; PPP, platelet-poor plasma. (Reproduced from Honn and Sloane 1983c, with permission of Academic Press.)

labeled tumor cells. We found (Honn 1983) that although some alteration of cell distribution may occur, once released from the lung these cells are not retained in the organ of secondary arrest (liver, spleen, etc.). In addition, PGI_2 had no effect on the initial entrapment of tumor cells in the lung following i.v. injection (Honn 1983); a decrease might be expected if the PGI_2 effect were due to vasodilation. The lack of PGI_2 effect on initial tumor cell arrest raises the question of whether TCIPA occurs while the tumor cell is circulating or alternatively whether the critical aggregation event occurs after tumor cell arrest and attachment to the endothelium.

The above results with exogenous PGI_2 demonstrate its efficacy as an anti-metastatic agent. We have also proposed that the production of PGI_2 by the vascular endothelium is a natural deterrent to metastasis (Honn et al. 1981b). To test this hypothesis, we perfused mice with a lipoxygenase product of arachidonic acid, 15-hydroperoxyeicosatetraenoic acid (15-HPETE), prior to tail-vein injection of B16a tumor cells. Hydroperoxy fatty acids in general are potent inhibitors ($K_i \sim 10^{-7}$ M) of prostacyclin synthase (Salmon et al. 1978). Little structural specificity is evident in the inhibition, since a number of isomeric hydroperoxides are equally effective (Salmon et al. 1978). If mice were treated with 15-HPETE (100–200 μg/animal) approximately 20 min prior to tail-vein injection of B16a cells, 300–500% more pulmonary metastatic lesions were

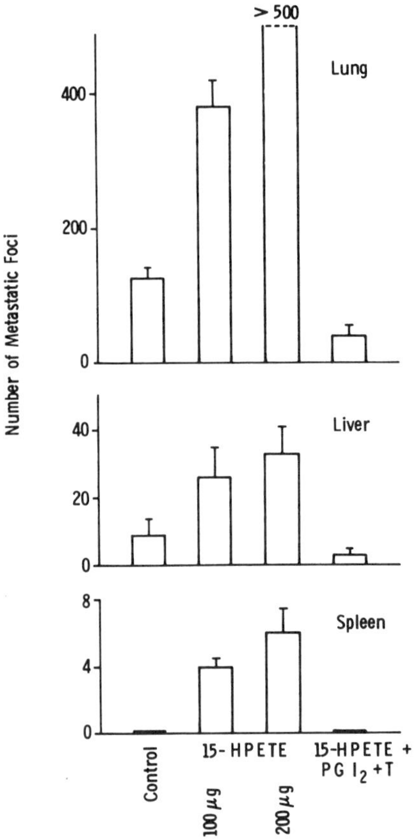

FIG. 8. Increased lung colony formation of B16a cells by prior administration of the PGI_2 synthase inhibitor, 15-HPETE. Exogenous PGI_2 reverses this effect. T, theophylline.

observed 26 days later (Figure 8). Increased macroscopic tumors were also found in the liver and spleen of 15-HPETE-treated animals (Figure 8). Infusion of 15-HPETE followed by PGI_2 plus theophylline significantly reduced the number of metastases compared to 15-HPETE infusion alone (Figure 8). Collectively, these results suggest that endogenous PGI_2 production may function as a natural deterrent to metastasis, possibly by limiting tumor cell–platelet–vessel wall interactions.

Effect of Agents That Stimulate or Syngergize with Endogenous PGI_2 Production

The use of PGI_2 as a clinical therapeutic entity is still in its infancy (Moncada 1982), although several studies report therapeutic efficacy with PGI_2 infusion for advanced atherosclerotic lower limb peripheral vascular disease (Szczeklik et al. 1979), peripheral artery disease (Szczeklik and Gryglewski 1981), idiopathic pulmonary artery hypertension (Watkins et al. 1980), coronary artery disease (Bergman et al. 1981), and unstable angina (Hall and Dewar 1981). Nevertheless,

PGI_2 infusion is clinically impractical for use as an antimetastatic agent. We had originally proposed that long-lived analogs of PGI_2 could be used as antimetastatic agents (Honn et al. 1981b). Numerous analogs have been developed (Aristoff and Harrison 1982, Hall and Dewar 1981, Morton and Brokow 1979, Nishiyama and Ohno 1979, Pike and Bundy 1982, Whittle et al. 1980). Although some of these analogs have interesting and promising biological effects (Whittle et al. 1980), none is more potent than native PGI_2, and the most effective of these must be administered by vascular infusion.

We therefore propose that agents that stimulate endogenous PGI_2 production or inhibit its metabolism may be clinically useful as antimetastatic agents.

Agents that alter PGI_2 metabolism

One compound that alters PGI_2 metabolism may represent the prototype of a new class of pharmacologically active agents—nafazatrom (Bay g 6575; 2,4-dihydro-5-methyl-2[2-(2napthyloxy)ethyl]-3H-pyrazol-3-one). Seuter et al. (1979) first reported significant antithrombotic activity of nafazatrom in several rat and rabbit models of thrombosis. These authors reported that nafazatrom was devoid of direct effects on platelet TXA_2 production, aggregation in vitro and ex vivo, and ADP- and collagen-induced platelet aggregation. Recently, Buchanan et al. (1982) reinvestigated the antithrombotic effects of nafazatrom and reported it had no effect on venous thrombosis and yet inhibited arterial thrombosis. Differences in the model systems used for venous thrombosis could account for this discrepancy. In addition, Buchanan et al. (1982) reported that nafazatrom inhibited ADP-induced platelet aggregation in vivo and prolonged platelet survival time.

The mechanism(s) responsible for the antithrombotic effects of nafazatrom is a matter of current debate. It centers on nafazatrom's ability to stimulate vascular wall PGI_2 production or prolong its biological half-life. Vermylen et al. (1979) first presented evidence for increased PGI_2 production. Plasma obtained from human volunteers after they ingested a single dose (1.2 g) of nafazatrom stimulated PGI_2 release from slices of rat aorta. Others also have reported increased PGI_2 production (Carreras et al. 1980, Chamone et al. 1981). Recently, nafazatrom has been reported to stimulate PGI_2 biosynthesis from arachidonic acid by ram seminal vesicle microsomes (Eling et al. 1982), cultured endothelial cells, and B16a cells (K. V. Honn, L. J. Marnett and T. E. Eling, unpublished observation).

Three biochemical mechanisms have been proposed to explain the PGI_2-stimulating effects of nafazatrom (Figure 2). First, (Figure 2, part 1), nafazatrom has been found to inhibit the cytosolic lipoxygenase (generation of HPETE) of B16a cells (Honn and Dunn 1982), as well as that of human and rabbit neutrophils (Busse et al. 1982). Since vascular endothelial cells have been found to produce 12-HPETE by lipoxygenation of arachidonic acid (Herman et al. 1979) and hydroperoxy fatty acid has been proposed as an endogenous regulator of PGI_2 biosynthesis, nafazatrom may interfere with PGI_2 synthase inhibition. Second, nafazatrom may act as a reducing co-factor for the hydroperoxidase activity (Figure 2, part 2) of prostaglandin endoperoxide synthase (Eling et al. 1982, L. J. Marnett, T. E. Eling, and K. V. Honn, unpublished observation). Third, (Figure 2, part 3) nafazatrom has been reported to inhibit the enzymatic degradation of PGI_2 to 15-keto-PGI_2 by 15 hydroxy prostaglandin dehydrogenase (Wong et al. 1982). This is the major route of PGI_2 catabolism in the cat (Machleidt et al. 1981) and man (Rosenkranz et al. 1980). Any or all of the above mechanisms would increase endogenous PGI_2 levels.

Nafazatrom has been evaluated for its antimetastatic activity against elutriated B16a and 3LL tumor cells injected into the tail vein. It inhibited lung colony formation by >70% (Honn and Sloane 1983b, Honn et al. 1982, 1983a). In addition, this compound significantly reduces spontaneous pulmonary metastasis from subcutaneous B16a and 3LL tumors (Honn et al. 1982). Ambrus et al. (1982) have also reported antimetastatic activity of nafazatrom in three of four tumor lines tested. Collectively, these results point to significant antimetastatic properties of this PGI_2-enhancing agent.

Thromboxane synthase inhibitors

TXA_2 synthase inhibitors result in decreased platelet adhesion to injured vascular wall (Hall et al. 1982) and increased platelet sensitivity to PGI_2 inhibition (Bertele et al. 1982), presumably because the lower the platelet TXA_2 biosynthetic capability the lower the dose of PGI_2 required for inhibition of aggregation (Aiken et al. 1981). In addition, TX synthase inhibitors have been reported to reorient platelet endoperoxide (PGH_2, Figure 2) metabolism towards PGI_2 biosynthesis by the vessel wall (Defreyn et al. 1982). This hypothesis was originally termed the "steal hypothesis" when first proposed by Gryglewski et al. (1976). It states that under conditions in which aggregating platelets are juxtaposed to the endothelium (in a narrow vessel lumen), platelet PGH_2 may be utilized by vessel wall PGI_2 synthase to augment basal PGI_2 production (Figure 9). These results are consistent with the work of Needleman et al. (1979), which suggested that normally the "steal" of precursor by the vessel wall may not be an important pathway for PGI_2 biosynthesis. However, under conditions of a strong stimulus for platelet aggregation (i.e., circulating tumor cells), the selective blockade of TXA_2 synthase could drive platelet PGH_2 metabolism into PGI_2 biosynthesis by the vessel wall (Figure 9). In vivo evidence for the "steal hypothesis" has been recently provided by the experiments of Aiken et al. (1981).

We had initially proposed that, in addition to PGI_2, TXA_2 synthase inhibitors would also function as antimetastatic agents (Honn et al. 1981a,b). This prediction was based on the working hypothesis that circulating tumor cells disrupt the intravascular balance between PGI_2 and TXA_2. We initially investigated a series of endoperoxide analogs that were TX synthase inhibitors (Menter et

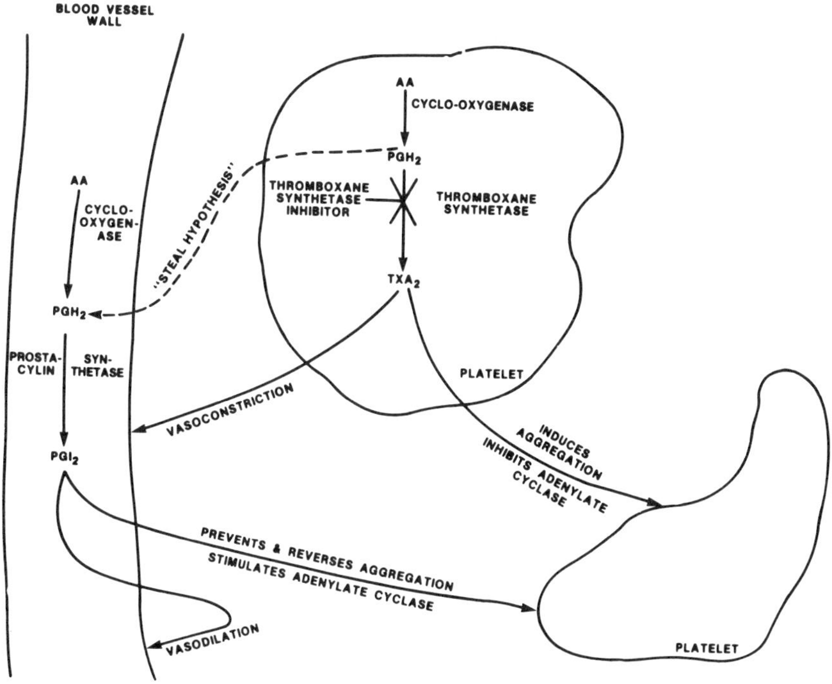

FIG. 9. The "steal hypothesis." See text for details. (Reproduced with permission of R. R. Gorman, Upjohn Co.)

al. 1982, Honn et al. 1983b). One endoperoxide analog, TX synthase inhibitor U54701 (9,11-iminoepoxy-prosta-5,13-dienoic acid; Fitzpatrick et al. 1979), completely inhibited TXA_2 production by human platelets in response to elutriated Lewis lung carcinoma cells concomitant with an inhibition of platelet aggregation (Honn et al. 1983b). However, W256 TCIPA was only inhibited 25% by a comparable dose of U54701, even though TXA_2 biosynthesis was almost completely inhibited (Honn et al. 1983b). Furthermore, TX synthase inhibitors that are imidazole derivatives [i.e., 1-(7-carboxyheptyl)imidazole] did not inhibit in vitro TCIPA even in the presence of inhibited platelet TXA_2 production. These unexpected results suggest that tumor cells can initiate platelet aggregation by a mechanism independent of TXA_2 biosynthesis (see discussion by Honn et al. 1983a). Nevertheless, both endoperoxide analogs and imidazole derivatives possess antimetastatic activity in vivo (Honn 1983, Honn, unpublished observation).

We propose that the discrepancy between lack of consistent inhibition of TCIPA by TX synthase inhibitors in vitro and their antimetastatic activity in vivo is due to the operation of the "steal hypothesis" in vivo. In vitro, TCIPA may proceed by pathways independent of TXA_2 biosynthesis. Thus, the antimetastatic activity of TX synthase inhibitors in vivo may ultimately be due to augmented endogenous PGI_2 biosynthesis.

Calcium channel blocker compounds

A number of vascular and myocardial disorders can be alleviated by inducing vasodilation with calcium channel blocker compounds (CCBC), including vasospastic angina, acute myocardial infarction, arrhythmias, and pulmonary hypertension. For recent reviews, see Braunwald (1982), Henry (1980), Godfraind (1981), Pedersen (1981), Flaim and Zelis (1981). In addition, CCBC have recently been found to inhibit platelet aggregation (Ribeiro et al. 1980, Addonizio et al. 1980, Schmunk and Lefer 1982). Therefore, we evaluated the effects of one CCBC of the dihydropyridine class (nimodipine; Bay e 9736) on TCIPA and spontaneous pulmonary metastasis of B16a. Nimodipine effected a dose-dependent inhibition of B16a TCIPA over a dose range of 4–400 μg/ml (K. V. Honn and J. M. Onoda, unpublished observation). In addition, the platelet-stimulated adhesion of [^{125}I]Udr-labeled W256 cells to cultured rat endothelial cells was inhibited 60% with 40 μg/ml nimodipine (K. V. Honn and J. M. Onoda, unpub-

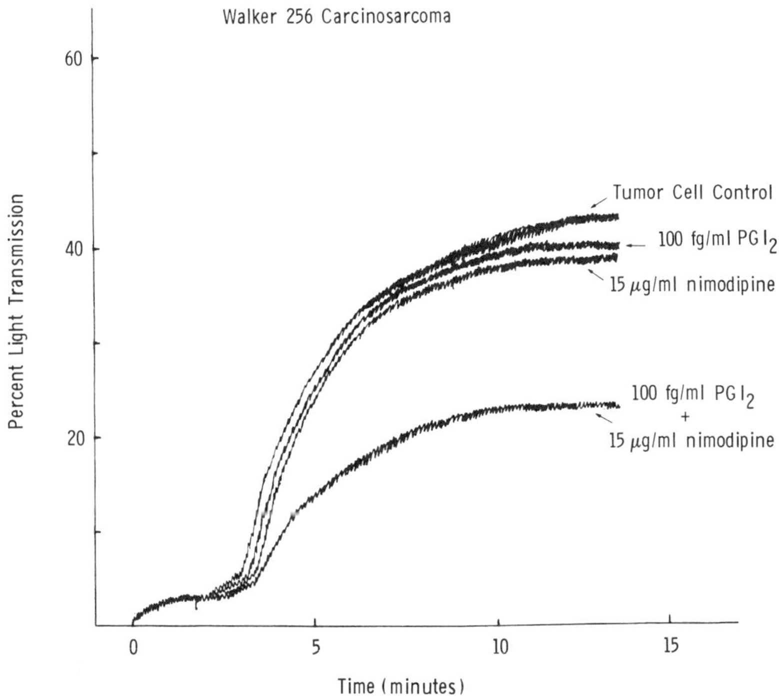

FIG. 10. Synergism between PGI_2 and the calcium channel blocker nimodipine on inhibition of platelet aggregation induced by W256 cells.

lished observation). In vivo, the daily administration of nimodipine (80 mg/kg) to C57BL/6J mice bearing subcutaneous B16a tumors inhibited spontaneous pulmonary metastasis >81% (K. V. Honn and J. M. Onoda, unpublished observation).

We next examined the possibility of a synergism between CCBC and PGI_2 in inhibition of TCIPA in vitro. PGI_2 at a dose of 100 fg/ml does not significantly affect TCIPA induced by W256 cells (Figure 10). Similarly, nimodipine (15 μg/ml) produces only a 15% inhibition of TCIPA (Figure 10). However, the combination of PGI_2 (100 fg/ml) plus nimodipine (15 μg/ml) results in a >50% inhibition of W256 TCIPA (Figure 10). Although preliminary, these in vitro results suggest a possible synergism between CCBC and PGI_2 for inhibition of tumor cell metastasis in vivo.

CONCLUSIONS

It is intuitive that for hematogenous metastasis to occur, the tumor cell must arrest in the microvasculature and attach to the vessel wall prior to extravasation and growth into a metastatic focus. Indirect evidence supports the concept that tumor cells interact with platelets during this process as discussed above.

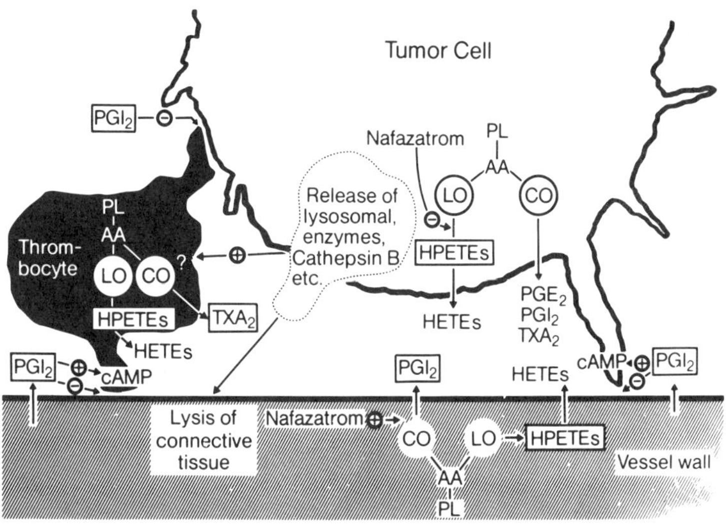

FIG. 11. Interactions among tumor cells, platelets (thrombocytes), and blood vessel wall. Direct interactions are possible between the platelet and the vessel wall, the tumor cell and vessel wall, and the platelets and tumor cells. Any one or all of the above may enhance tumor cell arrest and metastasis. Prostacyclin may prevent attachment of tumor cells to platelets or to vessel wall. PL, phospholipids; AA, arachidonic acid; CO, cyclooxygenase; LO, lipoxygenase; HPETE, hydroperoxyeicosatetraenoic acid; HETE, hydroxyeicosatetraenoic acid; PGI_2, prostacyclin; and TXA_2, thromboxane A_2. (Reproduced from Honn et al. 1983a, with permission of Pergamon Press.)

We propose that the metabolism of arachidonic acid in the tumor cell, the platelet, and the vessel wall plays an essential role in the sum total of these interactions (Figure 11). For example, the production of PGI_2 by the vessel wall and of TXA_2 by the platelet is thought to play a key (although possibly not an exclusive) role in thrombosis.

Exogenous PGI_2 may function as an antimetastatic agent by inhibiting the association of the tumor cell with the vessel wall (Figure 11). The interactions between the vessel wall and tumor cells or platelets may be inhibited by stimulation of platelet cAMP or tumor cell cAMP by exogenous PGI_2. Similarly, vessel wall PGI_2 may serve as a natural deterrent to metastasis by inhibiting these interactions (Figure 6). A new class of antimetastatic agents have the ability to stimulate endogenous PGI_2 production or prolong the half-life of PGI_2 (e.g., nafazatrom). A new proposal for the antimetastatic activity of TX synthase inhibitors ("steal hypothesis") may also center around enhanced endogenous PGI_2 production. Finally, a heretofore unsuspected class of pharmacological agents (CCBC) are reported by us to have potent antimetastatic activity, which in part may result from a synergism with PGI_2.

ACKNOWLEDGMENTS

This investigation was supported by grant numbers CA29405 and CA29997 awarded by the National Cancer Institute, Department of Health and Human Services and by American Cancer Society Grant BC-356, Miles Institute for Preclinical Pharmacology and Bayer AG. The excellent technical assistance of Marjorie Carufel, Deborah Moilanen, Gregory Neagos, and Kim Pampalona is appreciated. The expert typing of Susan Lyman is greatly appreciated.

REFERENCES

Addonizio, V. P., C. A. Fisher, and L. H. Edmunds. 1980. Effects of verapamil and nifedipine on platelet activation. (Abstract) Circulation 62:326.

Aiken, J. W., R. J. Shebuski, O. V. Miller, and R. R. Gorman. 1981. Endogenous prostacyclin contributes to the efficacy of a thromboxane synthetase inhibitor for preventing coronary artery thrombosis. J. Pharmacol. Exp. Ther. 219:299–308.

Ambrus, J. L., C. M. Ambrus, H. Gastpar, and P. Williams. 1982. Study of platelet aggregation in vivo. IX. Effect of nafazatrom on in vivo platelet aggregation and spontaneous tumor metastasis. J. Med. 13:35–47.

Aristoff, P. A., and A. W. Harrison. 1982. Synthesis of benzindene prostaglandins: A novel potent class of stable prostacyclin analogs. Tetrahed. Lett. 23:2067–2070.

Bastida, E., A. Ordinas, and G. A. Jamieson. 1981. Idiosyncratic platelet responses to human tumor cells. Nature 291:661–662.

Bastida, E., A. Ordinas, S. L. Giardina, and G. A. Jamieson. 1982. Differentiation of platelet-aggregating effects of human tumor cell lines based on inhibition studies with apyrase, hirudin, and phospholipase. Cancer Res. 42:4348–4352.

Bergman, G., R. Daly, L. Atkinson, M. Rothman, P. J. Richardson, G. Jackson, and D. E. Jewitt. 1981. Prostacyclin: Haemodynamic and metabolic effects in patients with coronary artery disease. Lancet 1:569–572.

Bertele, V., A. Falanga, M. C. Roncaglioni, C. Cerletti, and G. de Gaetano. 1982. Thromboxane synthetase inhibition results in increased sensitivity to prostacyclin. Thromb. Haemost. 47:294.

Black, P. H. 1980. Shedding from the cell surface of normal and cancer cells. Adv. Cancer Res. 32:75–199.

Brain, M. C., J. G. Azzopardi, L. R. I. Baker, G. F. Pinco, P. D. Roberts, and J. V. Dacie. 1970. Microangiopathic haemolytic anemia: The possible role of vascular lesions in pathogenesis. Br. J. Haematol. 18:183–193.

Braunwald, E. 1982. Mechanism of action of calcium-channel-blocking agents. N. Engl. J. Med. 307:1618–1627.

Buchanan, M. R., M. Blajchman, and J. Hirsch. 1982. Inhibition of arterial thrombosis and platelet function by nafazatrom. Thromb. Res. 28:157–170.

Busse, W. D., M. Mardin, R. Grutzmann, J. R. Dunn, M. Theodoreau, B. F. Sloane, and K. V. Honn. 1982. Nafazatrom (Bay g 6575): An inhibitor of cellular lipoxygenase. (Abstract) Fed. Proc. 41:1717.

Carreras, L. O., D. A. F. Chamone, P. Klerckx, and J. Vermylen. 1980. Decreased vascular prostacyclin (PGI_2) in diabetic rats. Stimulation of PGI_2 release in normal and diabetic rats by the antithrombotic compound Bay g 6575. Thromb. Res. 19:663–670.

Chamone, D. A. F., B. van Damme, L. O. Carreras, and J. Vermylen. 1981. Increased release of vascular prostacyclin-like activity after long-term treatment of diabetic rats with Bay g 6575. Haemostasis 10:297–303.

Cowan, D. H., and J. Graham. 1982. Effect of platelet growth factor(s) on growth of human tumor colonies, *in* Interactions of Platelets and Tumor Cells, G. A. Jamieson, ed. Alan R. Liss, New York, pp. 249–268.

Curatolo, L., M. Colucci, A. L. Cambini, A. Poggi, L. Morasca, M. B. Donati, and N. Semeraro. 1979. Evidence that cells from experimental tumours can activate coagulation factor X. Br. J. Cancer 40:228–233.

Defreyn, G., H. Deckmyn, and J. Vermylen. 1982. A thromboxane synthetase inhibitor reorients endoperoxide metabolism in whole blood towards prostacyclin and prostaglandin E_2. Thromb. Res. 26:389–400.

del Regato, J. A. 1977. Pathways of metastatic spread of malignant tumors. Semin. Oncol. 4:33–38.

Donati, M. B., and A. Poggi. 1980. Malignancy and haemostasis. Br. J. Haematol. 44:173–182.

Dvorak, H. F., S. C. Quay, N. S. Orenstein, A. M. Dvorak, P. Hahn, A. M. Bitzer, and A. C. Carvalho. 1981. Tumor shedding and coagulation. Science 212:923–924.

Edwards, R. L., F. R. Rickles, and M. Cronlund. 1981. Abnormalities of blood coagulation in patients with cancer. Mononuclear cell tissue factor generation. J. Lab. Clin. Med. 98:917–928.

Elias, E. G., F. Sepulveda, and I. B. Mink. 1973. Increasing the efficiency of cancer chemotherapy with heparin: Clinical study. J. Surg. Oncol. 5:189–193.

Eling, T. E., K. V. Honn, W. D. Busse, F. Seuter, and L. J. Marnett. 1982. Stimulation of PGI_2 biosynthesis by nafazatrom (Bay g 6575), *in* Prostaglandins and Cancer, T. J. Powles, R. S. Bockman, K. V. Honn, and P. Ramwell, eds. Alan R. Liss, New York, pp. 783–787.

Fantone, J., S. Kunkel, and J. Varani. 1982. Inhibition of tumor cell adherence by prostaglandins, *in* Prostaglandins and Cancer, T. J. Powles, R. S. Bockman, K. V. Honn, and P. Ramwell, eds. Alan R. Liss, New York, pp. 673–677.

Fidler, I. J. 1973. The relationship of embolic homogeneity, number, size, and viability to the incidence of experimental metastasis. Eur. J. Cancer 9:223–227.

Fidler, I. J., D. M. Gersten, and I. Hart. 1978. The biology of cancer invasion and metastasis. Adv. Cancer Res. 28:149–250.

Fisher, E. R., and B. Fisher. 1967. Recent observations on concepts of metastasis. Arch. Pathol. 83:321–324.

Fitzpatrick, F., G. Bundy, R. Gorman, T. Honohan, J. McGuire, and F. Sun. 1979. 9,11-Iminoepoxyprosta-5,13-dienoic acid is a selective thromboxane A_2 synthetase inhibitor. Biochim. Biophys. Acta 573:238–244.

Flaim, S. F., and R. Zelis. 1981. Clinical use of calcium entry blockers. Fed. Proc. 40:2877–2881.

Fogel, M., P. Altevogt and V. Schirrmacher. 1983. Metastatic potential severely altered by changes in tumor cell adhesiveness and cell-surface sialylation. J. Exp. Med. 157:371–376.

Gasic, G. J., D. Boettiger, J. L. Catalfamo, T. B. Gasic, and G. J. Stewart. 1978. Aggregation of platelets and cell membrane vesiculation by rat cells transformed in vitro by Rous sarcoma virus. Cancer Res. 38:2950–2955.

Gasic, G. J., J. L. Catalfamo, T. B. Gasic, and N. Avdalovic. 1981. In vitro mechanism of platelet aggregation by purified plasma membrane vesicles shed by mouse 15091A tumor cells, *in* Malignancy and the Hemostatic System, M. B. Donati, J. F. Davidson and S. Garattini, eds. Raven Press, New York, pp. 27–35.

Gasic, G. J., T. B. Gasic, N. Galanti, T. Johnson, and J. Murphy. 1973. Platelet tumor-cell interactions in mice. The role of platelets in the spread of malignant disease. Int. J. Cancer 11:704–718.

Gasic, G. J., T. B. Gasic, and C. C. Stewart. 1968. Antimetastatic effects associated with platelet reaction. Proc. Natl. Acad. Sci. USA 61:46–52.

Gasic, G. J., P. A. G. Koch, B. Hsu, T. B. Gasic, and S. Niewiarowski. 1976. Thrombogenic activity of mouse and human tumors: Effects on platelets, coagulation and fibrinolysis, and possible significance for metastasis. Z. Krebsforsch. 86:263–277.

Gastpar, H. 1977. Platelet cancer cell interaction in metastasis formation: A possible therapeutic approach to metastasis prophylaxis. J. Med. 8:103–114.

Gastpar, H., J. Ambrus, and L. E. Thurber. 1977. Study of platelet aggregation in vivo. II. Effect of bencyclane on circulating metastatic tumor cells. J. Med. 8:53–56.

George, J. W., L. L. Thoi, and R. K. Morgan. 1981. Quantitative analysis of platelet membrane glycoproteins: Effect of platelet washing procedures and isolation of platelet density subpopulations. Thromb. Res. 23:69–77.

Godfraind, T. 1981. Mechanisms of action of calcium entry blockers. Fed. Proc. 40:2866–2871.

Goodnight, S. H. 1974. Bleeding and intravascular clotting in malignancy: A review. Ann. N.Y. Acad. Sci. 230:271–288.

Gordon, J. L. 1975. Blood platelet lysosomes and their contribution to the pathophysiological role of platelets, *in* Lysosomes in Biology and Pathology, vol. 4, J. T. Dingle and R. T. Dean, eds. Elsevier/North Holland, Amsterdam, pp. 3–31.

Gordon, S. G., and B. A. Cross. 1981. A factor X activating cysteine protease from malignant tissue. J. Clin. Invest. 67:1665–1671.

Gordon, S. G., J. J. Franks, and B. Lewis. 1975. Cancer procoagulant A: A factor X activating procoagulant from malignant tissue. Thromb. Res. 6:127–137.

Gorman, R. R. 1979. Modulation of human platelet function by prostacyclin and thromboxane A_2. Fed. Proc. 38:83–88.

Gryglewski, R. J., S. Bunting, S. Moncada, R. J. Flower, and J. R. Vane. 1976. Arterial walls are protected against deposition of platelet thrombi by a substance (prostaglandin X) which they make from prostaglandin endoperoxides. Prostaglandins 12:685–713.

Hall, E. R., Y. C. Chen, T. Ho, and K. K. Wu. 1982. The reduction of platelet thrombi on damaged vessel wall by a thromboxane synthetase inhibitor in platelets. Thromb. Res. 27:501–511.

Hall, R. J. C., and H. A. Dewar. 1981. Safety of coronary arterial prostacyclin infusion. Lancet 1:949.

Hamberg, M., J. Svensson, and B. Samuelsson. 1975. Thromboxanes: A new group of biologically active compounds derived from prostaglandin endoperoxides. Proc. Natl. Acad. Sci. USA 72:2994–2998.

Hara, Y., M. Steiner, and M. G. Baldini. 1980. Characterization of the platelet aggregating activity of tumor cells. Cancer Res. 40:1217–1222.

Harker, L. A., and S. J. Slichter. 1972. Platelet and fibrinogen consumption in man. N. Engl. J. Med. 287:999–1005.

Henry. P. D. 1980. Comparative pharmacology of calcium antagonists nifedipine, verapamil, and diltiazem. Am. J. Cardiol. 46:1047–1058.

Heptinstall, S., J. Bevan, S. R. Cockbill, S. P. Hanley, and M. J. Parry. 1980. Effects of a selective inhibitor of thromboxane synthetase on human blood platelet behaviour. Thromb. Res. 20:219–230.

Herman, A. G., M. Claeys, S. Moncada, and J. R. Vane. 1979. Biosynthesis of prostacyclin (PGI_2) and 12L-hydroxy-5,8,10,14-eicosatetraenoic acid (HETE) by pericardium, pleura, peritoneum and aorta of the rabbit. Prostaglandins 18:439–452.

Hilgard, P. 1973. The role of blood platelets in experimental metastases. Br. J. Cancer 28:429–435.

Hilgard, P., L. Beyerle, R. Hohage, V. Hiemeyer, and M. Kubler. 1972. The effect of heparin on the initial phase of metastasis formation. Eur. J. Cancer 8:347–352.

Holmsen, H., and H. J. Day. 1970. The selectivity of the thrombin-induced platelet release reaction: Subcellular localization of released and retained constituents. J. Lab. Clin. Med. 75:840–855.

Holmsen, H., and H. J. Weiss. 1979. Secretable storage pools in platelets. Annu. Rev. Med. 30:119–134.

Honn, K. V. 1983. Inhibition of tumor cell metastasis by modulation of the vascular prostacyclin/thromboxane A_2 system. Clin. Exp. Metastasis 1:103–114.

Honn, K. V., R. S. Bockman, and L. J. Marnett. 1981a. Prostaglandins and cancer: A review of tumor initiation through tumor metastasis. Prostaglandins 21:833–864.

Honn, K. V., W. D. Busse, and B. F. Sloane. 1983a. Commentary. Prostacyclin and thromboxanes. Implications for their role in tumor cell metastasis. Biochem. Pharmacol. 32:1–11.

Honn, K. V., B. Cicone, and A. Skoff. 1981b. Prostacyclin: A potent antimetastatic agent. Science 212:1270–1272.

Honn, K. V., and J. R. Dunn. 1982. Nafazatrom (Bay g 6575) inhibition of tumor cell lipoxygenase activity and cellular proliferation. FEBS Lett. 139:65–68.

Honn, K. V., D. Menter, P. G. Cavanaugh, G. Neagos, D. Moilanen, J. D. Taylor, and B. F. Sloane. 1983b. A review of prostaglandins and the treatment of tumor metastasis. Acta Clin. Belg. 38:53–67.

Honn, K. V., D. Menter, D. Moilanen, P. G. Cavanaugh, J. D. Taylor and B. F. Sloane. 1983c. Role of prostacyclin and thromboxanes in tumor cell-platelet-vessel wall interactions, *in* Protective Agents in Cancer, D. C. H. McBrian, and T. F. Slater, eds. Academic Press, New York, pp. 57–79.

Honn, K. V., J. Meyer, G. Neagos, T. Henderson, C. Westley, and V. Ratanatharathorm. 1982. Control of tumor growth and metastasis with prostacyclin and thromboxane synthetase inhibitors: Evidence for a new antitumor and antimetastatic agent (Bay g 6575), *in* Interaction of Platelets and Tumor Cells, G. A. Jamieson, ed. Alan R. Liss, New York, pp. 295–331.

Honn, K. V., and B. F. Sloane, eds. 1983a. Hemostatic Mechanisms and Metastasis. Martinus Nijhoff, The Hague (in press).

Honn, K. V., and B. F. Sloane. 1983b. Prostacyclin, thromboxanes, and hematogenous metastasis. Adv. Prostaglandin Thromboxane Leukotriene Res. 12:313–318.

Honn, K. V., and B. F. Sloane. 1983c. Prostaglandins in tumor cell metastasis, *in* Basic Mechanisms and Clinical Treatments of Tumor Metastasis, M. Torisu and Y. Yoshida, eds. Academic Press, New York (in press).

Hope, W., T. J. Martin, C. N. Chesterman, and F. J. Morgan. 1979. Human β-thromboglobulin inhibits PGI_2 production and binds to a specific site in bovine aortic endothelial cells. Nature 282:210–212.

Irimura, T., R. Gonzalez, and G. L. Nicolson. 1981. Effects of tunicamycin on B16 metastatic melanoma cell surface glycoproteins and blood-borne arrest and survival properties. Cancer Res. 41:3411–3418.

Irimura, T., and G. L. Nicolson. 1981. The role of glycoconjugates in metastatic melanoma blood-borne arrest and cell surface properties. J. Supramol. Struct. Cell. Biochem. 17:325–336.

Jamieson, G. A., ed. 1982. Interaction of Platelets and Tumor Cells. Alan R. Liss, New York.

Kaplan, K. L. 1981. Platelet granule proteins: Localization and secretion, *in* Platelets in Biology and Pathology, vol. 2, J. L. Gordon, ed. Elsevier/North Holland, Amsterdam, pp. 77–90.

Karpatkin, S., and E. Pearlstein. 1981. Role of platelets in tumor cell metastases. Ann. Intern. Med. 95:636–641.

Karpatkin, S., A. Smerling, and E. Pearlstein. 1980. Plasma requirement for the aggregation of rabbit platelets by an aggregating material derived from SV40-transformed 3T3 fibroblasts. J. Lab. Clin. Med. 96:994–1001.

Kramer, R. H., R. Gonzalez, and G. L. Nicolson. 1980. Metastatic tumor cells adhere preferentially to the extracellular matrix underlying vascular endothelial cells. Int. J. Cancer 26:639–645.

Kramer, R. H., and G. L. Nicolson. 1979. Interactions of tumor cells with vascular endothelial cell monolayers: A model for metastatic invasion. Proc. Natl. Acad. Sci. USA 76:5704–5706.

Kramer, R. H., and G. L. Nicolson. 1981. Invasion of vascular endothelial cell monolayers and underlying matrix by metastatic human cancer cells, *in* International Cell Biology, S. Schweiger, ed. Springer Verlag, Heidelberg, pp. 794–799.

Liepins, A., and E. de Harven. 1982. Effects of cyclic nucleotides on the shedding of tumor cell surface molecules. Exp. Cell Res. 139:265–273.

Liepins, A., and A. J. Hillman. 1981. Shedding of tumor cell surface membranes. Cell Biol. Int. Rep. 5:15–26.

Lione, A., and H. B. Bosmann. 1978. The inhibitory effect of heparin and warfarin treatments on the intravascular survival of B16 melanoma cells in syngeneic C57 mice. Cell Biol. Int. Rep. 2:81–86.

Liotta, L. A., J. Kleinerman, and G. M. Saidel. 1974. Quantitative relationships of intravascular tumor cells, tumor vessels, and pulmonary metastases following tumor implantation. Cancer Res. 34:997–1004.

Liotta, L. A., J. Kleinerman, and G. M. Saidel. 1976. The significance of hematogenous tumor cell clumps in the metastatic process. Cancer Res. 36:889–894.

Lipton, A., N. Kepner, C. Rogers, E. Witkoski, and K. Leitzel. 1982. A mitogenic factor for transformed cells from human platelets, *in* Interactions of Platelets and Tumor Cells, G. A. Jamieson, ed. Alan R. Liss, New York, pp. 233–248.

Maat, B., and P. Hilgard. 1981. Anticoagulant and experimental metastases—Evaluation of anti-metastatic effects in different model systems. J. Cancer Res. Clin. Oncol. 101:275–283.

Machleidt, C., U. Forstermann, H. Anhut, and G. Hertting. 1981. Formation and elimination of prostacyclin metabolites in the cat in vivo as determined by radioimmunoassay of unextracted plasma. Eur. J. Pharmacol. 74:19–26.

Marcum, J. M., M. McGill, E. Bastida, A. Ordinas, and G. A. Jamieson. 1980. The interaction of platelets, tumor cells, and vascular subendothelium. J. Lab. Clin. Med. 96:1048–1053.

Menter, D., G. Neagos, J. Dunn, R. Palazzo, T. T. Tchen, J. D. Taylor, and K. V. Honn. 1982. Tumor cell induced platelet aggregation: Inhibition by prostacyclin, thromboxane A_2, and phosphodiesterase inhibitors, *in* Prostaglandins and Cancer, T. J. Powles, R. S. Bockman, K. V. Honn, and P. Ramwell, eds. Alan R. Liss, New York, pp. 809–813.

Moncada, S. 1982. Biological importance of prostacyclin. Br. J. Pharmacol. 76:3–31.

Moncada, S., R. J. Gryglewski, S. Bunting, and J. R. Vane. 1976a. A lipid peroxide inhibits the enzyme in blood vessel microsomes that generates from prostaglandin endoperoxides the substance (Prostaglandin X) which prevents platelet aggregation. Prostaglandins 12:715–733.

Moncada, S., R. J. Gryglewski, S. Bunting, and J. R. Vane. 1976b. An enzyme isolated from arteries transforms prostaglandin endoperoxides to an unstable substance that inhibits platelet aggregation. Nature 263:663–665.

Moncada, S., and J. R. Vane. 1977. The discovery of prostacyclin (PGX); a fresh insight into arachidonic acid metabolism, *in* Biochemical Aspects of Prostaglandins and Thromboxanes, N. Kharasch and J. Fried, eds. Academic Press, New York, pp. 155–177.

Moncada, S., and J. R. Vane. 1980. Prostacyclin in the cardiovascular system, *in* Advances in Prostaglandin and Thromboxane Research, vol. 6, B. Samuelsson, P. W. Ramwell, and R. Paoletti, eds. Raven Press, New York, pp. 43–60.

Morton, D. R., and F. C. Brokow. 1979. Total synthesis of 6a-carbaprostaglandin I_2 and related isomers. J. Org. Chem. 44:2880–2887.

Mullane, K. M., G. J. Dusting, J. A. Salmon, S. Moncada, and J. R. Vane. 1979. Biotransformation and cardiovascular effects of arachidonic acid in the dog. Eur. J. Pharmacol. 54:217–228.

Murray, J. C., L. Liotta, S. I. Rennard, and G. R. Martin. 1980. Adhesion characteristics of murine metastatic and nonmetastatic tumor cells in vitro. Cancer Res. 40:347–351.

Needleman, P., A. Wyche, and A. Raz. 1979. Platelet and blood vessel arachidonate metabolism and interactions. J. Clin. Invest. 63:345–349.

Nicolson, G. L. 1982. Cancer metastasis. Organ colonization and the cell-surface properties of malignant cells. Biochim. Biophys. Acta 695:113–176.

Nicolson, G. L., T. Irimura, R. Gonzalez, and E. Ruoslahti. 1981. The role of fibronectin in adhesion of metastatic melanoma cells to endothelial cells and their basal lamina. Exp. Cell Res. 135:461–465.

Nishiyama, H., and K. Ohno. 1979. Synthesis of 6,7-dehydro-5-oxo-prostaglandin I_1: A stable analog of prostacyclin. Tetrahed. Lett. 36:3481–3484.

Paschen, W., H. Patscheke, and P. Worner. 1979. Aggregation of activated platelets with Walker 256 carcinoma cells. Blut 38:17–24.

Pearlstein, E., C. Ambrogio, G. Gasic, and S. Karpatkin. 1981. Inhibition of the platelet-aggregating activity of two human adenocarcinomas of the colon and an anaplastic murine tumor with a specific thrombin inhibitor, dansylarginine N-(3-ethyl-1,5-pentanediyl)amide. Cancer Res. 41:4535–4539.

Pearlstein, E., L. B. Cooper, and S. Karpatkin. 1979. Extraction and characterization of a platelet-aggregating material from SV40-transformed mouse 3T3 fibroblasts. J. Lab. Clin. Med. 93:332–344.

Pearlstein, E., P. L. Salk, G. Yogeeswaran, and S. Karpatkin. 1980. Correlation between spontaneous metastatic potential, platelet-aggregating activity of cell surface extracts, and cell surface sialylation in 10 metastatic-variant derivatives of rat renal sarcoma cell line. Proc. Natl. Acad. Sci. USA 77:4336–4339.

Pedersen, O. L. 1981. Calcium blockade as a therapeutic principle in arterial hypertension. Acta Pharmacol. Toxicol. 49:(Suppl 2) 1–31.

Pike, J. E., and G. L. Bundy. 1982. Prostaglandin analogues, *in* Prostaglandins and Cancer, T. J. Powles, R. S. Bockman, K. V. Honn and P. Ramwell, eds. Alan R. Liss, New York, pp. 67–77.

Poste, G., and I. J. Fidler. 1980. The pathogenesis of cancer metastasis. Nature 283:139–146.

Poste, G., and G. L. Nicolson. 1980. Arrest and metastasis of blood-borne tumor cells are modified by fusion of plasma membrane vesicles from highly metastatic cells. Proc. Natl. Acad. Sci. USA 77:399–403.

Raz, A., W. L. McLellan, I. R. Hart, C. D. Bucana, L. C. Hoyer, B. A. Sela, P. Dragsten, and I. J. Fidler. 1980. Cell surface properties of B16 melanoma variants with differing metastatic potential. Cancer Res. 40:1645–1651.

Ribeiro, L. G. T., T. A. Brandon, J. K. Horak, R. T. Solis, and R. R. Miller. 1980. Inhibition of platelet aggregation by verapamil: Further rationale for the use of calcium antagonists in coronary artery disease. (Abstract) Circulation 62:293.

Rosenkranz, B., C. Fischer, K. E. Weimer, and J. C. Frolich. 1980. Metabolism of prostacyclin and 6-keto-prostaglandin $F_{1\alpha}$ in man. J. Biol. Chem. 255:10194–10198.

Salmon, J. A., D. R. Smith, R. S. Flower, S. Moncada, and J. R. Vane. 1978. Further studies on the enzymatic conversion of prostaglandin endoperoxide into prostacyclin by porcine aortic microsomes. Biochim. Biophys. Acta 523:250–262.

Salsbury, A. J. 1975. The significance of the circulating cancer cell. Cancer Treat. Rev. 2:55–72.

Santoro, S. A., and L. W. Cunningham. 1981. The interaction of platelets with collagen, *in* Platelets in Biology and Pathology, J. L. Gordon, ed. Elsevier/North Holland, Amsterdam, pp. 249–264.

Schmunk, G. A., and A. M. Lefer. 1982. Anti-aggregatory actions of calcium channel blockers in cat platelets. Res. Commun. Chem. Pathol. Pharmacol. 35:179–187.

Seuter, F., W. D. Busse, K. Meng, F. Hoffmeister, E. Moller, and H. Horstmann. 1979. The antithrombotic activity of Bay g 6575. Arzneim.-Forsch./Drug Res. 29:54–59.

Skolnik, G., M. Alpsten, and L. Ivarsson. 1980. Studies on mechanisms involved in metastasis formation from circulating tumor cells. J. Cancer Res. Clin. Oncol. 97:249–256.

Sloane, B. F., J. R. Dunn, and K. V. Honn. 1981. Lysosomal cathepsin B: Correlation with metastatic potential. Science 212:1151–1153.

Stringfellow, D. A., and F. A. Fitzpatrick. 1979. Prostaglandin D_2 controls pulmonary metastasis of malignant melanoma cells. Nature 282:76–78.

Szczeklik, A., and R. J. Gryglewski. 1981. Treatment of vascular disease with prostacyclin, *in* Clinical Pharmacology of Prostacyclin, P. J. Lewis and J. O'Grady, eds. Raven Press, New York, pp. 159–167.

Szczeklik, A., R. J. Gryglewski, R. Nizankowski, J. Musial, R. Pieton, and J. Mruk. 1978. Circulatory and anti-platelet effects of intravenous prostacyclin in healthy men. Pharmacol. Res. Commun. 10:545–556.

Szczeklik, A., R. Nizankowski, S. Skawinski, J. Szczeklik, P. Gluszko, and R. J. Gryglewski. 1979. Successful therapy of advanced arteriosclerosis obliterans with prostacyclin. Lancet 1:1111–1114.

Takacz, J. S., and J. O. Lampen. 1975. Tunicamycin inhibition of polyisoprenyl N-acetylglucosaminylpyrophosphate formation in calf-liver microsomes. Biochem. Biophys. Res. Commun. 65:248–257.

Takatsuki, A., K. Kohno, and G. Tamura. 1975. Inhibition of biosynthesis of polyisoprenol sugars in chick embryo microsomes by tunicamycin. Agr. Biol. Chem. 39:2089–2091.

Tanaka, N., S-I Ashida, A. Tohgo, and H. Ogawa. 1982. Platelet-aggregating activities of metastasizing tumor cells. Invasion Metastasis 2:289–298.

Terranova, V. P., L. A. Liotta, R. G. Russo, and G. R. Martin. 1982. Role of laminin in the attachment and metastasis of murine tumor cells. Cancer Res. 42:2265–2269.

Thompson, C. B., K. Eaton, S. M. Princiotta, C. A. Rushin, and C. R. Valleri. 1982. Size dependent platelet subpopulations: Relationship of platelet volume to ultrastructure, enzymatic activity and function. Br. J. Haematol. 50:509–519.

Turner, W. A., D. G. Menter, K. V. Honn, and J. D. Taylor. 1983. Tumor cell induced platelet fibronectin release. (Abstract) Proc. Am. Assoc. Cancer Res. 24:25.
Vane, J. R., S. Bunting, and S. Moncada. 1982. Prostacyclin in physiology and pathophysiology. Int. Rev. Exp. Pathol. 23:161–207.
Vargaftig, B. B., M. Chignard, and J. Benveniste. 1981. Present concepts on the mechanism of platelet aggregation. Biochem. Pharmacol. 30:263–271.
Vermylen, J., D. A. F. Chamone, and M. Verstraete. 1979. Stimulation of prostacyclin release from vessel wall by Bay g 6575, an antithrombotic compound. Lancet 1:518–520.
Vilarem, M. J., J. Jouanneau, and R. Bourrillon. 1981. Differences in sialic acid contents of low cancer cells, high cancer cells and normal mouse lung counterparts. Biochem. Biophys. Res. Commun. 98:7–14.
Vlodavsky, I., and D. Gospodarowicz. 1981. Respective roles of laminin and fibronectin in adhesion of human carcinoma and sarcoma cells. Nature 289:304–306.
Watanabe, S. 1954. Metastasizability of tumor cells. Cancer 7:215–223.
Watkins, W. D., M. B. Peterson, R. K. Crone, D. C. Shannon, and L. Levine. 1980. Prostacyclin and prostaglandin E_1 for severe idiopathic pulmonary artery hypertension. Lancet 1:1083.
Weiss, L. 1977. A pathobiologic overview of metastasis. Semin. Oncol. 4:5–17.
Weiss, L. 1980. Cancer cell traffic from the lungs to the liver: An example of metastatic inefficiency. Int. J. Cancer 25:385–392.
Weiss, L. 1982. Metastatic inefficiency, *in* Tumor Invasion and Metastasis, L. A. Liotta and I. R. Hart, eds. Martinus Nijhoff, The Hague, pp. 81–98.
Weiss, L. 1983. Overview of the metastatic cascade, *in* Hemostatic Mechanisms and Metastasis, K. V. Honn and B. F. Sloane, eds. Martinus Nijhoff, The Hague (in press).
Whittle, B. J. R., S. Moncada, F. Whiting, and J. R. Vane. 1980. Carbacyclin—A potent stable prostacyclin analogue for the inhibition of platelet aggregation. Prostaglandins 19:605–627.
Willmott, N., A. Malcolm, T. McLeod, A. Gracie, and K. C. Calman. 1983. Changes in anatomical distribution of tumour lesions induced by platelet-active drugs. Invasion Metastasis 3:32–51.
Wong, P. Y-K, P. H-W Chao, and J. C. McGiff. 1982. Nafazatrom (Bay g 6575), an antithrombotic and antimetastatic agent, inhibits 15-hydroxyprostaglandin dehydrogenase. J. Pharmacol. Exp. Ther. 223:757–760.
Yahara, Y., S. Okawa, Y. Onozawa, T. Motomiya, K. Tanoue, and H. Yamazaki. 1983. Activation of platelets in cancer, especially with reference to genesis of disseminated intravascular coagulation. Thromb. Res. 29:27–35.
Zacharski, L. R., W. G. Henderson, F. R. Rickles, W. B. Forman, C. J. Cornell, R. J. Forcier, H. W. Harrower, and R. O. Johnson. 1979. Rationale and experimental design for the VA cooperative study of anticoagulation (Warfarin) in the treatment of cancer. Cancer 44:732–741.
Zamora, P. O., K. G. Danielson, and H. L. Hosick. 1980. Invasion of endothelial cell monolayers on collagen gels by cells from mammary tumor spheroids. Cancer Res. 40:4631–4639.

Therapy of Metastasis

Cancer Invasion and Metastasis: Biologic and Therapeutic Aspects edited by Garth L. Nicolson and Luka Milas. Raven Press, New York © 1984.

Concepts for the Treatment of Tumor Metastasis

Daniel P. Griswold, Jr., Frank M. Schabel, Jr., Donald J. Dykes, Mary W. Trader, and W. Russell Laster, Jr.

Chemotherapy Department, Southern Research Institute, Birmingham, Alabama 35205

In the past few years, considerable progress has been made toward achieving a better understanding of tumor biology and, in particular, the metastatic process. This new and growing body of knowledge has in turn led to reconsideration of some cancer chemotherapeutic concepts, particularly those involving the treatment of metastatic disease.

Not only have new views emerged in regard to the manner of treatment of metastatic cancer, but serious questions have been raised concerning the validity of drug development programs and anticancer drug sensitivity assays. In brief, the questions have arisen from those observations that any cancer cell population may be heterogeneous in regard to metastatic potential (Fidler and Hart 1981) and in regard to drug sensitivity or resistance (Schabel et al. 1980) (perhaps the two most important among many other characteristics).

Our understanding of some current thinking, simply stated, is:

1. The major part of the cancer problem in man is related to metastatic disease, and chemotherapy of most human solid tumors is directed toward the metastatic cancer.
2. There is now considerable evidence that primary tumors are heterogeneous and that metastases are derived from a subpopulation of cells within the primary tumor that possesses a unique propensity for metastasis.
3. It is further believed by some that the metastatic cohort, a distinct, homogeneous cell population, has a different spectrum of chemotherapeutic sensitivity than the parent primary from which it was derived.
4. This premise is based on the assumption that metastatic potential and drug resistance (or drug insensitivity) conferred by cell transformation are not mutually exclusive events, or that a drug-resistant or insensitive tumor cell *may* be selected, with some unknown degree of probability, by the metastatic event.

If the first assumption is correct, then many of the models we have used and are now using for the selection of new anticancer chemotherapeutic agents should be expected to be inappropriate, and the selection/rejection, drug-screening program, as we know it, could reject those agents that could be active against metastatic tumors and select for clinical trial agents that may be inactive against the metastatic disease. However, if the second assumption is correct, then probability becomes the overriding issue. In that case, the possibility that drug resistance or insensitivity is a characteristic of metastatic tumor cell populations would become of increasing importance only as the probability of its occurrence increased.

A complicating problem arises from the view that much of the observed variability in the response of tumors to drug treatment results from host differences in metabolic capability and rates, leading to variable drug concentrations at the target site. This problem would apply to metastatic as well as primary tumors.

These concerns may be briefly summarized by three questions. Do variable tumor responses result from (1) tumor-associated factors, e.g., drug-resistant cells derived from a heterogeneous tumor cell population, (2) host differences that result in the attainment of variable drug concentrations (3) or both?

DIFFERENTIAL DRUG SENSITIVITY

Resistance of a tumor cell or a subpopulation of cells to the cytotoxic action of a drug may result from a variety of conditions. There is the true, biochemical drug resistance that is perhaps best recognized and has been shown to be a contributing factor to drug treatment failures in tumors of both animal and man. Based on the earlier work of Luria and Delbrück (1943) and that of Law (1952), we know that mutation to resistance may occur spontaneously and independently of the agent to which resistance is developed. Although the mutational event is in a sense random, the mathematical model described by Goldie and Coldman (1979) "predicts that there will be a variation in the size of the resistant fraction (of cells) within tumor colonies of the same size for any given value of the mutation rate, and furthermore that there will be a sudden decline in the expectation for cure as the (total) cell number increases." Although the mutation rate cannot be decreased, treatment at the earliest possible indication has the effect of avoiding subsequent spontaneous mutations.

If the rates of cell proliferation and cell loss for both the drug-sensitive and -resistant cell subpopulations within a tumor may be considered constant, then the resistant fraction will remain the smaller unless and until the resistant fraction is *selected* and allowed to overgrow the drug-sensitive fraction. This selection is routinely achieved by drug treatment to develop experimental drug-resistant cell lines and is done unintentionally by drug treatment of animal and human cancers. Mathematical relationships derived by Lloyd (1977) and Skipper et al. (1978) have helped in the study of the variables that affect the rate of selection and overgrowth of drug-resistant tumor cell populations. An alternative method of selection involves cloning by dilution and transplantation. Differential drug sensitivities of sublines of tumors have been demonstrated both in vivo and in vitro (Barranco et al. 1972, Heppner et al. 1978).

Another type of drug resistance may result from natural barriers associated with tumor site and tumor growth characteristics. For example, there is the pharmacokinetic barrier that may occur due to poor vasculature in some areas of the tumor, disallowing the establishment of an effective product of drug concentration and time of maintenance of the minimal effective dose level (Cxt). Reports by Tannock and Steel (1969) and by Jirtle and Clifton (1971) suggest a relationship not only between tumor growth and vasculature but to chemotherapeutic responsiveness as well. Furthermore, it has been reported that some metastases preferentially take up greater concentrations of certain drugs than does the primary tumor and coincidentally have a greater sensitivity to those drugs (Donelli et al. 1977).

The growth kinetics of a tumor cell population may also lead to apparent drug resistance. Such resistance could occur in tumors in which some cells have unusually long cell-cycle times. Even if drug delivery were otherwise adequate to kill the cell, the long cell-cycle transit time might allow repair prior to division and cell death.

Finally, there is the anatomic barrier. It has been adequately documented in animals and man in the case of the blood-brain barrier, which precludes (except with special techniques) the delivery of effective concentrations of certain drugs to tumors of the brain.

There is another type of resistance, or perhaps it should be called drug insensitivity, that is not at all understood. Examples are those cancers of man, e.g., colorectal cancer and carcinoma of the pancreas, that respond poorly if at all to any currently known anticancer agents. Interestingly, a pancreatic carcinoma of mice developed by Corbett also has been shown to be unresponsive, or marginally responsive at best, to all the known classes of anticancer agents (unpublished data of Southern Research Institute).

The point is that resistance to drug treatment may have a variety of causes. Studies of differential sensitivities to drugs, however, have not been simple. Furthermore, proper interpretation of the results of some studies is made difficult by the occasional lack of *pure* drug-resistant cell lines (e.g., a mixed population of drug-sensitive and -resistant cells), the narrow range of effective concentrations (low therapeutic indices) of available drugs, poor ability to measure quantitatively the in vivo tumor cell killing effects of drugs, and the many biologic and therapeutic variables.

BIOLOGIC AND THERAPEUTIC VARIABLES

The drug effects that are seen in in vivo tumors are functions of the interaction of drug, tumor, and host. Proper interpretation of the results of tumor treatment can only be made if the variables that affect or result from these interactions are recognized. Since the interest here is in the potential drug resistance of metastatic tumor cell populations, it should be first understood that the cytotoxicity of drugs to spontaneously metastatic tumors is difficult to quantitate. Although there is a trend toward a direct relationship between the size of a primary tumor and the extent of metastasis within any group of animals bearing potentially metastasizing primary tumors, the extent of metastasis at any given time in a single animal correlates poorly with the size or age of the primary tumor. This poor correlation apparently results primarily from the variability of the time of metastasis, an observation that has been well documented (Schabel et al. 1979, Griswold et al. 1981) and is supported by the data in Table 1.

Similar variability may be observed in the relationship between drug and host. Robert et al. (1982) evaluated the correlation between the plasma clearance rate of Adriamycin (doxorubicin) and tumor response among a group of patients, and the two parameters varied widely from patient to patient. Although the study was somewhat compromised by the subsequent use of additional drugs, the results clearly show the pharmacokinetic variability from patient to patient. Variation in the ability of animals to metabolize or clear drugs may also be inferred from the data in Figure 1. Those results show the variability in lethality in groups of 10 mice treated with the same dose of the same drug at the same time, even though these hybrid mice were as nearly identical as possible (same strain, source, size, sex, and age).

Variability in the response of apparently similar tumors to a given drug has often been observed (Schabel et al. 1981) and may be expected on the basis of any of a number of proved or theoretical grounds. These would include differential uptake of drug by tumors (Donelli et al. 1977), differences in the ratios of drug-sensitive to drug-resistant cell populations from tumor to tumor (Skipper et al. 1978), and differences in the population kinetics of tumors (DeWys 1972).

Still another variable is the drug itself. Montgomery (1980) has shown that tumor responses can differ because of almost imperceptible differences in the physical state of CCNU. Differences in the formulation of a drug for administration might also be expected to produce differential effects on tumor and host.

In the tumor-drug-host relationship, it is evident that any number of variables,

TABLE 1. *Metastasis of Lewis lung carcinoma*

Group no.	Tumor wt. (mg) at surgery	Median day of death (dying only)	113th-day tumor-free survivors
1	1080–1930	29	6/12
2	1110–1830	31	5/10
3	1140–1580	31	2/11
4	1110–1510	29	7/10
5	1070–1820	31	1/10

BDFI (C57BL/6 × DBA/2) mice were implanted i.m. in the right back leg with 0.02 ml of a 20% w/v tumor brei prepared from pooled donor tumors. Mice were randomized to the five groups. The entire leg of each tumor-bearing mouse was surgically removed, from one-half the mice on day 7 and from the others on day 8, by one operator. These mice were again randomized. All mice were autopsied at death or sacrifice and grossly examined for evidence of metastasis. Additionally, lungs were preserved in formalin for subsequent microscopic examination.

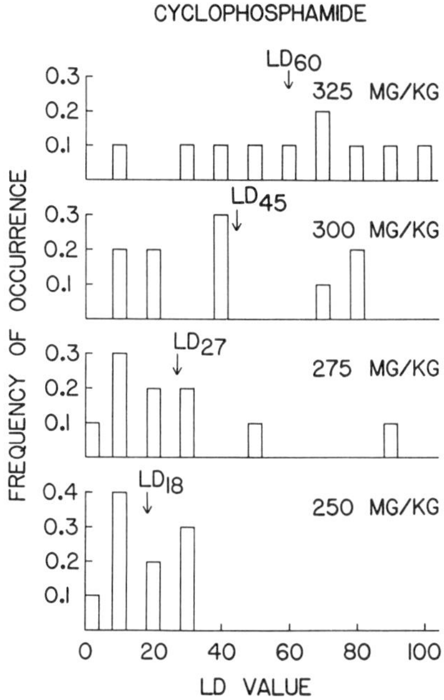

FIG. 1. Variable toxicity of cyclophosphamide in CDFI (BALB/c × DBA/2) mice. Female mice were implanted i.p. with 10^7 L1210 leukemia cells on day 0 and randomized into 10 cages of 10 mice each for a single i.p. treatment on day 1 with one of four doses of cyclophosphamide. Thus, 100 mice were treated with 325 mg/kg, another 100 with 275 mg/kg, etc. Drug-related deaths were based on the absence of leukemia determined by the absence of ascites and splenomegaly at autopsy.

often interrelated and compounded, may influence the outcome of drug treatment in both host and tumor. Schabel et al. (1981), reporting on the response to drug treatment of a variety of in vivo tumors, suggested that host variability was a major contributing factor in observed different tumor responses. They did not, however, discount the potential effect of tumor heterogeneity. Fisher and Saffer (1981), using bilateral implants of C3H mammary tumors, observed differential responses between two tumors in the same host following treatment with cyclophosphamide and *Corynebacterium parvum* and concluded that the differential effects observed were due to heterogeneity of the tumors. Nelson et al. (1982), also using bilateral implants, but of Ridgway osteogenic sarcoma, likewise found differential tumor responses to drug treatment. Not only did they observe different response patterns between two tumors in the same host, but they found differential tumor responses from mouse to mouse. These authors concluded that the observed differential tumor responses were due to both host and tumor factors, although host variability was apparently the major contributing factor.

Finally, consideration must be given to the pharmacokinetic characteristics of the drugs available for use today. The cell killing capability of cytotoxic agents is a function of the duration of exposure of target cells to an effective concentration. These drugs kill normal cells and tumor cells, although to different degrees. The differential, expressed as the therapeutic index, is unfortunately low for most, if not all, of the clinically effective cytotoxic agents available today. As a result, these drugs can be used only over a very narrow range of dosages, and the narrower the range, the greater is the chance for variable tumor response rates (Griswold et al. 1981). Aggressive, individualized drug treatment of patients with breast cancer has been reported to provide a highly significant correlation between drug-induced leukopenia and freedom from recurrence (Carpenter et al. 1982). Thus, it appears that some variability can be overcome and greater antitumor effect obtained if drug dose level is individualized by basing it on an observed toxicity end point.

CONCLUSION

It seems evident that variability of tumor response, including treatment failure, may result from any of the biologic and therapeutic variables discussed. These would include host differences, tumor heterogeneity, and the interaction of tumor, host, and drug. No single factor can be isolated as the only cause of treatment failure. However, one of the greatest remaining problems facing clinical oncologists in planning chemotherapy for metastatic cancer is the notable lack of chemotherapeutic agents with marked cytotoxic specificity. One of the striking differences between systemic chemotherapy for cancer and that for infectious diseases is that most antibacterial antibiotics have unusually large margins of safety. The differential cytotoxicity for infectious agents and normal tissue cell populations is sufficiently high that curative dosages may be given without fear of toxicity, and in the case of stubborn infections treatment can often be maintained for long periods. In spite of the fact that several chemical classes of chemotherapeutic agents have been developed, the identification or development of agents with marked cytotoxic specificity remains an elusive goal.

A further complicating problem in the treatment of metastatic cancer results from current diagnostic capability. With few exceptions (principally choriocarcinoma, Burkitt's lymphoma, and certain leukemias and lymphomas), the size of a metastatic tumor cell population that can be destroyed by chemotherapy is smaller than can be identified by conventional diagnostic techniques. The great promise of adjuvant immunotherapy or chemotherapy for metastatic cancer is based on the reduction of the total body burden of tumor stem cells by surgical removal or radiation reduction of detectable and accessible tumor masses, leaving a residual body burden within the curative potential of available chemo- or immunotherapy. Furthermore, recognition that most currently available cancer chemotherapeutic agents suppress immune responses further weakens the oncologist's approach since both primary and metastatic cancer can arise or recur from a small number of, and possible only one, surviving cancer cells that may not be controlled by natural immunity that is weakened or suppressed by cytotoxic chemotherapy.

In spite of the obstacles noted above, however, progress has been made in chemotherapy for metastatic cancer. This progress has resulted to a great extent from a better understanding of the mechanism of action of the various anticancer drugs, allowing improved agent selection and manipulation of dose regimens to take advantage of tumor and normal cell population characteristics.

Specifically, combination chemotherapy is now routinely employed to kill specific, drug-resistant tumor cells; to enhance cytotoxic specificity through overlapping sites of biochemical activity within the tumor cell; and to take advantage of cell population kinetic changes. A better understanding of the toxicology of these cytotoxic agents has provided a basis for selection of agents for use in combinations to avoid overlapping organ toxicities. And aggressive treatment with appropriate supportive care has been shown to be a feasible way to achieve and maintain effective serum and tissue levels of cytotoxic agents without lethal host toxicity. These and other therapeutic concepts, many of which have now become principles, have improved chemotherapy for metastatic cancer and, I hope, will lead to still greater progress in the future.

ACKNOWLEDGMENTS

Work from Southern Research Institute reported herein was supported by Contract NO1-CM9-7309 from the Division of Cancer Treatment, National Cancer Institute, Department of Health and Human Services.

REFERENCES

Barranco, S. C., B. Drewinko, D. Ho, R. M. Humphrey, and M. M. Romsdahl. 1972. Differential sensitivities of human melanoma cells grown in vitro to arabinosylcytosine. Cancer Res. 32:2733–2736.

Carpenter, J. T., Jr., W. A. Maddox, H. L. Laws, D. D. Wirtschafter, and S. J. Soong. 1982. Favorable factors in the adjuvant therapy of breast cancer. Cancer 50:18–23.

Donelli, M. G., T. Columbo, M. Broggini, and S. Garattini. 1977. Differential distribution of antitumor agents in primary and secondary tumors. Cancer Treat. Rep. 61:1319–1324.

DeWys, W. D. 1972. A quantitative model for the study of the growth and treatment of a tumor and its metastases with correlation between proliferative state and sensitivity to cyclophosphamide. Cancer Res. 32:367–373.

Fidler, I. J., and I. R. Hart. 1981. The origin of metastatic heterogeneity in tumors. Eur. J. Cancer 17:487–494.

Fisher, B., and E. A. Saffer. 1981. Heterogeneity of tumor growth during chemo-immunotherapy: Observations in a murine model, *in* Design of Models for Testing Cancer Therapeutic Agents, I. Fidler and R. White, eds. Van Nostrand Reinhold Co., New York, pp. 114–135.

Goldie, J. H., and A. J. Coldman. 1979. A mathematic model for relating the drug sensitivity of tumors to their spontaneous mutation rate. Cancer Treat. Rep. 63:1727–1733.

Griswold, D. P., Jr., T. H. Corbett, and F. M. Schabel, Jr. 1981. Pharmacology and development of new therapeutic agents, *in* Gastrointestinal Cancer, J. R. Stroehlein and M. M. Romsdahl, eds. Raven Press, New York, pp. 443–455.

Heppner, G. H., D. L. Dexter, T. DeNucci, F. R. Miller, and P. Calabresi. 1978. Heterogeneity in drug sensitivity among tumor cell subpopulations of a single mammary tumor. Cancer Res. 38:3758–3763.

Jirtle, R., and K. H. Clifton. 1971. On carcinoma growth and vascular supply: A study of mouse mammary tumor strain MTG-B. Proc. Soc. Exp. Biol. Med. 138:267–269.

Law, L. W. 1952. Origin of the resistance of leukemic cells to folic acid antagonists. Nature 159:628–629.

Lloyd, H. H. 1977. Application of tumor models toward the design of treatment schedules for cancer chemotherapy, *in* Growth Kinetics and Biochemical Regulation of Normal and Malignant Cells, B. Drewinko and R. M. Humphrey, eds. Williams & Wilkins Co., Baltimore, pp. 455–469.

Luria, S. E., and M. Delbrück. 1943. Mutations of bacteria from virus sensitivity to virus resistance. Genetics 28:421–511.

Montgomery, J. A. 1980. Cause of variability in activity of samples of CCNU against P388 leukemia in vivo. Cancer Treat. Rep. 64:987–988.

Nelson, J. A., J. A. Hokanson, and V. K. Jenkins. 1982. Role of the host in the variable chemotherapeutic response of advanced Ridgway osteogenic sarcoma. Cancer Chemother. Pharmacol. 9:148–155.

Robert, J., A. Illiadis, B. Hoerni, J-P Cano, M. Durand, and C. Lagarde. 1982. Pharmacokinetics of Adriamycin in patients with breast cancer: Correlation between pharmacokinetic parameters and clinical short-term response. Eur. J. Cancer Clin. Oncol. 18:739–745.

Schabel, F. M., Jr., D. P. Griswold, Jr., T. H. Corbett, W. R. Laster, Jr., D. J. Dykes, and W. C. Rose. 1979. Recent studies with surgical adjuvant chemotherapy or immunotherapy of metastatic solid tumors of mice, *in* Adjuvant Therapy of Cancer II, S. E. Jones and S. E. Salmon, eds. Grune & Stratton, Inc., New York, pp. 3–17.

Schabel, F. M., Jr., H. E. Skipper, M. W. Trader, W. R. Laster, Jr., T. H. Corbett, and D. P. Griswold, Jr. 1980. Concepts for controlling drug-resistant tumor cells, *in* Breast Cancer. Experimental and Clinical Aspects, H. T. Mouridsen and T. Palshof, eds. Pergamon Press, Oxford, pp. 199–211.

Schabel, F. M., Jr., D. P. Griswold, Jr., T. H. Corbett, W. R. Laster, Jr., H. H. Lloyd, and W. C. Rose. 1981. Variable responses of advanced solid tumors of mice to treatment with anticancer drugs, *in* Design of Models for Testing Cancer Therapeutic Agents, I. Fidler and R. White, eds. Van Nostrand Reinhold Co., New York, pp. 95–113.

Skipper, H. E., F. M. Schabel, Jr., and H. H. Lloyd. 1978. Experimental therapeutics and kinetics: Selection and overgrowth of specifically and permanently drug-resistant tumor cells. Semin. Hematol. 15:207–219.

Tannock, I. F., and G. G. Steel. 1969. Quantitative techniques for study of the anatomy and function of small blood vessels in tumors. JNCI 42:771–782.

Cancer Invasion and Metastasis: Biologic and Therapeutic Aspects edited by Garth L. Nicolson and Luka Milas. Raven Press, New York © 1984.

Chemotherapy for Metastatic Disease

Stephen K. Carter

Pharmaceutical Research and Development Division, Bristol-Myers Company, New York, New York 10022

The roles of cancer chemotherapy in the treatment of metastatic tumors are manifold (Carter et al. 1981) with the diversity being dependent on: (1) whether the target is macroscopic (clinically evident) disease or microscopic disease; (2) the site of the primary tumor from which the metastases arose; and (3) the clinical and pathologic stage of the disease at the time of treatment. The intent of treatment can be curative or palliative depending upon the three factors just elucidated. Chemotherapy can be administered as single-agent treatment, as combination chemotherapy, or within a combined modality setting with irradiation or surgery.

The choice of drugs for use against metastatic tumor is again exquisitely dependent upon the primary site of origin. Over the years, a data base has been established that links specific primary tumor types with drugs that have demonstrated reproducible clinical activity. This data base is far from complete and is replete with examples of differences of opinion among clinical investigators. Few, if any, of the commercially available anticancer agents have a data base for every type of malignancy for which treatment of metastatic disease would be indicated adequate to determine whether they are active or not.

The most successful chemotherapy of clinically evident metastatic disease has been combination chemotherapy (Carter and Livingston 1982). The choice of drugs to be included in a disease-specific combination regimen has generally followed some empirically developed guidelines: (1) the drugs should be active when used alone against the disease in question; (2) the drugs should have different postulated or known mechanisms of action; and (3) the drugs should not have overlapping toxicity patterns to the degree possible.

Since most drugs cause myelosuppression, the last aspect cannot be perfectly followed. This last aspect has made drugs that do not cause significant myelosuppression, e.g., vincristine and bleomycin, highly popular in combination regimens when even a hint of possible disease-specific activity can be found.

Activity against macroscopic metastatic disease is generally defined as some minimal rate of objective regression in a cohort of treated patients. An objective regression is either a complete or partial regression of measurable or evaluable tumor masses by criteria that are generally accepted in only a broad sense and open to wide variations in interpretation. The wide variation has led to a great lack of consistency in the chemotherapy literature and a major interpretive challenge for a busy clinican or clinical investigator.

A complete regression is defined as complete disappearance of all clinical evidence of metastatic disease. In essence, a patient in complete remission should be clinically indistinguishable from an individual without cancer. The validity of this determination is dependent upon how vigorous and complete is the search for residual metastatic disease. As a generalization, the harder the search the more that is uncovered. The vigor of the search is limited by the cost of the search to the patient in physical, psychosocial, and socioeconomic terms. In some diseases the definition of complete regression is subdivided into a clinical and pathologic variety. In ovarian cancer, a pathologic complete remission is defined as no residual disease in the abdomen after a second-look laparotomy. The morbidity, risks, and costs of the procedure are deemed justifiable because further therapy is determined by the procedure and the procedure itself may have therapeutic benefit, as any residual disease found is resected, if possible. Other tumors in which the concept of pathologic complete regression has gained credence are the malignant lymphomas and testicular cancer.

Partial regression is open to a much broader range of interpretations. The most generally accepted criterion is a 50% or greater shrinkage of the product of the two longest perpendicular diameters of a measurable lesion, lasting a minimum of 4 weeks, with no evidence of new tumor growth. Among the areas of interpretational variability with this criterion is how to handle multiple lesions that are either measurable or only evaluable in a less-specific sense. Areas of metastatic disease that do not lend themselves easily to measurement include bone metastases, hepatic metastases, central nervous system mestastases, and metastases to serosal surfaces that produce malignant effusions. Unfortunately, these are some of the most common areas for metastatic spread. If clinical trials are restricted to patients with only fully measurable lesions, perhaps only a minority of the total patient population will be treated and will therefore be potentially unrepresentative. This factor must be weighed against the greater potential reproducibility of the data that will result. If patients with poorly measurable or unevaluable lesions are used in clinical trials, then survival becomes the best criterion to use. The problem with using survival is that it is open to a range of influences besides the treatment under test, and a survival advantage is a more stringent criterion than an objective regression rate in 25% to 40% of patients treated. In addition, because of the various influences on survival, the use of the historical data base as a control is less defensible than it is with objective regression.

Another difficulty in interpreting partial response data is that some investigators allow the use of less stringent criteria than the greater than 50% shrinkage. These investigators will use stability of disease or a minor regression, of less than 50%, as a criterion. The less rigorous the criteria the higher the response rate, which is a major cause of the heterogeneity within the oncology literature.

It is common in medical oncology to accept a 20% partial regression as the minimum level for activity. On this basis, 5-fluorouracil is considered to be active in metastatic large bowel cancer and decarbazine (DTIC) is considered active in metastatic malignant melanoma. The value of this level of activity can be viewed in several ways: (1) will it achieve meaningful palliation of symptoms; (2) will it improve survival; and (3) will it elucidate a meaningful building block for combination approaches.

There is a growing body of evidence and opinion that drugs that just barely meet the 20% response rate activity level are not valuable by any of the above criteria. To the extent that this is true, there needs to be a reevaluation of how: (1) therapy is generally recommended; (2) drugs for combination chemotherapy and combined modality investigative studies are selected; and (3) the criteria within drug development programs are selected.

Chemotherapy can lead to prolonged disease-free survival in some percentage of patients with some stages of 11 different malignancies (see chapter appendix). For some of these, chemotherapy can eradicate all malignancy by itself in advanced stages when macroscopic metastatic disease is present. For the three pediatric solid tumors on the list, chemotherapy is used as an adjuvant to surgery or irradiation to eradicate microscopic metastatic disease after the local modalities have ablated the primary local and residual disease.

The hematological malignancies are among the most responsive to cancer chemotherapy. They are prominently included in the curative group of ten and, in the remaining group of tumors, e.g. adult acute leukemia, multiple myeloma, and the chronic leukemias, high response rates are observed. These hematologic malignancies are disseminated at the time of diagnosis and therefore the dichotomy of primary lesion and metastatic disease does not exist. In a semantic sense they can be viewed as metastatic at the time of diagnosis. Various explanations can be put forth as to why the hematologic malignancies are more responsive to drugs than are most of the so-called solid tumors.

1. The peak drug concentration achieved in the blood is the concentration to which the tumor cells in the blood are exposed.
2. Solid tumor masses many times consist of a core of hypoxic cells that are poorly perfused by drug concentrations adequate for effective cell kill.
3. Solid tumors, again to some degree because of their hypoxic compartment, contain a large number of cells not kinetically active (in the Go phase) and therefore are less responsive to chemotherapy.
4. In solid tumors, drugs attack metastatic cells that are likely to be genetically more unstable than primary malignancies and therefore have a greater probability of having developed a mutation toward drug resistance.
5. In hematologic malignancies drugs attack what is more the primary neoplasm, in a disseminated state, and therefore one more genetically stable than the selected population of cells of the established foci of metastatic disease from solid tumor primaries.

6. It is likely that the malignant state being treated by drugs in hematologic malignancies has been clinically evident in the host for a shorter period of time than the metastases from a primary solid tumor.

It is difficult to evaluate fully the impact of chemotherapy on survival when chemotherapy is not dramatically successful. The positive impact of chemotherapy on survival is easy to observe in tumors such as the leukemias, lymphomas, and testicular cancer when the older historical data base showed short survival and few patients were induced into complete remission. What is hard to gauge is the survival benefit from a 20% to 50% partial response rate, which is commonly reported for the majority of advanced solid tumors. Survival is influenced by a range of prognostic variables that also tend to be prognostic variables for response as well. These include performance status, extent of metastatic disease, prior therapy, nutritional status linked to weight loss, and comorbidity. It is often shown that responders live longer than nonresponders, the implication being that the therapeutically induced response is the sole cause. Since responders tend to have a better mix of positive prognostic variables for survival, it is more reasonable at best to assume that the therapy is only partially involved in the survival advantage over nonresponders. The clinical trial that is rarely performed is one that randomizes patients to therapy versus no therapy, properly stratified for important prognostic variables. It is my opinion that if such a trial were performed with regimens that result in only 15–30% partial response rates, no significant survival advantage to treatment would be demonstrated. It therefore would be reasonable to use these types of patients for phase II studies of new drugs or regimens without requiring prior exposure to so-called standard therapy.

Traditional pharmacokinetic studies are often performed with cancer drugs, but the value of the data obtained is not as obvious as it is with drugs of other classes. The peak blood level and concentration over time curve in the blood may not reflect what is critical to drug effectiveness, namely the concentration of the active moiety of the drug at the tumor cell level. The tissue pharmacology may be significantly different from what is observed in the plasma and not extrapolatable from the classic pharmacokinetic curves. While pharmacology studies are now routine in phase I trials, their influence in the more rational design of phase II studies is negligible at present. What is also forgotten is that pharmacology by itself cannot explain the therapeutic dilemma of partial responsiveness in a cohort of patients studied. The tissue pharmacology must interact with the tumor cell burden, the kinetics of the tumor cells exposed, and the mutations to drug resistance that have occurred in the population. Without that context, the evaluation of pharmacological data becomes an academic exercise best suited for publishing papers and satisfying the requirements of the regulatory agencies. Animal pharmacology and its value for human treatment design is even more difficult to evaluate.

Animal pharmacology can only be compared to human pharmacology within the comparative context of tumor burden, tumor kinetics, and intrinsic drug resistance in both animal and man. While these variables are feasibly measured in animals, they are not currently measurable in patients with deep-seated metastatic disease. This correlation is even more tenuous when the animal tumor evaluated is a primary tumor rather than the metastases since the metastases are almost always the drug target in man. For these reasons, the challenge of predicting whether new drug delivery systems, which enable easy continuous infusions, will be valuable is extremely difficult. That continuous infusions improve the therapeutic index, or fail to do so, in rodent tumor systems may not be relevant to the treatment of humans.

A new concept that is now receiving increased research interest is that drug-resistant neoplastic stem cells often arise from mutations and that the drug-resistant phenotype is inherited and propogated. In cell culture studies, three major mechanisms of genetic resistance have been delineated and characterized: (1) overproduction of the drug target (e.g. gene amplification); (2) reduced drug permeability; and (3) altered interaction of the drug with its target. The evidence in support of a genetic origin for a drug-resistant phenotype found in cell culture studies include: (1) the phenotype is stably inherited in the absence of selection; (2) it is spontaneously generated at a rate consistent with mutation rates in natural populations; (3) known mutagens can increase the frequency of appearance of resistant phenotypes; (4) an altered gene product can be demonstrated; (5) chromosomal localization of the determinant is associated with the drug-resistance trait; and (6) an altered gene can be demonstrated at the DNA level.

If within a given population of tumor cells mutation to resistance occurs spontaneously, then a fluctuation among subclonal populations is to be expected and will probably be large. Therefore, the ratio of variance compared with the mean number of resistant colonies will be large. A reasonable extrapolation is that the larger the population of cells the greater the proportion or frequency of mutants in each subclonal population will be. Eventually, it can be expected that some equilibrium level will occur. This will depend on the mutation rate, the relative growth rate of the mutants compared with the rest of the population, and the reversion rate.

It can be hypothesized that the evolution of a tumor results in genetic instability, which is the major cause of tumor cell heterogeneity. It is known that malignant neoplasms are heterogeneous in a range of critical factors such as metabolic patterns, growth rate, karyotypes, antigenicity, immunogenicity, susceptibility to cytotoxic drugs, and invasion and metastasis potential. There are many practical implications of this heterogeneity for the clinical cancer researcher (Table 1).

One of the important unanswered questions relates to the differences between the metastatic tumor cells and the cells residing within the primary neoplasm. It has been estimated that perhaps only 0.1% of the cells in a primary tumor will metastasize. In addition, the spontaneous metastases produced from a parent neoplasm are heterogeneous in growth rate, growth fraction, antigenicity, and

TABLE 1. *Practical implication of tumor heterogeneity*

Growth rate	Initial kinetic sensitivity to effective cytotoxic therapy followed by relative kinetic resistance.
Sensitivity	It is unlikely that a single agent will be effective equally against all tumor cells, either interactive with or independent of kinetics.
Metastatic potential	Studies on primary tumors may dilute the specific needed effects on the metastatic clones.
Differentiation	Probably (but not definitely) strongly interrelated to growth rate, sensitivity, and metastatic potential.
Antigenic components	It is unlikely that a single antibody would interact with all tumor cells, which has both therapeutic and diagnostic implications.
Tumor marker production	It is unlikely that a single marker (based on tumor cell production and a measurable material) will correlate with the total tumor cell burden.

sensitivity to drugs, as are the cells in the primary. It has been postulated that the cells populating metastases have a higher rate of spontaneous mutation than those populating the primary tumor. The possible reasons why metastases are genetically unstable include error-prone DNA replication, poor DNA repair mechanisms in the face of errors in DNA replication, and the production of a mutagenic factor by metastatic cells. Among the potential implications of the genetic instability of metastasis is the critically important one that experiments on primary tumors will not be relevant to metastasis, the target of clinical chemotherapy the great majority of the time.

Anticancer drug development is currently a balance between the search for new structures and the search for analogues with an improved therapeutic index in comparison to established active structures. The strategy for the clinical evaluation of new drugs needs to be elucidated in relationship to whether the compound is a new structure or an analogue. With an analogue, the major difference is that activity per se is not as critically important as it is with a new structure. With an analogue, activity superior to the parent structure is the essential factor. Therefore, the results with an analogue must always be viewed in direct comparison to the parent structure. On the other hand, for a new compound results need only be viewed against the broad historical data base for chemotherapy against specific malignancies.

While the pharmaceutical industry tends to view the evaluation of new drugs in predominantly drug-oriented terms, the clinical research establishment gives significant emphasis to a disease-oriented strategy that, at times, is in direct conflict with a drug-oriented strategy. This conflict begins to manifest itself in phase II studies but is most acute in phase III studies. The phase I protocol is clearly a drug-oriented study in which patients with a range of different diseases are studied. The phase II protocol, on the other hand, becomes a disease-oriented study in which the end result must be evaluated in terms of both drug and disease.

The success of cancer chemotherapy has made the clinical testing of new drugs more difficult. The best chance for observing responses to a new drug exists when the patients treated have had no prior exposure to cytotoxic drugs. This possibility is lost for tumors that are significantly responsive to chemotherapy and exists only for the more-resistant solid tumors. Therefore, a drug found to be active 20 years ago might not be discovered as being so today due to the change in the population available for phase II studies.

It is now well established that the response rate in any tumor to a given effective therapy is lower in patients who have received prior chemotherapy. This is due in significant part to the fact that patients who develop progressive disease after initial treatment have a more extensive tumor cell burden and, in general, have a poorer mix of prognostic response variables. Additional factors may include the development of partial resistance and a greater sensitivity of the bone marrow to myelosuppressive drugs.

In developing clinical trial strategies, it is of paramount importance to test new drugs in the most favorable patient populations consistent with the delivery of optimal care. These are predominantly patients in whom there has been no prior exposure to chemotherapy. New guidelines are required for the appropriateness of testing new drugs in previously untreated populations. This is particularly crucial for phase II studies. It is highly likely that some recent drugs failed to show effectiveness because of poor case selection and suboptimally designed phase II studies.

Still another problem for cytotoxic drug development are approaches that compete with cancer chemotherapy for drug development resources—biologic response modifiers, radiation sensitizers, radiation protectors, hyperthermia, and monoclonal antibodies. Each of these competitive approaches requires preclinical studies as well as extensive clinical trial resources. Any drug development program must wrestle with the determination of what is the optimal balance of resources appropriated for traditional cytotoxic drugs and these alternatives.

The noncytotoxic approach to cancer therapy is a current glamour stock in the cancer treatment arena. As with all glamour issues, it is currently being over-publicized as having a faster payoff than is realistic. The major thrust in the noncytotoxic approach falls under the rubric of biologic response modifiers (BRM). This broad term encompasses nonspecific immune modulators, interferons, thymic hormones, lymphokines, and redifferentiation drugs. Other noncytotoxic approaches that receive less current publicity include hormone therapy, radiation sensitizers and protectors, and antimetastatic drugs.

The BRM approach to cancer therapy should be viewed as a long-term development process with only a small probability of short-term success in terms of a marketable product. BRM have the following important characteristics that differ from cytotoxics and will make their development more difficult, time consuming, and expensive: (1) They are less likely to be patentable, defined chemical entities. (2) What may be patentable will be the process of making the material. (3) A clinically successful BRM will be more rapidly copied by another company for marketing. (4) BRMs do not have an empirical base or history of clinical success. (5) Since BRM will be unlikely to be able to shrink clinically evident metastatic disease, their value will have to be established as adjuvant therapy. Adjuvant trials require large numbers of patients and many years of follow-up before giving definitive results. (6) BRM trials will require laboratory correlates of their effectiveness, which will make the cost of trials significantly higher.

The concept of biologic response modification is based on the hypothesis that cancer elicits from the host a reaction which, if stimulated or modulated in some way, will be able to attack the neoplastic process. This reaction, in its natural state, has obviously been overwhelmed as evidenced by a clinically obvious cancerous process. The assumption in BRM therapy is that if this reaction can be boosted, the neoplasm will be attacked at a level of intensity to be of clinical benefit to the patient.

The majority of BRM approaches available today are spin-offs and dissections of the immunological approach to cancer therapy. The immunological approach assumes that tumor cells have antigens that elicit from the host an antibody response that can be stimulated or modulated in a way that destroys a significant number of cancer cells. It is now understood that cancer immunology is a much more complex problem than was previously thought. The following facts are now recognized: (1) tumor-specific antigens probably do not exist; at best, they are tumor-associated antigens; (2) tumors are heterogeneous and, therefore, their antigenic activity, to the extent that it exists, is also heterogeneous; and (3) the cellular and humoral response to tumor-associated antigens is a highly complex one with a mixture of helper, suppressor, and effector mechanisms interacting. With the above facts in mind, it is now easy to understand the massive failure of the past approach of nonspecific immune stimulation with materials such as BCG, *Corynebacterium parvum,* and levamisole. For the same reason, it is also unlikely that the newer approaches to nonspecific immune stimulation will be successful.

The interferons and thymic hormones must also be viewed as materials that are stimulating a mixture of responses that, at the current time, are still poorly understood. While appearing to be more specific than the crude vaccines of the past, their stimulation may come too early in the process and be so generalized as to lead to little therapeutic benefit. It is highly unlikely that interferons, by themselves, will have a positive therapeutic index for cancer patients.

Lymphokines, or cytokines, are biologic materials excreted by cells to mediate specific effects. The potential promise of lymphokines is that they will ultimately enable us dissect out the complex host response to cancer in such a way that beneficial responses can be specifically boosted in a pharmacologic way. This promise must be viewed as a relatively long-term one with small likelihood of immediate commercial success. Specific lymphokines are only now being identified and purified along with the development of reliable assays. Initially, these lymphokines are derived from cell preparations. With their purification, the next step has to be a genetically engineered approach to the production of large quantities. The recent breakthroughs in gene cloning finally enable us to think realistically of a specific lymphokine development activity. What still remains unknown is what lymphokine will specifically attack the neoplastic process in a therapeutic way. Several lymphokines have been isolated and purified and their biologic effects are being evaluated. To date, these effects appear to be predominantly immunological, and their specificity for cancer cells is undetermined.

REFERENCES

Carter, S. K., M. Bakowski, and K. Hellman. 1981. Chemotherapy of Cancer, 2nd Ed. John Wiley and Sons, New York, 379 pp.

Carter, S. K. and R. B. Livingston. 1982. Principles of Cancer Chemotherapy, *in* Principles of Cancer Treatment, S. K. Carter, E. Glatstein, and R. B. Livingston, eds. McGraw-Hill, New York, pp 95–111.

APPENDIX

The Varying Roles of Cancer Chemotherapy

TABLE 1. *Tumors in which chemotherapy used alone has a curative potential*

Tumor	Stage	Representative regimens	Comments
Acute lymphocytic leukemia	NA	Induction Vincristine + prednisone + daunorubicin CNS prophylaxis Intrathecal methotrexate ± craniospinal irradiation Maintenance Methotrexate and 6-mercaptopurine with periodic reinduction	Curative potential in children under age 15. Complete remission induction about 90% but long-term maintenance required.
Hodgkin's disease	III–IV	MOPP Nitrogen mustard Oncovin (vincristine) Procarbazine Prednisone	Complete remission induction 65–80%. Maintenance of no proved value. Important to pathologically restage.

continued

TABLE 1. (*Cont.*)

Tumor	Stage	Representative regimens	Comments
Diffuse histiocytic lymphomas	III–IV	CHOP Cyclophosphamide Doxorubicin Oncovin (vincristine) Prednisone *or* BACOP Bleomycin Doxorubicin Cyclophosphamide Oncovin Prednisone	Complete remission 50–60%. Maintenance of no proved value. Important to pathologically restage complete remissions.
Testicular carcinoma	III (disseminated disease)	PVB Cisplatin Vinblastine Bleomycin	Complete remission in about 75%. Can use surgery in patients with partial response to further induce complete remission. Long-term maintenance of no proved value. Data predominantly in nonseminomatous histologies.
Burkitt's tumor	IV	Cyclophosphamide	—
Uterine choriocarcinoma	Metastatic	Methotrexate *or* actinomycin D + methotrexate + alkylating agent	Single agents give 95% cure in low-risk patients, while combinations give 70–80% complete remission in high-risk patients.

TABLE 2. *Tumors in which chemotherapy increases the cure rates when used as adjuvant to surgery and/or X-ray therapy*

Tumor	Stage	Local control therapy	Representative regimens	Comments
Breast cancer	II	Surgery ± X-ray	CMF Cyclophos-phamide Methotrexate 5-Fluorouracil CMFVP Above 3 drugs + vincristine + prednisone	Data most persuasive for premenopausal women and suggestive for postmenopausal women.
Osteogenic sarcoma	Clinically localized	Radical amputation	High-dose methotrexate + vincristine ± doxorubicin	Data suggestive from historically controlled studies but not proved in prospective randomized studies.
Wilms' tumor	Local or regional spread	Surgery and X-ray	Actinomycin D ± vincristine	
Embryonal rhabdomyosarcoma	Local or regional spread	Surgery and X-ray	Cyclophosphamide + actinomycin D + vincristine	
Ewing's sarcoma	Localized disease	X-ray	Cyclophosphamide + vincristine ± actinomycin D	

TABLE 3. *Tumors in which chemotherapy can achieve complete remissions in more than one quarter of patients treated, with resultant significant prolongation of survival and occasional long-term disease-free survival*

Tumor	Representative Regimens	Comments
Small cell anaplastic lung cancer	Cyclophosphamide + doxorubicin + vincristine *or* Cyclophosphamide + doxorubicin + etoposide (VP-16) *or*	In limited disease, combination chemotherapy plus irradiation gives complete response in > 50% with 2-year disease-free survival of about 20%.

continued

TABLE 3. (*Cont.*)

Tumor	Representative Regimens	Comments
	POCC Procarbazine Oncovin Cyclophosphamide Lomustine (CCNU)	
Ovarian cancer	Doxorubicin + cyclophosphamide + cisplatin *or* Cisplatin + doxorubicin	High complete response rate in patients with minimal residual cancer after surgery. Cytoreductive surgery may be helpful. Pathologic determination of complete response with surgery indicates those with long-term survival benefit.
Nodular lymphomas	CVP Cyclophos-phamide Vincristine Prednisone *or* Chlorambucil *or* Cyclophosphamide	Aggressive chemotherapy may have curative potential in nodular mixed lymphomas. In nodular lymphocytic, conservative therapy with single agents may be preferable.
Acute nonlympho-cytic leukemia	Arabinosyl cytosine + either dauno-rubicin *or* Doxorubicin ± thioguanine *or* Vincristine+ prednisone	Complete remissions in more than half the patients treated. Bone marrow transplantation in remission may offer curative potential.

TABLE 4. *Tumors in which chemotherapy can give high response rates with survival prolongation and significant palliation*

Tumor	Representative regimens	Comments
Breast cancer	CMF ± VP Cyclophosphamide Methotrexate 5-Fluorouracil Vincristine Prednisone *or* Doxorubicin + cyclophosphamide ± 5-fluorouracil	Objective response rate in 50–70% of patients with complete responses in 10–20%.

continued

TABLE 4. (*Cont.*)

Tumor	Representative regimens	Comments
Multiple myeloma	Melphalan + prednisone ± vincristine cyclophosphamide *or* ± vincristine doxorubicin	Objective response rates in 50–60% of patients treated with median survival > 2 years.
Chronic lymphocytic leukemia	Chlorambucil + prednisone	High response rates in patients with active disease. In patients with indolent disease, supportive care is best.
Chronic myelocytic leukemia	Busulfan	Diminishment of leukemic cells observed in most patients. Median survival is about 3.3 years. Chemotherapy may not actually prolong survival but is significantly palliative.

TABLE 5. *Tumors in which chemotherapy achieves objective regression in 30–50% of patients treated with drugs for the first time*

Tumor	Representative regimens	Comments
Squamous cell carcinomas of head and neck	Cisplatin ± bleomycin *or* Methotrexate	Response rates nearly 50% with occasional complete response.
Soft tissue and bone sarcomas	Doxorubicin ± dacarbazine vincristine cyclophosphamide	Response rates close to 50% with complete response in 10–20%.
Gastric cancer	5-Fluorouracil + doxorubicin + mitomycin C	Response rates in about 40% of patients.
Transitional cell bladder cancer	Cisplatin ± adriamycin cyclophosphamide	Response rates in about 40% of patients.
Malignant gliomas	Carmustine (BCNU)	Response rates in about 30% of patients.
Adrenocortical carcinoma	Mitotane (Ortho para'DDD)	Response rates in about 30% of patients.
Uterine cervix carcinoma	Cisplatin	Preliminary evidence of response rates in 40% range.

continued

TABLE 5. (*Cont.*)

Tumor	Representative regimens	Comments
Islet cell tumors of the pancreas	Streptozotocin ± 5-fluorouracil	Objective response rates in about 50%. In functioning tumors, more than 50% have symptomatic improvement.
Prostate cancer	Doxorubicin *or* Cisplatin *or* Estramustine	Symptomatic improvement and stability of disease in nearly 50%. Actual objective response lower, but the majority of patients do not have measurable disease.
Neuroblastoma	Cyclophosphamide + vincristine ± dacarbazine + doxorubicin	Response in about 40% with 2 drugs. More aggressive combinations may give higher response rates.
Endometrial adenocarcinoma	Progestational agents	Response rates in about 30%.

TABLE 6. *Tumors in which chemotherapy gives response rates in only 10–25% of patients with minimal survival benefit*

Tumor	Comments
Non-oat cell carcinoma of the lung	Some combinations in adenocarcinoma give higher response rates, but survival benefit in large scale studies not yet shown.
Colorectal adenocarcinoma	5-Fluorouracil will give about 20% response rate.
Malignant melanoma	Dacarbazine will give about 20% response rate.
Pancreatic adenocarcinoma	5-Fluorouracil will give about 10–20% response rates. Some combinations give higher response rates in small series.
Renal cell carcinoma	Progestational agents give 0–15% response rates. No active drugs to date.
Esophageal cancer	Preliminary evidence that cisplatin may have activity. Further studies needed.

Cancer Invasion and Metastasis: Biologic and Therapeutic Aspects edited by Garth L. Nicolson and Luka Milas. Raven Press, New York © 1984.

The Role of Radiation Therapy in the Curative Treatment of Metastatic Disease

Lester J. Peters, Luka Milas, and Gilbert H. Fletcher

Division of Radiotherapy, The University of Texas M.D. Anderson Hospital and Tumor Institute at Houston, Houston, Texas 77030

The value of radiation therapy in the palliative treatment of symptomatic metastatic disease is generally well known and will not be reviewed in this paper. Rather, we will focus on the curative role of radiotherapy for metastases and possible ways in which this role might be expanded.

RADIOBIOLOGICAL PRINCIPLES

Energy deposition by irradiation is a random and discrete process, and to a first approximation cell survival is an exponential function of dose. Although single-dose radiation survival curves are characterized by an initial shoulder region representing the accumulation of reparable injury, the repetition of this shoulder with each dose in a fractionated treatment regimen effectively results in a simple exponential survival curve for a fractionated dose (Withers and Peters 1980). Factors other than repair of sublethal injury are important in determining response to fractionated treatment. However, provided these influences are in a dynamic equilibrium, a net exponential survival curve is maintained. Rigorous analysis of fractionated dose-response relationships for the stem cells of the intestinal crypts of the mouse is consistent with a simple exponential relationship, i.e., equal effect per fraction (Thames and Withers 1980).

If the same dose-response relationship applies to tumors, it follows that if the dose required for a certain cure probability of a given-size tumor is known, the dose required for the same probability of control of different-size foci of the same tumor can be estimated (Figure 1). Certain assumptions must be made for this type of calculation: e.g., that the growth fraction and percent of hypoxic cells either remain constant in tumors of different sizes, or that if, as is more likely, the growth fraction is higher and the percentage of hypoxic cells lower in smaller tumor foci, these influences counteract one another. In any case, clinical data, outlined below, support the general concept that subclinical disease is controllable with radiation doses substantially lower than those required for control of gross tumor aggregates and that the probability of control is related to the "density of infestation" of subclinical disease in the area to be treated (Fletcher 1983).

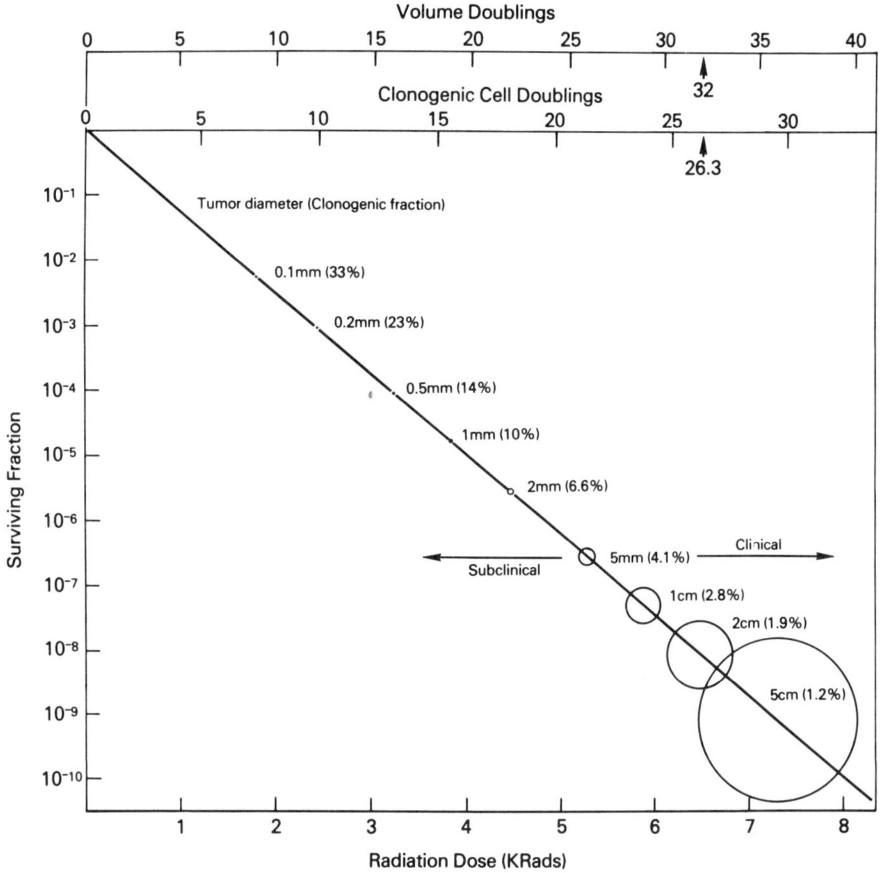

FIG. 1. Relationship between the fractionated radiation dose required for a given tumor control probability and tumor size or number of clonogenic cell doublings, assuming equal effect per fraction. (Reproduced from Withers and Peters 1980, with permission of Lea & Febiger.)

In addition to the tumor cell burden, the major factors influencing the ability of radiation to control metastatic disease are the sites of involvement (which dictate the total dose that can be given without producing unacceptable normal tissue injury) and the radiation sensitivity of the tumor. For example, while large cervical lymph node metastases from certain squamous carcinomas of the head and neck region are curable by radiotherapy because high doses can safely be given to the surrounding normal tissues, the same volume of metastatic cancer in the lung would be far beyond control by irradiation because of the dose limitation imposed by normal lung tolerance.

Only a few tumor types, such as Wilms' tumors, seminomas, and lymphomas, are responsive enough to ionizing radiation that gross pulmonary metastases can be controlled by doses within lung tolerance. The challenge for radiobiological research is to develop ways of increasing the therapeutic margins so that more tumor types fall into this category. At present, however, the main value of radiation therapy for metastatic disease lies in its ability to sterilize microscopic metastases of all histological types with doses lower than those required to control gross disease. This principle underlies the increasing integration of radiotherapy into combined modality therapy.

CLINICAL DATA

Radiation therapy has been shown to be effective in eradicating subclinical metastatic disease disseminated along all pathways of spread from a variety of primary sites. The following examples may be cited: regional lymphatic metastases, e.g. from head and neck and breast primary sites (Table 1) (Fletcher 1974); blood-borne metastases, e.g., to the brain from lung cancer (Cox et al. 1978); transcelomic metastases, e.g., peritoneal seeding by ovarian cancer (Dembo et al. 1979); subarachnoid metastases, e.g., from medulloblastoma (Bloom 1982); perineural spread, e.g., by adenoid cystic carcinoma (McNaney et al. 1983); spread along fascial planes, e.g., from soft tissue sarcomas (Lindberg et al. 1981); and surgical implants, e.g., from urothelial carcinoma (van der Werf-Messing et al. 1983).

Of particular interest in illustrating the radiobiological concepts involved are the results of the European Organization for Research and Treatment of Cancer trial to assess the value of elective lung irradiation following locally ablative therapy for osteogenic sarcoma (Breur et al. 1978). The susceptibility of the lungs to radiation injury limits the dose that can safely be given to about 20 Gy in 10 fractions over 2 weeks. This dose might be expected to control only very small metastatic foci, of perhaps no more than 0.1–0.2 mm in diameter (Figure 1). From an analysis of the time of appearance of overt lung metastases and their subsequent growth rate, Breur et al. (1978) estimated that approxi-

TABLE 1. *Percentage of eradication of expected occult infestation in the lymphatics of the neck as function of dose**

Adenocarcinoma of the breast		Squamous cell carcinoma of upper respiratory and digestive tracts	
Dose	Percent eradicated	Dose	Percent eradicated
3,000–3,500 rad (89 pts)	60–70	3,000–4,000 rad (50 pts)	60–70
4,000 rad (121 pts)	80–90		
5,000 rad (273) pts)	90	5,000 rad (356 pts)	90

* 1,000 rad per week, 5 days a week.
(Adapted from Fletcher 1974, with permission from Charles C. Thomas, Publishers.)

mately 25% of patients would have micrometastases in this size range at the time of primary tumor treatment. The results of the trial (which was most unfortunately terminated prematurely because of excessive enthusiasm for the chemotherapy of osteosarcoma) showed the prediction to be true, and a statistically significant improvement in both absolute and disease-free survival for patients under 17 receiving elective lung irradiation was demonstrated (Figure 2).

Combination with Surgery

Radiation may be combined with surgery either to treat different anatomical areas or for mutual reinforcement in the treatment of essentially the same areas. An example of the first application is the combination of definitive surgery for a primary cancer of the oral cavity with elective irradiation to the neck to obviate neck dissection. With respect to the second type of combination, surgical failures occur because not all microscopic disease is removed in many patients despite the most radical procedures; conversely, radiation failures are highest with gross tumor masses, the frequency increasing as the volume of cancer increases. Thus, the two modalities are complementary: surgery is used to remove gross tumor masses with limited margins and irradiation is delivered to eradicate microscopic extensions and regional metastatic foci. It is important to emphasize

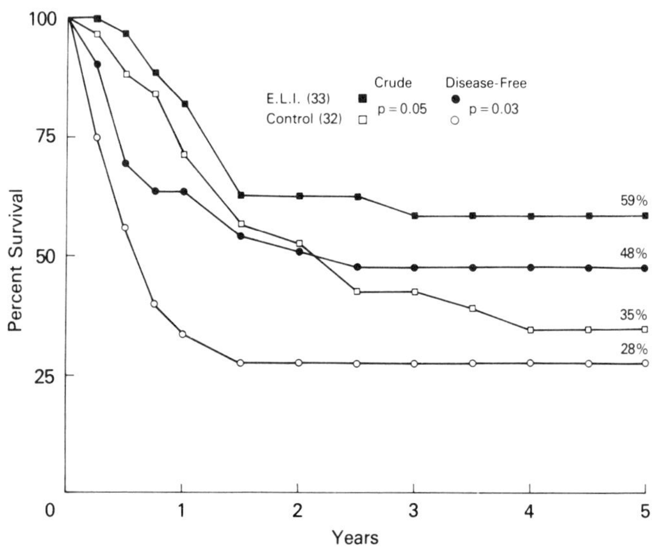

FIG. 2. EORTC osteosarcoma-O_2 trial. Crude and disease-free survival curves for patients under 17 years of age randomized to receive either elective lung irradiation (E.L.I.) or no further treatment after local therapy for osteosarcoma.

that all gross tumor must be excised for this approach to have any significant advantage. For example, "debulking" a tumor by removing 90% of its mass represents the equivalent of only a 1-log cell kill in radiation dose, and this may be more than offset by perturbation of the tumor bed and increased radioresistance resulting from tumor cell hypoxia (Figure 3). When these criteria are respected, exploiting the complementary roles of surgery and radiation therapy has permitted increasing use of function-preserving, nondisfiguring surgical techniques with equal, or improved, rates of tumor control (Fletcher 1979).

Combination with Chemotherapy

Radiotherapy has two important roles in combination with cytotoxic chemotherapy in the attempted cure of metastatic disease: treatment of sanctuary sites and "consolidation" of areas at highest risk of relapse.

The treatment of sanctuary sites is best illustrated by the success of radiotherapy in preventing central nervous system relapse in patients with acute leukemia (Simone et al. 1978) and lung cancer as discussed above.

The rationale for consolidation therapy is illustrated in Figure 4. If both gross and subclinical metastatic disease are treated with an effective cytotoxic drug to produce a complete regression of the measurable disease, it is logical

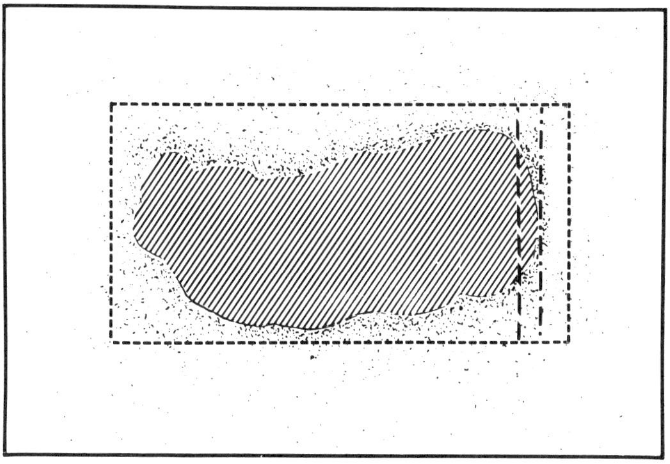

FIG. 3. Optimal exploitation of the complementary roles of surgery and radiotherapy requires that all gross disease be removed, with a clear margin. (Reproduced from Fletcher 1983, with permission of Harper & Row.)

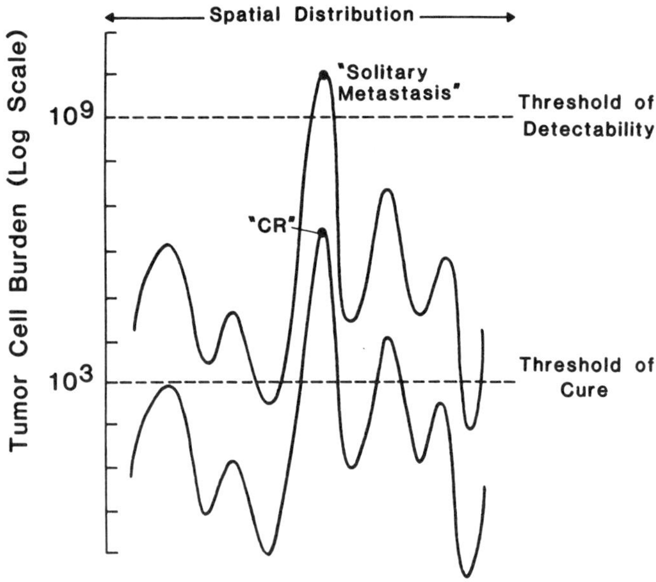

FIG. 4. The spatial distribution of cancer cells in the body of a hypothetical patient with a "solitary" clinical metastasis. Effective systemic therapy, capable of a 3-log cell kill, would produce a complete regression of the clinically detectable lesion and would sterilize foci of subclinical disease not larger than 3 logs above the cure threshold. If all subclinical disease were sterilized without local consolidation therapy, however, cure would be limited by relapse at the originally involved site. Even if, as in this example, all other sites were not sterilized, relapse would most likely occur first at the original site of overt metastasis.

to anticipate that if the treatment is noncurative, relapse will occur first at the originally involved sites. This was demonstrated clinically by Legha et al. (1979) in a study of patients with metastatic breast cancer treated by aggressive systemic therapy alone. Of 116 patients achieving a complete remission, 81 relapsed in 3–44 months, and 62 of these relapses (76.5%) included the original sites of overt metastatic disease.

The closer one approaches the threshold of curability with systemic therapy, the greater is the need to prevent this pattern of relapse with local consolidation therapy. This rationale underlies the treatment policies evolved at U.T. M. D. Anderson Hospital for the treatment of patients with apparently isolated metastatic breast cancer. These call for radiation therapy, with or without surgical excision of sites of clinically overt disease, either before aggressive chemotherapy or after it achieves complete regression. The most recent results of this study (Buzdar 1983) show that with a median follow-up of 73 months, only 20% of these patients have had relapses at the initial sites of involvement. Furthermore, the survival pattern of these patients is significantly improved over that of similar patients treated with systemic therapy alone. However, the fact that of the patients who did relapse 53% had local recurrences indicates that the consolidation therapy was not intensive enough. More aggressive local therapy is now being tested.

FUTURE PROSPECTS

Several experimental approaches aimed at extending the role of radiotherapy in the treatment of metastatic disease are the subject of ongoing laboratory and clinical research. We will confine our consideration to three of these areas of research.

Total Body Irradiation and Bone Marrow Transplantation

The success of bone marrow transplantation in the treatment of acute leukemia (Gale et al. 1982) has led to the hope that intensive marrow-ablating chemotherapy, together with total body irradiation, might be effective in eradicating disseminated disease from selected solid tumors. In this context, depending on the chemotherapy regimen used, the maximum dose of total body irradiation that can be given without a prohibitive incidence of interstitial pneumonitis is around 16 Gy in 8 fractions (Clift et al. 1982). For most epithelial tumors, this dose would be expected to achieve no more than a 2–3-log cell kill. However, it is conceivable that this level is sufficient to reach the threshold of cure in certain circumstances, depending on the initial tumor cell burden and the efficacy of the cytotoxic chemotherapy available. As discussed above, any sites of overt metastatic disease should receive boosts of local irradiation in addition to systemic therapy. To avoid impairing marrow engraftment, this boost therapy should be given prior to total body irradiation.

Targeted Radionuclide Therapy

^{131}I has long been established as effective treatment for differentiated thyroid cancers that have a natural avidity for the isotope, resulting in selective concentration of the radiation dose in the metastatic lesions. Unfortunately, no other types of cancers are sufficiently selective in their natural uptake of a specific element for this approach to be used. However, the raising of antibodies to tumor surface markers or secretion products offers the possibility of using such antibodies to target cytotoxic radionuclides selectively to tumor cells of all types. For this purpose, it is not necessary for the antibody to have any cytolytic activities, but the antigenic determinant must be in sufficient concentration on the tumor cell surface and the antigen-antibody complex sufficiently stable to achieve a satisfactory radiation dose to the tumor cells. Preliminary work by Order et al. (1981) has shown that in selected cases of hepatoma, these conditions can be met with polyclonal antiferritin antibodies. Whether this approach will find more general applicability to the treatment of metastatic disease is at present uncertain.

Radioprotectors

The compound WR-2721 (S-2- (3 aminopropylamino)-ethylphosphorothioic acid) is a radioprotective drug currently undergoing laboratory and preliminary clinical evaluation. The WR-2721 protects all normal tissues (with the exception of the central nervous system) to a varying degree (Yuhas and Spellman 1980) by scavenging free radicals or depleting intracellular oxygen (Durand 1983). Protection of solid experimental tumors, however, is generally less efficient, possibly because of poor drug access to tumors, deficient active transport mechanisms in tumor cell membranes, or severe intratumoral hypoxia. This preferential protection of normal tissues offers the prospect of achieving a therapeutic gain clinically by the delivery of higher effective tumor doses.

With regard to the treatment of metastatic disease, we have recently reported that the degree of protection afforded to tumors of the same type is greater for microaggregates than for larger cell masses (Milas et al. 1983). For example WR-2721 protected 4-day-old lung micrometastases of a murine fibrosarcoma against both single and fractionated irradiation (with dose fractions in the clinical range) by factors of 1.26 and 1.19 respectively (Figure 5). By comparison, protection against death from radiation pneumonitis or from late lung fibrosis after single doses of radiation was by factors of 1.34 and 1.50, respectively. The fact that the protection factors for tumor sterilization and lethal pneumonitis are not significantly different would appear to exclude any advantage from the use of WR-2721 in the treatment of occult lung metastases of this tumor.

However, it is too simplistic merely to compare protection factors in assessing a therapeutic ratio. What must be considered is the absolute dose required for

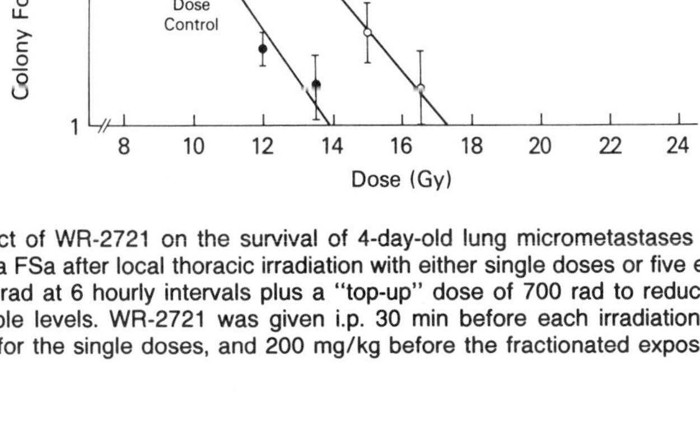

FIG. 5. Effect of WR-2721 on the survival of 4-day-old lung micrometastases of the murine fibrosarcoma FSa after local thoracic irradiation with either single doses or five equal fractions of 180–340 rad at 6 hourly intervals plus a "top-up" dose of 700 rad to reduce cell survival to measurable levels. WR-2721 was given i.p. 30 min before each irradiation at a dose of 400 mg/kg for the single doses, and 200 mg/kg before the fractionated exposures.

TABLE 2. *Effect of WR-2721 on LD_{50} values for mice following single dose whole-lung irradiation*

WR-2721*	Pneumonitis (95% confidence limits) (Rad)	Lung fibrosis (95% confidence limits) (Rad)
+	1650 (1610–1680)	1600 ± (1550–1650)
–	1225 (1200–1250)	1010 ± (960–1060)

* 400 mg/kg i.p. 30 min. before irradiation.
(From Travis, E. L., unpublished data.)

tumor sterilization in relation to dose-limiting normal tissue toxicity with and without the protector. In the case of the lung, the LD_{50} values for penumonitis and lung fibrosis are set out in Table 2. These data show that lung fibrosis is the dose-limiting normal tissue toxicity, and that the absolute dose tolerated by the lung is considerably increased by the use of WR-2721. Conversely, for tumor sterilization, although microaggregates of tumor cells are better protected than large tumors masses, the latter nonetheless require higher absolute doses for their eradication because of the larger number of tumor clonogens to be eliminated. Thus, provided the same degree of protection against lung fibrosis after fractionated irradiation is maintained with WR-2721, there may well be a therapeutic advantage in its use in elective treatment of occult metastatic lung disease.

CONCLUSIONS

From this brief review, it is apparent that radiation therapy does have an important role in the curative treatment of metastatic disease. We predict that this role will increase as more effective use of combined modality treatment evolves and as experimental techniques to increase the effective dose of radiation that can be safely delivered to metastatic foci are developed.

ACKNOWLEDGMENTS

This investigation was supported in part by grants CA06294 and CA16672 from the National Cancer Institute, Department of Health and Human Services.

REFERENCES

Bloom, H. J. G. 1982. Medulloblastoma in children: Increasing survival rates and further prospects. (Editorial) Int. J. Radiat. Oncol. Biol. Phys. 8:2023–2027.

Breur, K., P. Cohen, O. Schweisguth, and A. M. M. Hart. 1978. Irradiation of the lungs as an adjuvant therapy in the treatment of osteosarcoma of the limbs: An E.O.R.T.C. randomized study. Eur. J. Cancer 14:461–471.

Buzdar, A. U. 1983. Combined modality approach in breast cancer with isolated or multiple metastases. Clin. Oncol. (in press).

Clift, R. A., C. D. Buckner, E. D. Thomas, J. E. Sanders, P. S. Stewart, K. M. Sullivan, R. McGuffin, J. Hersman, G. E. Sale, and R. Strob. 1982. Allogeneic marrow transplantation using fractionated total body irradiation in patients with acute lymphoblastic leukemia in relapse. Leukemia Res. 6:401–407.

Cox, J. D., Z. Petrovich, C. Paig, and K. Stanley. 1978. Prophylactic cranial irradiation in patients with inoperable carcinoma of the lung. Cancer 42:1135–1140.

Dembo, A. J., J. Van Dyk, B. Japp, H. A. Bean, F. A. Beale, J. F. Pringle, and R. S. Bush. 1979. Irradiation by a moving-strip technique for patients with ovarian cancer. Int. J. Radiat. Oncol. Biol. Phys. 5:1933–1942.

Durand, R. E. 1983. Radioprotection by WR-2721 in vitro at low oxygen tensions: Implications for its mechanisms of action. Br. J. Cancer 47:387–392.

Fletcher, G. H. 1974. Clinical dose response curve of subclinical aggregates of epithelial cells and its practical application in the management of human cancer, *in* Biological and Clinical Basis of Radiosensitivity, M. Friedman, ed. Charles C Thomas, Springfield, Illinois, pp. 485–501.

Fletcher, G. H. 1979. Combination of irradiation and surgery. Int. Adv. Surg. Oncol. 2:55–98.

Fletcher, G. H. 1983. Combined treatment, *in* Modern Radiation Oncology, Classic Literature and Current Management, Vol. II, H. A. Gilbert, ed. Harper & Row Publishers, Hagerstown, Maryland (in press).

Gale, R. P., H. E. M. Kay, A. A. Rimm, and M. M. Bortin. 1982. Bone marrow transplantation for acute leukemia in first remission. Lancet 2:1006–1008.

Legha, S. S., A. U. Buzdar, T. L. Smith, G. N. Hortobagyi, K. D. Swenerton, G. R. Blumenschein, E. A. Gehan, G. P. Bodey, and E. J Freireich. 1979. Complete remissions in metastatic breast cancer treated with combination drug therapy. Ann. Intern. Med. 91:847–852.

Lindberg, R. D., R. G. Martin, M. M. Romsdahl, and H. T. Barkley, Jr. 1981. Conservative surgery and postoperative radiotherapy in 300 adults with soft tissue sarcomas. Cancer 47:2391–2397.

McNaney, D., M. D. McNeese, O. M. Guillamondegui, G. H. Fletcher, and M. J. Oswald. 1983. Postoperative irradiation in malignant epithelial tumors of the parotid. Int. J. Radiat. Oncol. Biol. Phys. (in press).

Milas, L., N. Hunter, H. Ito, E. L. Travis, and L. J. Peters. 1983. Factors influencing radioprotection of tumors by WR-2721, *in* Radioprotectors and Anticarcinogens, O. F. Nygaard and M. Simic, eds. Academic Press, New York, pp. 695–718.

Order, S. E., J. L. Lein, and P. K. Leichner. 1981. Antiferritin IgG antibody for isotopic cancer therapy. Oncology 38:154–160.

Simone, J. V., J. A. Aur, H. O. Hustu, M. S. Verzosa, and D. Pinkel. 1978. Three to ten years after cessation of therapy in children with leukemia. Cancer 42 (suppl):839–844.

Thames, H. D., Jr., and H. R. Withers. 1980. Tests of equal effect per fraction and estimation of clonogen number in microcolony assays of survival after fractionated irradiation. Br. J. Radiol. 53:1071–1077.

van der Werf-Messing, B., R. S. Menon, and W. C. J. Hop. 1983. Carcinoma of the urinary bladder category $T_3N_xM_0$ treated by the combination of radium implant and external irradiation: Second report. Int J. Radiat. Oncol. Biol. Phys. 9:177–180.

Withers, H. R., and L. J. Peters. 1980. Biologic aspect of radiation therapy, *in* Textbook of Radiotherapy, Ed. 3, G. H. Fletcher, ed. Lea & Febiger, Philadelphia, pp. 103–181.

Yuhas, J. M., and C. F. Spellman. 1980. The role of WR2721 in radiotherapy and/or chemotherapy. Cancer Clin. Trials 3:211–216.

Cancer Invasion and Metastasis: Biologic and Therapeutic Aspects edited by Garth L. Nicolson and Luka Milas. Raven Press, New York © 1984.

The Generation of Tumoricidal Activity in Macrophages for the Treatment of Established Metastases

Isaiah J. Fidler

Cancer Metastasis and Treatment Laboratory, NCI-Frederick Cancer Research Facility, Frederick, Maryland 21701

Metastasis—the spread of malignant tumor cells from a primary site to other parts of the body where they multiply to form new growths—is a major cause of death from cancer. Treatment of metastases poses formidable problems to clinical oncologists. By the time many cancers are diagnosed, metastases are already present in many organs of the patient's body, making surgical removal or destruction by radiation or drugs impossible. Exacerbating the problem of treating metastatic disease is the fact that cancer cells in different metastases, and in some cases, even different regions within an individual metastatic tumor, may respond entirely differently to treatment. Although promising anticancer drugs have been developed, their effectiveness is still hindered by the all-too-common presence of drug-resistant cells within tumors. Tumor cell resistance to conventional therapeutic modalities is the single most important reason for the lack of success in treating many types of solid neoplasms. A tumor mass at the lower limit of clinical detection may reach a size of 1 cm^3. This size tumor could well contain up to a billion cells. Even the destruction of 99.9% of these cells would still leave a million cells to proliferate and kill the host (Fidler and Hart 1982).

Pathologists have been aware for years that malignant neoplasms are pleomorphic, i.e., their morphology is heterogeneous. Recent studies suggest that cells obtained from human and animal neoplasms exhibit an almost endless diversity with regard to growth rate, antigenic or immunogenic properties, membrane receptors, ability to invade and metastasize, and response to a variety of cytotoxic agents (reviews, Poste and Fidler 1980; Hart and Fidler 1981). The complex nature of the pathogenesis of cancer metastasis has been discussed in detail elsewhere in this volume (Fidler 1984, see pages 5–26). Suffice it to say that the development of secondary tumor growths is dependent on an interplay between host factors and intrinsic characteristics of the metastatic cells. The process is highly selective, and metastases represent the end point of several highly lethal events that few cells survive. The demonstrations that metastases result from the nonrandom proliferation of specialized subpopulations of cells that preexist within the primary tumor (Fidler and Kripke 1977), that metastases can be clonal in their origin, and that different metastases can originate from different progenitor cells (Talmadge et al. 1982) provide explanations for the clinical observations that the response to cancer therapy can vary greatly among different metastases. The implication of the varied responses of tumor cells to chemotherapy and other treatment modalities is that, to be successful, therapy for disseminated metastases will have to circumvent the problems of biological heterogeneity and the development of resistance by tumor cells.

In this chapter, I shall present some of the evidence to support the hypothesis that macrophages activated to the tumoricidal state can fulfill these demanding tasks. In addition, I shall summarize work from our laboratory and many others dealing with methods to achieve the in vivo activation of macrophages.

RECOGNITION AND DESTRUCTION OF TUMORIGENIC CELLS BY ACTIVATED MACROPHAGES

Macrophages can be activated to become tumoricidal by two major pathways: (1) by direct interaction with parasites, microorganisms, and cell wall components isolated from these organisms (Hibbs 1974a, Russell and McIntosh 1977, Chedid et al. 1979, Lederer 1980), and (2) by an indirect mechanism involving a lymphokine, called macrophage-activating factor (MAF). that is released from antigen-sensitized and mitogen-stimulated lymphocytes. MAF first binds to a macrophage surface receptor and then is internalized to elicit tumoricidal properties in the macrophages (Fidler and Raz 1981).

Regardless of the method of their activation, rodent and human tumoricidal macrophages acquire the ability to recognize and destroy neoplastic cells both in vitro and in vivo while leaving nonneoplastic cells unharmed. The mechanism for this selective cytotoxicity is not known, but appears to be nonimmunological in nature and to require intimate cell-to-cell contact (Hibbs 1974b, Bucana et al. 1976, Marino and Adams 1980a,b) (Figure 1). The results of investigations in diverse mammalian systems suggest that macrophage-mediated cytolysis of tumor cells occurs independently of such tumor cell characteristics as metastatic potential, antigenicity and immunogenicity, and drug sensitivity (review, Fidler and Poste 1982). For example, regardless of whether murine melanoma lines are nonmetastatic or metastatic, resistant or susceptible to T-cell-mediated lysis, or resistant or susceptible to natural killer (NK)-cell-mediated lysis, they are all lysed by tumoricidal macrophages. Even more important, tumoricidal macrophages can lyse in vitro both drug-sensitive and drug-resistant tumor cells (Fidler 1978, Fidler and Poste 1982).

The major limitations of many cancer therapies are their lack of selectivity and their toxicity. The ability of tumoricidal macrophages to distinguish tumorigenic from normal cells presents an attractive possibility for treatment of disseminated cancer. Because most studies on the interaction of macrophages with

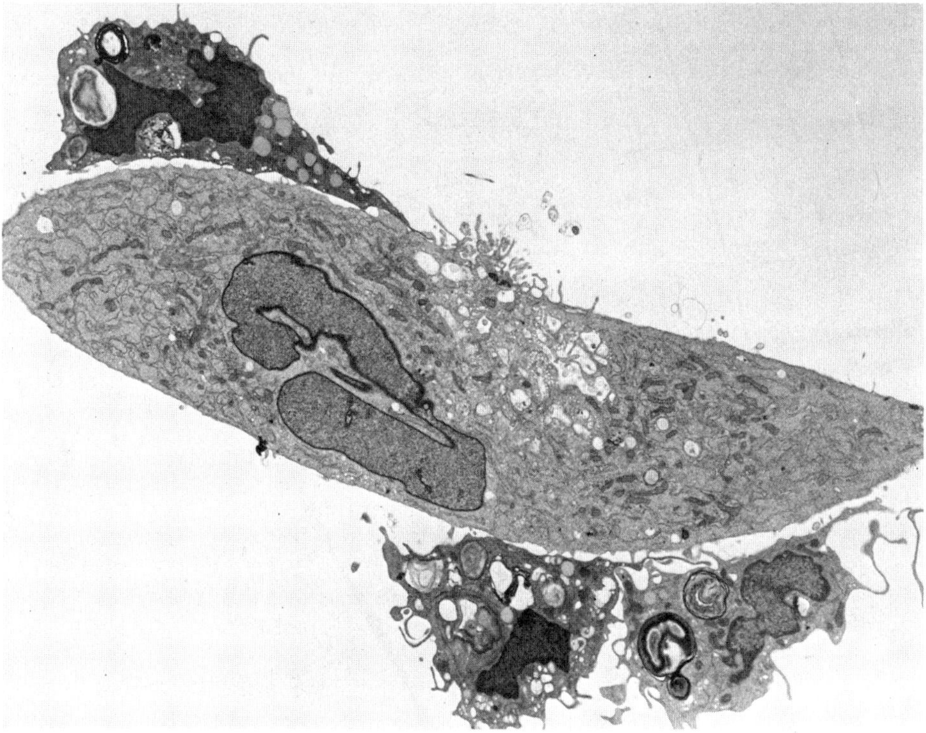

FIG. 1. The interaction of human blood monocytes activated by liposomes containing muramyl dipeptide with human melanoma target cell (× 3,400).

tumor cells have been carried out in rodent systems using individual cultures of tumorigenic or nontumorigenic cells, we recently examined whether human blood monocytes that had been activated to the tumoricidal state by their interaction with liposomes containing MAF (see below) could also discriminate in vitro between tumorigenic and nontumorigenic human target cells under cocultivation conditions, which are more relevant to the situation encountered in vivo. Highly homogeneous preparations of peripheral blood monocytes isolated from normal human donors were activated in vitro by incubation with human MAF encapsulated within multilamellar liposomes. The cytotoxic properties of these monocytes against several tumorigenic and nontumorigenic allogeneic targets were assessed by an in vitro radioisotope-release assay. Various combinations of three tumorigenic and three nontumorigenic targets labeled with either [^{3}H]thymidine or [^{14}C]thymidine were mixed and plated onto monolayers of blood monocytes. Three days later, macrophage-mediated lysis was determined. Assay results of representative mixtures of target cells are shown in Table 1. At any combination used, activated monocytes specifically lysed allogeneic neoplastic cells but not allogeneic nontumorigenic cells. In contrast, mitogen-stimu-

TABLE 1. *Selective cytotoxicity mediated by activated human blood monocytes against allogeneic tumorigenic cells cocultivated with allogeneic nontumorigenic targets**

Target cells labeled with [^{3}H]thymidine (%)	Target cells labeled with [^{14}C]thymidine (%)	Target cells labeled with [^{3}H]thymidine (%)	Target cells labeled with [^{14}C]thymidine (%)
A375 melanoma (58)	Skin cells (0)	Lung cells (−1)	NAT-glioblastoma (41)
Skin cells (1)	A375 melanoma (33)	Lung cells (−2)	Kidney cells (0)
HT-24 carcinoma (44)	Kidney cells (−1)	A375 melanoma (48)	HT-29 carcinoma (39)
Kidney cells (0)	HT-29 carcinoma (46)	A375 melanoma (48)	NAT-glioblastoma (47)
NAT-glioblastoma (38)	Lung cells (0)		

* In these experiments target cells were cultured alone, with monocytes incubated with liposomes containing medium, or with liposomes containing MAF. Control monocytes were not cytotoxic against any of the targets. The number in parentheses is percentage of target cell lysis as compared with control monocytes and target cells ($P < 0.001$).

lated human peripheral blood mononuclear cells killed both tumorigenic and nontumorigenic targets (Kleinerman et al. 1983).

Taken together, the data generated in rodent and human systems indicate that, at least in vitro, tumoricidal macrophages can discriminate between neoplastic and nonneoplastic cells by a process independent of transplantation antigens, species-specific antigens, tumor-specific antigens, cell cycle time, or various phenotypes associated with transformation. Again, although the exact mechanism by which macrophages recognize and lyse tumor cells is still unclear, it is probably regulated by a tumor cell characteristic that is linked with the tumorigenic capacity of tumor cells (Fidler et al. 1978).

ATTEMPTS TO SELECT TUMOR CELL VARIANTS RESISTANT TO MACROPHAGE-MEDIATED LYSIS

The second criterion that a successful approach for treatment of metastases must fulfill is that it avoid the problem of cellular resistance. We therefore set out to determine whether macrophage-resistant tumor cell variants could emerge under severe selection pressures. We used an in vitro selection technique that had been developed by our laboratory and used successfully to isolate tumor cells resistant to killing by syngeneic lymphocytes (Fidler et al. 1976) or NK cells (Hanna and Fidler 1981). Cells from eight different murine tumor cell lines were incubated with tumoricidal macrophages for 3–4 days. After this incubation, the cultures were washed twice to remove nonadherent tumor cells. The remaining viable tumor cells were recovered by trypsinization of the monolayer for 3–5 min. Viable tumor cells were replated onto fresh culture and allowed to grow to provide target cells for the next selection cycle. The cultures of surviving tumor cells were also frozen. The selection cycle was repeated six times. All frozen cultures were recovered simultaneously, grown in culture, and labeled with [^{125}I]iododeoxyuridine. The susceptibility of the parent tumor (starting population) and the six selected lines (lines that survived the successive interactions with murine tumoricidal macrophages) to macrophage-mediated lysis was determined in two independent assays. Regardless of the tumor system used, the results were strikingly similar. The data from one representative experiment are summarized in Table 2 and clearly demonstrate that we failed to select tumor cells with increased resistance to macrophage-mediated lysis. This failure was observed in both highly antigenic and moderately antigenic tumors and could not be attributed to the heterogeneous nature of the parent tumor. These types of studies suggest that the development of tumor cell resistance to destruction by macrophages, if it occurs, is not a common event. Thus, treatment with activated tumoricidal macrophages is likely to circumvent the problem of treatment-resistant metastatic lesions.

HOMING OF MACROPHAGES TO METASTASES

Many primary neoplasms are infiltrated by macrophages, but the exact role of these macrophages has been controversial. In rats, the macrophage content

TABLE 2. *Macrophage-mediated lysis of cells from parent neoplasms and variants exposed to successive selection cycles*

	% Macrophage-mediated cytotoxicity against							
Source of cells	K-1735	SR-149	UV-1422	UV-1316	UV-1591	UV-2240	UV-2237	Osteo-J
Parent tumor (starting population)	70	93	58	68	69	63	89	87
Variant 1	81	75	66	73	84	45	85	88
Variant 2	87	90	62	67	54	50	58	91
Variant 3	74	85	65	70	75	48	84	80
Variant 4	63	75	63	78	81	53	87	87
Variant 5	75	84	58	71	71	50	83	87
Variant 6	73	87	59	N.D.	76	54	75	N.D.

of several carcinogen-induced fibrosarcomas correlated directly with their immunogenicity and inversely with their metastatic potential (Eccles and Alexander 1974a,b, Eccles 1978), suggesting that some tumors do not produce metastases because they contain a large number of macrophages (Alexander et al. 1976).

This correlation is not the usual case. We examined the macrophage content of 16 different rodent tumors and did not find a correlation between the extent of macrophage infiltration into neoplasms and the metastatic behavior of these tumors (Talmadge et al. 1981). Moreover, in our study and in those of Evans and Lawler (1980) and Evans and Eidlen (1981), who examined the macrophage content of 33 different methylcholanthrene-induced murine fibrosarcomas and rhabdomyosarcomas, no relationship between macrophage content and the immunogenicity of the tumors was observed. More recently, we examined the macrophage content of three different spontaneously occurring mouse lymph node and lung metastasis systems to determine whether the lesions represent selected tumor populations that are not infiltrated by macrophages to the same extent as their parent tumors. All lung and lymph node metastases in the three different tumor systems contained macrophages. Some metastases had fewer and others had the same or even more infiltrating macrophages than their parent tumors, suggesting that the survival and growth of metastases are unlikely to be contingent on the absence of infiltrating macrophages (Key et al. 1982a).

In several experimental systems, progressively growing tumors are accompanied by suppression of the migration or chemotactic response of macrophages from the peritoneal cavity or the site of tumor growth (Bernstein et al. 1972, Eccles and Alexander 1974b, Snyderman et al. 1976). For this reason, we examined whether the presence of progressively growing pulmonary metastases influences the number and function of alveolar macrophages. Female F344 rats were given i.v. injections of cells from a metastatic variant line of the syngeneic mammary adenocarcinoma. Normal and metastasis-bearing rats were also given i.v. injections of *Nocardia rubra* cell wall skeleton to determine whether the presence of large pulmonary metastases would interfere with the activation of alveolar macrophages in situ. At days 7, 14, 21, and 28 after injection, normal and tumor-bearing animals were killed, and their alveolar macrophages harvested by lavage. The functional integrity of the macrophages was determined by their capacity to phagocytose opsonized erythrocytes and by their ability to respond to a variety of activating agents in vitro.

The data in Table 3 clearly demonstrate that the presence of progressively growing lesions in the lung led to a slight increase in the number of macrophages harvested and that these macrophages from tumor-bearing rats were as phagocytic as those obtained from normal rats. Most important, macrophages harvested from rats with metastases became tumoricidal against syngeneic tumor target cells in response to activation stimuli in vitro and in vivo. Therefore, at least in this tumor system, the presence of progressively growing lung metastases does not suppress the number or function of alveolar macrophages. The use of agents known to activate macrophages could, therefore, be of benefit in the therapy for pulmonary metastases (Sone and Fidler 1981a).

TABLE 3. *In situ activation of tumoricidal properties of alveolar macrophages in normal and metastasis-bearing rats following the i.v. injection of a preparation of* Nocardia *cell wall skeleton (N-CWS)*

Days after establishment of lung metastases	Donor rats (n = 3)	% Macrophage-mediated cytotoxicity None	Placebo (300 μg/rat)	N-CWS (300 μg/rat)
7	Normal	0	0	80
	Tumor bearing	0	0	76
14	Normal	0	0	65
	Tumor bearing	0	2	70
21	Normal	0	0	54
	Tumor bearing	2	4	45
28	Normal	0	0	55
	Tumor bearing	0	0	44

IN VIVO ACTIVATION OF MACROPHAGES BY LIPOSOMES CONTAINING IMMUNOMODULATORS

In general, attempts to activate macrophages in vivo to enhance host defense against metastases have been unsuccessful. Systemic administration of MAF is hindered by the lack of purified preparations of this lymphokine and by the fact that lymphokines injected i.v. have a very short half-life and do not activate macrophages in vivo. The systemic activation of macrophages by microorganisms or their products has also suffered from major drawbacks. For instance, administration of whole bacteria such as bacillus Calmette-Guérin activates various effector cells and is accompanied by serious toxicity problems such as allergic reactions and granuloma formation (Allison 1979). Little progress was made until the discovery of muramyl dipeptide (*N*-acetylmuramyl-L-alanyl-D-isoglutamine; MDP), a small component of the bacterial cell wall (Chedid et al. 1979, Matter 1979, Lederer 1980) that is capable of activating macrophages. However, water-soluble synthetic MDP has not been of use in therapy because, after parenteral administration, this agent is rapidly cleared (<60 min) from the body to be excreted in the urine (Parant et al. 1979). This brief period is insufficient to activate macrophages even under ideal in vitro conditions (Sone and Fidler 1981b).

Advances in liposome technology have suggested a way in which immunomodulators might be used to activate macrophages in vivo. This involves encapsulating the agent in liposomes. There are several advantages to this approach: first, when injected i.v. most liposomes localize in phagocytic cells of the reticuloendothelial system, cells responsible for the rapid clearance of particulate matter from the circulation. Second, encapsulation of macrophage activators within liposomes prevents their rapid degradation or clearance. Third, many macrophage-activating agents such as MAF can be antigenic, and repeated systemic administration can lead to adverse reactions. Liposomes consisting of natural phospholipids are nonimmunogenic and thus should not elicit the allergic reactions commonly associated with the systemic administration of immune adjuvants (Allison 1979, Allison and Gregoriadis 1974).

Numerous studies have recently shown that both MAF and MDP entrapped in liposomes are very efficient in activating macrophages to become tumoricidal in vitro (reviews, Fidler and Poste, 1981, 1982). Unlike free MAF, which requires binding to a macrophage surface receptor (Poste et al. 1979a), liposome-entrapped MAF enters the cytoplasm via phagocytosis and can activate macrophages that lack receptors for MAF (Poste and Kirsh 1979). Moreover, for activators such as MAF and MDP that are ordinarily degraded or cleared from the body too rapidly to be effective, encapsulation in liposomes extends active half-life within the body and enables these agents to activate macrophages in vivo (Fidler and Fogler 1982).

We examined whether the in situ activation of macrophages by i.v. administration of liposomes containing MDP resulted from the direct interaction of MDP and macrophages or whether it occurred indirectly by the action of lymphokines released by sensitized T cells. We used three groups of mice with impaired T-cell function: mice exposed to UV radiation, adult thymectomized X-irradiated mice, and athymic nude mice. Mice were given i.v. injections of multilamellar liposomes containing MDP or placebo preparations. Their alveolar macrophages were harvested 24 h later and assessed for cytotoxic properties against syngeneic tumor targets. Macrophages harvested from all groups of mice became tumoricidal in response to liposome-encapsulated MDP, demonstrating that liposome-MDP activation of macrophages occurred directly and was a thymus-independent process (Fidler 1981).

ERADICATION OF SPONTANEOUS ESTABLISHED LUNG AND LYMPH NODE METASTASES BY THE I.V. INJECTION OF LIPOSOMES CONTAINING MAF OR MDP

The B16-BL6 melanoma cell line, which is syngeneic to C57BL/6 mice, was used to determine the effectiveness of liposome-encapsulated immunomodulators in the treatment of metastases. After implantation into the footpad, this tumor metastasizes to lymph nodes and the lungs in over 90% of recipient mice (Hart 1979). C57BL/6 mice were given s.c. injections of 5×10^4 viable cells in 0.05 ml of calcium-magnesium–free phosphate-buffered saline (PBS). Four to five weeks later, when tumors reached 10–15 mm, the tumor-bearing legs and the popliteal lymph nodes were amputated. Intravenous injections with liposome preparations began 3 days after the surgery. Each treatment consisted of an i.v. injection into the tail vein of 2.5 or 5 μmoles of phospholipid multilamellar liposomes suspended in 0.2 ml PBS. Liposomes were prepared from a chromatographically pure egg phosphatidylcholine and beef brain phosphatidylserine (7:3 mole ratio) by mechanical shaking of the mixture on a Vortex mixer, as described elsewhere (Poste et al. 1979b). Encapsulation of MDP, MAF, or PBS within liposomes was achieved using methods similar to those described previously (Schroit and Fidler 1982). We have used these phospholipid liposomes as carriers because they are not toxic at the dose used here (Hart et al. 1981) and because they are arrested efficiently in the lungs as well as organs of the reticuloendothelial system following i.v. injection (Fidler et al. 1980). The internal volume of the liposomes has been determined to be 2.4 ± 0.3 μl/μmole phospholipid. Thus, for the in vivo studies reported here, mice injected i.v. with 5 μmole of liposomes received 12 μl of entrapped suspension.

In experiments designed to evaluate the efficacy of liposome-encapsulated MAF for eradication of spontaneous metastases, control groups of animals were injected i.v. with PBS, with free MAF (200 μl), or with liposomes that contained PBS but were suspended in 200 μl of free MAF. (The lymphokine MAF was obtained from cultures of rat lymphocytes sensitized in vitro to concanavalin A.) In experiments to evaluate the efficacy of liposome-encapsulated MDP in eradicating spontaneous metastases, mice were injected with liposomes containing 2.5 μg MDP. Control groups were injected i.v. with PBS, with free MDP (100 μg/mouse), or with liposomes that contained PBS and were suspended in PBS containing 2.5 μg MDP/mouse. In all experiments, treatments were administered twice weekly for 4 weeks.

Two major types of experiments were carried out. In the first set of experiments, mice were killed 2 weeks after the final treatment and necropsied; the presence of metastases was determined by the use of a dissecting microscope. All suspected pulmonary and extrapulmonary metastases were confirmed by microscopic examination of fixed histological sections. In a second set of experiments, mice were not killed at a predetermined time, but were allowed to survive. The animals were monitored daily, and dead or moribund mice were necropsied. Animals surviving at least 120 days after the last treatment were considered disease free. The in vivo data were analyzed by the Mann-Whitney U-test and Chi square analysis.

Spontaneous pulmonary and lymph node metastases were well established at the time liposome treatment began, and many individual metastases could be seen macroscopically (Fidler 1980, Fidler et al. 1981). Without therapy, these metastases developed into nodules 1–3 mm in diameter, and the growth or lack of growth of lung metastases could be readily determined by the end of the experiment. The results of several experiments are shown in Table 4. Metastases were present in 41 of 48 PBS-treated control mice, and a similar incidence was observed for mice given i.v. injections of free MAF or of liposomes containing PBS suspended in free MAF. However, multiple i.v. injections of liposome-encapsulated MAF significantly reduced the incidence of spontaneous metastases ($P < 0.001$, Chi square analysis), and metastases were found in only five of 20 mice. Moreover, the median number of metastases in the five mice was significantly lower than in the other treatment groups. Similar data were obtained by treating mice with liposomes containing MDP. Here again, treatment

TABLE 4. *Treatment of spontaneous metastases in mice by the i.v. injection of liposome-encapsulated MAF or MDP*

Treatment group	Pulmonary metastasis: Mice with metastases/total mice	Median	Range	P
PBS, control mice	41/48	20	0–107	
Liposomes containing PBS suspended in free MAF	16/18	12	0–65	
Free MAF	8/10	13	0–38	
Liposome-encapsulated MAF	5/20	0	0–10	< 0.001
Free MDP (100 μg)	8/10	55	0–94	
Liposomes containing PBS suspended in 2.5 μg free MDP	23/26	68	0–308	
Liposomes containing 2.5 μg MDP	7/27	0	0–7	< 0.001

of mice with PBS, free MDP (100 μg/dose), or liposomes containing PBS had no effect on the number of pulmonary metastases. In sharp contrast, treatment of mice with liposomes containing MDP significantly reduced both the incidence of pulmonary metastasis (20/27 mice were tumor free, P <0.001) and the median number of metastases in the few tumor-positive mice (Table 4).

In the next set of experiments with the B16-BL6 tumor, mice were not killed at a predetermined time but were allowed to survive. As shown in Table 5, virtually all of the mice injected i.v. with PBS, free MAF, free MDP, or liposomes containing PBS were dead by day 90 of the experiment, i.e. 60 days after the amputation of the tumor-bearing leg. In marked contrast, 66% of mice injected i.v. with liposome-encapsulated MAF and 60% of mice injected with liposome-encapsulated MDP were alive when the experiment was terminated at 200 days.

In this tumor system, at the time of first liposome treatment, spontaneous lung and lymph node metastases were well established and contained an estimated 10^7 cells. Since the median survival time of mice injected with 10 viable

TABLE 5. *Eradication of metastases by the i.v. injection of liposomes containing MAF or MDP: survival studies*

Treatment group	Survival* on day 40	60	90	200
PBS, control mice	30/30	14/30	1/30	1/30
Free MDP (100 μg)	15/15	9/15	1/15	1/15
Liposomes containing PBS suspended in 0.2 μg MDP	15/15	7/15	1/15	1/15
Liposomes containing 0.2 μg MDP	15/15	9/15	9/15	9/15
Free MAF	14/14	10/14	2/14	1/14
Liposomes containing MAF	15/15	13/15	10/15	10/15

* Survival: number of live mice/total number of mice. The differences in median life span are highly significant (P <0.001).

B16 cells (admixed with 10^6 dead cells) is 40–50 days (Griswold 1972, Schabel et al. 1977), we speculate that the tumor burden in the successfully treated mice (alive on day 200) must have been reduced to less than 10 viable cells. Similar data on the successful treatment of a murine fibrosarcoma metastasis have now been published (Deodhar et al. 1982).

Studies on mice treated with liposome-encapsulated MDP that have residual metastatic disease (albeit reduced compared with untreated control mice) have revealed that the tumor cells in these lesions are still fully susceptible to destruction by activated macrophages. This result is consistent with the evidence discussed earlier, which suggests that tumor cell resistance to killing by activated macrophages is not likely to be a rate-limiting factor in the effectiveness of liposome-encapsulated macrophage activators. The more challenging problem will be the extent of the tumor burden at the time therapy is initiated.

THE MECHANISM RESPONSIBLE FOR THE DESTRUCTION OF METASTASES FOLLOWING I.V. INJECTION OF LIPOSOMES CONTAINING MACROPHAGE ACTIVATORS

The mechanisms responsible for the regression of established metastases after the systemic administration of liposomes containing MAF probably involved the activation of macrophages to become tumoricidal. Several lines of evidence tend to support this conclusion. First, administration of macrophage-activating agents encapsulated within liposomes that are not retained in the lung fails to activate lung macrophages and produces no regression of lung metastases (Fidler et al. 1982). Second, the pretreatment of tumor-bearing animals with agents that are toxic for macrophages (silica, carageenan, hyperchlorinated drinking water) before systemic therapy with liposome-encapsulated lymphokines abrogates the response to liposome therapy, and such animals rapidly die of metastatic disease (Fidler et al. 1982). Third, i.v. injection of macrophages activated in vitro by incubation with liposomes containing MAF effects a reduction in metastatic burden comparable to that achieved by systemic administration of liposome-encapsulated activators (Fidler et al. 1982).

Although these data strongly suggested that tumoricidal macrophages were involved in the destruction of metastases in this tumor system, their precise role remained unclear. Direct evidence that tumoricidal macrophages are the effector cells responsible for the destruction of established metastases in mice treated systemically with liposome-entrapped MDP was recently obtained (Key et al. 1982b). Morphological and functional analysis of macrophages isolated from pulmonary metastases of mice given i.v. injections of liposomes containing an MDP derivative, muramyl tripeptide phosphatidylethanolamine (MTP-PE), showed that macrophages containing phagocytosed liposomes infiltrate and localize within pulmonary metastases. Furthermore, once localized, macrophages that have engulfed liposomes containing MDP, but not macrophages that have engulfed liposomes containing a placebo, cytotoxic against the metastatic tumor cells.

CONCLUSIONS

The heterogeneous response of metastases to conventional therapy is a major cause of failure in cancer treatment. Evidence that activated macrophages can recognize and destroy neoplastic cells in vitro without regard to their phenotypic diversity has stimulated a significant effort in many laboratories to develop effective approaches for the activation of macrophages in situ. Systemic administration of liposomes containing immunomodulators, such as lymphokines or MDP, has been shown to activate rodent macrophages in situ and thereby to augment host resistance against spontaneous metastases. The stimulation of host antitumor responses by liposome-encapsulated lymphokines or MDP did not require the participation of functional T lymphocytes or NK cells. Rather, the destruction of established metastases after the multiple systemic administration of liposome-encapsulated immunomodulators was mediated by activated macrophages.

Although the initial results reported from our laboratory regarding the use of macrophages for destruction of metastases are encouraging, it is unlikely that this approach could serve for treatment of large tumor burdens. For example, in a murine melanoma system, the tumor burden in spontaneous metastases that are amenable to treatment by macrophages has been estimated to be $<10^7$ cells. Tumor burdens frequently exceed this level before the disease is even diagnosed. For this reason, potential therapeutic regimens designed to stimulate host immunity must be used in combination with other treatment modalities such as chemotherapy in order to first reduce the tumor burden; the activated macrophages can then lyse tumor cells that have survived destruction by other agents.

ACKNOWLEDGMENTS

I wish to thank Ms. Vickie Koogle for help in preparation of this manuscript and Dr. Cora Bucana for Figure 1.

Research sponsored by the National Cancer Institute, DHHS, under contract No. N01-C0-23909 with Litton Bionetics, Inc. The contents of this publication do not necessarily reflect the views or policies of the Department of Health and Human Services, nor does mention of trade names, commercial products, or organizations imply endorsement by the U.S. Government.

REFERENCES

Alexander, P., S. A. Eccles, and C. L. L. Gauci. 1976. The significance of macrophages in human and experimental tumors. Ann. N.Y. Acad. Sci. 276:124–129.

Allison, A. C. 1979. Mode of action of immunological adjuvants. J. Reticuloendothel. Soc. 26:619–630.

Allison, A. C., and G. Gregoriadis. 1974. Liposomes as immunological adjuvants. Nature 252:252–254.

Bernstein, I. D., B. Zbar, and H. Rapp. 1972. Impaired inflammatory response in tumor-bearing guinea pigs. JNCI 49:1641–1647.

Bucana, C., L. L. Hoyer, B. Hobbs, S. Breesman, M. McDaniel, and M. G. Hanna, Jr. 1976.

Morphological evidence for the translocation of lysosomal organelles from cytotoxic macrophages into the cytoplasm of tumor target cells. Cancer Res. 36:4444–4458.

Chedid, L., L. Carelli, and F. Audibert. 1979. Recent developments concerning muramyl dipeptide, a synthetic immunoregulating molecule. J. Reticuloendothel. Soc. 26:631–641.

Deodhar, S. D., B. P. Borna, M. Edinger, and T. Chiang. 1982. Inhibition of lung metastases by liposomal immunotherapy in a murine fibrosarcoma model. Journal of Biological Response Modifiers 1:27–34.

Eccles, S. A. 1978. Macrophages and cancer, *in* Immunological Aspects of Cancer, J. E. Castro, ed. MTP Press, Lancaster, England, pp. 123–154.

Eccles, S. A., and P. Alexander. 1974a. Macrophage content of tumors in relationship to metastatic spread. Nature 250:667–669.

Eccles, S. A., and P. Alexander. 1974b. Sequestration of macrophages in growing tumors and its effect on the immunological capacity of the host. Br. J. Cancer 30:42–49.

Evans, R., and D. M. Eidlen. 1981. Macrophage accumulation in transplanted tumors is not dependent on host immune responsiveness or presence of tumor-associated rejection antigens. J. Reticuloendothel. Soc. 30:425–430.

Evans, R., and E. M. Lawler. 1980. Macrophage content and immunogenicity of C57BL/6J and BALB/cByJ methylcholanthrene-induced sarcomas. Int. J. Cancer 26:831–835.

Fidler, I. J. 1978. Recognition and destruction of target cells by tumoricidal macrophages. Isr. J. Med. Sci. 14:177–191.

Fidler, I. J. 1980. Therapy of spontaneous metastases by intravenous injection of liposomes containing lymphokines. Science 208:1469–1471.

Fidler, I. J. 1981. The in situ induction of tumoricidal activity in alveolar macrophages by liposomes containing muramyl dipeptide is a thymus-independent process. J. Immunol. 127:1719–1720.

Fidler, I. J., Z. Barnes, W. E. Fogler, R. Kirsh, P. Bugelski, and G. Poste. 1982. Involvement of macrophages in the eradication of established metastases following intravenous injection of liposomes containing macrophage activators. Cancer Res. 42:496–501.

Fidler, I. J., and W. E. Fogler. 1982. Activation of tumoricidal properties in macrophages by lymphokines encapsulated in liposomes. Lymphokine Res. 1:73–77.

Fidler, I. J., D. M. Gersten, and M. B. Budmen. 1976. Characterization in vivo and in vitro of tumor cells selected for resistance to syngeneic lymphocyte-mediated cytotoxicity. Cancer Res. 36:3160–3165.

Fidler, I. J., and I. R. Hart. 1982. Biological diversity in metastatic neoplasms: origins and implications. Science 217:998–1003.

Fidler, I. J., and M. L. Kripke. 1977. Metastasis results from preexisting variant cells within a malignant tumor. Science 197:893–895.

Fidler, I. J., and G. Poste. 1981. Treatment of spontaneous murine metastases by the systemic administration of liposomes containing macrophage-activating agents, *in* Cancer: Achievements, Challenges, and Prospects. Proceedings of the 1980 International Symposium on Cancer, vol. 2, J. H. Burchenal, ed. Grune & Stratton, New York, pp. 77–89.

Fidler, I. J., and G. Poste. 1982. Macrophage-mediated destruction of malignant tumor cells and new strategies for the therapy of metastatic disease. Springer Semin. Immunopathol. 5:161–174.

Fidler, I. J., and A. Raz. 1981. The induction of tumoricidal capacities in mouse and rat macrophages by lymphokines, *in* Lymphokines, vol. 3, E. Pick, ed. Academic Press, New York, pp. 345–363.

Fidler, I. J., A. Raz, W. E. Fogler, R. Kirsh, P. Bugelski, and G. Poste. 1980. The design of liposomes to improve delivery of macrophage-augmenting agents to alveolar macrophages. Cancer Res. 40:4460–4466.

Fidler, I. J., R. O. Roblin, and G. Poste. 1978. In vitro tumoricidal activity of macrophages against virus-transformed lines with temperature-dependent transformed phenotypic characteristics. Cell. Immunol. 38:131–146.

Fidler, I. J., S. Sone, W. E. Fogler, and Z. L. Barnes. 1981. Eradication of spontaneous metastases and activation of alveolar macrophages by intravenous injection of liposomes containing muramyl dipeptide. Proc. Natl. Acad. Sci. USA 78:1680–1684.

Griswold, D. P., Jr. 1972. Consideration of the subcutaneously implanted B16 melanoma as a screening model for potential anticancer agents. Cancer Chemother. Rep. 3:315–323.

Hanna, N., and I. J. Fidler. 1981. Relationship between metastatic potential and resistance to natural killer cell-mediated cytotoxicity in three murine tumor systems. JNCI 66:1183–1190.

Hart, I. R. 1979. The selection and characterization of an invasive variant of the B16 melanoma. Am. J. Pathol. 97:587–600.
Hart, I. R., and I. J. Fidler. 1981. The implications of tumor heterogeneity for studies on the biology and therapy of cancer metastasis. Biochim. Biophys. Acta 651:37–50.
Hart, I. R., W. E. Fogler, G. Poste, and I. J. Fidler. 1981. Toxicity studies of liposome-encapsulated immunomodulators administered intravenously into dogs and mice. Cancer Immunol. Immunother. 10:157–166.
Hibbs, J. B., Jr. 1974a. Discrimination between neoplastic and non-neoplastic cells in vitro by activated macrophages. JNCI 53:1487–1492.
Hibbs, J. B., Jr. 1974b. Heterocytolysis by macrophages activated by bacillus Calmette-Guérin: Lysosome exocytosis into tumor cells. Science 184:468–471.
Key, M., J. E. Talmadge, and I. J. Fidler. 1982a. Lack of correlation between the progressive growth of spontaneous metastases and their content of infiltrating macrophages. J. Reticuloendothel. Soc. 32:387–396.
Key, M. E., J. E. Talmadge, W. E. Fogler, C. Bucana, and I. J. Fidler. 1982b. Isolation of tumoricidal macrophages from lung melanoma metastases of mice treated systemically with liposomes containing a lipophilic derivative of muramyl dipeptide. JNCI 69:1189–1198.
Kleinerman, E. S., K. L. Erickson, A. J. Schroit, W. E. Fogler, and I. J. Fidler. 1983. Activation of tumoricidal properties in human blood monocytes by liposomes containing lipophilic muramyl tripeptide. Cancer Res. 43:2010–2014.
Lederer, E. 1980. Synthetic immunostimulants derived from the bacterial cell wall. J. Med. Chem. 23:819–825.
Marino, P. A., and D. O. Adams. 1980a. Interaction of bacillus Calmette-Guérin-activated macrophages and neoplastic cells in vitro. I. Conditions of binding and its selectivity. Cell. Immunol. 54:11–25.
Marino, P. A., and D. O. Adams. 1980b. Interaction of bacillus Calmette-Guérin-activated macrophages and neoplastic cells in vitro. II. The relationship of selective binding to cytolysis. Cell. Immunol. 54:26–35.
Matter, A. 1979. The effects of muramyl dipeptide (MDP) in cell-mediated immunity. A comparison between in vitro and in vivo systems. Cancer Immunol. Immunother. 6:201–210.
Parant, M., F. Parant, L. Chedid, A. Yapo, J. F. Petit, and E. Lederer. 1979. Fate of the synthetic immunoadjuvant, muramyl dipeptide (14C-labelled) in the mouse. Int. J. Immunopharmacol. 1:35–41.
Poste, G., and I. J. Fidler. 1980. The pathogenesis of cancer metastasis. Nature 283:139–146.
Poste, G., and R. Kirsh. 1979. Rapid decay of tumoricidal activity and loss of responsiveness to lymphokines in inflammatory macrophages. Cancer Res. 39:2582–2590.
Poste, G., R. Kirsh, and I. J. Fidler. 1979a. Cell surface receptors for lymphokines. Cell. Immunol. 44:71–88.
Poste, G., R. Kirsh, W. Fogler, and I. J. Fidler. 1979b. Activation of tumoricidal properties in mouse macrophages by lymphokines encapsulated in liposomes. Cancer Res. 39:881–892.
Russell, S. W., and A. T. McIntosh. 1977. Macrophages isolated from regressing Moloney sarcomas are more cytotoxic than those recovered from progressing sarcoma. Nature (Lond.) 268:69–71.
Schabel, F. M., Jr., D. R. Griswold, Jr., T. H. Corbett, and H. H. Lloyd. 1977. Quantitative evaluation of anticancer agent activity in experimental animals. Pharmacol. Ther.[A] 1:411–435.
Schroit, A. J., and I. J. Fidler. 1982. Effects of liposome structure and lipid composition on the activation of the tumoricidal properties of macrophages by liposomes containing muramyl dipeptide. Cancer Res. 42:161–167.
Snyderman, R., M. C. Pike, B. L. Blaylock, and P. Weinstein. 1976. Effect of neoplasms on inflammation: Depression of macrophage accumulation after tumor implantation. J. Immunol. 116:585–589.
Sone, S., and I. J. Fidler. 1981a. Activation of rat alveolar macrophages to the tumoricidal state in the presence of progressively growing pulmonary metastasis. Cancer Res. 41:2401–2406.
Sone, S., and I. J. Fidler. 1981b. In vitro activation of tumoricidal properties in rat alveolar macrophages by synthetic muramyl dipeptide encapsulated in liposomes. Cell. Immunol. 57:42–50.
Talmadge, J. E., M. E. Key, and I. J. Fidler. 1981. Macrophage content of metastatic and nonmetastatic rodent neoplasms. J. Immunol. 126:2245–2248.
Talmadge, J. E., S. R. Wolman, and I. J. Fidler. 1982. Evidence for the clonal origin of spontaneous metastases. Science 217:361–363.

Cancer Invasion and Metastasis: Biologic and Therapeutic Aspects edited by Garth L. Nicolson and Luka Milas. Raven Press, New York © 1984.

Monoclonal Antibody 791T/36 for Tumor Detection and Therapy for Metastases

Robert W. Baldwin, Malcolm V. Pimm, M. Jim Embleton, Nicholas M. Armitage,* Paul A. Farrands,* Jack D. Hardcastle,* and Alan Perkins†

*Cancer Research Campaign Laboratories, *Department of Surgery, and †Medical Physics Department, University of Nottingham, Nottingham NG7 2RD, England*

The management of and therapy for metastatic cancer could be materially improved if noninvasive diagnostic techniques were available. To this end, the idea of using antibodies to target diagnostic agents to tumors has been under consideration for some years, and in 1978 Goldenberg reported the successful scanning of colorectal carcinoma patients imaged with ^{131}I-labeled anti-CEA antibodies (Goldenberg et al. 1978). The source of antibodies hitherto has been xenogeneic antisera produced against tumor cells or fractions, and several studies have been reported in which successful tumor localization has been achieved with such radiolabeled antibodies, notably those prepared against CEA (Goldenberg et al. 1978, Mach et al. 1981, Begent et al. 1982) and alphafetoprotein (Halsall et al. 1981). But in many cases, xenogeneic antisera prepared against tumor cells and adsorbed with normal tissues have proved to be unsatisfactory. Therefore, the development of techniques for producing monoclonal antibodies by constructing somatic cell hybrids between antibody-producing cells and myeloma cells (Kohler and Milstein 1975) has provided a considerable stimulus to developing techniques for radioimmunodetection of tumors (Farrands et al. 1982, 1983, Epenetos et al. 1982, Berche et al. 1982).

In addition to their potential for detecting primary and metastatic tumors, tumor-localizing monoclonal antibodies can be used for targeting antitumor agents. Cytotoxic agents already conjugated to antibodies include plant and bacterial toxins (Thorpe and Ross 1982), as well as cytotoxic drugs such as Adriamycin (Pimm et al. 1982a), vindesine (Embleton et al. 1983), and methotrexate (Garnett et al. 1983). Antibody conjugation to interferon (Baldwin et al. 1982a,b) is also under investigation as part of research aimed at targeting immunomodulating agents to tumors for the local activation of host antitumor responses. This latter approach is especially pertinent in developing immunotherapy for metastases since intratumoral activation of host cells such as macrophages enhances the therapeutic response (Fidler and Poste 1982).

These developments are considered with respect to the application of an anti-human tumor monoclonal antibody designated 791T/36. This monoclonal antibody (subclass IgG2b) is produced by a hybridoma obtained following fusion of splenocytes from a mouse immunized against cells of an osteogenic sarcoma cell line designated 791T and mouse myeloma P3NS1 (Embleton et al. 1981). This antibody was found to react with 7 of 13 osteogenic sarcoma cell lines, but is not osteogenic sarcoma–specific since cells from 6 of 26 unrelated tumors were also reactive (Embleton et al. 1981). It does not react with a range of normal fibroblasts, blood mononuclear cells, or erythrocytes. Biochemical studies have identified the antigen on osteogenic sarcoma cells as a glycoprotein with molecular mass of 72,000 daltons (Price et al. 1983). This p72 receptor is expressed to differing degrees on tumor cells. On the most reactive osteogenic sarcomas (791T and 788T), there are 2.2×10^6 antibody-binding sites/cell.

TUMOR LOCALIZATION OF 791T/36 MONOCLONAL ANTIBODY IN HUMAN TUMOR XENOGRAFTS

The tumor localizing properties of anti–human tumor monoclonal antibody 791T/36 has been evaluated by studying the organ distribution of radioiodine-labeled preparations in xenografts of human tumors in CBA mice immunodeprived by thymectomy, whole-body irradiation, and cytosine arabinoside treatment (Pimm et al. 1982b). Following injection of ^{131}I-labeled 791T/36, there was preferential localization of radioactivity in osteogenic sarcoma 791T xenografts as assessed by the tissue:blood ratios of tumor tissues and normal organs (Figure 1). This localization was not due to an abnormal blood distribution in the tumor since simultaneously injected normal mouse IgG2b (labeled with ^{125}I) did not localize preferentially in tumor (Figure 1). The simultaneous injection of ^{131}I-labeled antibody and ^{125}I-labeled normal IgG2b into tumor-bearing mice allows one to calculate the extent of specific:nonspecific binding of immunoglobulins. This is expressed as a localization index calculated as the ratios of tissue:blood (antibody) and tissue:blood (normal IgG2b) levels. In the experiment illustrated in Figure 1, the localization index is 6.1 for tumor compared to a value of 1.1 for liver. It was further established that localization of 791T/36 in osteogenic sarcoma xenografts was a specific reaction, since no such localization was observed with tumors such as bladder carcinoma T24 and colon carcinoma HCT8, which do not express the 791T/36 antibody-defined antigen (Pimm et al. 1982b).

These organ distribution studies conclusively demonstrate that radioiodine-labeled 791T/36 antibody specifically localizes in appropriate target tumors growing as xenografts in immunodeprived mice. Furthermore, tumors could be detected by external imaging of tumor-bearing mice following injection of ^{131}I-labeled antibody and image enhancement after blood pool labeling with ^{113m}In or ^{99m}Tc (Pimm et al. 1982b, Baldwin 1982).

These tumor xenograft studies provide the basis for developing clinical trials

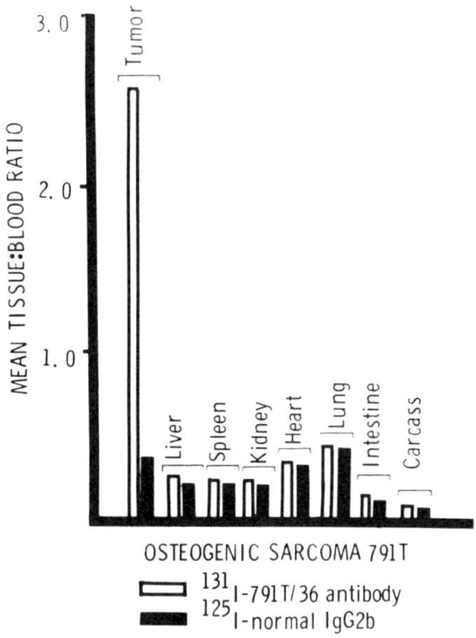

FIG. 1. Distribution of ^{131}I-791T/36 antibody and ^{125}I-normal IgG2b (5 μg each) injected simultaneously into mice bearing osteogenic sarcoma 791T xenografts. Organ distribution of radioactivity was determined two days after antibody injection (mean of four mice). Tissue: blood ratio = cpm/g radioactivity in tissue ÷ cpm/g radioactivity in blood.

for tumor imaging and in addition provide useful animal models for evaluating factors influencing antibody localization (Baldwin and Pimm 1983). For example, the experiments illustrated in Figure 2 were designed to compare the relative uptake of ^{131}I-labeled 791T/36 antibody with ^{125}I-labeled normal mouse Ig in 791T xenografts over a time course of 7 days. Antibody was detectable in tumors within 24 h, reaching peak levels 2 to 4 days after injection. In comparison, normal mouse IgG levels in tumors showed very little variation over the 7 days. These time course studies also show that the increasing tumor-to-blood ratio of the ^{131}I-antibody label and the relatively static ratio of the ^{125}I-labeled normal IgG increases the localization index (2.16 on day 1 and 6.48 on day 7).

The relationship between tumor mass and localization of 791T/36 monoclonal antibody is also important both with respect to defining the size of tumors that can be detected by external imaging and the potential for targeting antitumor agents attached to antibody. As shown in Figure 3, there was a statistically significant correlation ($r^2 = 0.88$; $p < 0.001$) between the proportion of the total body count of ^{131}I (the 791T/36 antibody label) within tumors and their mass. From the slope of the regression line, it can be calculated that 0.034% of the total body radioactivity was present in each milligram of tumor tissue. There was also a significant correlation ($r^2 = 0.62$; $p < 0.001$) between the proportion of the total body count of normal IgG2b (^{125}I-labeled) within tumors and their masses, but only 0.007% of the total body radioactivity was present in each milligram of tumor tissue (Pimm and Baldwin 1983).

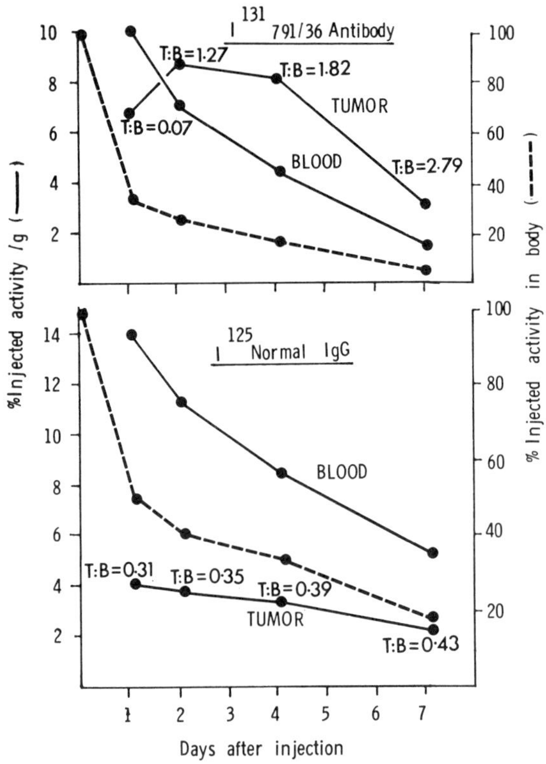

FIG. 2. Kinetics of tumor localization and blood and body survival of radioisotope-labeled 791T/36 antibody and normal IgG in osteogenic sarcoma 791T-bearing mice. Mice were injected simultaneously with a mixture of ^{131}I-labeled 791T/36 antibody and ^{125}I-labeled normal IgG2b. Groups of four or five mice were killed and radioactivity counted in tumor, blood, and whole carcass. Tumor localization index is calculated as T:B ratio ^{131}I 791T/36 antibody ÷ T:B ratio ^{125}I normal IgG (T:B = tumor:blood ratio).

CLINICAL STUDIES

Clinical trials have been established to determine whether 791T/36 monoclonal antibody localizes in primary and metastatic human tumors, based on the experience gained from the tests with human tumor xenografts. The tumors studied to date include osteogenic sarcomas, colorectal carcinomas, and ovarian tumors.

Osteogenic Sarcoma

Immunoscintigraphy using ^{131}I-labeled 791T/36 antibody has been used to detect a primary osteogenic sarcoma in a young girl who presented with pain and swelling in her right knee (Farrands et al. 1983). One, 2, and 3 days after intravenous administration of ^{131}I-labeled antibody (200 μg protein, 70 MBq

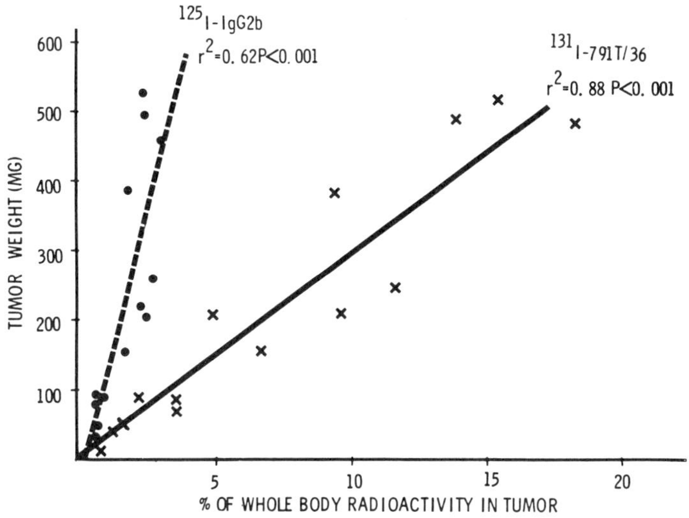

FIG. 3. Correlation between tumor mass and tumor uptake of ^{131}I-labeled 791T/36 antibody and ^{125}I-labeled normal IgG2b. Tumor-bearing mice receiving a mixture of the two radiolabeled preparations were killed two days later and organ distribution of radioactivity determined. The radioactivity in tumor is expressed as a percentage of the total body radioactivity.

^{131}I), anterior and posterior images of the legs, abdomen, and chest were taken with a gamma camera and images recorded by computer. Image enhancement was then achieved by subtraction of blood pool images acquired following in vivo labeling of the patient's red blood cells with ^{99m}Tc. The results of these images (Figure 4) show uptake of radioactivity into the tumor in the right leg following infusion of ^{131}I-labeled antibody (view 1). View 2 shows the blood

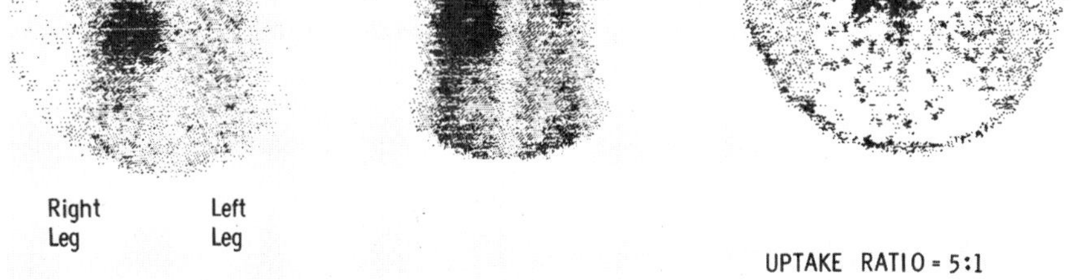

FIG. 4. Gamma camera images of the legs of an osteogenic sarcoma patient infused 24 h before with ^{131}I-labeled 791T/36 antibody. View 1—^{131}I image. View 2—^{99M}Tc image. View 3—subtracted image showing ^{131}I antibody localization (Farrands et al. 1983).

pool image obtained with ^{99m}Tc indicating abnormal uptake into the right leg, but after subtraction (view 3) obvious activity, representing ^{131}I-labeled antibody, is seen in the area of the tumor. No metastatic lesions were detected in the lungs or elsewhere in the patient.

Colorectal Carcinoma

Clinical studies have been developed using the imaging procedures outlined with the osteogenic sarcoma patient to examine the potential of 791T/36 antibody for radioimmunodetection of primary and metastatic colorectal carcinomas. In the first trial (Farrands et al. 1982), 11 patients with primary and metastatic tumors were studied, and in nine of them accurate tumor localization was observed (Table 1). In one patient, postoperative imaging of the resected specimen was positive (Table 2), and failure to detect the tumor in the patient was thought to be due to its disposition behind the bladder, which itself produced an image because of excreted ^{131}I. The other patient in which imaging was not successful was examined 2 weeks after radiotherapy (30 Gy), and it is thought that radiotherapy may have contributed to the failure of the antibody to localize.

The patients in the first trial included five with primary colorectal cancers and five with extensive disseminated disease histologically confirmed at a previous laparotomy. As summarized in Table 1, positive images were obtained with metastases. In case 10, for example, a brain metastasis was clearly identified (Figure 5). This accorded with the patient's right hemiplegia and was confirmed at necropsy. This brain metastasis was the smallest tumor identified in the series, measuring 2 × 2 × 1 cm. The trial is being continued and extended to evaluate the potential of external imaging following injection of radiolabeled 791T/36 using a range of radionuclides, including ^{131}I, ^{123}I, ^{111}In, and ^{67}Ga. The immunoscintigraphy findings are being compared with those obtained using a range of other tests, including liver imaging following the injection of ^{99m}Tc-sulphur colloid and nuclear magnetic resonance scanning. These studies, together with improvements in gamma camera imaging techniques, particularly tomoscintigraphy, will establish the minimum size of tumor that can be detected and also evaluate the potential of antibody imaging for detecting metastases.

The opportunity to image primary colorectal cancer patients preoperatively has made possible analysis of the uptake of ^{131}I-labeled antibody (or degradation products) into tumor and nontumor tissues. First, resected specimens have been reimaged by gamma camera scanning, and second, tumor and nontumor tissue samples have been dissected and radioactivity counted in a γ spectrometer. The results of analyses of resected tissue specimens from five patients are shown in Table 2. In all of these samples, the images acquired in the gamma camera exactly matched the size and contours of the tumors. Also the tumor : nontumor ratio of ^{131}I radioactivity was comparable by the two assays (except for Case 2), indicating that gamma camera imaging gives a good indication of the proportion of antibody radioactivity that can be delivered to a tumor.

Specificity of 791T/36 Antibody Uptake

The specificity of localization of 791T/36 antibody in colorectal carcinomas has been examined by comparing the tumor uptake obtained in patients infused with ^{131}I-labeled 791T/36 antibody and ^{123}I-labeled normal mouse serum IgG2b. Figure 6 shows tissue:blood ratios of radioactivity in a patient whose tumor was resected 18 h after infusion of the differently labeled antibodies. The tumor:blood ratio of ^{131}I (the label for 791T/36 antibody) was 0.57:1 compared with 0.20:1 for normal colonic tissue taken adjacent to the tumor (localization index 2.8). The tumor:blood ratio of ^{123}I (the label for normal mouse IgG2b) was 0.14 and that of normal colonic tissue 0.11 (localization index 1.27). These results indicate that tumor localization of ^{131}I-labeled 791T/36 involves a specific interaction with tissue antigen rather than nonspecific accumulation of mouse immunoglobulin in the tumor.

Circulating 791T/36 Antibody Levels

The already discussed experimental studies of human tumor xenografts in immunodeprived mice indicate that, following infusion of radiolabeled 791T/36 mouse antibody, radioactivity is rapidly lost from blood over the first 24 h, and thereafter blood levels decay with a half-life of approximately 2.7 days (Baldwin and Pimm 1983). This parameter has also been examined in colorectal cancer patients since changes in blood levels of 791T/36 antibody influence the timing of imaging to obtain optimal resolution. As can be seen from the data illustrated in Figure 7, following intravenous infusion of ^{131}I-labeled 791T/36, blood radioactivity fell within 24 h to a level approximately 26% of that determined immediately after infusion. Thereafter, blood levels of radioactivity declined more slowly with a half-life of approximately 2 days. Blood-borne radioactivity was associated with plasma rather than cellular elements (95% $\pm$ 2.3, n = 9) in samples taken between 1 and 7 days after infusion, and the plasma-associated radioactivity was precipitable with 10% trichloroacetic acid (95% $\pm$ 1.7, n = 9). It was also established that the radioactivity present in plasma taken from patients up to 4 days after antibody infusion was precipitable with rabbit anti-mouse IgG (88% $\pm$ 2.2, n = 6). These experiments indicate that the radiolabel detected in patients' plasma was associated with mouse immunoglobulin, which was further demonstrated by Sephacryl S-300 chromatography of patients' plasma samples, which showed that radioactivity was associated exclusively with the IgG fraction (Figure 8).

Finally, plasma samples from patients infused with ^{131}I-labeled 791T/36 were assayed for circulating antibody, this being determined by its binding to osteogenic sarcoma 791T target cells or, in controls, to bladder carcinoma T24 cells. In the two examples illustrated in Figure 9, circulating 791T/36 antibody was demonstrable in the patients' plasma by its binding to osteogenic sarcoma 791T cells but not to bladder carcinoma T24 cells.

TABLE 1. *Immunoscintigraphy of colorectal carcinoma patients following infusion of ^{131}I-labeled 791T/36 monoclonal antibody*

		Tumor			Imaging			
							Tumor to nontumor ratio	
Patient	Age (sex)	Macroscopic	Stage	Grade/ differen- tiation	Background subtraction agent	Site of image	Before subtraction	After background subtraction
1	71 (M)	Primary: nodular Ca. of sigmoid 5 × 6 × 2 cm	B	Moderate	^{99m}Tc — RBC ^{113m}In-transferrin	Positive Primary in pelvis	1.5:1	8.0:1
2	66 (F)	Primary: nodular Ca. rectosigmoid 4 × 4 × 3 cm	B	Well	^{99m}Tc — RBC	Positive Primary in pelvis attached to bladder	1.5:1	2.1:1
3	75 (M)	Primary: nodular Ca. sigmoid	B	Moderate	^{99m}Tc — RBC	Not detected behind bladder	—*†	—*†
4	67 (M)	2 Primaries: transverse and rectum. 3 × 3 × 2 cm 4 × 3 × 4 cm	C	Moderate	^{99m}Tc — RBC	Positive for both epigastrium and pelvis	1.5:1	2.1:1
5	64 (M)	Primary ulcerating Ca. sigmoid 6 × 3 × 3 cm	B	Well	^{99m}Tc — RBC	Positive Primary in pelvis	1.2:1	1.5:1

6	58 (F)	Disseminated Ca. with omental 2° post-op. 10 × 15 × 3 cm	D	Moderate	^{99m}Tc — RBC	Positive Peritoneal and omental 2°	2.0:1	8.1:1
7	71 (M)	Disseminated Ca. with liver 2° post-op. 6 × 6 × 3 cm	D	Moderate	^{99m}Tc — RBC ^{113}In-transferrin	Positive Pelvis and liver	1.2:1	5.1:1
8	64 (M)	Post-op. ? 2° in liver at operation 2 × 2 × 1 cm 1 × 1 × 2 cm	D	Moderate	^{99m}Tc — RBC	Not detected	—	—
9	72 (M)	Inoperable Ca. rectum—Post-op. 4 × 3 × 4 cm	D	Moderate	^{99m}Tc — RBC ^{99m}Tc sulphur colloid ^{113}In-transferrin	Not detected†	—	—
10	44 (M)	Disseminated Ca. Cecum — 2° in liver and brain. Post-op. 2 × 2 × 1 cm (brain)	D	Moderate	^{99m}Tc — RBC ^{113m}In-transferrin	Positive Brain and liver	1.3:1	4.0:1
11	60 (F)	Disseminated Ca. sigmoid with pelvis recurrence 6 × 7 × 5 cm	D	Moderate	^{99m}Tc — RBC ^{113m}In-transferrin	Positive Mass anterior to rectum	1.9:1	4.3:1

* Positive on counting tumor.
† Imaging 2 weeks after radiotherapy.
(Reproduced from Farrands et al. 1982, with permission of *The Lancet.*)

TABLE 2. *Postoperative analyses of resected tumor specimens from colon carcinoma patients infused with ^{131}I-labeled 791T/36 antibody*

Patients	Tumor	Size of tumor resected	Tumor to nontumor ratio on image	Tumor to nontumor counts/gram of tissue
1	Primary nodular Ca. sigmoid	5 × 6 × 2 cm	2.3:1	2.2:1
2	Primary nodular Ca. rectosigmoid	4 × 4 × 5 cm	2.5:1	5.8:1
3	Primary nodular Ca. rectosigmoid	4 × 5 × 3 cm	Not counted	2.1:1
4	2 Primary ulcerating Ca.	3 × 3 × 2 cm	2.1:1	3.1:1
	Rectum and transverse colon*	4 × 4 × 2 cm	2.0:1	Not counted
5	Primary ulcerating Ca. sigmoid colon	6 × 3 × 3 cm	1.5:1	1:1

* Undiagnosed carcinoma identified on the patient's image.

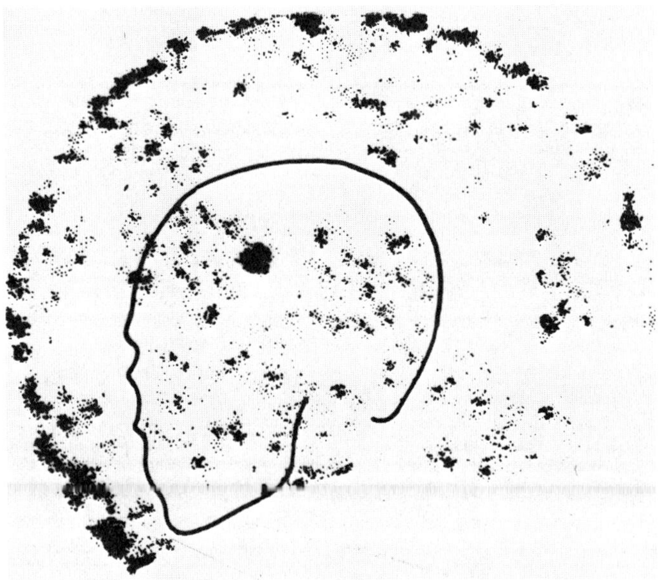

FIG. 5. Brain metastases detected in colorectal carcinoma patient (Case 10, Table 1) following imaging with ^{131}I-labeled 791T/36. (Reproduced from Farrands et al. 1982, with permission of *The Lancet.*)

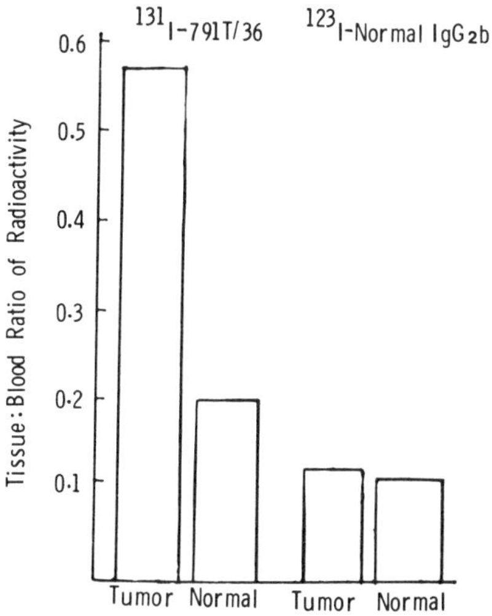

FIG. 6. Specificity of tumor uptake of 791T/36 monoclonal antibody. A patient with colon carcinoma was infused with a mixture of 200 μg of each of ^{131}I-labeled 791T/36 antibody and ^{123}I-labeled normal mouse IgG2b. Tissue was resected 18 hr later and the radioactivity of each isotope in blood, tumor, and normal colonic mucosa counted.

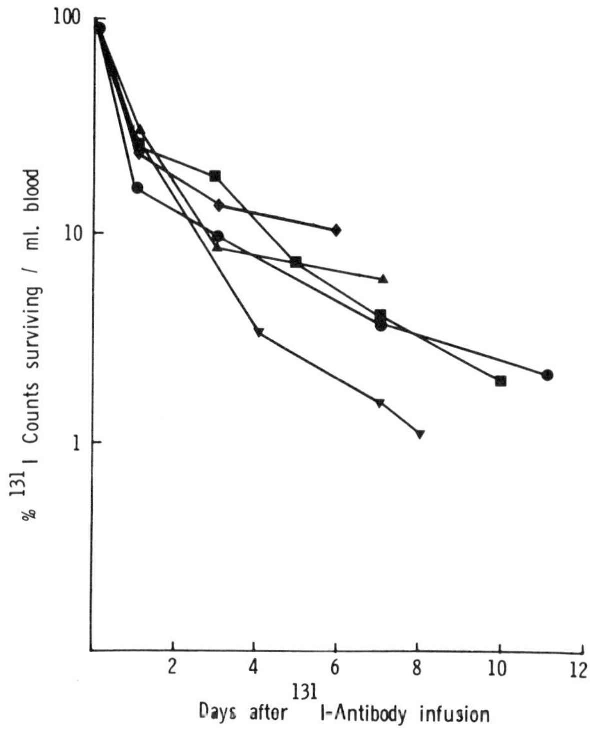

FIG. 7. Blood survival of ^{131}I-791T/36 monoclonal antibody in patients with colorectal carcinoma.

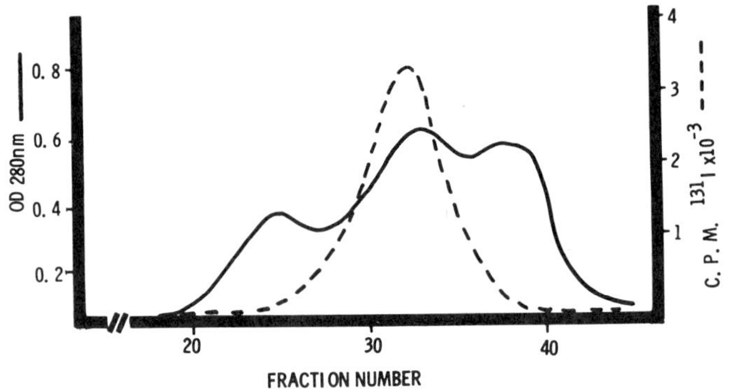

FIG. 8. Sephacryl S300 chromatography profile of plasma from a colorectal cancer patient infused with ^{131}I-791T/36 antibody.

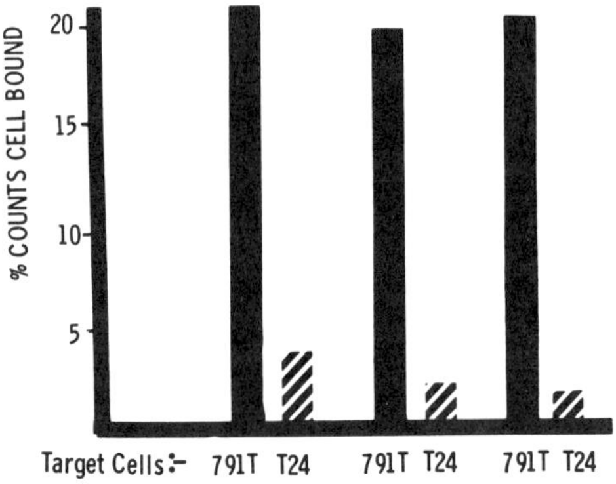

FIG. 9. Cell binding activity of ^{131}I-791T/36 antibody and radioactivity in plasma of colon carcinoma patients injected 1 day before with labeled antibody. Cells were incubated with 0.1 ml of the preparations and after extensive washing the bound ^{125}I was counted. Target cells: osteogenic sarcoma 791T bladder carcinoma T24 (Reproduced from Baldwin and Pimm 1983, with permission).

Development of Anti–Mouse Immunoglobulin Antibody

Since tumor imaging is carried out following infusion of mouse monoclonal antibody, the development by patients of antibodies to mouse immunoglobulin represents a potential problem for repeated imaging trials. This problem has been investigated by determining the production of anti-mouse antibodies in patients following infusion of ^{131}I-labeled 791T/36 (200 to 300 μg). The plasma from five patients was analyzed for anti–mouse immunoglobulin antibody by its capacity to interact with ^{131}I-labeled 791T/36 (Table 3). In these tests, plasma samples were incubated with ^{131}I-labeled 791T/36, and after incubation any complexes coprecipitated with excess goat anti–human IgG. The results indicate that the amount of radioactivity precipitated in patients' plasma was not greater than that observed for normal human plasma. These pilot studies indicate that a single infusion of ^{131}I-labeled 791T/36 monoclonal antibody into colorectal carcinoma patients does not lead to the development of a significant antibody response to mouse immunoglobulins. The pattern of response following further

TABLE 3. *Analysis of the development of anti-mouse immunoglobulin antibodies in colorectal carcinoma patients infused with 791T/36 monoclonal antibody*

Patient no.*	Days after antibody infusion†	Co-precipitation of ^{131}I-791T/36 antibody‡			
		Patients plasma		Normal plasma	
		cpm × 10^{-4}	% input	cpm × 10^{-4}	% input
8	120	0.68	7	1.49	12
9	70	1.63	12	1.49	12
11	300	4.70	18	3.32	12
12	7	0.82	8	1.49	12
15	45	1.24	13	1.49	12

* Case numbers refer to patients in Table 1 (except patient 15).
† 200 μg 791T/36 antibody.
‡ 200 ng 791T/36 antibody was incubated with 20μl plasma and subsequently human Ig precipitated by addition of goat anti-human Ig.

791T/36 antibody infusions is being determined in a trial evaluating the potential of immunoscintigraphy for the postoperative follow-up of colorectal cancer patients.

ANTIBODY TARGETING OF ANTITUMOR AGENTS

Tumor-localizing monoclonal antibodies have considerable potential for targeting antitumor agents, especially for treatment of metastatic tumors (Baldwin and Pimm 1983). Plant and bacterial toxins, or more particularly their A-chain fragments, have been conjugated to monoclonal antibodies to form immunotoxins with selectivity of action, at least in vitro, for target cells expressing the appropriate antigen (Thorpe and Ross 1982, Casellas et al. 1982). Immunotoxins in certain selected situations have also been used to suppress tumor growth in vivo (Krolick et al. 1982). There are, however, major problems with respect to the clinical applications of these immunotoxins (Mason et al. 1982), and consequently attention has been restricted to the conjugation of 791T/36 monoclonal antibody to cytotoxic drugs including vindesine (Embleton et al. 1983) and methotrexate (Garnett et al. 1983). In addition, 791T/36 antibody has been conjugated to interferon α as part of research developing methods for targeting immunomodulating agents for regional immunotherapy (Baldwin et al. 1982a, 1982b).

The former approach is illustrated by the development of the conjugates with the vinca alkaloid analogue vindesine (VDS) (Embleton et al. 1983). These VDS-791T/36 antibody conjugates retain antibody activity and, as shown in Figure 10, are cytotoxic for tumor cells expressing the 791T/36 antibody-defined antigen. In these tests, conjugate and parent drug were assayed for their ability to inhibit the uptake of [^{75}Se]selenomethionine by the target cells, it having

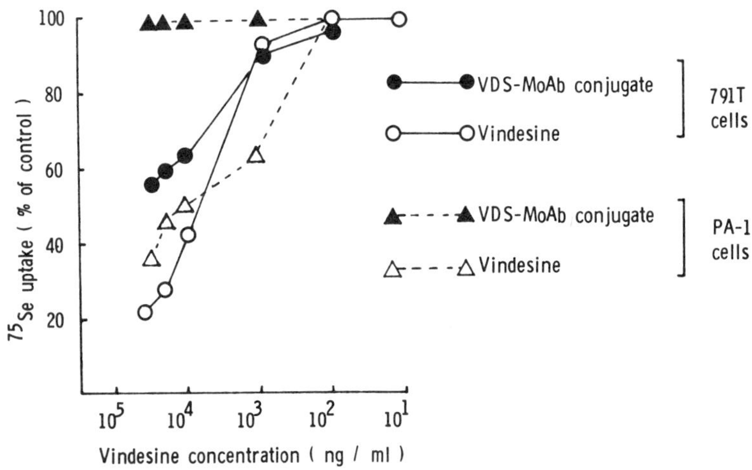

FIG. 10. Effect of vindesine (VDS) and VDS-791T/36 monoclonal antibody on survival of tumor cells in culture. Cells were treated with the agent for 15 min, then washed and cultured for 24 hr. They were then labeled for 16 hr with ^{75}Se-selenomethionine and washed three times. Uptake of ^{75}Se by treated cells is expressed as a percentage of that in controls (treated with phosphate-buffered saline). 791T/36, osteogenic sarcoma; PA1, ovarian carcinoma.

been established that ^{75}Se uptake correlates extremely well with tumor cell survival. In this representative experiment, 15-min exposure of osteogenic sarcoma 791T/36 cells to VDS-791T/36 antibody conjugate followed by extensive washing of the cells before plating markedly inhibited protein synthesis when assayed 24 h later ([^{75}Se]selenomethionine uptake). Similar treatment of ovarian carcinoma PA1 cells, which do not express the 791T/36 antibody-defined antigen, did not affect survival of these cells. That this difference is not due to inherent resistance of PA1 cells to VDS in comparison with 791T cells is indicated by the comparable susceptibility of both cell lines to free drug. These in vitro studies establish that VDS-791T/36 antibody conjugates retain antibody and drug cytotoxic activities (Embleton et al. 1983).

In extending these in vitro studies, we have initiated an evaluation of in vivo responses to the conjugates. Experiments were carried out initially to confirm that the VDS-antibody conjugates, like free 791T/36 antibody, localized in osteogenic sarcoma 791T xenografts in immunodeprived mice. Figure 11 shows the preferential tumor localization of a ^{125}I labeled VDS-791T/36 antibody conjugate compared with the levels in other organs in the tumor-bearing mouse.

As a result of the above studies, trials have been started to evaluate the in vivo effectiveness of VDS-antibody conjugates. In the initial trials, osteogenic sarcoma 791T cells were inoculated subcutaneously into immunodeprived mice, which then received a course of treatment with either VDS or VDS-791T/36 conjugates (Figure 12). The agents were administered intraperitoneally in seven equal doses on days 1,3,6,8,10,13, and 15 after tumor challenge, the total doses

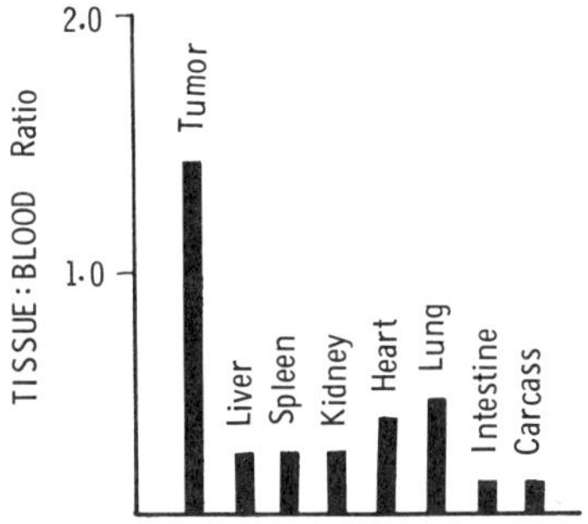

FIG. 11. Localization of ^{125}I-labeled VDS–791T/36 antibody conjugate in osteogenic sarcoma xenografts in immunodeprived mice.

being equivalent to 19.2 mg VDS and 500 mg antibody/kg body weight. Treatment with VDS-791T/36 antibody conjugate markedly suppressed tumor growth compared with untreated controls. Also, the conjugates were nontoxic when administered by this regime of treatment. Other studies have confirmed that a single dose of VDS-antibody at 50 mg/kg body weight with respect to VDS

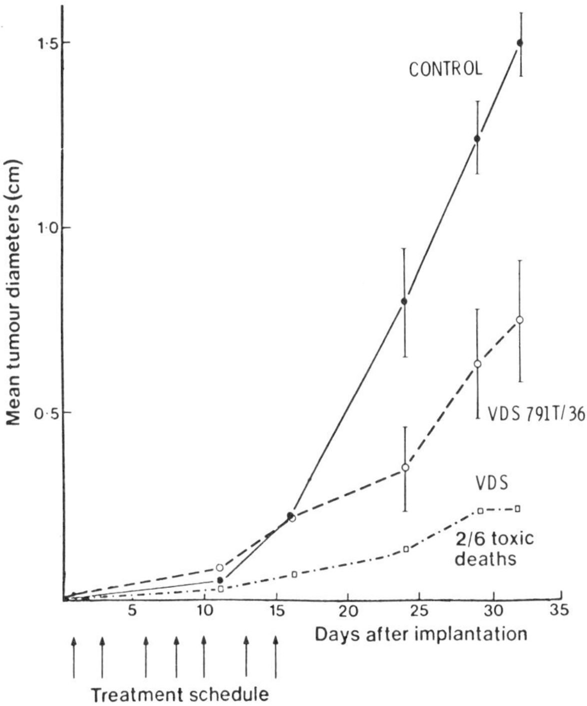

FIG. 12. Effect of vindesine (VDS) and VDS–791T/36 antibody conjugate on growth of xenografts of osteogenic sarcoma 791T. Each agent was given intraperitoneally according to the treatment schedule shown. Total dose/mouse was 19.2 mg/kg body weight of VDS alone; when conjugated to 791T/36 antibody it was 500 mg/kg.

is nontoxic, which can be compared with the LD50 of approximately 5 mg/kg for VDS (Rowland, personal communication). Although free VDS produced a more marked inhibition of tumor growth (Figure 12), the dose was above that which was tolerated, resulting in two deaths in the VDS group of six mice. Treatment with unconjugated 791T/36 antibody does not influence growth of 791T xenografts (Price et al. 1982).

Further trials with VDS-antibody conjugate against osteogenic sarcoma 791T are being developed to determine optimum dose and timing of treatment. In this respect, it is evident that the antibody conjugates behave in a fashion completely different from that of free VDS. For example, the greatly reduced toxicity of VDS-antibody conjugates indicates that higher doses may be given as either single or multiple treatments.

DISCUSSION

Immunoscintigraphy with radiolabeled monoclonal antibodies has considerable potential for the detection and localization of metastases. These approaches are still at an early stage of development, and there are many problems to be resolved. First, the range of monoclonal antibodies that react specifically, or, more realistically, preferentially with tumors must be increased. Despite considerable efforts in many laboratories, the number of monoclonal antibodies so far applied for immunoscintigraphy is still very limited, but includes anti-CEA monoclonal antibodies (Berche et al. 1982), 791T/36 antibody (Farrands et al. 1982, 1983), anti–milk fat globule membrane antibody (Epenetos et al. 1982), and anti–colon carcinoma antibodies including YPC2/R1 (Smedley et al. 1983), and 17–1A (Chatel et al. 1982). The choice of radionuclide and methods for labeling antibodies, as well as the use of intact antibodies or antibody fragments such as $F(ab)_2'$ also need to be evaluated. Finally the choice of gamma camera-imaging techniques including conventional scintigraphy or tomoscintigraphy (Berche et al. 1982) is important. Nevertheless, the studies carried out in colorectal cancer patients indicate that imaging following infusion of ^{131}I-labeled 791T/36 antibody is able to detect metastatic tumors. The single brain metastasis measuring 2 × 2 × 1 cm is the smallest tumor so far detected, but one expects this to be improved upon with refinements in technology.

All of the monoclonal antibodies so far used for patient imaging have been of mouse origin, apart from HPC2/R.1, which is a rat antibody (Smedley et al. 1983). Basically, therefore, it is likely that infusion of these immunoglobulins into patients will lead to the development of antirodent antibody responses against the infused protein. This has been observed in patients receiving large doses of mouse monoclonal antibody (up to 200 mg) for therapeutic applications (Sears et al., 1982), but has not yet proved to be a problem in the imaging of colorectal carcinoma in patients. As shown in Table 3, antibodies to mouse immunoglobulin were not detected in patients' plasma taken after infusion of ^{131}I-791T/36 monoclonal antibody. These studies are still limited since patients have not received multiple mouse antibody infusions for repeated imaging. This is desirable, however, when it is necessary to image at intervals for the detection of metastases, in, for example, patients with osteogenic sarcoma.

One of the long-term objectives in developing tumor-localizing monoclonal antibodies is to use them therapeutically for treatment of occult or established metastases. In some cases, antibody alone may exert a therapeutic effect through the mediation of host responses including complement-dependent or cell-dependent cytotoxic attack. The best example of this to date is the use of monoclonal anti-idiotype antibodies for the treatment of a B-cell lymphoma (Miller et al. 1982). A more general approach involves the conjugation of antitumor agents to antibody, so providing methods for targeting them to tumors (Rowland et al. 1982, Baldwin 1982, Baldwin et al. 1982a). The potential of this approach is emphasized by the studies described on the conjugation of VDS to 791T/36 monoclonal antibody to produce conjugates specifically cytotoxic for cells expressing the 791T/36-defined antigen (Figure 10). There are major problems to be resolved in this approach, particularly ones related to the capacity of drug-antibody conjugates to localize within tumors and then produce a therapeutic response. As illustrated in Figure 11, VDS-791T/36 antibody conjugates do localize in human osteogenic sarcoma xenografts; similarly, VDS conjugates with a polyclonal anti-CEA antibody localize in metastatic colon carcinomas (Ford et al. 1983). Therapeutic trials in progress already indicate that the conjugate suppresses growth of osteogenic sarcoma xenografts (Figure 12), and importantly are much less toxic than free drug. These features are now being examined in detail since they suggest that this approach may be of considerable use for treating metastatic tumors.

ACKNOWLEDGMENTS

This work was supported by a grant from the Cancer Research Campaign, U.K., and part of the work was carried out in collaboration with Dr. G. Rowland, Lilly Research, U.K.

REFERENCES

Baldwin, R. W. 1982. Monoclonal antibodies in the diagnosis, detection and therapy of cancer. Proc. R. Soc. Edinburgh 81b:261–276.

Baldwin, R. W., and M. V. Pimm. 1983. Antitumor monoclonal antibodies for radioimmunodetection of tumors and drug targeting. Cancer Metastases Reviews. 2:89–106.

Baldwin, R. W., M. J. Embleton, G. R. Flannery, J. M. Pelham, M. V. Pimm, M. R. Price, and R. A. Robins. 1982a. Diagnostic and therapeutic applications of a monoclonal antibody against human osteogenic sarcoma, *in:* Protides of the Biological Fluids, H. Peeters, ed. Vol. 30 Pergamon Press, London, pp. 381–386.

Baldwin, R. W., G. R. Flannery, J. M. Pelham, and J. D. Gray. 1982b. Immunomodulation by IFN-conjugated monoclonal antibody to human osteogenic sarcoma (abstract). Proc. Amer. Soc. Cancer Res. 23:254.

Begent, R. H. J., A. J. Green, K. D. Bagshaw, B. E. Jones, P. A. Keep, F. Searle, R. F. Jewkes,

G. M. Barratt, and B. E. Ryman. 1982. Lipsosomally entrapped second antibody improves tumour imagining with radiolabelled (first) antitumor antibody. Lancet i:739–741.

Berche, C., J.-P. Mach, J.-D. Lumbroso, C. Langlais, F. Aubry, F. Buchegger, S. Carrel, P. Rougier, C. Parmentier, and M. Tubiana. 1982. Tomoscintigraphy for detecting gastrointestinal and medullary thyroid cancers: first clinical results using radiolabelled monoclonal antibodies against carcinoembryonic antigen. Br. Med. J. 285:1147–1451.

Casellas, P., J. P. Brown, O. Gros, P. Gros, I. Hellstrom, F. K. Jansen, P. Poncelet, R. Roncucci, H. Vidal, and K. E. Hellstrom. 1982. Human melanoma cells can be killed in vitro by an immunotoxin specific for melanoma-associated antigen p97. Int. J. Cancer 30:437–443

Chatal, J. F., J. C. Saccavini, P. Fumoleau, A. Bardy, J. Y. Douillard, J. Aubry, and B. Le Mevel. 1982. Photoscanning localization of human tumors using radioiodinated monoclonal antibodies to colorectal carcinoma. (Abstract) J. Nucl. Med. 23:8.

Embleton, M. J., B. Gunn, V. S. Byers, and R. W. Baldwin. 1981. Antitumour reactions of monoclonal antibody against a human osteogenic sarcoma cell line. Br. J. Cancer 43:582–587.

Embleton, M. J., G. F. Rowland, R. G. Simmonds, E. Jacobs, C. H. Marsden, and R. W. Baldwin. 1983. Selective cytotoxicity against human tumour cells by a vindesine-monoclonal antibody conjugate. Br. J. Cancer 47:43–49.

Epenetos, A. A., S. Mather, M. Granowska, C. C. Nimmon, L. R. Hawkins, K. E. Britton, J. Shepherd, J. Taylor-Papadimitrious, H. Durbin, J. A. Malpas, and W. F. Bodmer. 1982. Targeting of iodine-123-labelled tumour-associated monoclonal antibodies to ovarian, breast and gastrointestinal tumours. Lancet ii:999–1006.

Farrands, P. A., A. C. Perkins, M. V. Pimm, M. J. Embleton, J. D. Hardy, R. W. Baldwin, and J. D. Hardcastle. 1982. Radioimmunodetection of human colorectal cancers by an anti-tumour monoclonal antibody. Lancet ii:397–400.

Farrands, P. A., A. Perkins, L. Sully, J. S. Hopkins, M. V. Pimm, R. W. Baldwin, and J. D. Hardcastle. 1983. Localisation of human osteosarcoma by anti-tumour monoclonal antibody (791T/36). J. Bone Joint Surg. (in press).

Fidler, I. J., and G. Poste. 1982. Macrophage-mediated destruction of malignant tumor cells and new strategies for the therapy of metastatic disease, *in:* Springer Siminars in Immunopathology, Vol. 5, R. W. Baldwin, P. A. Miescher, H. J. Muller-Erberhard, eds. Springer Verlag, New York, pp. 161–174.

Ford, C. H. J., C. E. Newman, J. R. Johnson, C. S. Woodhouse, T. A. Reeder, G. F. Rowland, and R. G. Simmonds. 1983. Localisation and toxicity study of a vindesine-anti-CEA conjugate in patients with advanced cancer. Br. J. Cancer 47:35–42.

Garnett, M. C., M. J. Embleton, E. Jacobs, and R. W. Baldwin. 1983. Preparation and properties of a drug-carrier-antibody conjugate showing selective antibody-directed cytotoxicity in vitro. Int. J. Cancer 31:661–670.

Goldenberg, D. M., F. Deland, E. Kimm, S. Bennett, F. J. Primus, J. R. Nagel, N. Esles, P. Desimore, and P. Rayburn. 1978. Use of radiolabelled antibodies to carcinoembryonic antigen for the detection of localization of diverse cancers by external photoscanning. N. Engl. J. Med. 298:1384–1388.

Halsall, A. K., D. S. Fairweather, A. R. Bradwell, J. C. Blackburn, P. W. Dykes, A. Howell, A. Reeder, and K. R. Hine. 1981. Localisation of malignant germ-cell tumours by external scanning after injection of radiolabelled anti-alpha-fetoprotein. Br. Med. J. 283:942–944.

Kohler, G., and C. Milstein. 1975. Continuous cultures of fused cells secreting antibody of predefined specificity. Nature 256:495–497

Krolick, K. A., J. Uhr, S. Slavin, and E. S. Vitetta. 1982. In vivo therapy of a murine B cell tumor (BCL_1) using antibody-ricin A chain immunotoxins. J. Exp. Med. 155:1797–1809.

Mach, J.-P., F. Buchegger, M. Forni, J. Ritschard, C. Berche, J.-D. Lumbroso, M. Schreyer, C. Girardet, R. S. Accolla, and S. Carrel. 1981. Use of radiolabelled monoclonal anti-CEA antibodies for the detection of human carcinomas by external photoscanning and tomoscintigraphy. Immunology Today 2:239–249.

Mason, D. W., P. E. Thorpe, and W. D. J. Ross. 1982. Elimination of leukaemic cells from rodent bone marrow in vitro with antibody-ricin conjugates: Implications for autologous marrow transplantation in man, *in:* Imperial Cancer Research Fund Cancer Surveys, Vol. 1, A. J. S. Davies and M. J. Crumpton, eds. Oxford University Press, Oxford, pp. 389–415.

Miller, R. A., D. G. Maloney, R. Warnke, and R. Levy. 1982. Treatment of B-cell lymphoma with monoclonal anti-idiotype antibody. N. Engl. J. Med. 306:517–522.

Pimm, M. V., J. A. Jones, M. R. Price, J. G. Middle, M. J. Embleton, and R. W. Baldwin. 1982a. Tumour localization of monoclonal antibody against a rat mammary carcinoma and suppression of tumour growth with adriamycin-antibody conjugates. Cancer Immunol. Immunother. 12:125–134.

Pimm, M. V., M. J. Embleton, A. C. Perkins, M. R. Price, R. A. Robins, G. R. Robinson, and R. W. Baldwin. 1982b. In vivo localization of antiosteogenic sarcoma 791T monoclonal antibody in osteogenic sarcoma xenografts. Int. J. Cancer 30:75–85.

Price, M. R., D. G. Campbell, R. A. Robins, and R. W. Baldwin. 1983. Characteristics of a cell surface antigen defined by an anti-human osteogenic sarcoma monoclonal antibody. Eur. J. Cancer Clin. Oncol. 19:81–90.

Price, M. R., M. V. Pimm, and R. W. Baldwin. 1982. Complement dependent cytotoxicity of anti-human osteogenic sarcoma monoclonal antibodies. Br. J. Cancer 46:601–610.

Rowland, G. F., R. G. Simmonds, J. R. F. Corvalan, R. W. Baldwin, J. P. Brown, M. J. Embleton, C. H. J. Ford, K. E. Hellstrom, I. Hellstrom, J. T. Kemshead, C. E. Newman, and C. S. Woodhouse. 1982. Monoclonal antibodies for targeted therapy with vindesine, *in:* Protides of the Biological Fluids, Vol. 30, H. Peeters, ed. Pergamon Press, London, pp. 375–379.

Sears, H. F., B. Atkinson, J. Mattis, C. Ernst, D. Herlyn, Z. Steplewski, P. Hayry, and H. Koprowski. 1982. Phase-1 clinical trial of monoclonal antibody in treatment of gastrointestinal tumours. Lancet i:762–765.

Smedley, H. M., P. Finan, E. S. Lennox, A. Ritson, F. Takei, P. Wraight, and K. Sikora. 1983. Localisation of metastatic carcinoma by a radiolabelled monoclonal antibody. Br. J. Cancer 47:253–259.

Thorpe, P. E., and W. C. J. Ross. 1982. The preparation and cytotoxic properties of antibody-toxin conjugates. Immunol. Rev. 62:119–158.

Cancer Invasion and Metastasis: Biologic and Therapeutic Aspects edited by Garth L. Nicolson and Luka Milas. Raven Press, New York © 1984.

Tumor Metastasis: Achievements, Dilemmas, and Future, a Summary of the Conference

Luka Milas

Department of Experimental Radiotherapy, The University of Texas M. D. Anderson Hospital and Tumor Institute at Houston, Houston, Texas 77030

Metastasis is a complex, multistep event in the progression of malignant tumors and is influenced by many systemic and local host factors, as well as by the properties of tumor cells. In order to establish metastatic growth, tumor cells leave the primary tumor and travel through the lymphatic and blood circulation to remote tissues and organs. On this journey, tumor cells face a multitude of perils that determine the final outcome of the metastatic process. Many factors that shape the metastatic process and influence the response of metastases to therapies are already known, and many are still awaiting discovery. Attempts to discover the latter have been enormous, especially during the past few decades. The most recent activities in this field were presented during this symposium.

It would be presumptuous of me to even attempt to recount in this short summary all the conclusions and comments contained in the many excellent presentations, masterly reviews, and posters. Instead, I shall try to highlight some of the main features of the symposium and present a few random comments condensed from the enormous number of ideas presented and discussed during the meeting. Naturally, the summary will also reflect my personal perception of the state of the art in metastasis. In fact, the meeting in itself can be considered to have been a summary of the knowledge that has been accumulated in the field of tumor metastasis during the past several years. The whole meeting was held in a dynamic and professional atmosphere beginning with the opening remarks of Dr. Charles A. LeMaistre, President of The University of Texas M. D. Anderson Hospital and Tumor Institute at Houston, followed by the impressive talks of the Bertner award recipient and the keynote speaker, and continued in the excellent presentations of the invited speakers.

BERTNER AWARD PRESENTATION AND KEYNOTE ADDRESS

In his presentation, the Bertner award recipient, Dr. Isaiah J. Fidler, briefly ventured through his remarkable research achievements in the field of experimental tumor metastasis. Dr. Fidler not only resurrected the "seed" portion of Paget's "seed and soil" hypothesis, but transformed it into a sweeping postulate of tumor heterogeneity. Since heterogeneity of metastases will be discussed in more detail further on in this text, here I shall mention only a few of the many conclusions Dr. Fidler made. Malignant neoplasms are heterogeneous in regard to metastatic and other phenotypic characteristics. Of the cells they contain, some clones are metastatic and some are not; consequently, metastases are generated by cells belonging only to metastatic clones. However, even in metastasis (which can be either clonal or originated by different progenitor cells) biological diversity develops because metastatic clones exhibit an increased rate of spontaneous mutation. This generation of biological diversity in malignant tumors, as well as in metastasis, has a profound implication for the therapy of metastatic disease, requiring new approaches in the therapeutic strategy. As Dr. Fidler stated, the hypotheses he advanced and the conclusions he reached were based on a single tumor system, the murine B16 melanoma, and may not be applicable to all tumor settings. Even if not universally applicable, his research has stimulated investigational activity that is bound to advance our understanding of the biology and therapy of tumor metastases.

A true veteran in experimental and clinical tumor metastasis research delivered the keynote address. Although Dr. Fisher did not intend to be philosophical, as he mentioned, his presentation was full of practical philosophy based on enormous personal research and clinical experience. He discussed the change in the treatment philosophy of human breast cancer over the past decades with surgery, radiation therapy, chemotherapy, hormonal therapy, and their combinations. Many examples were described to illustrate that this change has been the result of knowledge concerning tumors and their metastasis acquired in the laboratory. The overall message of Dr. Fisher's paper is that in order to achieve the final victory over cancer metastasis, there *must* be a close interdependence of laboratory and clinical research. Separation of the two would be tragic. It is needless to emphasize that one of the major objectives of this conference, as illustrated by the title of this book, was to promote close contact between the laboratory and clinic, research that should be considered and practiced as one.

TUMOR CELL FACTORS

Tumor cells are endowed with many properties needed to complete malignant growth. First of all, they carry genetic information for unlimited cell renewal. In addition, they are in constant interaction with each other and with host elements with which they come into contact, all of which influence the final outcome of the tumor cell. The first contact of a tumor cell with its microenvironment is via the external plasma membrane, which carries alterations acquired through neoplastic transformation. The membrane changes, both qualitative and quantitative, will determine the nature and the extent of tumor cell interactions with the microenvironment. While many alterations become recognized by host resistance mechanisms with consequent death of tumor cells, many other alterations will be conducive to tumor and metastatic growth.

The section on tumor cell factors covers only a part of the tumor cell factors important for the ability of tumors to metastasize. Separation and in vitro expansion of tumor cell variants that exhibit a broad range of metastatic propensity was a basic experimental approach in studies of tumor cell factors. These cell variants were then analyzed for different phenotypic characteristics, and properties responsible for metastatic behavior of cells were identified. Low and high metastatic cell variants of murine leukemia or lymphomas (Kerbel et al., Schirrmacher et al.) and solid tumors (Eisenbach et al.) exhibited great variability in cell membrane composition, alterations that were both structural and functional. Many examples were presented to support these observations.

Cell variants can exhibit differences in cell surface antigens, including histocompatibility antigens, tumor-associated transplantation antigens, viral antigens, differentiation antigens, and blood group–related antigens. For example, a low ratio of $H\text{-}2K^b$ to $H\text{-}2D^b$ determinants (irrespective of their absolute density) was associated with increased metastatic potential (Eisenbach et al.). Antigenic loss was a common property of highly metastatic variants (Schirrmacher et al.).

Cell variants exhibit differences in cell surface receptors for plant lectins (Kerbel et al., Schirrmacher et al.), hepatocyte lectins (Schirrmacher et al.), fibronectin, collagen, laminin (Liotta et al., Nicolson et al., Schirrmacher et al.), IgG (Schirrmacher et al.), etc. It appears that the expression of these receptors correlates well with the metastatic ability of cell clones. Some of the above receptors can be blocked by sialic acid, which was associated with the loss of the metastatic property.

Cell variants can differ in enzymatic activities, such as in glycosyl transferases and in enzymes degrading the basal lamina of blood vessels (Liotta et al., Nicolson et al., Schirrmacher et al.). (The enzymatic activity of tumor cells is discussed later in the text—see Tumor Invasion.) There can be a change in membrane fluidity and dynamics. For example, highly metastatic lymphoma cells spontaneously shed membrane vesicles, which carry degradative enzymes and tumor transplantation antigens, several times more often than cells of low metastatic lines (Schirrmacher et al.).

Using B16 melanoma cell variants, Stringfellow reported that tumor cells release prostaglandins, and that one of them, PGD_2, was produced in higher quantity by a low-metastatic tumor cell line. Suppression of prostaglandin synthesis by treatment of low-metastatic cells with indomethacin increased the metastatic ability of these cells. It was suggested that PGD_2 inhibited platelet aggregation, and by this mechanism influenced the metastatic process. However, prostaglandins could operate by other mechanisms, especially by modulation of antitumor resistance mechanisms.

Membrane changes in tumor cells can be the result of genetic instability, cell differentiation events, and epigenetic influences. Both Kerbel et al. and Eisenbach et al. provided evidence that tumor cells can fuse with normal bone marrow cells, followed by chromosome segregation, which promotes karyotypic heterogeneity and aneuploidy. The resulting hybrids exhibit different metastatic propensity and organ selectivity from the parent tumor cell line. Through all of these processes, tumor cells undergo constant dynamic change that results in a diversity of phenotypes.

TUMOR INVASION

Since secondary tumor growths are usually formed in extracapillary spaces, tumor cells must cross the vascular wall. The process of extravasation of tumor cells requires the interaction of these cells with endothelium and other components of capillary walls. Recently developed technical capabilities to grow endothelial cells in vitro has led to studies on extravasation processes in more depth, and our understanding of these events has increased. Three speakers reviewed their research on this aspect of metastasis formation (Jones et al., Liotta et al., Nicholson et al.) and their findings can be briefly summarized as follows. Tumor cells bind to endothelial cells and stimulate breakage of endothelial junctions, exposing the basal lamina matrix to which tumor cells adhere because they carry receptors for laminin, fibronectin, collagen, or other glycoproteins. This adherence is followed by destruction of capillary wall constituents by enzymes that the tumor cells secrete in order to make their way through the capillary wall. Several of these glycoprotein-degrading enzymes were isolated from both human and animal tumor cells, and they include collagenases, plasminogen activator, and elastase. The glycoprotein-degrading enzymes are also important during the entry of tumor cells into vascular beds of the primary tumor. Here, however, tumor cells may enter the circulation passively by the necrosis and hemorrhage that commonly occur within the growing tumor.

In order to sustain progressive growth, both primary tumors and metastatic foci must be supplied with oxygen and nutrients. This supply takes place via tumor blood vessels that originate from the tumor bed. Angiogenic stimulus initiated by tumor cells acts on small-venule endothelial cells of the tumor bed. A series of angiogenesis events follows (Folkman, Rifkin): endothelial cells secrete collagenase and plasminogen activator, and possibly other enzymes, which by virtue of their basal lamina degradative activities make openings in the basal membrane through which endothelial cells migrate out. Endothelial cells first form vascular sprouts, then loops, and then a mesh of capillary channels. Mast cells stimulate migration of endothelial cells through secretion of heparin. In contrast, protamin and platelet factor 4 are inhibitors of angiogenesis (Folkman).

TUMOR HETEROGENEITY

The most prominent feature of this symposium was undoubtedly heterogeneity of metastasis. To explain the anatomic distribution of metastasis from human breast cancer, Paget almost a century ago introduced the "seed and soil" hypothesis, according to which successful metastasis depended on both a fertile tumor cell "seed" and a supportive tissue "soil" in which to grow. The "seed" portion of Paget's hypothesis has recently attracted great investigational interest, and it has evolved into the heterogeneity postulate. Major aspects and findings of tumor heterogeneity in reference to metastasis were reviewed in depth at this meeting.

According to the tumor heterogeneity postulate, tumors, although most of them unicellular in origin, become composites of many cell subpopulations during their growth. These subpopulations vary among themselves in morphology, karyotype, antigenic composition, immunogenicity, growth properties, sensitivity to therapeutic agents, and *ability to metastasize.* Thus, metastases at remote sites are generated by cells "specialized" to so do, whereas other tumor cells within the same tumor are innocent in this respect. The phenotypic heterogeneity in the primary tumor is primarily the outcome of genetic instability of tumor cells (Nowell), but also the result of the ability of tumor cells to interact with themselves and with host normal cells (Hart, Heppner et al.). There is ample evidence that both animal and human tumors are composed of cell clones with different phenotypes. Dexter discussed heterogeneity in human colon cancer and Baylin et al. discussed heterogeneity in human lung cancer. Dexter established two cell lines from colon cancer, one anaplastic and the other moderately differentiated. Their antigenic composition, sensitivity to chemotherapy and other agents, and ability to grow and metastasize in nude mice were different. Baylin et al. presented evidence that in cell culture small (oat) cell lung carcinoma can change into large cell undifferentiated carcinoma. During that transition, oat cells lose their endocrine properties and become more resistant to treatments. They suggested that not only normal bronchial epithelial cells, but also all four major types of lung cancer (squamous, adeno-, oat cell, and large cell carcinomas) emerge from a common endodermal stem cell. Neoplastic transformation can occur at different stages of cell differentiation, but the final type of cancer will depend on the cell differentiation step at which transformation occurred; further continuation of the cell differentiation pathway and genetic instability can cause a constant emergence of cell phenotypes within the evolving tumor. Thus, the resulting tumors can be very heterogeneous in spite of the predominance of a particular cell type.

Long-established murine leukemia (and lymphoma) cell lines and their sublines are highly heterogeneous in their malignancy (Kamenov et al.). Cells of greater malignancy are less susceptible to lysis by complement-dependent natural antibody than less-malignant cells. The more-malignant cells have high affinity to adhere to adherent bone marrow cells that provide "microenvironmental" stimulus for proliferation of leukemic cells. Therefore, both the "seed" and the "soil" determine whether leukemic cells will be rejected or stimulated in their growth.

The changes that occur within the tumor and lead to phenotypic diversity are dynamic. Cells belonging to different clones interact among themselves and with host normal cells. Poste presented data showing that the stability of a metastatic phenotype and the rate at which new cell variants are formed are regulated by the degree of diversity of cell subpopulations within tumors. Formation of new metastatic variants appears to be greatest under conditions of limited subpopulation diversity. Interactions among cells lead to a constant change in phenotypic characteristics. For example, a nonmetastatic mammary carcinoma cell line will become metastatic in the presence of a metastatic cell line (Heppner et al.). Cell differentiation rather than genetic change was considered to be the mechanism of this diversification (Heppner et al.). Cells within the same tumor can even fuse to each other, resulting in hybrid cells (Eisenbach et al., Hart, Kerbel et al.). Fusion of two tumor cells with different metastatic capacities will result in the production of cells that are more metastatic tnan the parent cells. However, if a metastatic cell is fused with a normal cell, the progeny will not be metastatic but will exhibit the tumorigenic property only. This metastatic behavior of hybrids, however, cannot be taken as a general rule (Eisenbach et al., Kerbel et al.), since many different interactions may take place within the tumor that can lead to all sorts of phenotypes. Concluding her talk, Gloria Heppner stated that cancer should not be considered "as collections of individual cells, but rather as complex societies with unexpected capacity for interaction, change, and evolution."

The session on tumor heterogeneity was followed by vigorous and constructive discussion. The major criticism of the heterogeneity postulate was that most of the evidence on which this postulate is based was generated by in vitro studies (cell sublines were selected and expanded in vitro and then tested for their organ-colonizing ability by i.v. injection), which might not be the true reflection of the in vivo process of spontaneous metastasis. Since the evidence from in vivo studies in reference to the heterogeneity postulate is limited at present, the message of the discussion was that the role of heterogeneity should not be overstated. To overemphasize the "seed" portion of the Paget theory, as the tendency exists in this metastasis selection hypothesis, is to downplay the importance of the tissue factors conducive to growth at the site of tumor cell arrest, as well as systemic host influences. Therefore, the presented papers and the discussion they invoked clearly showed that this aspect of metastasis has enhanced greatly our understanding of metastases and opened new avenues for further research.

HOST FACTORS

Host factors that influence metastasis formation are many, and they have been attracting significant investigational interest for several decades. There can be systemic and local environment factors, and some of each were discussed at the symposium.

Host immune resistance factors were discussed by Alexander and Eccles, Hanna, Kim, and Milas and Peters, and we learned that immune resistance mechanisms, such as specific antitumor response mediated by T-lymphocytes, antibodies, natural killer (NK) cells, and macrophages, can influence the process of metastasis. They can interact with tumor cells in all phases of the metastatic process. Metastatic behavior of rodent sarcomas and lymphomas are controlled by antitumor immune response better than rodent carcinomas, most likely because the former are more immunogenic (Alexander and Eccles). There was an inverse correlation between the immunogenicity of tumors and their metastatic capacity. Lymphocytes and macrophages infiltrate tumors and react with tumor cells there or they can act alone or in cooperation with humoral antibodies to destroy circulating cells. Different immunosuppressive procedures affecting T-cell–dependent immune reactions greatly enhance the spread of immunogenic tumors.

NK cells have the natural ability to kill tumor cells of different tumor types. Hanna presented evidence that these cells are very important in the restriction of metastatic spread. It was suggested that they are most effective against tumor cells that are still in circulation, whereas their effect is small on cells that have already entered the extracapillary space. This implies that the role of NK cells is important in prevention rather than in therapy of metastases. A further limiting factor with NK cell antitumor activity is that only a certain proportion of tumors are sensitive to NK cells. Furthermore, resistance to NK cells can develop, but the evidence on whether it is due to selection or adaptation is lacking. Highly metastatic tumor cell variants were, in general, less sensitive to NK cells than low-metastatic variants (Eisenbach et al., Kerbel et al.).

It was clear from several presentations that nonimmunogenic tumors are more prone to spontaneously metastasize than immunogenic tumors. A very sound and interesting hypothesis was put forward (Kim) that all tumors, regardless of their cause, share a common pathogenetic pathway, which is a prolonged latent period during which there exists constant selection pressure on the tumor cells by the host immune surveillance mechanisms, whatever these mechanisms might have been. This, in the majority of cases, would lead to tumors that are nonimmunogenic, and since as such they are no longer under immune surveillance, their cells, once in circulation, have a better chance to develop into metastases. This suggestion could be very applicable to human tumors, most of which are likely to be nonimmunogenic. The important question that remains to be investigated is whether and which immune resistance mechanisms can control the spread of nonimmunogenic tumors.

It has been established that circulating tumor cells can be surrounded by platelets and fibrin. Particularly in capillaries, a thrombus formation around tumor cells adherent to the vascular capillaries is a frequent event, but short-lived, lasting only minutes to hours. Consequently, a logical assumption is that interference with processes leading to thrombus formation would result in a reduction of metastasis formation, since tumor cells would continue circulating and would die in the blood because of blood turbulence or other mechanisms. Reviewing the effect of anticoagulants on tumor metastasis, Hilgard presented evidence that heparin and classic anti-platelet-aggregating agents, such as aspirin, were often capable of reducing metastasis formation after i.v. injection of tumor cells, but their action in spontaneous metastasis situations was inconsistent, if they had any. However, Coumarin-type anticoagulants were quite effective in reducing spontaneous metastasis. Their mechanism seems to be independent of their influence on the coagulation mechanism, and yet it appears to be closely related to their vitamin K antagonistic activity.

Recent discoveries that certain products in arachidonic acid metabolism play an important role in platelet aggregation have led to attempts to prevent metastasis formation by manipulation of arachidonic acid metabolism. Specifically, thromboxane, which is secreted by platelets, promotes platelet aggregation, and prostacyclin, secreted by the wall of blood vessels, inhibits platelet aggregation. Whether platelet aggregation will take place depends on the balance between prostacyclin and thromboxane. Honn et al. presented evidence that tumor cells release cysteine proteinase cathepsin B, which induces aggregation of platelets through generation of thromboxane, which can then help them to be arrested in the capillaries. This action of thromboxane can be reduced or prevented by injection of prostacyclin into tumor cell recipients or by stimulation of production of endogenous prostacyclin via treatment of mice with the agent nafazatrom. Both prostacyclin and nafazatrom injections resulted in reduction of artificial (Honn et al., Milas and Peters) and spontaneous metastasis formation of tumors (Honn et al.). More studies are needed to establish the full potency of this approach in prevention of metastasis formation.

Local environment factors are also very important, and they can be modified in such a way that they can promote or inhibit the establishment and growth of metastases. For example, mechanical damage of tissues is associated with enhanced probability of metastatic growth in such tissues. Data were presented (Milas and Peters) that local thoracic irradiation (LTI) and treatment with cyclophosphamide (CY) can increase by manifold the metastasis formation of murine tumors generated by i.v. injected cells. Direct damage to the lung tissue seems to be the major mechanism by which these treatments promote metastasis formation. CY may act in part by suppressing host antitumor resistance mechanisms mediated by NK cells. The clinical implications of these findings are uncertain. It might be expected that damage to the lung by drugs or radiation could lead to promotion of spontaneous metastases if a source of circulating tumor cells persists. Several approaches have been tried to prevent or reduce the enhancement of metastasis. Approaches designed to interfere specifically with putative mechanisms of the CY and LTI effect were ineffective. However, a significant reduction of metastasis enhancement can be achieved by pretreatment with agents that activate macrophages or stimulate NK cell activity. It is quite possible that, in addition to agents reported herein, many other iatrogenic agents can under certain circumstances enhance metastatic formation. It is important for future research to identify such damaging agents, understand the mechanism of their effect, and develop means of prevention.

The occurrence of metastases does not entirely mirror the extent of the initial trapping of tumor cells in capillaries. Many tumor cells die even after being trapped. Alexander and Eccles advanced on attractive hypothesis by which they implicate oxygen as a cause for tumor cell death. They postulated that tumor cells die in capillary beds in which the oxygen concentration is in equilibrium with that of the atmosphere. Accordingly, hypoxic blood would favor tumor cell survival. This mechanism was advanced as a cause for the relatively frequent involvement of liver and bone by metastasis, because portal circulation and the sinusoidal circulation in the bone marrow are hypoxic. Among supportive evidence for the hypothesis were in vitro observations of enhanced cell plating in hypoxic conditions and in vivo reduction of lung colony formation by i.v. injected tumor cells if mice were breathing for some time under hyperbaric oxygen conditions. The hypothesis needs still more supportive evidence to attain recognition.

THERAPY OF METASTASIS

Five presentations dealt with therapy for metastatic disease: two discussed chemotherapy, one radiotherapy, and two therapy with biological response modifiers.

Treatment of systemic metastatic disease is the real domain of cancer chemotherapy. Traditionally, it has been used to eradicate clinically evident metastases; here, it mostly has a palliative role aimed at alleviation of symptoms and prolongation of patient survival. However, in a few selected malignancies such as childhood leukemia, testicular cancer, Hodgkin's disease, and diffuse lymphoma, chemotherapy has been quite successful. Adjuvant chemotherapy is another approach aimed at sterilizing nondetectable micrometastatic foci that remain in the host after the primary tumor has been removed by surgery or radiotherapy. Theoretically, this clinical setting should be ideal for the use of chemotherapy because of the proportional cell killing by chemotherapeutic drugs. This approach has had some positive results in the treatment of breast cancer and osteosarcoma, but overall "after earlier enthusiasm adjuvant chemotherapy has not lived up to its proposed potential" (Carter). The authors of the two chemotherapy presentations directed most of their efforts toward reviewing factors responsible for the poor success of tumor chemotherapy. Many factors were mentioned, but two of them were stressed: lack of cytotoxic specificity for tumor cells and development of drug-resistant tumor cell clones. Because of the lack of a significant cytotoxic specificity of currently available chemotherapeutic drugs, these drugs can be used only with narrow margins of safety and, consequently, tumor curative doses can rarely be achieved without producing nonacceptable normal tissue toxicity. A statement was made that ". . . the identification or development of agents with marked cytotoxic specificity remains an elusive goal" (Griswold et al.).

There is no doubt that the present art of cancer chemotherapy was pictured with pessimism, and it is likely that this pessimistic feeling is largely a result of overexpectation in the past. Research efforts toward uncovering the biological secrets of cancer coupled with diverse investigational activities in chemotherapy research should provide a more rational and effective approach to cancer cell destruction than presently available. The following are only a few of many research avenues already under way in experimental chemotherapy that have promise in improving tumor therapy with chemotherapeutic agents: searches for more-specific cytotoxic drugs, research directed at overcoming drug resistance, targeting of chemotherapeutic agents to micrometastases, and combination with radio(chemo)sensitizers and radio(chemo)protectors.

Radiotherapy is a powerful tumor treatment modality for both localized neoplasms and metastasis in many diverse clinical settings (Peters et al.). In a curative sense, radiotherapy if often used successfully for elective treatment of subclinical metastases, primarily within regional lymph nodes but also within another anatomical locations. Sterilization of small metastatic foci require lower doses of radiation than what is used in the treatment of large bulk disease. Use of elective radiotherapy in the treatment of occult metastatic disease has led to the abandonment of many elective surgical resections and it has resulted in the better quality of life for many patients. Radiotherapy also has an important role in the curative management of overt metastatic disease such as from seminoma. Isotopic radiotherapy is successfully used to treat metastatic thyroid cancer. There exists a significant research activity in experimental radiotherapy. For example, significant effort is under way to use monoclonal antibodies coupled with radioisotopes to treat metastatic disease. Research on combinations of radiotherapy with radio(chemo)sensitizers and radio(chemo)protectors in order to increase tumor cell kill and increase normal tissue tolerance is also prominent at present. Peters et al. illustrated the potential for the radioprotective agent WR-2721 to increase the therapeutic gain of radiotherapy for metastatic disease.

In setting the stage for his presentation, Fidler stated that "successful therapy of metastases will have to circumvent the problems of biological heterogeneity and the development of resistancy by tumor cells" and that macrophages could fulfill this requirement. The selection of macrophages for this task was based on evidence generated during the past decade that macrophages can be activated to become cytocidal for tumor cells in a reaction that is immunologically nonspecific and tumor selective. Therefore, activated macrophages can kill any type of tumor cells but cannot damage normal tissue even if the tissue is antigenically foreign. Macrophage-mediated tumor cell kill is not influenced by any known tumor cell phenotypes, and tumor cells cannot be resistant to macrophages. An elegant approach that results in a strong in vivo activation of macrophages was presented, consisting of encapsulation of muramyl dipeptide (MDP) into liposomes. Since liposomes are taken up by macrophages, they bring MDP along and strong activation ensues. Intravenous treatment of mice bearing spontaneous B16 melanoma metastases in the lung was associated with a remarkably high cure rate. Incorporation of macrophage-activating agents into liposomes obviates toxicities otherwise associated with most immunotherapeutic agents, and particularly bacteria. If this approach proves to be as effective in other tumor systems as it was in B16 melanoma, it may be an efficient modality in the treatment of cancer metastases.

Finally, the role of monoclonal antibodies in the detection and therapy of metastasis was discussed. Baldwin et al. presented their own research experience with an anti-human tumor monoclonal antibody 791T/36 produced by a hybridoma obtained by fusion of murine splenocytes sensitized to a human osteogenic sarcoma with a murine myeloma. Radioactively labeled monoclonal antibodies preferentially localized in xenografts of human osteogenic sarcomas growing in immunodeprived mice. In their initial clinical studies with this antibody, they found that radioactively labeled antibodies preferentially localized in osteogenic sarcomas and colorectal carcinomas. They detected brain metastasis of approximately 2 cm in diameter in a patient with colon cancer; this was the smallest tumor identified by monoclonal antibodies in their clinical study. Tumor-localizing monoclonal antibodies have great potential for therapy of metastatic disease through targeting of various anticancer agents conjugated with antibodies. These agents include radioactive materials, plant and bacterial toxins, chemotherapy drugs, and immunomodulating agents. A chemotherapeutic agent, vindesine, bound to monoclonal antibody exerted potent antitumor activity against human xenografts. An important and interesting observation was that this conjugate was less toxic than free vindesine. Monoclonal antibody research is in its infancy and there are many problems to be resolved. However, the future applicability of monoclonal antibody conjugates in both diagnosis and therapy of metastasis appears to be considerable.

CONCLUSION

There is no doubt that metastasis remains the principal killer of cancer patients. However, secrets of cancer cell metastasis are rapidly becoming understood. New discoveries are made virtually every day, spreading the optimism that this terrible disease may come under control. We have witnessed during this conference how much new knowledge on metastasis has been acquired within the past several years. In our quest for this final goal, conferences such as this one are of paramount importance. This conference has not only provided us with important discoveries and recent advances in biology and therapy of metastatic disease, but it also synthesized the acquired knowledge for us, presented current dilemmas, and identified some future directions. Many of the comments and conclusions offered should still be regarded as open, unanswered questions that await further investigation. The conference brought us together, offering the opportunity to exchange ideas and experiences, and I am sure that we are richer with new ideas to persist in our quest to conquer cancer, a task we owe to mankind.

Subject Index